2004 HCPCS

Level II

National Codes

1st Edition

Updated and Published Annually!

by
MedBooks
101 West Buckingham Road
Richardson, Texas 75081
1-800-443-7397
972-643-1809

www.medbooks.com
ISBN: 0923369945

2004 MedBooks *Select* Products:

CP"Teach" Expert Coding Made Easy! Textbook   **0923369864**

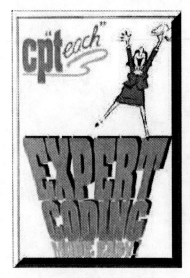

The CP"Teach" textbook reveals the coveted secrets of coding and explains classified details for all sections of the CPT book with emphasis on getting paid for the services you do. CP"Teach" explains ways to see, evaluate, and gain control over such things as the surgical package, starred procedures, evaluation and management services and modifier nuances and shows how to choose codes wisely and when to add the necessary components to these codes for optimum reimbursement. Unlike the competition, the CP"Teach" textbook is updated annually and goes way beyond merely paraphrasing the CPT book. CP"Teach" is essential reading and understanding for anyone who wants an easy way to blow through the jargon and master the truth behind proper coding. With a 30%+ rewrite for 2004 - CP"Teach" provides over 110 pages each in both the E/M and Surgery sections.

CP"Teach" Expert Coding Made Easy! Student Workbook   **0923369872**
CP"Teach" Expert Coding Made Easy! (w/Answers)   **0923369880**

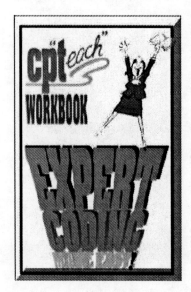

At last there is a resource that defines the study of how-to CPT coding. Unlike the competition, this superbly organized workbook presents the subject in practical, accessible language making how to understand CPT coding a breeze. Amply supplied with case studies, contemporary explanations, fun how-to exercises, anagrams, cross word puzzles, and matching this volume provides users of all specialties and levels of proficiency with the fool proof techniques to master coding. Contributors provide indispensable guidance for assessing, understanding and responding to unique coding situations and have made special efforts to represent nuances within the different sections of the CPT manual. With the addition of new cases and an approximate 30% rewrite for 2004 - CP"Teach" Workbook is perfect as a companion to the CP"Teach" textbook or usable as a stand-alone.

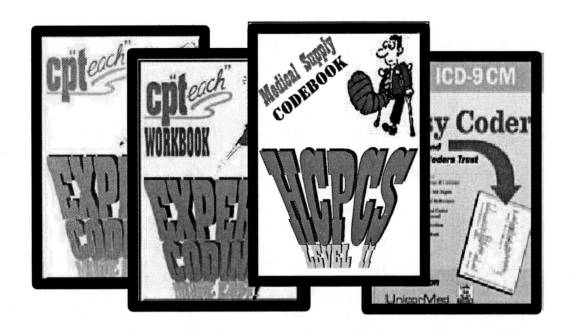

Select Pack! (Inc. 2004 HCPCS and CP"Teach" Textbook)   **0923369937**

For value conscience individuals and academic institutions. Select Pack: includes 2004 CP"Teach" and HCPCS. Since 10% of the income at the average physician's office is directly dependent on the HCPCS book having it available to your students is a must! But making it available at a price you can't refuse it even more important! Our Select Pack allows you to do just that and all at a price that fits right into your student's budgets! Nowhere else can you get the package deal at such an incredible price!

Deluxe Pack! (HCPCS plus our Textbook with Workbook)   **0923369953**

For value conscience individuals and academic institutions who want more than the Select Pack. The Deluxe Pack includes CP"Teach" text, workbook and HCPCS. Similar to the Select Pack only the addition is the CP"Teach" Workbook. What a great deal on either a self-learning tool or on a system that will help you optimize the students learning and all at such a great savings!

CP"Teach" Exclusive Pack! (All 3 products + the Unicor Easy Coder)   **0923369961**

For value conscience individuals and academic institutions who want it all. The Professional Pack includes CP"Teach" textbook and workbook, HCPCS and the ICD-9-CM Easy Coder! All the tools you need to be able to code like a professional and get guarantee the physician expert results! Nowhere else can you get the easy-to understand products at such an incredible value! Purchased individually these products would cost much more than this!

Advanced Case Study Workbook	**0923369570**
Advanced Case Study Workbook (w/Answers)	**0923369589**

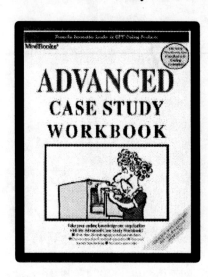

Hospitals, physician offices and experienced professionals have long understood that coding in an academic setting can only give the novice a rough imitation of what happens in real life. Yet how can the "real-coding world", with all its medical specialties and variables best be illustrated? Bridge the gap between books and real-life with the only advanced and one of a kind workbook that offers intriguing new ways of bringing the "real-world" into the classroom (or learning environment). With the use of real patient charts, there is finally a workbook that provides an advanced source for students to master their coding skills. The CP"Teach" Advanced Case Study workbook is the first place to turn for authoritative practice exercises on every area of the field and can provide a self-pacing, self-teaching source that can be used to gel all the CPT/HCPCS/ICD-9 concepts quickly and effectively.

Instructor's Manual with Mylar Transparencies	**0923369899**
Instructor's Manual with Paper Transparency Templates	**0923369902**
Instructor's Manual Refill with Mylar Transparencies	**0923369910**
Instructor's Manual Refill with Paper Transparency Templates	**0923369929**

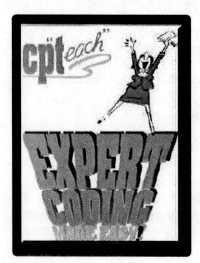

Teaching coding just got easier thanks to the CP"Teach" Instructor's Manual. Gone are the days when educators were forced to search through stacks of journals and books on coding for the best way to construct their CPT coding courses. With hundreds of questions and assessment techniques to choose from, the experienced professor of coding or even rookie educator will not have any trouble coming up with quick and accurate quizzes, homework assignments or final exam! From the author of the CP"Teach" text, the Instructor's Manual is the definitive guide to every area of CPT coding theory, practice and reimbursement techniques. Comes complete with more than 100 whimsical illustrations, 40+ ready to go overhead transparencies, homework assignments, quizzes and course agendas (from 1 to 60 hour programs) and of course the 2004 CP"Teach" textbook. EVERYTHING you need is provided – just add students, the classroom and teacher!

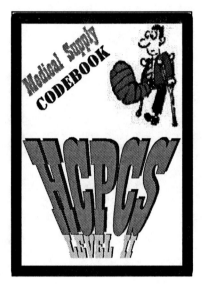

New for 2004, MedBooks delivers a simple, inexpensive and comprehensive version of the official Medicare codes in HCPCS. We list every Level II HCPCS code that the government as of November 1, 2003, the long description, payment indicators, multiple payment indicators and more! Other important information like statute, cross references, coverage and action codes plus ASC payment group and effective dates have been listed. All at a great price! If you have not been getting paid for casting supplies, blood draws, surgical trays, drugs and more, you need this book.

DOC Forms (Call for Prices)

Problem Focused, Detailed, Comprehensive, Straight Forward, 10 minutes. Who knows these days? MedBooks does! MedBooks DOC forms are the perfect solutions for Evaluation and Management coding issues. Selecting accurate visit codes is one of the major problems that faces physicians. Our form allows the physician to easily take an active part in the Evaluation and Management (E/M) coding decision, and allows the coder to work with greater speed.

MedBooks *Select* Services:

NATIONAL & INTERNATIONAL CODING AND REIMBURSEMENT SEMINARS

Wide in scope and comprehensive in coverage, our how-to coding seminars uncover the mysteries of:

1. Why physicians lose money,
2. How to help patients pay lower balances,
3. How to obtain payment for supplies and drugs
4. All about the fifth digit, and
5. Perils of mismatching diagnoses/procedures.

We provide indispensable guidance for understanding and responding to areas such as "red flags", carrier audits, what to do after the global fee period is over, surgical nuances, coding for supplies, starred procedures, as well as assessing claims and spotting problems. Our CPT and ICD-9 seminars are for anyone who wants to identify their coding deficiencies, significantly increase overall reimbursements, and learn more than they every have about coding.

NATIONAL & INTERNATIONAL CODING AND REIMBURSEMENT AUDITS

MedBooks offers a rare opportunity to sneak an objective and expert peek into what the insurance carriers and Medicare will look for once you have filled your claims. By looking at a broad sampling of your practice's submissions, we evaluate, grade and report back to you how to get paid for the services that you provide, what you may be doing wrong, AND how to stay clear (and safe) in an insurance audit. Our audits are for those who want to verify their coding accuracy, significantly improve reimbursements, lower their claims rejection rates, improve payment turn-around and avoid lost revenues and/or penalties due to untutored coding practices.

RETROACTIVE BILLING SERVICES

Why shouldn't you get it? With some statistics showing that fifty cents ($.50) of every dollar ($1.00) submitted to the insurance carriers is either rejected or denied, and only approximately twenty-five percent (25%) re-filed, your retirement date just got moved back five or more years. Our program searches for patterns, identifying them and more importantly notifies you of the errors. Don't continue to throw good money after bad. Computer programs and scrubbers are only as good as the person who has programmed them. We start with the basics, reviewing coding and billing errors, and have the expertise to resolve the problems.

ON-LINE WEBSITE OFFERING 100,000+ TITLES

Choose from over 100,000 different medical titles represented by over 500 of the top publishers in the world. Whether your needs are for one book or thousands, look to MedBooks to fill your needs.

EXPERT TESTIMONY/WITNESSING

MedBooks expert witnessing/testimony is for those law firms, insurance companies, CPA's and government entities who want straight-forward, no nonsense accurate facts presented in a professional manner. By reviewing the evidence, MedBooks will provide you and your client with accurate, concise and easy to understand professional testimony.

PHYSICIAN FEE ANALYSIS SERVICES

To arrive at values for physician's services, insurance companies, CPA's and medical managers use a relative value guide that attaches a certain value for time, skill, severity of illness, risk to patient, and risk to physicians to each and every CPT code. By using your current fees and running the mathematical equations with these relative values, new fees can be calculated giving you the most accurate set of charges possible for the services you provide.

SUPERBILL/FEE SLIP REVIEW

By utilizing MedBooks Fee Slip review service, all areas are carefully considered. The entire process, from patient arrival to filing of the claim form will be well thought-out. Having review hundreds of Fee Slips, MedBooks can put you on the fast track to solving some of your reimbursement issues.

Publisher's Notice

The Healthcare Common Procedure Coding System (HCPCS) is a collection of codes that represent procedures, supplies, products and services that may be provided to Medicare beneficiaries and to individuals enrolled in private health insurance programs.

All information contained herein, including HCPCS codes, alpha-numeric index and drug index are compiled from the official HCPCS Centers for Medicare and Medicaid Services (CMS), that are established by CMS's Alpha-Numeric Editorial Panel, primarily represent items and supplies and non-physician services not covered by the American Medical Association's CPT-4 codes. These files contain the Level II alphanumeric HCPCS procedure and modifier codes, their long descriptions and applicable Medicare administrative, coverage, and pricing data.

This MedBooks HCPCS codebook is designed to provide you with accurate information in regards to the current codes established by CMS. Every reasonable effort has been made to ensure that the information contained is accurate. The ultimate responsibility for correct usage of these codes lies with the provider of the services.

MedBooks, its employees, staff and agents make no representation, guarantee or warranty that the following codes and descriptions compiled in this 2004 HCPCS code book are error-free. Disputes or differences of opinion that may arise with Medicare or other third-party payers regarding code usage or amounts paid to the provider of services are at the sole responsibility of the user. MedBooks assumes no responsibility or liability for the results and/or consequences that may arise for usage of this 2004 HCPCS.

Information contained herein includes:

HCPCS Codes - Codes and descriptors approved and maintained jointly by the alphanumeric editorial panel (consisting of CMS, the Health Insurance Association of America, and the Blue Cross and Blue Shield Association).

Long Description - Contains all text of procedure or modifier long descriptions. The AMA owns the copyright on the CPT codes and descriptions; CPT codes and descriptions are not public property and must always be used in compliance with copyright law.

Pricing Indicators - Code used to identify the appropriate methodology for developing unique pricing amounts under part B. A procedure may have one to four pricing codes.

Multiple Pricing Indicators - Code used to identify instances where a procedure could be priced under multiple methodologies. Codes include:

9 = Not applicable as HCPCS not priced separately by part B (pricing indicator is 00) or value is not established (pricing indicator is '99')

A = Not applicable as HCPCS priced under one methodology

B = Professional component of HCPCS priced using RVU's, while technical component and global service priced by Medicare part B carriers interpretation of clinical lab service is priced under physician fee schedule using RVU's, while pricing of lab service is paid under clinical lab fee schedule

D = Service performed by physician is priced under physician fee schedule using RVU's, while service performed by clinical psychologist is priced under clinical psychologist fee schedule (not applicable as of January 1, 1998)

E = Service performed by physician is priced under physician fee schedule using RVU's, service performed by clinical psychologist is priced under clinical psychologist's fee schedule and service performed by clinical social worker is priced under clinical social worker fee schedule (not applicable as of January 1, 1998)

F = Service performed by physician is priced under physician fee schedule by carriers, service performed by clinical psychologist is priced under clinical psychologist's fee schedule and service performed by clinical social worker is priced under clinical social worker fee schedule (not applicable as of January 1, 1998)

G = Clinical lab service priced under reasonable charge when service is submitted on claim with blood products, while service is priced under clinical lab fee schedule when there are no blood products on claim.

Statute - Number identifying statute reference for coverage or non-coverage of procedure or service.

Cross Reference - An explicit reference cross-walking a deleted code or a code that is not valid for Medicare to a valid current code (or range of codes).

Coverage Codes - A code denoting Medicare coverage status. Codes include:

D = Special coverage instructions apply
I = Not payable by Medicare (no grace period)
G = Not payable by Medicare (90 day grace period)
M = Non-covered by Medicare
M = Non-covered by Medicare
S = Non-covered by Medicare statute
C = Carrier judgment

ASC Payment Group - The code that represents the dollar amount of the facility charge payable by Medicare for the procedure. Payment group rates, which are updated annually, (most recently on October 1, 2003), are as follows: Group 1 - $340; Group 2 - $455; Group 3 - $520; Group 4 - $643; Group 5 - $731; Group 6 - $840 ($690+$150 for intraocular lenses IOLS); Group 7 - $1015; Group 8 - $989 ($839+$150 for IOLS); Group 9 - $1366. The $150 payment allowance in groups 6 and 8 is for intraocular lenses.

ASC Payment Group Effective Date - The date the procedure is assigned to the ASC payment group. Listed as YYYYMMDD

Action Code - A code denoting the change made to a procedure or modifier code within the HCPCS system. Codes include:

A = Add procedure or modifier code
B = Change in both administrative data field and long description of procedure or modifier code
C = Change in long description of procedure or modifier code
D = Discontinue procedure or modifier code
F = Change in administrative data field of procedure or modifier code
N = No maintenance for this code
P = Payment change (MOG, pricing indicator codes, anesthesia base units)
R = Re-activate discontinued/deleted procedure or modifier code
S = Change in short description of procedure code
T = Miscellaneous change (BETOS, type of service)

Contents

HCPCS	Long Description	PH	MPI	Statute	X-Refl	Coverage	ASC Pay Grp	ASC Pay Grp Eff Date	Action Code
A1	DRESSING FOR ONE WOUND					C			N
A2	DRESSING FOR TWO WOUNDS					C			N
A3	DRESSING FOR THREE WOUNDS					C			N
A4	DRESSING FOR FOUR WOUNDS					C			N
A5	DRESSING FOR FIVE WOUNDS					C			N
A6	DRESSING FOR SIX WOUNDS					C			N
A7	DRESSING FOR SEVEN WOUNDS					C			N
A8	DRESSING FOR EIGHT WOUNDS					C			N
A9	DRESSING FOR NINE OR MORE WOUNDS					C			N
AA	ANESTHESIA SERVICES PERFORMED PERSONALLY BY ANESTHESIOLOGIST					D			N
AD	MEDICAL SUPERVISION BY A PHYSICIAN: MORE THAN FOUR CONCURRENT ANESTHESIA PROCEDURES					D			N
AH	CLINICAL PSYCHOLOGIST					D			N
AJ	CLINICAL SOCIAL WORKER					D			N
AM	PHYSICIAN, TEAM MEMBER SERVICE				QM	D			N
AP	DETERMINATION OF REFRACTIVE STATE WAS NOT PERFORMED IN THE COURSE OF DIAGNOSTIC OPHTHALMOLOGICAL EXAMINATION					C			N
AS	PHYSICIAN ASSISTANT, NURSE PRACTITIONER, OR CLINICAL NURSE SPECIALIST SERVICES FOR ASSISTANT AT SURGERY					C			N
AT	ACUTE TREATMENT (THIS MODIFIER SHOULD BE USED WHEN REPORTING SERVICE 98940, 98941, 98942)					C			N
AU	ITEM FURNISHED IN CONJUNCTION WITH A UROLOGICAL, OSTOMY, OR TRACHEOSTOMY SUPPLY					C			N
AV	ITEM FURNISHED IN CONJUNCTION WITH A PROSTHETIC DEVICE, PROSTHETIC OR ORTHOTIC					C			N
AW	ITEM FURNISHED IN CONJUNCTION WITH A SURGICAL DRESSING					C			N
AX	ITEM FURNISHED IN CONJUNCTION WITH DIALYSIS SERVICES					C			N
BA	ITEM FURNISHED IN CONJUNCTION WITH PARENTERAL ENTERAL NUTRITION (PEN) SERVICES					C			N
BO	ORALLY ADMINISTERED NUTRITION, NOT BY FEEDING TUBE					C			N
BP	THE BENEFICIARY HAS BEEN INFORMED OF THE PURCHASE AND RENTAL OPTIONS AND HAS ELECTED TO PURCHASE THE ITEM					C			N
BR	THE BENEFICIARY HAS BEEN INFORMED OF THE PURCHASE AND RENTAL OPTIONS AND HAS ELECTED TO RENT THE ITEM					C			N
BU	THE BENEFICIARY HAS BEEN INFORMED OF THE PURCHASE AND RENTAL OPTIONS AND AFTER 30 DAYS HAS NOT INFORMED THE SUPPLIER OF HIS/HER DECISION					C			N
CA	PROCEDURE PAYABLE ONLY IN THE INPATIENT SETTING WHEN PERFORMED EMERGENTLY ON AN OUTPATIENT WHO EXPIRES PRIOR TO ADMISSION					C			N
CB	SERVICE ORDERED BY A RENAL DIALYSIS FACILITY (RDF) PHYSICIAN AS PART OF THE ESRD BENEFICIARYS DIALYSIS BENEFIT, IS NOT PART OF THE COMPOSITE RATE, AND IS SEPARATELY REIMBURSABLE					C			F

HCPCS	Long Description	PI1	MPI	Statute	X-Ref1	Coverage	ASC Pay Grp	ASC Pay Grp Eff Date	Action Code
CC	PROCEDURE CODE CHANGE (USE CC WHEN THE PROCEDURE CODE SUBMITTED WAS CHANGED EITHER FOR ADMINISTRATIVE REASONS OR BECAUSE AN INCORRECT CODE WAS FILED)					C			N
E1	UPPER LEFT, EYELID					C			N
E2	LOWER LEFT, EYELID					C			N
E3	UPPER RIGHT, EYELID					C			N
E4	LOWER RIGHT, EYELID					C			N
EJ	SUBSEQUENT CLAIMS FOR A DEFINED COURSE OF THERAPY, E.G., EPO, SODIUM HYALURONATE, INFLIXIMAB					D			N
EM	EMERGENCY RESERVE SUPPLY (FOR ESRD BENEFIT ONLY)					D			N
EP	SERVICE PROVIDED AS PART OF MEDICAID EARLY PERIODIC SCREENING DIAGNOSIS AND TREATMENT (EPSDT) PROGRAM					C			N
ET	EMERGENCY SERVICES					C			N
EY	NO PHYSICIAN OR OTHER LICENSED HEALTH CARE PROVIDER ORDER FOR THIS ITEM OR SERVICE					C			N
F1	LEFT HAND, SECOND DIGIT					C			N
F2	LEFT HAND, THIRD DIGIT					C			N
F3	LEFT HAND, FOURTH DIGIT					C			N
F4	LEFT HAND, FIFTH DIGIT					C			N
F5	RIGHT HAND, THUMB					C			N
F6	RIGHT HAND, SECOND DIGIT					C			N
F7	RIGHT HAND, THIRD DIGIT					C			N
F8	RIGHT HAND, FOURTH DIGIT					C			N
F9	RIGHT HAND, FIFTH DIGIT					C			N
FA	LEFT HAND, THUMB					C			N
FP	SERVICE PROVIDED AS PART OF MEDICAID FAMILY PLANNING PROGRAM					C			N
G1	MOST RECENT URR READING OF LESS THAN 60					C			N
G2	MOST RECENT URR READING OF 60 TO 64.9					C			N
G3	MOST RECENT URR READING OF 65 TO 69.9					C			N
G4	MOST RECENT URR READING OF 70 TO 74.9					C			N
G5	MOST RECENT URR READING OF 75 OR GREATER					C			N
G6	ESRD PATIENT FOR WHOM LESS THAN SIX DIALYSIS SESSIONS HAVE BEEN PROVIDED IN A MONTH MONTH					C			N
G7	PREGNANCY RESULTED FROM RAPE OR INCEST OR PREGNANCY CERTIFIED BY PHYSICIAN AS LIFE THREATENING LIFE THREATENING					D			N
G8	MONITORED ANESTHESIA CARE (MAC) FOR DEEP COMPLEX, COMPLICATED, OR MARKEDLY INVASIVE SURGICAL PROCEDURE INVASIVE SURGICAL PROCEDURE					C			N
G9	MONITORED ANESTHESIA CARE FOR PATIENT WHO HAS HISTORY OF SEVERE CARDIO-PULMONARY CONDITION					C			N
GA	WAIVER OF LIABILITY STATEMENT ON FILE					C			N

HCPCS	Long Description	PH	MPI	Statute	X-Ref	Coverage	ASC Pay Grp	ASC Pay Grp Eff Date	Action Code
GB	CLAIM BEING RE-SUBMITTED FOR PAYMENT BECAUSE IT IS NO LONGER COVERED UNDER A GLOBAL PAYMENT DEMONSTRATION					C			N
GC	THIS SERVICE HAS BEEN PERFORMED IN PART BY A RESIDENT UNDER THE DIRECTION OF A TEACHING PHYSICIAN					D			N
GE	THIS SERVICE HAS BEEN PERFORMED BY A RESIDENT WITHOUT THE PRESENCE OF A TEACHING PHYSICIAN UNDER THE PRIMARY CARE EXCEPTION					D			N
GF	NON-PHYSICIAN (E.G. NURSE PRACTITIONER (NP), CERTIFIED REGISTERED NURSE ANAESTHETIST (CRNA), CERTIFIED REGISTERED NURSE (CRN), CLINICAL NURSE SPECIALIST (CNS), PHYSICIAN ASSISTANT (PA)) SERVICES IN A CRITICAL ACCESS HOSPITAL					C			N
GG	PERFORMANCE AND PAYMENT OF A SCREENING MAMMOGRAM AND DIAGNOSTIC MAMMOGRAM ON THE SAME PATIENT, SAME DAY					C			N
GH	DIAGNOSTIC MAMMOGRAM CONVERTED FROM SCREENING MAMMOGRAM ON SAME DAY					C			N
GJ	"OPT OUT" PHYSICIAN OR PRACTITIONER EMERGENCY OR URGENT SERVICE					C			N
GK	ACTUAL ITEM/SERVICE ORDERED BY PHYSICIAN, ITEM ASSOCIATED WITH GA OR GZ MODIFIER					C			N
GL	MEDICALLY UNNECESSARY UPGRADE PROVIDED INSTEAD OF STANDARD ITEM, NO CHARGE, NO ADVANCE BENEFICIARY NOTICE (ABN)					C			N
GM	MULTIPLE PATIENTS ON ONE AMBULANCE TRIP					C			N
GN	SERVICES DELIVERED UNDER AN OUTPATIENT SPEECH LANGUAGE PATHOLOGY PLAN OF CARE					C			N
GO	SERVICES DELIVERED UNDER AN OUTPATIENT OCCUPATIONAL THERAPY PLAN OF CARE					C			N
GP	SERVICES DELIVERED UNDER AN OUTPATIENT PHYSICAL THERAPY PLAN OF CARE					C			N
GQ	VIA ASYNCHRONOUS TELECOMMUNICATIONS SYSTEM					C			N
GT	VIA INTERACTIVE AUDIO AND VIDEO TELECOMMUNICATION SYSTEMS					D			N
GU	PROCEDURE PERFORMED IN NON FEE SCHEDULE PLACE OF SERVICE					C			N
GV	ATTENDING PHYSICIAN NOT EMPLOYED OR PAID UNDER ARRANGEMENT BY THE PATIENTS HOSPICE PROVIDER					D			N
GW	SERVICE NOT RELATED TO THE HOSPICE PATIENTS TERMINAL CONDITION					D			N
GX	SERVICE NOT COVERED BY MEDICARE					M			N
GY	ITEM OR SERVICE STATUTORILY EXCLUDED OR DOES NOT MEET THE DEFINITION OF ANY MEDICARE BENEFIT					S			N
GZ	ITEM OR SERVICE EXPECTED TO BE DENIED AS NOT REASONABLE AND NECESSARY					M			N
H9	COURT-ORDERED					I			N
HA	CHILD/ADOLESCENT PROGRAM					I			N
HB	ADULT PROGRAM, NON GERIATRIC					I			N
HC	ADULT PROGRAM, GERIATRIC					I			N

HCPCS	Long Description	PII	MPI	Statute	X-Ref	Coverage	ASC Pay Grp	ASC Pay Grp Eff Date	Action Code
HD	PREGNANT/PARENTING WOMENS PROGRAM					I			N
HE	MENTAL HEALTH PROGRAM					I			N
HF	SUBSTANCE ABUSE PROGRAM					I			N
HG	OPIOID ADDICTION TREATMENT PROGRAM					I			N
HH	INTEGRATED MENTAL HEALTH/SUBSTANCE ABUSE PROGRAM					I			N
HI	INTEGRATED MENTAL HEALTH AND MENTAL RETARDATION/DEVELOPMENTAL DISABILITIES PROGRAM					I			N
HJ	EMPLOYEE ASSISTANCE PROGRAM					I			N
HK	SPECIALIZED MENTAL HEALTH PROGRAMS FOR HIGH-RISK POPULATIONS					I			N
HL	INTERN					I			N
HM	LESS THAN BACHELOR DEGREE LEVEL					I			N
HN	BACHELORS DEGREE LEVEL					I			N
HO	MASTERS DEGREE LEVEL					I			N
HP	DOCTORAL LEVEL					I			N
HQ	GROUP SETTING					I			N
HR	FAMILY/COUPLE WITH CLIENT PRESENT					I			N
HS	FAMILY/COUPLE WITHOUT CLIENT PRESENT					I			N
HT	MULTI-DISCIPLINARY TEAM					I			N
HU	FUNDED BY CHILD WELFARE AGENCY					I			N
HV	FUNDED STATE ADDICTIONS AGENCY					I			N
HW	FUNDED BY STATE MENTAL HEALTH AGENCY					I			N
HX	FUNDED BY COUNTY/LOCAL AGENCY					I			N
HY	FUNDED BY JUVENILE JUSTICE AGENCY					I			N
HZ	FUNDED BY CRIMINAL JUSTICE AGENCY					I			N
JW	DRUG AMOUNT DISCARDED/NOT ADMINISTERED TO ANY PATIENT					C			N
K0	LOWER EXTREMITY PROSTHESIS FUNCTIONAL LEVEL 0 - DOES NOT HAVE THE ABILITY OR POTENTIAL TO AMBULATE OR TRANSFER SAFELY WITH OR WITHOUT ASSISTANCE AND A PROSTHESIS DOES NOT ENHANCE THEIR QUALITY OF LIFE OR MOBILITY.					C			N

HCPCS	Long Description	PII	MPI	Statute	X-Ref1	Coverage	ASC Pay Grp	ASC Pay Grp Eff Date	Action Code
K1	LOWER EXTREMITY PROSTHESIS FUNCTIONAL LEVEL 1 - HAS THE ABILITY OR POTENTIAL TO USE A PROSTHESIS FOR TRANSFERS OR AMBULATION ON LEVEL SURFACES AT FIXED CADENCE. TYPICAL OF THE LIMITED AND UNLIMITED HOUSEHOLD AMBULATOR.					C			N
K2	LOWER EXTREMITY PROSTHESIS FUNCTIONAL LEVEL 2 - HAS THE ABILITY OR POTENTIAL FOR AMBULATION WITH THE ABILITY TO TRAVERSE LOW LEVEL ENVIRONMENTAL BARRIERS SUCH AS CURBS, STAIRS OR UNEVEN SURFACES. TYPICAL OF THE LIMITED COMMUNITY AMBULATOR.					C			N
K3	LOWER EXTREMITY PROSTHESIS FUNCTIONAL LEVEL 3 - HAS THE ABILITY OR POTENTIAL FOR AMBULATION WITH VARIABLE CADENCE. TYPICAL OF THE COMMUNITY AMBULATOR WHO HAS THE ABILITY TO TRANSVERSE MOST ENVIRONMENTAL BARRIERS AND MAY HAVE VOCATIONAL, THERAPEUTIC, OR EXERCISE ACTIVITY THAT DEMANDS PROSTHETIC UTILIZATION BEYOND SIMPLE LOCOMOTION					C			N
K4	LOWER EXTREMITY PROSTHESIS FUNCTIONAL LEVEL 4 - HAS THE ABILITY OR POTENTIAL FOR PROSTHETIC AMBULATION THAT EXCEEDS THE BASIC AMBULATION SKILLS, EXHIBITING HIGH IMPACT, STRESS, OR ENERGY LEVELS, TYPICAL OF THE PROSTHETIC DEMANDS OF THE CHILD, ACTIVE ADULT, OR ATHLETE.					C			N
KA	ADD ON OPTION/ACCESSORY FOR WHEELCHAIR					C			N
KB	BENEFICIARY REQUESTED UPGRADE FOR ABN, MORE THAN 4 MODIFIERS IDENTIFIED ON CLAIM					C			N
KH	DMEPOS ITEM, INITIAL CLAIM, PURCHASE OR FIRST MONTH RENTAL					C			N
KI	DMEPOS ITEM, SECOND OR THIRD MONTH RENTAL					C			N
KJ	DMEPOS ITEM, PARENTERAL ENTERAL NUTRITION (PEN) PUMP OR CAPPED RENTAL, MONTHS FOUR TO FIFTEEN					C			N
KK	INHALATION SOLUTION COMPOUNDED FROM AN FDA APPROVED FORMULATION					C			N
KL	PRODUCT CHARACTERISTICS DEFINED IN MEDICAL POLICY ARE MET					C			N
KM	REPLACEMENT OF FACIAL PROSTHESIS INCLUDING NEW IMPRESSION/MOULAGE					C			N
KN	REPLACEMENT OF FACIAL PROSTHESIS USING PREVIOUS MASTER MODEL					C			N
KO	SINGLE DRUG UNIT DOSE FORMULATION					C			N
KP	FIRST DRUG OF A MULTIPLE DRUG UNIT DOSE FORMULATION					C			N
KQ	SECOND OR SUBSEQUENT DRUG OF A MULTIPLE DRUG UNIT DOSE FORMULATION					C			N
KR	RENTAL ITEM, BILLING FOR PARTIAL MONTH					C			N
KS	GLUCOSE MONITOR SUPPLY FOR DIABETIC BENEFICIARY NOT TREATED WITH INSULIN					D			N
KX	SPECIFIC REQUIRED DOCUMENTATION ON FILE					C			N
KZ	NEW COVERAGE NOT IMPLEMENTED BY MANAGED CARE					C			A
LC	LEFT CIRCUMFLEX CORONARY ARTERY					C			N
LD	LEFT ANTERIOR DESCENDING CORONARY ARTERY					C			N
LL	LEASE/RENTAL (USE THE LL MODIFIER WHEN DME EQUIPMENT RENTAL IS TO BE APPLIED AGAINST THE PURCHASE PRICE)					C			N

HCPCS	Long Description	PII	MPI	Statute	X-Refl	Coverage	ASC Pay Grp	ASC Pay Grp Eff Date	Action Code
LR	LABORATORY ROUND TRIP					C			N
LS	FDA-MONITORED INTRAOCULAR LENS IMPLANT					D			N
LT	LEFT SIDE (USED TO IDENTIFY PROCEDURES PERFORMED ON THE LEFT SIDE OF THE BODY)					C			N
MS	SIX MONTH MAINTENANCE AND SERVICING FEE FOR REASONABLE AND NECESSARY PARTS AND LABOR WHICH ARE NOT COVERED UNDER ANY MANUFACTURER OR SUPPLIER WARRANTY					C			N
NR	NEW WHEN RENTED (USE THE NR MODIFIER WHEN DME WHICH WAS NEW AT THE TIME OF RENTAL IS SUBSEQUENTLY PURCHASED)					C			N
NU	NEW EQUIPMENT					C			N
PL	PROGRESSIVE ADDITION LENSES					C			N
Q2	HCFA/ORD DEMONSTRATION PROJECT PROCEDURE/SERVICE					C			N
Q3	LIVE KIDNEY DONOR SURGERY AND RELATED SERVICES					C			N
Q4	SERVICE FOR ORDERING/REFERRING PHYSICIAN QUALIFIES AS A SERVICE EXEMPTION					C			N
Q5	SERVICE FURNISHED BY A SUBSTITUTE PHYSICIAN UNDER A RECIPROCAL BILLING ARRANGEMENT					D			N
Q6	SERVICE FURNISHED BY A LOCUM TENENS PHYSICIAN					D			N
Q7	ONE CLASS A FINDING					C			N
Q8	TWO CLASS B FINDINGS					C			N
Q9	ONE CLASS B AND TWO CLASS C FINDINGS					C			N
QA	FDA INVESTIGATIONAL DEVICE EXEMPTION					C			N
QB	PHYSICIAN PROVIDING SERVICE IN A RURAL HPSA					D			N
QC	SINGLE CHANNEL MONITORING					C			N
QD	RECORDING AND STORAGE IN SOLID STATE MEMORY BY A DIGITAL RECORDER					C			N
QE	PRESCRIBED AMOUNT OF OXYGEN IS LESS THAN 1 LITER PER MINUTE (LPM)					C			N
QF	PRESCRIBED AMOUNT OF OXYGEN EXCEEDS 4 LITERS PER MINUTE (LPM) AND PORTABLE OXYGEN IS PRESCRIBED					C			N
QG	PRESCRIBED AMOUNT OF OXYGEN IS GREATER THAN 4 LITERS PER MINUTE(LPM)					C			N
QH	OXYGEN CONSERVING DEVICE IS BEING USED WITH AN OXYGEN DELIVERY SYSTEM					C			N
QJ	SERVICES/ITEMS PROVIDED TO A PRISONER OR PATIENT IN STATE OR LOCAL CUSTODY, HOWEVER THE STATE OR LOCAL GOVERNMENT, AS APPLICABLE, MEETS THE REQUIREMENTS IN 42 CFR 411.4 (B)					D			N
QK	MEDICAL DIRECTION OF TWO, THREE, OR FOUR CONCURRENT ANESTHESIA PROCEDURES INVOLVING QUALIFIED INDIVIDUALS					D			N

HCPCS	Long Description	PH	MPI	Statute	X-Ref1	Coverage	ASC Pay Grp	ASC Pay Grp Eff Date	Action Code
QL	PATIENT PRONOUNCED DEAD AFTER AMBULANCE CALLED					C			N
QM	AMBULANCE SERVICE PROVIDED UNDER ARRANGEMENT BY A PROVIDER OF SERVICES					C			N
QN	AMBULANCE SERVICE FURNISHED DIRECTLY BY A PROVIDER OF SERVICES					C			N
QP	DOCUMENTATION IS ON FILE SHOWING THAT THE LABORATORY TEST(S) WAS ORDERED INDIVIDUALLY OR ORDERED AS A CPT-RECOGNIZED PANEL OTHER THAN AUTOMATED PROFILE CODES 80002-80019, G0058, G0059, AND G0060.					D			N
QQ	CLAIM SUBMITTED WITH A WRITTEN STATEMENT OF INTENT					C			N
QS	MONITORED ANESTHESIA CARE SERVICE					D			N
QT	RECORDING AND STORAGE ON TAPE BY AN ANALOG TAPE RECORDER					C			N
QU	PHYSICIAN PROVIDING SERVICE IN AN URBAN HPSA					D			N
QV	ITEM OR SERVICE PROVIDED AS ROUTINE CARE IN A MEDICARE QUALIFYING CLINICAL TRIAL					D			N
QW	CLIA WAIVED TEST					C			N
QX	CRNA SERVICE: WITH MEDICAL DIRECTION BY A PHYSICIAN					C			N
QY	MEDICAL DIRECTION OF ONE CERTIFIED REGISTERED NURSE ANESTHETIST (CRNA) BY AN ANESTHESIOLOGIST					D			N
QZ	CRNA SERVICE: WITHOUT MEDICAL DIRECTION BY A PHYSICIAN					C			N
RC	RIGHT CORONARY ARTERY					C			N
RP	REPLACEMENT AND REPAIR -RP MAY BE USED TO INDICATE REPLACEMENT OF DME, ORTHOTIC AND PROSTHETIC DEVICES WHICH HAVE BEEN IN USE FOR SOMETIME. THE CLAIM SHOWS THE CODE FOR THE PART, FOLLOWED BY THE RP MODIFIER AND THE CHARGE FOR THE PART.					C			N
RR	RENTAL (USE THE RR MODIFIER WHEN DME IS TO BE RENTED)					C			N
RT	RIGHT SIDE (USED TO IDENTIFY PROCEDURES PERFORMED ON THE RIGHT SIDE OF THE BODY)					C			N
SA	NURSE PRACTITIONER RENDERING SERVICE IN COLLABORATION WITH A PHYSICIAN					I			N
SB	NURSE MIDWIFE					I			N
SC	MEDICALLY NECESSARY SERVICE OR SUPPLY					I			N
SD	SERVICES PROVIDED BY REGISTERED NURSE WITH SPECIALIZED, HIGHLY TECHNICAL HOME INFUSION TRAINING					I			N
SE	STATE AND/OR FEDERALLY-FUNDED PROGRAMS/SERVICES					I			N
SF	SECOND OPINION ORDERED BY A PROFESSIONAL REVIEW ORGANIZATION (PRO) PER SECTION 9401, P.L. 99-272 (100% REIMBURSEMENT - NO MEDICARE DEDUCTIBLE OR COINSURANCE)					C			N
SG	AMBULATORY SURGICAL CENTER (ASC) FACILITY SERVICE					C			N
SH	SECOND CONCURRENTLY ADMINISTERED INFUSION THERAPY					I			N

HCPCS	Long Description	PTI	MPI	Statute	X-Ref	Coverage	ASC Pay Grp	ASC Pay Grp Eff Date	Action Code
SJ	THIRD OR MORE CONCURRENTLY ADMINISTERED INFUSION THERAPY					I			N
SK	MEMBER OF HIGH RISK POPULATION (USE ONLY WITH CODES FOR IMMUNIZATION)					I			N
SL	STATE SUPPLIED VACCINE					I			N
SM	SECOND SURGICAL OPINION					I			N
SN	THIRD SURGICAL OPINION					I			N
SQ	ITEM ORDERED BY HOME HEALTH					I			N
ST	RELATED TO TRAUMA OR INJURY					I			N
SU	PROCEDURE PERFORMED IN PHYSICIANS OFFICE (TO DENOTE USE OF FACILITY AND EQUIPMENT)					I			N
SV	PHARMACEUTICALS DELIVERED TO PATIENTS HOME BUT NOT UTILIZED					I			N
T1	LEFT FOOT, SECOND DIGIT					C			N
T2	LEFT FOOT, THIRD DIGIT					C			N
T3	LEFT FOOT, FOURTH DIGIT					C			N
T4	LEFT FOOT, FIFTH DIGIT					C			N
T5	RIGHT FOOT, GREAT TOE					C			N
T6	RIGHT FOOT, SECOND DIGIT					C			N
T7	RIGHT FOOT, THIRD DIGIT					C			N
T8	RIGHT FOOT, FOURTH DIGIT					C			N
T9	RIGHT FOOT, FIFTH DIGIT					C			N
TA	LEFT FOOT, GREAT TOE					C			N
TC	TECHNICAL COMPONENT. UNDER CERTAIN CIRCUMSTANCES, A CHARGE MAY BE MADE FOR THE TECHNICAL COMPONENT ALONE. UNDER THOSE CIRCUMSTANCES THE TECHNICAL COMPONENT CHARGE IS IDENTIFIED BY ADDING MODIFIER TC TO THE USUAL PROCEDURE NUMBER. TECHNICAL COMPONENT CHARGES ARE INSTITUTIONAL CHARGES AND NOT BILLED SEPARATELY BY PHYSICIANS. HOWEVER, PORTABLE X-RAY SUPPLIERS ONLY BILL FOR TECHNICAL COMPONENT AND SHOULD UTILIZE MODIFIER TC. THE CHARGE DATA FROM PORTABLE X-RAY SUPPLIERS WILL THEN BE USED TO BUILD CUSTOMARY AND PREVAILING PROFILES.					C			N
TD	RN					I			N
TE	LPN/LVN					I			N
TF	INTERMEDIATE LEVEL OF CARE					I			N
TG	COMPLEX/HIGH TECH LEVEL OF CARE					I			N
TH	OBSTETRICAL TREATMENT/SERVICES, PRENATAL OR POSTPARTUM					I			N
TJ	PROGRAM GROUP, CHILD AND/OR ADOLESCENT					I			N
TK	EXTRA PATIENT OR PASSENGER, NON-AMBULANCE					I			N
TL	EARLY INTERVENTION/INDIVIDUALIZED FAMILY SERVICE PLAN (IFSP)					I			N

HCPCS	Long Description	PH	MPI	Statute	X-Ref1	Coverage	ASC Pay Grp	ASC Pay Grp Eff Date	Action Code
TM	INDIVIDUALIZED EDUCATION PROGRAM (IEP)					I			N
TN	RURAL/OUTSIDE PROVIDERS CUSTOMARY SERVICE AREA					I			N
TP	MEDICAL TRANSPORT, UNLOADED VEHICLE					I			N
TQ	BASIC LIFE SUPPORT TRANSPORT BY A VOLUNTEER AMBULANCE PROVIDER					I			N
TR	SCHOOL-BASED INDIVIDUALIZED EDUCATION PROGRAM (IEP) SERVICES PROVIDED OUTSIDE THE PUBLIC SCHOOL DISTRICT RESPONSIBLE FOR THE STUDENT					I			N
TS	FOLLOW-UP SERVICE					I			N
TT	INDIVIDUALIZED SERVICE PROVIDED TO MORE THAN ONE PATIENT IN SAME SETTING					I			N
TU	SPECIAL PAYMENT RATE, OVERTIME					I			N
TV	SPECIAL PAYMENT RATES, HOLIDAYS/WEEKENDS					I			N
TW	BACK-UP EQUIPMENT					I			N
U1	MEDICAID LEVEL OF CARE 1, AS DEFINED BY EACH STATE					I			N
U2	MEDICAID LEVEL OF CARE 2, AS DEFINED BY EACH STATE					I			N
U3	MEDICAID LEVEL OF CARE 3, AS DEFINED BY EACH STATE					I			N
U4	MEDICAID LEVEL OF CARE 4, AS DEFINED BY EACH STATE					I			N
U5	MEDICAID LEVEL OF CARE 5, AS DEFINED BY EACH STATE					I			N
U6	MEDICAID LEVEL OF CARE 6, AS DEFINED BY EACH STATE					I			N
U7	MEDICAID LEVEL OF CARE 7, AS DEFINED BY EACH STATE					I			N
U8	MEDICAID LEVEL OF CARE 8, AS DEFINED BY EACH STATE					I			N
U9	MEDICAID LEVEL OF CARE 9, AS DEFINED BY EACH STATE					I			N
UA	MEDICAID LEVEL OF CARE 10, AS DEFINED BY EACH STATE					I			N
UB	MEDICAID LEVEL OF CARE 11, AS DEFINED BY EACH STATE					I			N
UC	MEDICAID LEVEL OF CARE 12, AS DEFINED BY EACH STATE					I			N
UD	MEDICAID LEVEL OF CARE 13, AS DEFINED BY EACH STATE					I			N
UE	USED DURABLE MEDICAL EQUIPMENT					C			N
UF	SERVICES PROVIDED IN THE MORNING					I			A
UG	SERVICES PROVIDED IN THE AFTERNOON					I			A
UH	SERVICES PROVIDED IN THE EVENING					I			A
UJ	SERVICES PROVIDED AT NIGHT					I			A
UK	SERVICES PROVIDED ON BEHALF OF THE CLIENT TO SOMEONE OTHER THAN THE CLIENT (COLLATERAL RELATIONSHIP)					I			A

HCPCS	Long Description	PTI	MPI	Statute	X-Ref	Coverage	ASC Pay Grp	ASC Pay Grp Eff Date	Action Code
UN	TWO PATIENTS SERVED					C			A
UP	THREE PATIENTS SERVED					C			A
UQ	FOUR PATIENTS SERVED					C			A
UR	FIVE PATIENTS SERVED					C			A
US	SIX OR MORE PATIENTS SERVED					C			A
VP	APHAKIC PATIENT					C			N
A0021	AMBULANCE SERVICE, OUTSIDE STATE PER MILE, TRANSPORT (MEDICAID ONLY)	00	9		A0030	I			N
A0030	AMBULANCE SERVICE, CONVENTIONAL AIR SERVICE, TRANSPORT, ONE WAY	00	9		A0430	I			N
A0040	AMBULANCE SERVICE, AIR, HELICOPTER SERVICE, TRANSPORT	00	9		A0431	I			N
A0050	AMBULANCE SERVICE, EMERGENCY, WATER, SPECIAL TRANSPORTATION SERVICES	00	9		A0429	I			N
A0080	NON-EMERGENCY TRANSPORTATION, PER MILE - VEHICLE PROVIDED BY VOLUNTEER (INDIVIDUAL OR ORGANIZATION), WITH NO VESTED INTEREST	00	9			I			N
A0090	NON-EMERGENCY TRANSPORTATION, PER MILE - VEHICLE PROVIDED BY INDIVIDUAL (FAMILY MEMBER, SELF, NEIGHBOR) WITH VESTED INTEREST	00	9			I			N
A0100	NON-EMERGENCY TRANSPORTATION; TAXI	00	9			I			N
A0110	NON-EMERGENCY TRANSPORTATION AND BUS, INTRA OR INTER STATE CARRIER	00	9			I			N
A0120	NON-EMERGENCY TRANSPORTATION: MINI-BUS, MOUNTAIN AREA TRANSPORTS, OR OTHER TRANSPORTATION SYSTEMS	00	9			I			N
A0130	NON-EMERGENCY TRANSPORTATION: WHEEL-CHAIR VAN	00	9			I			N
A0140	NON-EMERGENCY TRANSPORTATION AND AIR TRAVEL (PRIVATE OR COMMERCIAL) INTRA OR INTER STATE	00	9			I			N
A0160	NON-EMERGENCY TRANSPORTATION: PER MILE - CASE WORKER OR SOCIAL WORKER	00	9			I			N
A0170	TRANSPORTATION ANCILLARY: PARKING FEES, TOLLS, OTHER	00	9			I			N
A0180	NON-EMERGENCY TRANSPORTATION: ANCILLARY: LODGING-RECIPIENT	00	9			I			N
A0190	NON-EMERGENCY TRANSPORTATION: ANCILLARY: MEALS-RECIPIENT	00	9			I			N
A0200	NON-EMERGENCY TRANSPORTATION: ANCILLARY: LODGING ESCORT	00	9			I			N
A0210	NON-EMERGENCY TRANSPORTATION: ANCILLARY: MEALS-ESCORT	00	9			I			N
A0225	AMBULANCE SERVICE, NEONATAL TRANSPORT, BASE RATE, EMERGENCY TRANSPORT, ONE WAY	00	9			I			F
A0300	AMBULANCE SERVICE, BASIC LIFE SUPPORT (BLS), NON-EMERGENCY TRANSPORT, ALL INCLUSIVE (MILEAGE AND SUPPLIES)	00	9		A0428	I			N

HCPCS	Long Description	PB	MPI	Statute	X-Ref1	Coverage	ASC Pay Grp	ASC Pay Grp Eff Date	Action Code
A0302	AMBULANCE SERVICE, BLS, EMERGENCY TRANSPORT, ALL INCLUSIVE (MILEAGE AND SUPPLIES)	00	9		A0429	I			N
A0304	AMBULANCE SERVICE, ADVANCED LIFE SUPPORT (ALS), NON-EMERGENCY TRANSPORT, NO SPECIALIZED ALS SERVICES RENDERED, ALL INCLUSIVE (MILEAGE AND SUPPLIES)	00	9		A0428	I			N
A0306	AMBULANCE SERVICES, ALS, NON-EMERGENCY TRANSPORT, SPECIALIZED ALS SERVICES RENDERED, ALL INCLUSIVE (MILEAGE AND SUPPLIES)	00	9		A0426	I			N
A0308	AMBULANCE SERVICE, ALS, EMERGENCY TRANSPORT, NO SPECIALIZED ALS SERVICES RENDERED, ALL INCLUSIVE (MILEAGE AND SUPPLIES)	00	9		A0429	I			N
A0310	AMBULANCE SERVICE, ALS, EMERGENCY TRANSPORT, SPECIALIZED ALS SERVICES RENDERED, ALL INCLUSIVE (MILEAGE AND SUPPLIES)	00	9		A0427	I			N
A0320	AMBULANCE SERVICE, BLS, NON-EMERGENCY TRANSPORT, SUPPLIES INCLUDED, MILEAGE SEPARATELY BILLED	00	9		A0428	I			N
A0322	AMBULANCE SERVICE, BLS, EMERGENCY TRANSPORT, SUPPLIES INCLUDED, MILEAGE SEPARATELY BILLED	00	9		A0429	I			N
A0324	AMBULANCE SERVICE, ALS, NON-EMERGENCY TRANSPORT, NO SPECIALIZED ALS SERVICES RENDERED, SUPPLIES INCLUDED, MILEAGE SEPARATELY BILLED	00	9		A0428	I			N
A0326	AMBULANCE SERVICE, ALS, NON-EMERGENCY TRANSPORT, SPECIALIZED ALS SERVICES RENDERED, SUPPLIES INCLUDED, MILEAGE SEPARATELY BILLED	00	9		A0426	I			N
A0328	AMBULANCE SERVICE, ALS, EMERGENCY TRANSPORT, NO SPECIALIZED ALS SERVICES RENDERED, SUPPLIES INCLUDED, MILEAGE SEPARATELY BILLED	00	9		A0429	I			N
A0330	AMBULANCE SERVICE, ALS, EMERGENCY TRANSPORT, SPECIALIZED ALS SERVICES RENDERED, SUPPLIES INCLUDED, MILEAGE SEPARATELY BILLED	00	9		A0427	I			N
A0340	AMBULANCE SERVICE, BLS, NON-EMERGENCY TRANSPORT, MILEAGE INCLUDED, DISPOSABLE SUPPLIES SEPARATELY BILLED	00	9		A0428	I			N
A0342	AMBULANCE SERVICE, BLS, EMERGENCY TRANSPORT, MILEAGE INCLUDED, DISPOSABLE SUPPLIES SEPARATELY BILLED	00	9		A0429	I			N
A0344	AMBULANCE SERVICE, ALS, NON-EMERGENCY TRANSPORT, NO SPECIALIZED ALS SERVICES RENDERED, MILEAGE INCLUDED, DISPOSABLE SUPPLIES SEPARATELY BILLED	00	9		A0428	I			N
A0346	AMBULANCE SERVICE, ALS, NON-EMERGENCY TRANSPORT, SPECIALIZED ALS SERVICES RENDERED, MILEAGE INCLUDED, DISPOSABLE SUPPLIES SEPARATELY BILLED	00	9		A0426	I			N
A0348	AMBULANCE SERVICE, ALS, EMERGENCY TRANSPORT, NO SPECIALIZED ALS SERVICES RENDERED, MILEAGE INCLUDED, DISPOSABLE SUPPLIES SEPARATELY BILLED	00	9		A0429	I			N
A0350	AMBULANCE SERVICE, ALS, EMERGENCY TRANSPORT, SPECIALIZED ALS SERVICES RENDERED, MILEAGE INCLUDED, DISPOSABLE SUPPLIES SEPARATELY BILLED	00	9		A0427	I			N
A0360	AMBULANCE SERVICE, BLS, NON-EMERGENCY TRANSPORT, MILEAGE AND DISPOSABLE SUPPLIES SEPARATELY BILLED	00	9		A0428	I			N
A0362	AMBULANCE SERVICE, BLS, EMERGENCY TRANSPORT, MILEAGE AND DISPOSABLE SUPPLIES SEPARATELY BILLED	00	9		A0429	I			N
A0364	AMBULANCE SERVICE, ALS, NON-EMERGENCY TRANSPORT, NO SPECIALIZED ALS SERVICES RENDERED, MILEAGE AND DISPOSABLE SUPPLIES SEPARATELY BILLED	00	9		A0428	I			N
A0366	AMBULANCE SERVICE, ALS, NON-EMERGENCY TRANSPORT, SPECIALIZED ALS SERVICES RENDERED, MILEAGE AND DISPOSABLE SUPPLIES SEPARATELY BILLED	00	9		A0426	I			N
A0368	AMBULANCE SERVICE, ALS, EMERGENCY TRANSPORT, NO SPECIALIZED ALS SERVICES RENDERED, MILEAGE AND DISPOSABLE SUPPLIES SEPARATELY BILLED	00	9			I			N
A0370	AMBULANCE SERVICE, ALS, EMERGENCY TRANSPORT, SPECIALIZED ALS SERVICES RENDERED,	00	9		A0427	I			N
A0370	MILEAGE AND DISPOSABLE SUPPLIES SEPARATELY BILLED								

HCPCS	Long Description	PH	MPI	Statute	X-Ref1	Coverage	ASC Pay Grp	ASC Pay Grp Eff Date	Action Code
A0380	BLS MILEAGE (PER MILE)	00	9		A0425	I			N
A0382	BLS ROUTINE DISPOSABLE SUPPLIES	52	A			C			N
A0384	BLS SPECIALIZED SERVICE DISPOSABLE SUPPLIES; DEFIBRILLATION (USED BY ALS AMBULANCES AND BLS AMBULANCES IN JURISDICTIONS WHERE DEFIBRILLATION IS PERMITTED IN BLS AMBULANCES)	52	A			C			N
A0390	ALS MILEAGE (PER MILE)	00	9		A0425	I			N
A0392	ALS SPECIALIZED SERVICE DISPOSABLE SUPPLIES; DEFIBRILLATION (TO BE USED ONLY IN JURISDICTIONS WHERE DEFIBRILLATION CANNOT BE PERFORMED IN BLS AMBULANCES)	52	A			C			N
A0394	ALS SPECIALIZED SERVICE DISPOSABLE SUPPLIES; IV DRUG THERAPY	52	A			C			N
A0396	ALS SPECIALIZED SERVICE DISPOSABLE SUPPLIES; ESOPHAGEAL INTUBATION	52	A			C			N
A0398	ALS ROUTINE DISPOSABLE SUPPLIES	52	A			C			N
A0420	AMBULANCE WAITING TIME (ALS OR BLS), ONE HALF (1/2) HOUR INCREMENTS	52	A			C			N
A0422	AMBULANCE (ALS OR BLS) OXYGEN AND OXYGEN SUPPLIES, LIFE SUSTAINING SITUATION	52	A			C			N
A0424	EXTRA AMBULANCE ATTENDANT, GROUND (ALS OR BLS) OR AIR (FIXED OR ROTARY WINGED); (REQUIRES MEDICAL REVIEW)	52	A			C			N
A0425	GROUND MILEAGE, PER STATUTE MILE	52	A			C			N
A0426	AMBULANCE SERVICE, ADVANCED LIFE SUPPORT, NON-EMERGENCY TRANSPORT, LEVEL 1 (ALS 1)	52	A			C			N
A0427	AMBULANCE SERVICE, ADVANCED LIFE SUPPORT, EMERGENCY TRANSPORT, LEVEL 1 (ALS1-EMERGENCY)	52	A			C			N
A0428	AMBULANCE SERVICE, BASIC LIFE SUPPORT, NON-EMERGENCY TRANSPORT, (BLS)	52	A			C			N
A0429	AMBULANCE SERVICE, BASIC LIFE SUPPORT, EMERGENCY TRANSPORT (BLS-EMERGENCY)	52	A			C			N
A0430	AMBULANCE SERVICE, CONVENTIONAL AIR SERVICES, TRANSPORT, ONE WAY (FIXED WING)	52	A			C			N
A0431	AMBULANCE SERVICE, CONVENTIONAL AIR SERVICES, TRANSPORT, ONE WAY (ROTARY WING)	52	A			C			N
A0432	PARAMEDIC INTERCEPT (PI), RURAL AREA, TRANSPORT FURNISHED BY A VOLUNTEER AMBULANCE COMPANY WHICH IS PROHIBITED BY STATE LAW FROM BILLING THIRD PARTY PAYERS	52	A			C			N
A0433	ADVANCED LIFE SUPPORT, LEVEL 2 (ALS 2)	52	A			C			N
A0434	SPECIALTY CARE TRANSPORT (SCT)	52	A			C			N
A0435	FIXED WING AIR MILEAGE, PER STATUTE MILE	52	A			C			N
A0436	ROTARY WING AIR MILEAGE, PER STATUTE MILE	52	A			C			N
A0800	AMBULANCE TRANSPORT PROVIDED BETWEEN THE HOURS OF 7PM AND 7AM	52	A			C			A
A0888	NONCOVERED AMBULANCE MILEAGE, PER MILE (E.G., FOR MILES TRAVELED BEYOND CLOSEST APPROPRIATE FACILITY)	00	9			M			N
A0999	UNLISTED AMBULANCE SERVICE	57	A			D			N
A4206	SYRINGE WITH NEEDLE, STERILE 1CC, EACH	00	9			I			N
A4207	SYRINGE WITH NEEDLE, STERILE 2CC, EACH	00	9			I			T

HCPCS	Long Description	PH	MPI	Statute	X-Ref1	Coverage	ASC Pay Grp	ASC Pay Grp Eff Date	Action Code
A4208	SYRINGE WITH NEEDLE, STERILE 3CC, EACH	00	9			I			N
A4209	SYRINGE WITH NEEDLE, STERILE 5CC OR GREATER, EACH	00	9			I			N
A4210	NEEDLE-FREE INJECTION DEVICE, EACH	00	9			M			N
A4211	SUPPLIES FOR SELF-ADMINISTERED INJECTIONS	00	9			D			N
A4212	NON-CORING NEEDLE OR STYLET WITH OR WITHOUT CATHETER	57	A			C			N
A4213	SYRINGE, STERILE, 20 CC OR GREATER, EACH	00	9			I			N
A4214	STERILE SALINE OR WATER, 30 CC VIAL	37	A			C			D
A4215	NEEDLES ONLY, STERILE, ANY SIZE, EACH	00	9			I			N
A4216	STERILE WATER/SALINE, 10 ML	37	A			D			A
A4217	STERILE WATER/SALINE, 500 ML	37	A			D			A
A4220	REFILL KIT FOR IMPLANTABLE INFUSION PUMP	57	A			D			N
A4221	SUPPLIES FOR MAINTENANCE OF DRUG INFUSION CATHETER, PER WEEK (LIST DRUG SEPARATELY)	34	A			C			N
A4222	SUPPLIES FOR EXTERNAL DRUG INFUSION PUMP, PER CASSETTE OR BAG (LIST DRUG SEPARATELY)	34	A			C			N
A4230	INFUSION SET FOR EXTERNAL INSULIN PUMP, NON NEEDLE CANNULA TYPE	34	A			D			N
A4231	INFUSION SET FOR EXTERNAL INSULIN PUMP, NEEDLE TYPE	34	A			D			N
A4232	SYRINGE WITH NEEDLE FOR EXTERNAL INSULIN PUMP, STERILE, 3CC	00	9			I			F
A4244	ALCOHOL OR PEROXIDE, PER PINT	00	9			I			N
A4245	ALCOHOL WIPES, PER BOX	00	9			I			N
A4246	BETADINE OR PHISOHEX SOLUTION, PER PINT	00	9			I			N
A4247	BETADINE OR IODINE SWABS/WIPES, PER BOX	00	9			I			N
A4248	CHLORHEXIDINE CONTAINING ANTISEPTIC, 1 ML	52	A			C			A
A4250	URINE TEST OR REAGENT STRIPS OR TABLETS (100 TABLETS OR STRIPS)	00	9			M			N
A4253	BLOOD GLUCOSE TEST OR REAGENT STRIPS FOR HOME BLOOD GLUCOSE MONITOR, PER 50 STRIPS	32	A			D			N
A4254	REPLACEMENT BATTERY, ANY TYPE, FOR USE WITH MEDICALLY NECESSARY HOME BLOOD GLUCOSE MONITOR OWNED BY PATIENT, EACH	32	A			D			N
A4255	PLATFORMS FOR HOME BLOOD GLUCOSE MONITOR, 50 PER BOX	34	A			D			N
A4256	NORMAL, LOW AND HIGH CALIBRATOR SOLUTION / CHIPS	34	A			D			N

HCPCS	Long Description	PH	MPI	Statute	X-Ref1	Coverage	ASC Pay Grp	ASC Pay Grp Eff Date	Action Code
A4257	REPLACEMENT LENS SHIELD CARTRIDGE FOR USE WITH LASER SKIN PIERCING DEVICE, EACH	34	A			C			N
A4258	SPRING-POWERED DEVICE FOR LANCET, EACH	34	A			D			N
A4259	LANCETS, PER BOX OF 100	34	A			D			N
A4260	LEVONORGESTREL (CONTRACEPTIVE) IMPLANTS SYSTEM, INCLUDING IMPLANTS AND SUPPLIES	00	9	1862a1A		S			N
A4261	CERVICAL CAP FOR CONTRACEPTIVE USE	00	9	1862a1		S			N
A4262	TEMPORARY, ABSORBABLE LACRIMAL DUCT IMPLANT, EACH	00	9			D			N
A4263	PERMANENT, LONG TERM, NON-DISSOLVABLE LACRIMAL DUCT IMPLANT, EACH	11	A			D			N
A4265	PARAFFIN, PER POUND	34	A			D			N
A4266	DIAPHRAGM FOR CONTRACEPTIVE USE	00	9			I			N
A4267	CONTRACEPTIVE SUPPLY, CONDOM, MALE, EACH	00	9			I			N
A4268	CONTRACEPTIVE SUPPLY, CONDOM, FEMALE, EACH	00	9			I			N
A4269	CONTRACEPTIVE SUPPLY, SPERMICIDE (E.G., FOAM, GEL), EACH	00	9			I			N
A4270	DISPOSABLE ENDOSCOPE SHEATH, EACH	00	9			C			N
A4280	ADHESIVE SKIN SUPPORT ATTACHMENT FOR USE WITH EXTERNAL BREAST PROSTHESIS, EACH	38	A			C			N
A4281	TUBING FOR BREAST PUMP, REPLACEMENT	00	9			I			N
A4282	ADAPTER FOR BREAST PUMP, REPLACEMENT	00	9			I			N
A4283	CAP FOR BREAST PUMP BOTTLE, REPLACEMENT	00	9			I			N
A4284	BREAST SHIELD AND SPLASH PROTECTOR FOR USE WITH BREAST PUMP, REPLACEMENT	00	9			I			N
A4285	POLYCARBONATE BOTTLE FOR USE WITH BREAST PUMP, REPLACEMENT	00	9			I			N
A4286	LOCKING RING FOR BREAST PUMP, REPLACEMENT	00	9			I			N
A4290	SACRAL NERVE STIMULATION TEST LEAD, EACH	38	A			C			N
A4300	IMPLANTABLE ACCESS CATHETER, (E,G., VENOUS, ARTERIAL, EPIDURAL SUBARACHNOID, OR PERITONEAL, ETC.) EXTERNAL ACCESS	11	A			D			N
A4301	IMPLANTABLE ACCESS TOTAL CATHETER, PORT/RESERVOIR (E.G., VENOUS, ARTERIAL, EPIDURAL, SUBARACHNOID, PERITONEAL, ETC.)	00	9			C			N
A4305	DISPOSABLE DRUG DELIVERY SYSTEM, FLOW RATE OF 50 ML OR GREATER PER HOUR	00	9			C			N
A4306	DISPOSABLE DRUG DELIVERY SYSTEM, FLOW RATE OF 5 ML OR LESS PER HOUR	00	9			C			N
A4310	INSERTION TRAY WITHOUT DRAINAGE BAG AND WITHOUT CATHETER (ACCESSORIES ONLY)	37	A			D			N
A4311	INSERTION TRAY WITHOUT DRAINAGE BAG WITH INDWELLING CATHETER, FOLEY TYPE, TWO-WAY LATEX WITH COATING (TEFLON, SILICONE, SILICONE ELASTOMER OR HYDROPHILIC, ETC.)	37	A			D			N
A4312	INSERTION TRAY WITHOUT DRAINAGE BAG WITH INDWELLING CATHETER, FOLEY TYPE, TWO-WAY, ALL SILICONE	37	A			D			N
A4313	INSERTION TRAY WITHOUT DRAINAGE BAG WITH INDWELLING CATHETER, FOLEY TYPE, THREE-WAY, FOR CONTINUOUS IRRIGATION	37	A			D			N

HCPCS	Long Description	PH	MPI	Statute	X-Reff	Coverage	ASC Pay Grp	ASC Pay Grp Eff Date	Action Code
A4314	INSERTION TRAY WITH DRAINAGE BAG WITH INDWELLING CATHETER, FOLEY TYPE, TWO-WAY LATEX WITH COATING (TEFLON, SILICONE, SILICONE ELASTOMER OR HYDROPHILIC, ETC.)	37	A			D			N
A4315	INSERTION TRAY WITH DRAINAGE BAG WITH INDWELLING CATHETER, FOLEY TYPE, TWO-WAY, ALL SILICONE	37	A			D			N
A4316	INSERTION TRAY WITH DRAINAGE BAG WITH INDWELLING CATHETER, FOLEY TYPE, THREE-WAY, FOR CONTINUOUS IRRIGATION	37	A			D			N
A4319	STERILE WATER IRRIGATION SOLUTION, 1000 ML	37	A			D			D
A4320	IRRIGATION TRAY WITH BULB OR PISTON SYRINGE, ANY PURPOSE	37	A			D			N
A4321	THERAPEUTIC AGENT FOR URINARY CATHETER IRRIGATION	37	A			D			N
A4322	IRRIGATION SYRINGE, BULB OR PISTON, EACH	37	A			D			N
A4323	STERILE SALINE IRRIGATION SOLUTION, 1000 ML.	37	A			D			D
A4324	MALE EXTERNAL CATHETER, WITH ADHESIVE COATING, EACH	37	A			D			N
A4325	MALE EXTERNAL CATHETER, WITH ADHESIVE STRIP, EACH	37	A			D			N
A4326	MALE EXTERNAL CATHETER SPECIALTY TYPE WITH INTEGRAL COLLECTION CHAMBER, EACH	37	A			D			C
A4327	FEMALE EXTERNAL URINARY COLLECTION DEVICE; MEATAL CUP, EACH	37	A			D			N
A4328	FEMALE EXTERNAL URINARY COLLECTION DEVICE; POUCH, EACH	37	A			D			N
A4329	EXTERNAL CATHETER STARTER SET, MALE/FEMALE, INCLUDES CATHETERS/URINARY COLLECTION DEVICE, BAG/POUCH AND ACCESSORIES (TUBING, CLAMPS, ETC.), 7 DAY SUPPLY	37	A			D			N
A4330	PERIANAL FECAL COLLECTION POUCH WITH ADHESIVE, EACH	37	A			D			N
A4331	EXTENSION DRAINAGE TUBING, ANY TYPE, ANY LENGTH, WITH CONNECTOR/ADAPTOR, FOR USE WITH URINARY LEG BAG OR UROSTOMY POUCH, EACH	37	A			D			N
A4332	LUBRICANT, INDIVIDUAL STERILE PACKET, FOR INSERTION OF URINARY CATHETER, EACH	37	A			D			N
A4333	URINARY CATHETER ANCHORING DEVICE, ADHESIVE SKIN ATTACHMENT, EACH	37	A			D			N
A4334	URINARY CATHETER ANCHORING DEVICE, LEG STRAP, EACH	37	A			D			N
A4335	INCONTINENCE SUPPLY; MISCELLANEOUS	46	A			D			N
A4338	INDWELLING CATHETER; FOLEY TYPE, TWO-WAY LATEX WITH COATING (TEFLON, SILICONE, SILICONE ELASTOMER, OR HYDROPHILIC, ETC.), EACH	37	A			D			N
A4340	INDWELLING CATHETER; SPECIALTY TYPE, EG; COUDE, MUSHROOM, WING, ETC.), EACH	37	A			D			N
A4344	INDWELLING CATHETER, FOLEY TYPE, TWO-WAY, ALL SILICONE, EACH	37	A			D			N
A4346	INDWELLING CATHETER; FOLEY TYPE, THREE WAY FOR CONTINUOUS IRRIGATION, EACH	37	A			D			N
A4347	MALE EXTERNAL CATHETER WITH OR WITHOUT ADHESIVE, WITH OR WITHOUT ANTI-REFLUX DEVICE; PER DOZEN	37	A			D			N
A4348	MALE EXTERNAL CATHETER WITH INTEGRAL COLLECTION COMPARTMENT, EXTENDED WEAR, EACH (E.G., 2 PER MONTH)	37	A			D			N
A4351	INTERMITTENT URINARY CATHETER; STRAIGHT TIP, WITH OR WITHOUT COATING (TEFLON, SILICONE, SILICONE ELASTOMER, OR HYDROPHILIC, ETC.), EACH	37	A			D			N

HCPCS	Long Description	PII	MPI	Statute	X-Ref	Coverage	ASC Pay Grp	ASC Pay Grp Eff Date	Action Code
A4352	INTERMITTENT URINARY CATHETER; COUDE (CURVED) TIP, WITH OR WITHOUT COATING (TEFLON, SILICONE, SILICONE ELASTOMERIC, OR HYDROPHILIC, ETC.), EACH	37	A			D			N
A4353	INTERMITTENT URINARY CATHETER, WITH INSERTION SUPPLIES	37	A			D			N
A4354	INSERTION TRAY WITH DRAINAGE BAG BUT WITHOUT CATHETER	37	A			D			N
A4355	IRRIGATION TUBING SET FOR CONTINUOUS BLADDER IRRIGATION THROUGH A THREE-WAY INDWELLING FOLEY CATHETER, EACH	37	A			D			N
A4356	EXTERNAL URETHRAL CLAMP OR COMPRESSION DEVICE (NOT TO BE USED FOR CATHETER CLAMP), EACH	37	A			D			N
A4357	BEDSIDE DRAINAGE BAG, DAY OR NIGHT, WITH OR WITHOUT ANTI-REFLUX DEVICE, WITH OR WITHOUT TUBE, EACH	37	A			D			N
A4358	URINARY DRAINAGE BAG, LEG OR ABDOMEN, VINYL, WITH OR WITHOUT TUBE, WITH STRAPS, EACH	37	A			D			N
A4359	URINARY SUSPENSORY WITHOUT LEG BAG, EACH	37	A			D			N
A4360	ADULT INCONTINENCE GARMENT (E.G. BRIEF, DIAPER), EACH	00	9			M			N
A4361	OSTOMY FACEPLATE, EACH	37	A			D			N
A4362	SKIN BARRIER; SOLID, 4 X 4 OR EQUIVALENT; EACH	37	A			D			N
A4364	ADHESIVE, LIQUID OR EQUAL, ANY TYPE, PER OZ	37	A			D			N
A4365	ADHESIVE REMOVER WIPES, ANY TYPE, PER 50	37	A			D			N
A4366	OSTOMY VENT, ANY TYPE, EACH	37	A			C			A
A4367	OSTOMY BELT, EACH	37	A			D			N
A4368	OSTOMY FILTER, ANY TYPE, EACH	37	A			C			N
A4369	OSTOMY SKIN BARRIER, LIQUID (SPRAY, BRUSH, ETC), PER OZ	37	A			D			N
A4370	OSTOMY SKIN BARRIER, PASTE, PER OZ	37	A			C			N
A4371	OSTOMY SKIN BARRIER, POWDER, PER OZ	37	A			D			N
A4372	OSTOMY SKIN BARRIER, SOLID 4X4 OR EQUIVALENT, WITH BUILT-IN CONVEXITY, EACH	37	A			D			N
A4373	OSTOMY SKIN BARRIER, WITH FLANGE (SOLID, FLEXIBLE OR ACCORDIAN), WITH BUILT-IN	37	A			D			N
A4373	CONVEXITY, ANY SIZE, EACH								
A4374	OSTOMY SKIN BARRIER, WITH FLANGE (SOLID, FLEXIBLE OR ACCORDION), EXTENDED WEAR, WITH BUILT-IN CONVEXITY, ANY SIZE, EACH	37	A			C			N
A4375	OSTOMY POUCH, DRAINABLE, WITH FACEPLATE ATTACHED, PLASTIC, EACH	37	A			D			N
A4376	OSTOMY POUCH, DRAINABLE, WITH FACEPLATE ATTACHED, RUBBER, EACH	37	A			D			N
A4377	OSTOMY POUCH, DRAINABLE, FOR USE ON FACEPLATE, PLASTIC, EACH	37	A			D			N
A4378	OSTOMY POUCH, DRAINABLE, FOR USE ON FACEPLATE, RUBBER, EACH	37	A			D			N
A4379	OSTOMY POUCH, URINARY, WITH FACEPLATE ATTACHED, PLASTIC, EACH	37	A			D			N
A4380	OSTOMY POUCH, URINARY, WITH FACEPLATE ATTACHED, RUBBER, EACH	37	A			D			N
A4381	OSTOMY POUCH, URINARY, FOR USE ON FACEPLATE, PLASTIC, EACH	37	A			D			N

HCPCS	Long Description	PTI	MPI	Statute	X-Refl	Coverage	ASC Pay Grp	ASC Pay Grp Eff Date	Action Code
A4382	OSTOMY POUCH, URINARY, FOR USE ON FACEPLATE, HEAVY PLASTIC, EACH	37	A			D			N
A4383	OSTOMY POUCH, URINARY, FOR USE ON FACEPLATE, RUBBER, EACH	37	A			D			N
A4384	OSTOMY FACEPLATE EQUIVALENT, SILICONE RING, EACH	37	A			D			N
A4385	OSTOMY SKIN BARRIER, SOLID 4X4 OR EQUIVALENT, EXTENDED WEAR, WITHOUT BUILT-IN CONVEXITY, EACH	37	A			D			N
A4386	OSTOMY SKIN BARRIER, WITH FLANGE (SOLID, FLEXIBLE OR ACCORDION), EXTENDED WEAR, WITHOUT BUILT-IN CONVEXITY, ANY SIZE, EACH	37	A			C			N
A4387	OSTOMY POUCH, CLOSED, WITH BARRIER ATTACHED, WITH BUILT-IN CONVEXITY (1 PIECE), EACH	37	A			D			N
A4388	OSTOMY POUCH, DRAINABLE, WITH EXTENDED WEAR BARRIER ATTACHED, (1 PIECE), EACH	37	A			D			N
A4389	OSTOMY POUCH, DRAINABLE, WITH BARRIER ATTACHED, WITH BUILT-IN CONVEXITY (1 PIECE), EACH	37	A			D			N
A4390	OSTOMY POUCH, DRAINABLE, WITH EXTENDED WEAR BARRIER ATTACHED, WITH BUILT-IN CONVEXITY (1 PIECE), EACH	37	A			D			N
A4391	OSTOMY POUCH, URINARY, WITH EXTENDED WEAR BARRIER ATTACHED (1 PIECE), EACH	37	A			D			N
A4392	OSTOMY POUCH, URINARY, WITH STANDARD WEAR BARRIER ATTACHED, WITH BUILT-IN CONVEXITY (1 PIECE), EACH	37	A			D			N
A4393	OSTOMY POUCH, URINARY, WITH EXTENDED WEAR BARRIER ATTACHED, WITH BUILT-IN CONVEXITY (1 PIECE), EACH	37	A			D			N
A4394	OSTOMY DEODORANT FOR USE IN OSTOMY POUCH, LIQUID, PER FLUID OUNCE	37	A			D			N
A4395	OSTOMY DEODORANT FOR USE IN OSTOMY POUCH, SOLID, PER TABLET	37	A			D			N
A4396	OSTOMY BELT WITH PERISTOMAL HERNIA SUPPORT	37	A			D			N
A4397	IRRIGATION SUPPLY; SLEEVE, EACH	37	A			D			N
A4398	OSTOMY IRRIGATION SUPPLY; BAG, EACH	37	A			D			N
A4399	OSTOMY IRRIGATION SUPPLY; CONE/CATHETER, INCLUDING BRUSH	37	A			D			N
A4400	OSTOMY IRRIGATION SET	37	A			D			N
A4402	LUBRICANT, PER OUNCE	37	A			D			N
A4404	OSTOMY RING, EACH	37	A			D			N
A4405	OSTOMY SKIN BARRIER, NON-PECTIN BASED, PASTE, PER OUNCE	37	A			D			N
A4406	OSTOMY SKIN BARRIER, PECTIN-BASED, PASTE, PER OUNCE	37	A			D			N
A4407	OSTOMY SKIN BARRIER, WITH FLANGE (SOLID, FLEXIBLE, OR ACCORDION), EXTENDED WEAR, WITH BUILT-IN CONVEXITY, 4 X 4 INCHES OR SMALLER, EACH	37	A			D			N
A4408	OSTOMY SKIN BARRIER, WTIH FLANGE (SOLID, FLEXIBLE OR ACCORDION), EXTENDED WEAR, WITH BUILT-IN CONVEXITY, LARGER THAN 4 X 4 INCHES, EACH	37	A			D			N
A4409	OSTOMY SKIN BARRIER, WITH FLANGE (SOLID, FLEXIBLE OR ACCORDION), EXTENDED WEAR, WITHOUT BUILT-IN CONVEXITY, 4 X 4 INCHES OR SMALLER, EACH	37	A			D			N
A4410	OSTOMY SKIN BARRIER, WITH FLANGE (SOLID, FLEXIBLE OR ACCORDION), EXTENDED WEAR, WITHOUT BUILT-IN CONVEXITY, LARGER THAN 4 X 4 INCHES, EACH	37	A			D			N
A4413	OSTOMY POUCH, DRAINABLE, HIGH OUTPUT, FOR USE ON A BARRIER WITH FLANGE (2 PIECE SYSTEM), WITH FILTER, EACH	37	A			D			N

HCPCS	Long Description	PTI	MPI	Statute	X-Reff	Coverage	ASC Pay Grp	ASC Pay Grp Eff Date	Action Code
A4414	OSTOMY SKIN BARRIER, WITH FLANGE (SOLID, FLEXIBLE OR ACCORDION), WITHOUT BUILT-IN CONVEXITY, 4 X 4 INCHES OR SMALLER, EACH	37	A			D			N
A4415	OSTOMY SKIN BARRIER, WITH FLANGE (SOLID, FLEXIBLE OR ACCORDION), WITHOUT BUILT-IN CONVEXITY, LARGER THAN 4X4 INCHES, EACH	37	A			D			N
A4416	OSTOMY POUCH, CLOSED, WITH BARRIER ATTACHED, WITH FILTER (1 PIECE), EACH	37	A			C			A
A4417	OSTOMY POUCH, CLOSED, WITH BARRIER ATTACHED, WITH BUILT-IN CONVEXITY, WITH FILTER (1 PIECE), EACH	37	A			C			A
A4418	OSTOMY POUCH, CLOSED; WITHOUT BARRIER ATTACHED, WITH FILTER (1 PIECE), EACH	37	A			C			A
A4419	OSTOMY POUCH, CLOSED; FOR USE ON BARRIER WITH NON-LOCKING FLANGE, WITH FILTER (2 PIECE), EACH	37	A			C			A
A4420	OSTOMY POUCH, CLOSED; FOR USE ON BARRIER WITH LOCKING FLANGE (2 PIECE), EACH	37	A			C			A
A4421	OSTOMY SUPPLY; MISCELLANEOUS	00	9			I			F
A4422	OSTOMY ABSORBENT MATERIAL (SHEET/PAD/CRYSTAL PACKET) FOR USE IN OSTOMY POUCH TO THICKEN LIQUID STOMAL OUTPUT, EACH	37	A			D			N
A4423	OSTOMY POUCH, CLOSED; FOR USE ON BARRIER WITH LOCKING FLANGE, WITH FILTER (2 PIECE), EACH	37	A			C			A
A4424	OSTOMY POUCH, DRAINABLE, WITH BARRIER ATTACHED, WITH FILTER (1 PIECE), EACH	37	A			C			A
A4425	OSTOMY POUCH, DRAINABLE; FOR USE ON BARRIER WITH NON-LOCKING FLANGE, WITH FILTER (2 PIECE SYSTEM), EACH	37	A			C			A
A4426	OSTOMY POUCH, DRAINABLE; FOR USE ON BARRIER WITH LOCKING FLANGE (2 PIECE SYSTEM), EACH	37	A			C			A
A4427	OSTOMY POUCH, DRAINABLE; FOR USE ON BARRIER WITH LOCKING FLANGE, WITH FILTER (2 PIECE SYSTEM), EACH	37	A			C			A
A4428	OSTOMY POUCH, URINARY, WITH EXTENDED WEAR BARRIER ATTACHED, WITH FAUCET-TYPE TAP WITH VALVE (1 PIECE), EACH	37	A			C			A
A4429	OSTOMY POUCH, URINARY, WITH BARRIER ATTACHED, WITH BUILT-IN CONVEXITY, WITH FAUCET-TYPE TAP WITH VALVE (1 PIECE), EACH	37	A			C			A
A4430	OSTOMY POUCH, URINARY, WITH EXTENDED WEAR BARRIER ATTACHED, WITH BUILT-IN CONVEXITY, WITH FAUCET-TYPE TAP WITH VALVE (1 PIECE), EACH	37	A			C			A
A4431	OSTOMY POUCH, URINARY; WITH BARRIER ATTACHED, WITH FAUCET-TYPE TAP WITH VALVE (1 PIECE), EACH	37	A			C			A
A4432	OSTOMY POUCH, URINARY; FOR USE ON BARRIER WITH NON-LOCKING FLANGE, WITH FAUCET-TYPE TAP WITH VALVE (2 PIECE), EACH	37	A			C			A
A4433	OSTOMY POUCH, URINARY; FOR USE ON BARRIER WITH LOCKING FLANGE (2 PIECE), EACH	37	A			C			A
A4434	OSTOMY POUCH, URINARY; FOR USE ON BARRIER WITH LOCKING FLANGE, WITH FAUCET-TYPE TAP WITH VALVE (2 PIECE), EACH	37	A			C			A
A4450	TAPE, NON-WATERPROOF, PER 18 SQUARE INCHES	37	A			D			N
A4452	TAPE, WATERPROOF, PER 18 SQUARE INCHES	37	A			D			N
A4454	TAPE, ALL TYPES, ALL SIZES	37	A			D			N
A4455	ADHESIVE REMOVER OR SOLVENT (FOR TAPE, CEMENT OR OTHER ADHESIVE), PER OUNCE	37	A			D			N
A4458	ENEMA BAG WITH TUBING, REUSABLE	00	9			I			N
A4460	ELASTIC BANDAGE, PER ROLL (E.G. COMPRESSION BANDAGE)	35	A			D			N
A4462	ABDOMINAL DRESSING HOLDER, EACH	35	A			D			N

HCPCS	Long Description	PTI	MPI	Statute	X-Ref1	Coverage	ASC Pay Grp	ASC Pay Grp Eff Date	Action Code
A4464	JOINT SUPPORTIVE DEVICE/GARMENT, ELASTIC OR EQUAL, EACH	00	9			M			N
A4465	NON-ELASTIC BINDER FOR EXTREMITY	00	9			C			N
A4470	GRAVLEE JET WASHER	00	9			D			N
A4480	VABRA ASPIRATOR	00	9			D			N
A4481	TRACHEOSTOMA FILTER, ANY TYPE, ANY SIZE, EACH	37	A			D			N
A4483	MOISTURE EXCHANGER, DISPOSABLE, FOR USE WITH INVASIVE MECHANICAL VENTILATION	37	A			D			N
A4490	SURGICAL STOCKINGS ABOVE KNEE LENGTH, EACH	00	9			M			N
A4495	SURGICAL STOCKINGS THIGH LENGTH, EACH	00	9			M			N
A4500	SURGICAL STOCKINGS BELOW KNEE LENGTH, EACH	00	9			M			N
A4510	SURGICAL STOCKINGS FULL LENGTH, EACH	00	9			M			N
A4521	ADULT-SIZED INCONTINENCE PRODUCT, DIAPER, SMALL SIZE, EACH	00	9			M			N
A4522	ADULT-SIZED INCONTINENCE PRODUCT, DIAPER, MEDIUM SIZE, EACH	00	9			M			N
A4523	ADULT-SIZED INCONTINENCE PRODUCT, DIAPER, LARGE SIZE, EACH	00	9			M			N
A4524	ADULT-SIZED INCONTINENCE PRODUCT, DIAPER, EXTRA LARGE SIZE, EACH	00	9			M			N
A4525	ADULT-SIZED INCONTINENCE PRODUCT, BRIEF, SMALL SIZE, EACH	00	9			M			N
A4526	ADULT-SIZED INCONTINENCE PRODUCT, BRIEF, MEDIUM SIZE, EACH	00	9			M			N
A4527	ADULT-SIZED INCONTINENCE PRODUCT, BRIEF, LARGE SIZE, EACH	00	9			M			N
A4528	ADULT-SIZED INCONTINENCE PRODUCT, BRIEF, EXTRA-LARGE SIZE, EACH	00	9			M			N
A4529	CHILD-SIZED INCONTINENCE PRODUCT, DIAPER, SMALL/MEDIUM SIZE, EACH	00	9			M			N
A4530	CHILD-SIZED INCONTINENCE PRODUCT, DIAPER, LARGE SIZE, EACH	00	9			M			N
A4531	CHILD-SIZED INCONTINENCE PRODUCT, BRIEF, SMALL/MEDIUM SIZE, EACH	00	9			M			N
A4532	CHILD-SIZED INCONTINENCE PRODUCT, BRIEF, LARGE SIZE, EACH	00	9			M			N
A4533	YOUTH-SIZED INCONTINENCE PRODUCT, DIAPER, EACH	00	9			M			N
A4534	YOUTH-SIZED INCONTINENCE PRODUCT, BRIEF, EACH	00	9			M			N
A4535	DISPOSABLE LINER/SHIELD FOR INCONTINENCE, EACH	00	9			M			N
A4536	PROTECTIVE UNDERWEAR, WASHABLE, ANY SIZE, EACH	00	9			M			N
A4537	UNDER PAD, REUSABLE/WASHABLE, ANY SIZE, EACH	00	9			M			N
A4538	DIAPER, REUSABLE, PROVIDED BY A DIAPER SERVICE, EACH DIAPER	00	9			M			C
A4550	SURGICAL TRAYS	11	A			D			N
A4554	DISPOSABLE UNDERPADS, ALL SIZES, (E.G., CHUXS)	00	9			I			N

HCPCS	Long Description	PII	MPI	Statute	X-Reff	Coverage	ASC Pay Grp	ASC Pay Grp Eff Date	Action Code
A4556	ELECTRODES, (E.G., APNEA MONITOR), PER PAIR	34	A			C			N
A4557	LEAD WIRES, (E.G., APNEA MONITOR), PER PAIR	34	A			C			N
A4558	CONDUCTIVE PASTE OR GEL	34	A			C			N
A4560	PESSARY	38	A			C			N
A4561	PESSARY, RUBBER, ANY TYPE	38	A			C			N
A4562	PESSARY, NON RUBBER, ANY TYPE	38	A			C			N
A4565	SLINGS	52	A			C			N
A4570	SPLINT	52	A			I			N
A4572	RIB BELT	52	A		L0210	C			N
A4575	TOPICAL HYPERBARIC OXYGEN CHAMBER, DISPOSABLE	00	9			M			N
A4580	CAST SUPPLIES (E.G. PLASTER)	00	9			I			N
A4590	SPECIAL CASTING MATERIAL (E.G. FIBERGLASS)	00	9			I			N
A4595	ELECTRICAL STIMULATOR SUPPLIES, 2 LEAD, PER MONTH, (E.G. TENS, NMES)	34	A			D			N
A4606	OXYGEN PROBE FOR USE WITH OXIMETER DEVICE, REPLACEMENT	00	9			C			N
A4608	TRANSTRACHEAL OXYGEN CATHETER, EACH	32	A			C			N
A4609	TRACHEAL SUCTION CATHETER, CLOSED SYSTEM, FOR LESS THAN 72 HOURS OF USE, EACH	32	A			C			N
A4610	TRACHEAL SUCTION CATHETER, CLOSED SYSTEM, FOR 72 OR MORE HOURS OF USE, EACH	32	A			C			N
A4611	BATTERY, HEAVY DUTY; REPLACEMENT FOR PATIENT OWNED VENTILATOR	32	A			C			N
A4612	BATTERY CABLES; REPLACEMENT FOR PATIENT-OWNED VENTILATOR	32	A			C			N
A4613	BATTERY CHARGER; REPLACEMENT FOR PATIENT-OWNED VENTILATOR	32	A			C			N
A4614	PEAK EXPIRATORY FLOW RATE METER, HAND HELD	46	A			C			N
A4615	CANNULA, NASAL	33	A			D			N
A4616	TUBING (OXYGEN), PER FOOT	33	A			D			N
A4617	MOUTH PIECE	33	A			D			N
A4618	BREATHING CIRCUITS	32	A			D			N
A4619	FACE TENT	33	A			D			N
A4620	VARIABLE CONCENTRATION MASK	33	A			D			N
A4621	TRACHEOTOMY MASK OR COLLAR	33	A			D			D
A4622	TRACHEOSTOMY OR LARYNGECTOMY TUBE	37	A			D			D
A4623	TRACHEOSTOMY, INNER CANNULA	37	A			D			C

HCPCS	Long Description	PTI	MPI	Statute	X-Refl	Coverage	ASC Pay Grp	ASC Pay Grp Eff Date	Action Code
A4624	TRACHEAL SUCTION CATHETER, ANY TYPE OTHER THAN CLOSED SYSTEM, EACH	32	A			C			N
A4625	TRACHEOSTOMY CARE KIT FOR NEW TRACHEOSTOMY	37	A			D			N
A4626	TRACHEOSTOMY CLEANING BRUSH, EACH	37	A			D			N
A4627	SPACER, BAG OR RESERVOIR, WITH OR WITHOUT MASK, FOR USE WITH METERED DOSE	00	9			M			N
A4627	INHALER								
A4628	OROPHARYNGEAL SUCTION CATHETER, EACH	32	A			C			N
A4629	TRACHEOSTOMY CARE KIT FOR ESTABLISHED TRACHEOSTOMY	37	A			D			N
A4630	REPLACEMENT BATTERIES. MEDICALLY NECESSARY T.E.N.S. OWNED BY PATIENT	32	A			D			N
A4631	REPLACEMENT, BATTERIES FOR MEDICALLY NECESSARY ELECTRONIC WHEEL CHAIR OWNED BY PATIENT	32	A		E2360	D			D
A4632	REPLACEMENT BATTERY FOR EXTERNAL INFUSION PUMP, ANY TYPE, EACH	00	9			I			F
A4633	REPLACEMENT BULB/LAMP FOR ULTRAVIOLET LIGHT THERAPY SYSTEM, EACH	32	A			C			N
A4634	REPLACEMENT BULB FOR THERAPEUTIC LIGHT BOX, TABLETOP MODEL	00	9			C			N
A4635	UNDERARM PAD, CRUTCH, REPLACEMENT, EACH	32	A			D			N
A4636	REPLACEMENT, HANDGRIP, CANE, CRUTCH, OR WALKER, EACH	32	A			D			N
A4637	REPLACEMENT, TIP, CANE, CRUTCH, WALKER, EACH.	32	A			D			N
A4638	REPLACEMENT BATTERY FOR PATIENT-OWNED EAR PULSE GENERATOR, EACH	32	A			C			A
A4639	REPLACEMENT PAD FOR INFRARED HEATING PAD SYSTEM, EACH	32	A			C			N
A4640	REPLACEMENT PAD FOR USE WITH MEDICALLY NECESSARY ALTERNATING PRESSURE PAD OWNED BY PATIENT	32	A			D			N
A4641	SUPPLY OF RADIOPHARMACEUTICAL DIAGNOSTIC IMAGING AGENT, NOT OTHERWISE CLASSIFIED	51	A			C			N
A4642	SUPPLY OF SATUMOMAB PENDETIDE, RADIOPHARMACEUTICAL DIAGNOSTIC IMAGING AGENT, PER DOSE	51	A			C			N
A4643	SUPPLY OF ADDITIONAL HIGH DOSE CONTRAST MATERIAL(S) DURING MAGNETIC RESONANCE	51	A			C			N
A4643	IMAGING, E.G., GADOTERIDOL INJECTION								
A4644	SUPPLY OF LOW OSMOLAR CONTRAST MATERIAL (100-199 MGS OF IODINE)	51	A			D			D
A4645	SUPPLY OF LOW OSMOLAR CONTRAST MATERIAL (200-299 MGS OF IODINE)	51	A			D			D
A4646	SUPPLY OF LOW OSMOLAR CONTRAST MATERIAL (300-399 MGS OF IODINE)	51	A			D			D
A4647	SUPPLY OF PARAMAGNETIC CONTRAST MATERIAL, EG., GADOLINIUM	00	9			D			N
A4649	SURGICAL SUPPLY; MISCELLANEOUS	46	A			C			N
A4650	CENTRIFUGE (INCLUDES CALIBRATED MICROCAPILLARY TUBES AND SEALEASE)	52	A			D			N
A4651	CALIBRATED MICROCAPILLARY TUBE, EACH	52	A			D			N

HCPCS	Long Description	PII	MPI	Statute	X-Ref	Coverage	ASC Pay Grp	ASC Pay Grp Eff Date	Action Code
A4652	MICROCAPILLARY TUBE SEALANT	52	A			D			N
A4653	PERITONEAL DIALYSIS CATHETER ANCHORING DEVICE, BELT, EACH	52	A			C			N
A4655	NEEDLES AND SYRINGES FOR DIALYSIS	52	A			D			N
A4656	NEEDLE, ANY SIZE, EACH	52	A			D			N
A4657	SYRINGE, WITH OR WITHOUT NEEDLE, EACH	52	A			D			N
A4660	SPHYGMOMANOMETER/BLOOD PRESSURE APPARATUS WITH CUFF AND STETHOSCOPE	52	A			D			N
A4663	BLOOD PRESSURE CUFF ONLY	52	A			D			N
A4670	AUTOMATIC BLOOD PRESSURE MONITOR	00	9			M			N
A4671	DISPOSABLE CYCLER SET USED WITH CYCLER DIALYSIS MACHINE, EACH	52	A			D			A
A4672	DRAINAGE EXTENSION LINE, STERILE, FOR DIALYSIS, EACH	52	A			D			A
A4673	EXTENSION LINE WITH EASY LOCK CONNECTORS, USED WITH DIALYSIS	52	A			D			A
A4674	CHEMICALS/ANTISEPTICS SOLUTION USED TO CLEAN/STERILIZE DIALYSIS EQUIPMENT, PER 8 OZ	52	A			D			A
A4680	ACTIVATED CARBON FILTER FOR HEMODIALYSIS, EACH	52	A			D			N
A4690	DIALYZER (ARTIFICIAL KIDNEYS), ALL TYPES, ALL SIZES, FOR HEMODIALYSIS, EACH	52	A			D			N
A4700	STANDARD DIALYSATE SOLUTION, EACH	52	A			D			N
A4705	BICARBONATE DIALYSATE SOLUTION, EACH	52	A			D			N
A4706	BICARBONATE CONCENTRATE, SOLUTION, FOR HEMODIALYSIS, PER GALLON	52	A			D			N
A4707	BICARBONATE CONCENTRATE, POWDER, FOR HEMODIALYSIS, PER PACKET	52	A			D			N
A4708	ACETATE CONCENTRATE SOLUTION, FOR HEMODIALYSIS, PER GALLON	52	A			D			N
A4709	ACID CONCENTRATE, SOLUTION, FOR HEMODIALYSIS, PER GALLON	52	A			D			N
A4712	WATER, STERILE, FOR INJECTION, PER 10 ML	52	A			D			D
A4714	TREATED WATER (DEIONIZED, DISTILLED, OR REVERSE OSMOSIS) FOR PERITONEAL DIALYSIS, PER GALLON	52	A			D			N
A4719	"Y SET" TUBING FOR PERITONEAL DIALYSIS	52	A			D			N
A4720	DIALYSATE SOLUTION, ANY CONCENTRATION OF DEXTROSE, FLUID VOLUME GREATER THAN 249CC, BUT LESS THAN OR EQUAL TO 999CC, FOR PERITONEAL DIALYSIS	52	A			D			N
A4721	DIALYSATE SOLUTION, ANY CONCENTRATION OF DEXTROSE, FLUID VOLUME GREATER THAN 999CC BUT LESS THAN OR EQUAL TO 1999CC, FOR PERITONEAL DIALYSIS	52	A			D			N
A4722	DIALYSATE SOLUTION, ANY CONCENTRATION OF DEXTROSE, FLUID VOLUME GREATER THAN 1999CC BUT LESS THAN OR EQUAL TO 2999CC, FOR PERITONEAL DIALYSIS	52	A			D			N
A4723	DIALYSATE SOLUTION, ANY CONCENTRATION OF DEXTROSE, FLUID VOLUME GREATER THAN 2999CC BUT LESS THAN OR EQUAL TO 3999CC, FOR PERITONEAL DIALYSIS	52	A			D			N
A4724	DIALYSATE SOLUTION, ANY CONCENTRATION OF DEXTROSE, FLUID VOLUME GREATER THAN 3999CC BUT LESS THAN OR EQUAL TO 4999CC, FOR PERITONEAL DIALYSIS	52	A			D			N

HCPCS	Long Description	PI	MPI	Statute	X-Ref	Coverage	ASC Pay Grp	ASC Pay Grp Eff Date	Action Code
A4725	DIALYSATE SOLUTION, ANY CONCENTRATION OF DEXTROSE, FLUID VOLUME GREATER THAN 4999CC BUT LESS THAN OR EQUAL TO 5999CC, FOR PERITONEAL DIALYSIS	52	A			D			N
A4726	DIALYSATE SOLUTION, ANY CONCENTRATION OF DEXTROSE, FLUID VOLUME GREATER THAN 5999CC, FOR PERITONEAL DIALYSIS	52	A			D			N
A4728	DIALYSATE SOLUTION, NON-DEXTROSE CONTAINING, 500 ML	52	A			C			A
A4730	FISTULA CANNULATION SET FOR HEMODIALYSIS, EACH	52	A			D			N
A4735	LOCAL/TOPICAL ANESTHETICS FOR DIALYSIS ONLY	52	A			D			N
A4736	TOPICAL ANESTHETIC, FOR DIALYSIS, PER GRAM	52	A			D			N
A4737	INJECTABLE ANESTHETIC, FOR DIALYSIS, PER 10 ML	52	A			D			N
A4740	SHUNT ACCESSORY, FOR HEMODIALYSIS, ANY TYPE, EACH	52	A			D			N
A4750	BLOOD TUBING, ARTERIAL OR VENOUS, FOR HEMODIALYSIS, EACH	52	A			D			N
A4755	BLOOD TUBING, ARTERIAL AND VENOUS COMBINED, FOR HEMODIALYSIS, EACH	52	A			D			N
A4760	DIALYSATE SOLUTION TEST KIT, FOR PERITONEAL DIALYSIS, ANY TYPE, EACH	52	A			D			N
A4765	DIALYSATE CONCENTRATE, POWDER, ADDITIVE FOR PERITONEAL DIALYSIS, PER PACKET	52	A			D			N
A4766	DIALYSATE CONCENTRATE, SOLUTION, ADDITIVE FOR PERITONEAL DIALYSIS, PER 10 ML	52	A			D			N
A4770	BLOOD COLLECTION TUBE, VACUUM, FOR DIALYSIS, PER 50	52	A			D			N
A4771	SERUM CLOTTING TIME TUBE, FOR DIALYSIS, PER 50	52	A			D			N
A4772	BLOOD GLUCOSE TEST STRIPS, FOR DIALYSIS, PER 50	52	A			D			N
A4773	OCCULT BLOOD TEST STRIPS, FOR DIALYSIS, PER 50	52	A			D			N
A4774	AMMONIA TEST STRIPS, FOR DIALYSIS, PER 50	52	A			D			N
A4780	STERILIZING AGENT FOR DIALYSIS EQUIPMENT, PER GALLON	52	A			D			N
A4790	CLEANSING AGENTS FOR EQUIPMENT FOR DIALYSIS ONLY	52	A			D			N
A4800	HEPARIN FOR DIALYSIS AND ANTIDOTE, ANY STRENGTH, PORCINE OR BEEF, UP TO 1000 UNITS, 10-30 ML (FOR PARENTERAL USE SEE B4216)	57	A		A4801	D			N
A4801	HEPARIN, ANY TYPE, FOR HEMODIALYSIS, PER 1000 UNITS	52	A		J1644	D			N
A4802	PROTAMINE SULFATE, FOR HEMODIALYSIS, PER 50 MG	52	A			D			N
A4820	HEMODIALYSIS KIT SUPPLIES	52	A			D			N
A4850	HEMOSTATS WITH RUBBER TIPS FOR DIALYSIS	52	A		E1637	D			N
A4860	DISPOSABLE CATHETER TIPS FOR PERITONEAL DIALYSIS, PER 10	52	A			D			N
A4870	PLUMBING AND/OR ELECTRICAL WORK FOR HOME HEMODIALYSIS EQUIPMENT	52	A			D			N
A4880	STORAGE TANKS UTILIZED IN CONNECTION WITH WATER PURIFICATION SYSTEM, REPLACEMENT TANKS FOR DIALYSIS	52	A			D			N

HCPCS	Long Description	PII	MPI	Statute	X-Ref1	Coverage	ASC Pay Grp	ASC Pay Grp Eff Date	Action Code
A4890	CONTRACTS, REPAIR AND MAINTENANCE, FOR HEMODIALYSIS EQUIPMENT	52	A			D			N
A4900	CONTINUOUS AMBULATORY PERITONEAL DIALYSIS (CAPD) SUPPLY KIT	52	A			D			N
A4901	CONTINUOUS CYCLING PERITONEAL DIALYSIS (CCPD) SUPPLY KIT	52	A			D			N
A4905	INTERMITTENT PERITONEAL DIALYSIS (IPD) SUPPLY KIT	52	A			D			N
A4910	NON-MEDICAL SUPPLIES FOR DIALYSIS, (I.E., SCALE, SCISSORS, STOPWATCH, ETC.)	52	A			D			N
A4911	DRAIN BAG/BOTTLE, FOR DIALYSIS, EACH	52	A			D			N
A4912	GOMCO DRAIN BOTTLE	52	A		A4911	D			N
A4913	MISCELLANEOUS DIALYSIS SUPPLIES, NOT OTHERWISE SPECIFIED	52	A			D			N
A4914	PREPARATION KITS	52	A			D			N
A4918	VENOUS PRESSURE CLAMP, FOR HEMODIALYSIS, EACH	52	A			D			N
A4919	DIALYZER HOLDER, EACH	52	A			D			N
A4920	HARVARD PRESSURE CLAMP, EACH	52	A			D			N
A4921	MEASURING CYLINDER, ANY SIZE, EACH	52	A			D			N
A4927	GLOVES, NON-STERILE, PER 100	52	A			D			N
A4928	SURGICAL MASK, PER 20	52	A			D			N
A4929	TOURNIQUET FOR DIALYSIS, EACH	52	A			D			N
A4930	GLOVES, STERILE, PER PAIR	52	A			D			N
A4931	ORAL THERMOMETER, REUSABLE, ANY TYPE, EACH	52	A			C			N
A4932	RECTAL THERMOMETER, REUSABLE, ANY TYPE, EACH	00	9			I			N
A5051	OSTOMY POUCH, CLOSED; WITH BARRIER ATTACHED (1 PIECE), EACH	37	A			D			N
A5052	OSTOMY POUCH, CLOSED; WITHOUT BARRIER ATTACHED (1 PIECE), EACH	37	A			D			N
A5053	OSTOMY POUCH, CLOSED; FOR USE ON FACEPLATE, EACH	37	A			D			N
A5054	OSTOMY POUCH, CLOSED; FOR USE ON BARRIER WITH FLANGE (2 PIECE), EACH	37	A			D			N
A5055	STOMA CAP	37	A			D			N
A5061	OSTOMY POUCH, DRAINABLE; WITH BARRIER ATTACHED, (1 PIECE), EACH	37	A			C			N
A5062	OSTOMY POUCH, DRAINABLE; WITHOUT BARRIER ATTACHED (1 PIECE), EACH	37	A			D			N
A5063	OSTOMY POUCH, DRAINABLE; FOR USE ON BARRIER WITH FLANGE (2 PIECE SYSTEM), EACH	37	A			D			N
A5064	POUCH, DRAINABLE, WITH FACEPLATE ATTACHED; PLASTIC OR RUBBER	00	9			I			N

HCPCS	Long Description	PI1	MPI	Statute	X-Refl	Coverage	ASC Pay Grp	ASC Pay Grp Eff Date	Action Code
A5065	POUCH, DRAINABLE, FOR USE ON FACEPLATE; PLASTIC OR RUBBER	00	9			I			N
A5071	OSTOMY POUCH, URINARY; WITH BARRIER ATTACHED (1 PIECE), EACH	37	A			D			N
A5072	OSTOMY POUCH, URINARY; WITHOUT BARRIER ATTACHED (1 PIECE), EACH	37	A			D			N
A5073	OSTOMY POUCH, URINARY; FOR USE ON BARRIER WITH FLANGE (2 PIECE), EACH	37	A			D			N
A5074	POUCH, URINARY, WITH FACEPLATE ATTACHED; PLASTIC OR RUBBER	00	9			I			N
A5075	POUCH, URINARY, FOR USE ON FACEPLATE; PLASTIC OR RUBBER	00	9			I			N
A5081	CONTINENT DEVICE; PLUG FOR CONTINENT STOMA	37	A			D			N
A5082	CONTINENT DEVICE; CATHETER FOR CONTINENT STOMA	37	A			D			N
A5093	OSTOMY ACCESSORY; CONVEX INSERT	37	A			D			N
A5102	BEDSIDE DRAINAGE BOTTLE WITH OR WITHOUT TUBING, RIGID OR EXPANDABLE, EACH	37	A			D			N
A5105	URINARY SUSPENSORY; WITH LEG BAG, WITH OR WITHOUT TUBE	37	A			D			N
A5112	URINARY LEG BAG; LATEX	37	A			D			N
A5113	LEG STRAP; LATEX, REPLACEMENT ONLY, PER SET	37	A			D			N
A5114	LEG STRAP; FOAM OR FABRIC, REPLACEMENT ONLY, PER SET	37	A			D			N
A5119	SKIN BARRIER; WIPES, BOX PER 50	37	A			D			N
A5121	SKIN BARRIER; SOLID, 6 X 6 OR EQUIVALENT, EACH	37	A			D			N
A5122	SKIN BARRIER; SOLID, 8 X 8 OR EQUIVALENT, EACH	37	A			D			N
A5123	SKIN BARRIER; WITH FLANGE (SOLID, FLEXIBLE OR ACCORDION), ANY SIZE, EACH	37	A			D			N
A5126	ADHESIVE OR NON-ADHESIVE; DISK OR FOAM PAD	37	A			D			N
A5131	APPLIANCE CLEANER, INCONTINENCE AND OSTOMY APPLIANCES, PER 16 OZ.	37	A			D			N
A5149	INCONTINENCE/OSTOMY SUPPLY; MISCELLANEOUS	46	A		A4335, A4421	D			N
A5200	PERCUTANEOUS CATHETER/TUBE ANCHORING DEVICE, ADHESIVE SKIN ATTACHMENT	37	A			D			N
A5500	FOR DIABETICS ONLY, FITTING (INCLUDING FOLLOW-UP), CUSTOM PREPARATION AND SUPPLY OF OFF-THE-SHELF DEPTH-INLAY SHOE MANUFACTURED TO ACCOMMODATE MULTI-DENSITY INSERT(S), PER SHOE.	52	A			D			N
A5501	FOR DIABETICS ONLY, FITTING (INCLUDING FOLLOW-UP), CUSTOM PREPARATION AND SUPPLY OF SHOE MOLDED FROM CAST(S) OF PATIENTS FOOT (CUSTOM MOLDED SHOE), PER SHOE	52	A			D			N
A5502	FOR DIABETICS ONLY, MULTIPLE DENSITY INSERT(S), PER SHOE	52	A			D			N
A5503	FOR DIABETICS ONLY, MODIFICATION (INCLUDING FITTING) OF OFF-THE-SHELF DEPTH-INLAY SHOE OR CUSTOM-MOLDED SHOE WITH ROLLER OR RIGID ROCKER BOTTOM, PER SHOE	52	A			D			N
A5504	FOR DIABETICS ONLY, MODIFICATION (INCLUDING FITTING) OF OFF-THE-SHELF DEPTH-INLAY SHOE OR CUSTOM-MOLDED SHOE WITH WEDGE(S), PER SHOE	52	A			D			N
A5505	FOR DIABETICS ONLY, MODIFICATION (INCLUDING FITTING) OF OFF-THE-SHELF DEPTH-INLAY SHOE OR CUSTOM-MOLDED SHOE WITH METATARSAL BAR, PER SHOE	52	A			D			N

HCPCS	Long Description	PII	VPI	Statute	X-Ref	Coverage	ASC Pay Grp	ASC Pay Grp Eff Date	Action Code
A5506	FOR DIABETICS ONLY, MODIFICATION (INCLUDING FITTING) OF OFF-THE-SHELF DEPTH-INLAY SHOE OR CUSTOM-MOLDED SHOE WITH OFF-SET HEEL(S), PER SHOE	52	A			D			N
A5507	FOR DIABETICS ONLY, NOT OTHERWISE SPECIFIED MODIFICATION (INCLUDING FITTING) OF OFF-THE-SHELF DEPTH-INLAY SHOE OR CUSTOM-MOLDED SHOE, PER SHOE	52	A			D			N
A5508	FOR DIABETICS ONLY, DELUXE FEATURE OF OFF-THE-SHELF DEPTH-INLAY SHOE OR CUSTOM-MOLDED SHOE, PER SHOE	00	9			D			N
A5509	FOR DIABETICS ONLY, DIRECT FORMED, MOLDED TO FOOT WITH EXTERNAL HEAT SOURCE (I.E. HEAT GUN) MULTIPLE DENSITY INSERT (S), PREFABRICATED, PER SHOE	52	A			D			N
A5510	FOR DIABETICS ONLY, DIRECT FORMED, COMPRESSION MOLDED TO PATIENTS FOOT WITHOUT EXTERNAL HEAT SOURCE, MULTIPLE-DENSITY INSERT(S) PREFABRICATED, PER SHOE	52	A			D			N
A5511	FOR DIABETICS ONLY, CUSTOM-MOLDED FROM MODEL OF PATIENTS FOOT, MULTIPLE DENSITY INSERT(S), CUSTOM-FABRICATED, PER SHOE	52	A			D			N
A6000	NON-CONTACT WOUND WARMING WOUND COVER FOR USE WITH THE NON-CONTACT WOUND WARMING DEVICE AND WARMING CARD	00	9			M			N
A6010	COLLAGEN BASED WOUND FILLER, DRY FORM, PER GRAM OF COLLAGEN	35	A			D			N
A6011	COLLAGEN BASED WOUND FILLER, GEL/PASTE, PER GRAM OF COLLAGEN	35	A			D			N
A6020	COLLAGEN BASED WOUND DRESSING, EACH DRESSING	35	A			C			N
A6021	COLLAGEN DRESSING, PAD SIZE 16 SQ. IN. OR LESS, EACH	35	A			D			N
A6022	COLLAGEN DRESSING, PAD SIZE MORE THAN 16 SQ. IN. BUT LESS THAN OR EQUAL TO 48 SQ. IN., EACH	35	A			D			N
A6023	COLLAGEN DRESSING, PAD SIZE MORE THAN 48 SQ. IN., EACH	35	A			D			N
A6024	COLLAGEN DRESSING WOUND FILLER, PER 6 INCHES	35	A			D			N
A6025	GEL SHEET FOR DERMAL OR EPIDERMAL APPLICATION, (E.G., SILICONE, HYDROGEL, OTHER), EACH	00	9			I			C
A6154	WOUND POUCH, EACH	35	A			D			N
A6196	ALGINATE OR OTHER FIBER GELLING DRESSING, WOUND COVER, PAD SIZE 16 SQ. IN. OR LESS, EACH DRESSING	35	A			D			N
A6197	ALGINATE OR OTHER FIBER GELLING DRESSING, WOUND COVER, PAD SIZE MORE THAN 16 SQ. IN. BUT LESS THAN OR EQUAL TO 48 SQ. IN., EACH DRESSING	35	A			D			N
A6198	ALGINATE OR OTHER FIBER GELLING DRESSING, WOUND COVER, PAD SIZE MORE THAN 48 SQ. IN., EACH DRESSING	46	A			D			N
A6199	ALGINATE OR OTHER FIBER GELLING DRESSING, WOUND FILLER, PER 6 INCHES	35	A			D			N
A6200	COMPOSITE DRESSING, PAD SIZE 16 SQ. IN. OR LESS, WITHOUT ADHESIVE BORDER, EACH DRESSING	35	A			D			N
A6201	COMPOSITE DRESSING, PAD SIZE MORE THAN 16 SQ. IN. BUT LESS THAN OR EQUAL TO 48 SQ. IN., WITHOUT ADHESIVE BORDER, EACH DRESSING	35	A			D			N
A6202	COMPOSITE DRESSING, PAD SIZE MORE THAN 48 SQ. IN., WITHOUT ADHESIVE BORDER, EACH DRESSING	46	A			D			N
A6203	COMPOSITE DRESSING, PAD SIZE 16 SQ. IN. OR LESS, WITH ANY SIZE ADHESIVE BORDER, EACH DRESSING	35	A			D			N
A6204	COMPOSITE DRESSING, PAD SIZE MORE THAN 16 SQ. IN. BUT LESS THAN OR EQUAL TO 48 SQ. IN., WITH ANY SIZE ADHESIVE BORDER, EACH DRESSING	35	A			D			N

HCPCS	Long Description	PI1	MPI	Statute	X-Reff	Coverage	ASC Pay Grp	ASC Pay Grp Eff Date	Action Code
A6205	COMPOSITE DRESSING, PAD SIZE MORE THAN 48 SQ. IN., WITH ANY SIZE ADHESIVE BORDER, EACH DRESSING	46	A			D			N
A6206	CONTACT LAYER, 16 SQ. IN. OR LESS, EACH DRESSING	46	A			D			N
A6207	CONTACT LAYER, MORE THAN 16 SQ. IN. BUT LESS THAN OR EQUAL TO 48 SQ. IN., EACH DRESSING	35	A			D			N
A6208	CONTACT LAYER, MORE THAN 48 SQ. IN., EACH DRESSING	46	A			D			N
A6209	FOAM DRESSING, WOUND COVER, PAD SIZE 16 SQ. IN. OR LESS, WITHOUT ADHESIVE BORDER, EACH DRESSING	35	A			D			N
A6210	FOAM DRESSING, WOUND COVER, PAD SIZE MORE THAN 16 SQ. IN. BUT LESS THAN OR EQUAL TO 48 SQ. IN., WITHOUT ADHESIVE BORDER, EACH DRESSING	35	A			D			N
A6211	FOAM DRESSING, WOUND COVER, PAD SIZE MORE THAN 48 SQ. IN., WITHOUT ADHESIVE BORDER, EACH DRESSING	35	A			D			N
A6212	FOAM DRESSING, WOUND COVER, PAD SIZE 16 SQ. IN. OR LESS, WITH ANY SIZE ADHESIVE BORDER, EACH DRESSING	35	A			D			N
A6213	FOAM DRESSING, WOUND COVER, PAD SIZE MORE THAN 16 SQ. IN. BUT LESS THAN OR EQUAL TO 48 SQ. IN., WITH ANY SIZE ADHESIVE BORDER, EACH DRESSING	46	A			D			N
A6214	FOAM DRESSING, WOUND COVER, PAD SIZE MORE THAN 48 SQ. IN., WITH ANY SIZE ADHESIVE BORDER, EACH DRESSING	35	A			D			N
A6215	FOAM DRESSING, WOUND FILLER, PER GRAM	46	A			D			N
A6216	GAUZE, NON-IMPREGNATED, NON-STERILE, PAD SIZE 16 SQ. IN. OR LESS, WITHOUT ADHESIVE BORDER, EACH DRESSING	35	A			D			N
A6217	GAUZE, NON-IMPREGNATED, NON-STERILE, PAD SIZE MORE THAN 16 SQ. IN. BUT LESS THAN OR EQUAL TO 48 SQ. IN., WITHOUT ADHESIVE BORDER, EACH DRESSING	35	A			D			N
A6218	GAUZE, NON-IMPREGNATED, NON-STERILE, PAD SIZE MORE THAN 48 SQ. IN., WITHOUT ADHESIVE BORDER, EACH DRESSING	46	A			D			N
A6219	GAUZE, NON-IMPREGNATED, PAD SIZE 16 SQ. IN. OR LESS, WITH ANY SIZE ADHESIVE BORDER, EACH DRESSING	35	A			D			N
A6220	GAUZE, NON-IMPREGNATED, PAD SIZE MORE THAN 16 SQ. IN. BUT LESS THAN OR EQUAL TO 48 SQ. IN., WITH ANY SIZE ADHESIVE BORDER, EACH DRESSING	35	A			D			N
A6221	GAUZE, NON-IMPREGNATED, PAD SIZE MORE THAN 48 SQ. IN., WITH ANY SIZE ADHESIVE BORDER, EACH DRESSING	46	A			D			N
A6222	GAUZE, IMPREGNATED WITH OTHER THAN WATER, NORMAL SALINE, OR HYDROGEL, PAD SIZE 16 SQ. IN. OR LESS, WITHOUT ADHESIVE BORDER, EACH DRESSING	35	A			D			N
A6223	GAUZE, IMPREGNATED WITH OTHER THAN WATER, NORMAL SALINE, OR HYDROGEL, PAD SIZE MORE THAN 16 SQUARE INCHES, BUT LESS THAN OR EQUAL TO 48 SQUARE INCHES, WITHOUT ADHESIVE BORDER, EACH DRESSING	35	A			D			N
A6224	GAUZE, IMPREGNATED WITH OTHER THAN WATER, NORMAL SALINE, OR HYDROGEL, PAD SIZE MORE THAN 48 SQUARE INCHES, WITHOUT ADHESIVE BORDER, EACH DRESSING	35	A			D			N
A6228	GAUZE, IMPREGNATED, WATER OR NORMAL SALINE, PAD SIZE 16 SQ. IN. OR LESS, WITHOUT ADHESIVE BORDER, EACH DRESSING	46	A			D			N
A6229	GAUZE, IMPREGNATED, WATER OR NORMAL SALINE, PAD SIZE MORE THAT 16 SQ. IN. BUT LESS THAN OR EQUAL TO 48 SQ. IN., WITHOUT ADHESIVE BORDER, EACH DRESSING	35	A			D			N
A6230	GAUZE, IMPREGNATED, WATER OR NORMAL SALINE, PAD SIZE MORE THAN 48 SQ. IN., WITHOUT ADHESIVE BORDER, EACH DRESSING	46	A			D			N
A6231	GAUZE, IMPREGNATED, HYDROGEL, FOR DIRECT WOUND CONTACT, PAD SIZE 16 SQ. IN. OR LESS, EACH DRESSING	35	A			D			N
A6232	GAUZE, IMPREGNATED, HYDROGEL, FOR DIRECT WOUND CONTACT, PAD SIZE GREATER THAN 16 SQ. IN., BUT LESS THAN OR EQUAL TO 48 SQ. IN., EACH DRESSING	35	A			D			N

HCPCS	Long Description	PTI	MPI	Statute	X-Ref	Coverage	ASC Pay Grp	ASC Pay Grp Eff Date	Action Code
A6233	GAUZE, IMPREGNATED, HYDROGEL FOR DIRECT WOUND CONTACT, PAD SIZE MORE THAN 48 SQ. IN., EACH DRESSING	35	A			D			N
A6234	HYDROCOLLOID DRESSING, WOUND COVER, PAD SIZE 16 SQ. IN. OR LESS, WITHOUT ADHESIVE BORDER, EACH DRESSING	35	A			D			N
A6235	HYDROCOLLOID DRESSING, WOUND COVER, PAD SIZE MORE THAN 16 SQ. IN. BUT LESS THAN OR EQUAL TO 48 SQ. IN., WITHOUT ADHESIVE BORDER, EACH DRESSING	35	A			D			N
A6236	HYDROCOLLOID DRESSING, WOUND COVER, PAD SIZE MORE THAN 48 SQ. IN., WITHOUT ADHESIVE BORDER, EACH DRESSING	35	A			D			N
A6237	HYDROCOLLOID DRESSING, WOUND COVER, PAD SIZE 16 SQ. IN. OR LESS, WITH ANY SIZE ADHESIVE BORDER, EACH DRESSING	35	A			D			N
A6238	HYDROCOLLOID DRESSING, WOUND COVER, PAD SIZE MORE THAN 16 SQ. IN. BUT LESS THAN OR EQUAL TO 48 SQ. IN., WITH ANY SIZE ADHESIVE BORDER, EACH DRESSING	35	A			D			N
A6239	HYDROCOLLOID DRESSING, WOUND COVER, PAD SIZE MORE THAN 48 SQ. IN., WITH ANY SIZE ADHESIVE BORDER, EACH DRESSING	46	A			D			N
A6240	HYDROCOLLOID DRESSING, WOUND FILLER, PASTE, PER FLUID OUNCE	35	A			D			N
A6241	HYDROCOLLOID DRESSING, WOUND FILLER, DRY FORM, PER GRAM	35	A			D			N
A6242	HYDROGEL DRESSING, WOUND COVER, PAD SIZE 16 SQ. IN. OR LESS, WITHOUT ADHESIVE BORDER, EACH DRESSING	35	A			D			N
A6243	HYDROGEL DRESSING, WOUND COVER, PAD SIZE MORE THAN 16 SQ. IN. BUT LESS THAN OR EQUAL TO 48 SQ. IN., WITHOUT ADHESIVE BORDER, EACH DRESSING	35	A			D			N
A6244	HYDROGEL DRESSING, WOUND COVER, PAD SIZE MORE THAN 48 SQ. IN., WITHOUT ADHESIVE BORDER, EACH DRESSING	35	A			D			N
A6245	HYDROGEL DRESSING, WOUND COVER, PAD SIZE 16 SQ. IN. OR LESS, WITH ANY SIZE ADHESIVE BORDER, EACH DRESSING	35	A			D			N
A6246	HYDROGEL DRESSING, WOUND COVER, PAD SIZE MORE THAN 16 SQ. IN. BUT LESS THAN OR EQUAL TO 48 SQ. IN., WITH ANY SIZE ADHESIVE BORDER, EACH DRESSING	35	A			D			N
A6247	HYDROGEL DRESSING, WOUND COVER, PAD SIZE MORE THAN 48 SQ. IN., WITH ANY SIZE ADHESIVE BORDER, EACH DRESSING	35	A			D			N
A6248	HYDROGEL DRESSING, WOUND FILLER, GEL, PER FLUID OUNCE	35	A			D			N
A6250	SKIN SEALANTS, PROTECTANTS, MOISTURIZERS, OINTMENTS, ANY TYPE, ANY SIZE	00	9			D			N
A6251	SPECIALTY ABSORPTIVE DRESSING, WOUND COVER, PAD SIZE 16 SQ. IN. OR LESS, WITHOUT ADHESIVE BORDER, EACH DRESSING	35	A			D			N
A6252	SPECIALTY ABSORPTIVE DRESSING, WOUND COVER, PAD SIZE MORE THAN 16 SQ. IN. BUT LESS THAN OR EQUAL TO 48 SQ. IN., WITHOUT ADHESIVE BORDER, EACH DRESSING	35	A			D			N
A6253	SPECIALTY ABSORPTIVE DRESSING, WOUND COVER, PAD SIZE MORE THAN 48 SQ. IN., WITHOUT ADHESIVE BORDER, EACH DRESSING	35	A			D			N
A6254	SPECIALTY ABSORPTIVE DRESSING, WOUND COVER, PAD SIZE 16 SQ. IN. OR LESS, WITH ANY SIZE ADHESIVE BORDER, EACH DRESSING	35	A			D			N
A6255	SPECIALTY ABSORPTIVE DRESSING, WOUND COVER, PAD SIZE MORE THAN 16 SQ. IN. BUT LESS THAN OR EQUAL TO 48 SQ. IN., WITH ANY SIZE ADHESIVE BORDER, EACH DRESSING	35	A			D			N
A6256	SPECIALTY ABSORPTIVE DRESSING, WOUND COVER, PAD SIZE MORE THAN 48 SQ. IN., WITH ANY SIZE ADHESIVE BORDER, EACH DRESSING	46	A			D			N
A6257	TRANSPARENT FILM, 16 SQ. IN. OR LESS, EACH DRESSING	35	A			D			N
A6258	TRANSPARENT FILM, MORE THAN 16 SQ. IN. BUT LESS THAN OR EQUAL TO 48 SQ. IN., EACH DRESSING	35	A			D			N
A6259	TRANSPARENT FILM, MORE THAN 48 SQ. IN., EACH DRESSING	35	A			D			N

HCPCS	Long Description	PH	MPI	Statute	X-Ref1	Coverage	ASC Pay Grp	ASC Pay Grp Eff Date	Action Code
A6260	WOUND CLEANSERS, ANY TYPE, ANY SIZE	00	9			D			N
A6261	WOUND FILLER, GEL/PASTE, PER FLUID OUNCE, NOT ELSEWHERE CLASSIFIED	46	A			D			N
A6262	WOUND FILLER, DRY FORM, PER GRAM, NOT ELSEWHERE CLASSIFIED	46	A			D			N
A6263	GAUZE, ELASTIC, NON-STERILE, ALL TYPES, PER LINEAR YARD	35	A			D			N
A6264	GAUZE, NON-ELASTIC, NON-STERILE, PER LINEAR YARD	35	A			D			N
A6265	TAPE, ALL TYPES, PER 18 SQUARE INCHES	35	A			C			N
A6266	GAUZE, IMPREGNATED, OTHER THAN WATER, NORMAL SALINE, OR ZINC PASTE, ANY WIDTH, PER LINEAR YARD	35	A			D			N
A6402	GAUZE, NON-IMPREGNATED, STERILE, PAD SIZE 16 SQ. IN. OR LESS, WITHOUT ADHESIVE BORDER, EACH DRESSING	35	A			D			N
A6403	GAUZE, NON-IMPREGNATED, STERILE, PAD SIZE MORE THAN 16 SQ. IN. LESS THAN OR EQUAL TO 48 SQ. IN., WITHOUT ADHESIVE BORDER, EACH DRESSING	35	A			D			N
A6404	GAUZE, NON-IMPREGNATED, STERILE, PAD SIZE MORE THAN 48 SQ. IN., WITHOUT ADHESIVE BORDER, EACH DRESSING	35	A			D			N
A6405	GAUZE, ELASTIC, STERILE, ALL TYPES, PER LINEAR YARD	35	A			D			N
A6406	GAUZE, NON-ELASTIC, STERILE, ALL TYPES, PER LINEAR YARD	35	A			D			N
A6407	PACKING STRIPS, NON-IMPREGNATED, UP TO 2 INCHES IN WIDTH, PER LINEAR YARD	35	A			C			A
A6410	EYE PAD, STERILE, EACH	35	A			D			N
A6411	EYE PAD, NON-STERILE, EACH	35	A			D			N
A6412	EYE PATCH, OCCLUSIVE, EACH	00	9			I			N
A6421	PADDING BANDAGE, NON-ELASTIC, NON-WOVEN/NON-KNITTED, WIDTH GREATER THAN OR EQUAL TO 3 INCHES AND LESS THAN 5 INCHES, PER ROLL (AT LEAST 3 YARDS, UNSTRETCHED)	35	A			C			D
A6422	CONFORMING BANDAGE, NON-ELASTIC, KNITTED/WOVEN, NON-STERILE, WIDTH GREATER THAN OR EQUAL TO 3 INCHES AND LESS THAN 5 INCHES PER ROLL (AT LEAST 3 YARDS, UNSTRETCHED)	35	A			C			D
A6424	CONFORMING BANDAGE, NON-ELASTIC, KNITTED/WOVEN, NON-STERILE, WIDTH GREATER THAN OR EQUAL TO 5 INCHES, PER ROLL (AT LEAST 3 YARDS, UNSTRETCHED)	35	A			C			D
A6426	CONFORMING BANDAGE, NON-ELASTIC, KNITTED/WOVEN, STERILE WIDTH GREATER THAN OR EQUAL TO 3 INCHES AND LESS THAN 5 INCHES, PER ROLL (AT LEAST 3 YARDS, UNSTRETCHED)	35	A			C			D
A6428	CONFORMING BANDAGE, NON-ELASTIC, KNITTED/WOVEN, STERILE, WIDTH GREATER THAN OR EQUAL TO 5 INCHES, PER ROLL (AT LEAST 3 YARDS, UNSTRETCHED)	35	A			C			D
A6430	LIGHT COMPRESSION BANDAGE, ELASTIC, KNITTED/WOVEN, LOAD RESISTANCE LESS THAN 1.25 FOOT POUNDS AT 50% MAXIMUM STRETCH, WIDTH GREATER THAN OR EQUAL TO 3 INCHES AND LESS THAN 5 INCHES, PER ROLL (AT LEAST 3 YARDS, UNSTRETCHED)	35	A			C			D
A6432	LIGHT COMPRESSION BANDAGE, ELASTIC, KNITTED/WOVEN, LOAD RESISTANCE LESS THAN 1.25 FOOT POUNDS AT 50% MAXIMUM STRETCH, WIDTH GREATER THAN OR EQUAL TO 5 INCHES, PER ROLL (AT LEAST 3 YARDS, UNSTRETCHED)	35	A			C			D
A6434	MODERATE COMPRESSION BANDAGE, ELASTIC, KNITTED /WOVEN, LOAD RESISTANCE OF 1.25 TO 1.34 FOOT POUNDS AT 50% MAXIMUM STRETCH, WIDTH GREATER THAN OR EQUAL TO 3 INCHES OR LESS THAN 5 INCHES, PER ROLL (AT LEAST 3 YARDS, UNSTRETCHED)	35	A			C			D

HCPCS	Long Description	PTT	MPI	Statute	X-Ref	Coverage	ASC Pay Grp	ASC Pay Grp Eff Date	Action Code
A6436	HIGH COMPRESSION BANDAGE, ELASTIC, KNITTED/WOVEN, LOAD RESISTANCE GREATER THAN OR EQUAL TO 1.35 FOOT POUNDS AT 50% MAXIMUM STRETCH, WIDTH GREATER THAN OR EQUAL TO 3 INCHES AND LESS THAN 5 INCHES, PER ROLL (AT LEAST 3 YARDS, UNSTRETCHED)	35	A			C			D
A6438	SELF-ADHERENT BANDAGE, ELASTIC, NON-KNITTED/NON-WOVEN, LOAD RESISTANCE GREATER THAN OR EQUAL TO 0.55 FOOT POUNDS AT 50% MAXIMUM STRETCH, WIDTH GREATER THAN OR EQUAL TO 3 INCHES AND LESS THAN 5 INCHES, PER ROLL (AT LEAST 3 YARDS, UNSTRETCHED)	35	A			C			D
A6440	ZINC PASTE IMPREGNATED BANDAGE, NON-ELASTIC, KNITTED/WOVEN, WIDTH GREATER THAN OR EQUAL TO 3 INCHES AND LESS THAN 5 INCHES, PER ROLL (AT LEAST 10 YARDS, UNSTRETCHED)	35	A			C			D
A6441	PADDING BANDAGE, NON-ELASTIC, NON-WOVEN/NON-KNITTED, WIDTH GREATER THAN OR EQUAL TO THREE INCHES AND LESS THAN FIVE INCHES, PER YARD	35	A			C			A
A6442	CONFORMING BANDAGE, NON-ELASTIC, KNITTED/WOVEN, NON-STERILE, WIDTH LESS THAN THREE INCHES, PER YARD	35	A			C			A
A6443	CONFORMING BANDAGE, NON-ELASTIC, KNITTED/WOVEN, NON-STERILE, WIDTH GREATER THAN OR EQUAL TO THREE INCHES AND LESS THAN FIVE INCHES, PER YARD	35	A			C			A
A6444	CONFORMING BANDAGE, NON-ELASTIC, KNITTED/WOVEN, NON-STERILE, WIDTH GREATER THAN OR EQUAL TO 5 INCHES, PER YARD	35	A			C			A
A6445	CONFORMING BANDAGE, NON-ELASTIC, KNITTED/WOVEN, STERILE, WIDTH LESS THAN THREE INCHES, PER YARD	35	A			C			A
A6446	CONFORMING BANDAGE, NON-ELASTIC, KNITTED/WOVEN, STERILE, WIDTH GREATER THAN OR EQUAL TO THREE INCHES AND LESS THAN FIVE INCHES, PER YARD	35	A			C			A
A6447	CONFORMING BANDAGE, NON-ELASTIC, KNITTED/WOVEN, STERILE, WIDTH GREATER THAN OR EQUAL TO FIVE INCHES, PER YARD	35	A			C			A
A6448	LIGHT COMPRESSION BANDAGE, ELASTIC, KNITTED/WOVEN, WIDTH LESS THAN THREE INCHES, PER YARD	35	A			C			A
A6449	LIGHT COMPRESSION BANDAGE, ELASTIC, KNITTED/WOVEN, WIDTH GREATER THAN OR EQUAL TO THREE INCHES AND LESS THAN FIVE INCHES, PER YARD	35	A			C			A
A6450	LIGHT COMPRESSION BANDAGE, ELASTIC, KNITTED/WOVEN, WIDTH GREATER THAN OR EQUAL TO FIVE INCHES, PER YARD	35	A			C			A
A6451	MODERATE COMPRESSION BANDAGE, ELASTIC, KNITTED /WOVEN, LOAD RESISTANCE OF 1.25 TO 1.34 FOOT POUNDS AT 50% MAXIMUM STRETCH, WIDTH GREATER THAN OR EQUAL TO THREE INCHES AND LESS THAN FIVE INCHES, PER YARD	35	A			C			A
A6452	HIGH COMPRESSION BANDAGE, ELASTIC, KNITTED/WOVEN, LOAD RESISTANCE GREATER THAN OR EQUAL TO 1.35 FOOT POUNDS AT 50% MAXIMUM STRETCH, WIDTH GREATER THAN OR EQUAL TO THREE INCHES AND LESS THAN FIVE INCHES, PER YARD	35	A			C			A
A6453	SELF-ADHERENT BANDAGE, ELASTIC, NON-KNITTED/NON-WOVEN, WIDTH LESS THAN THREE INCHES, PER YARD	35	A			C			A
A6454	SELF-ADHERENT BANDAGE, ELASTIC, NON-KNITTED/NON-WOVEN, WIDTH GREATER THAN OR EQUAL TO THREE INCHES AND LESS THAN FIVE INCHES, PER YARD	35	A			C			A
A6455	SELF-ADHERENT BANDAGE, ELASTIC, NON-KNITTED/NON-WOVEN, WIDTH GREATER THAN OR EQUAL TO FIVE INCHES, PER YARD	35	A			C			A
A6456	ZINC PASTE IMPREGNATED BANDAGE, NON-ELASTIC, KNITTED/WOVEN, WIDTH GREATER THAN OR EQUAL TO THREE INCHES AND LESS THAN FIVE INCHES, PER YARD	35	A			C			A
A6501	COMPRESSION BURN GARMENT, BODYSUIT (HEAD TO FOOT), CUSTOM FABRICATED	35	A			D			N
A6502	COMPRESSION BURN GARMENT, CHIN STRAP, CUSTOM FABRICATED	35	A			D			N
A6503	COMPRESSION BURN GARMENT, FACIAL HOOD, CUSTOM FABRICATED	35	A			D			N
A6504	COMPRESSION BURN GARMENT, GLOVE TO WRIST, CUSTOM FABRICATED	35	A			D			N

HCPCS	Long Description	PI	MPI	Statute	X-Refl	Coverage	ASC Pay Grp	ASC Pay Grp Eff Date	Action Code
A6505	COMPRESSION BURN GARMENT, GLOVE TO ELBOW, CUSTOM FABRICATED	35	A			D			N
A6506	COMPRESSION BURN GARMENT, GLOVE TO AXILLA, CUSTOM FABRICATED	35	A			D			N
A6507	COMPRESSION BURN GARMENT, FOOT TO KNEE LENGTH, CUSTOM FABRICATED	35	A			D			N
A6508	COMPRESSION BURN GARMENT, FOOT TO THIGH LENGTH, CUSTOM FABRICATED	35	A			D			N
A6509	COMPRESSION BURN GARMENT, UPPER TRUNK TO WAIST INCLUDING ARM OPENINGS (VEST), CUSTOM FABRICATED	35	A			D			N
A6510	COMPRESSION BURN GARMENT, TRUNK, INCLUDING ARMS DOWN TO LEG OPENINGS (LEOTARD), CUSTOM FABRICATED	35	A			D			N
A6511	COMPRESSION BURN GARMENT, LOWER TRUNK INCLUDING LEG OPENINGS (PANTY), CUSTOM FABRICATED	35	A			D			N
A6512	COMPRESSION BURN GARMENT, NOT OTHERWISE CLASSIFIED	35	A			D			N
A6550	DRESSING SET FOR NEGATIVE PRESSURE WOUND THERAPY ELECTRICAL PUMP, STATIONARY OR PORTABLE, EACH	34	A			C			A
A6551	CANISTER SET FOR NEGATIVE PRESSURE WOUND THERAPY ELECTRICAL PUMP, STATIONARY OR PORTABLE, EACH	34	A			C			A
A7000	CANISTER, DISPOSABLE, USED WITH SUCTION PUMP, EACH	32	A			C			N
A7001	CANISTER, NON-DISPOSABLE, USED WITH SUCTION PUMP, EACH	32	A			C			N
A7002	TUBING, USED WITH SUCTION PUMP, EACH	32	A			C			N
A7003	ADMINISTRATION SET, WITH SMALL VOLUME NONFILTERED PNEUMATIC NEBULIZER, DISPOSABLE	32	A			C			N
A7004	SMALL VOLUME NONFILTERED PNEUMATIC NEBULIZER, DISPOSABLE	32	A			C			N
A7005	ADMINISTRATION SET, WITH SMALL VOLUME NONFILTERED PNEUMATIC NEBULIZER, NON-DISPOSABLE	32	A			C			N
A7006	ADMINISTRATION SET, WITH SMALL VOLUME FILTERED PNEUMATIC NEBULIZER	32	A			C			N
A7007	LARGE VOLUME NEBULIZER, DISPOSABLE, UNFILLED, USED WITH AEROSOL COMPRESSOR	32	A			C			N
A7008	LARGE VOLUME NEBULIZER, DISPOSABLE, PREFILLED, USED WITH AEROSOL COMPRESSOR	32	A			C			N
A7009	RESERVOIR BOTTLE, NON-DISPOSABLE, USED WITH LARGE VOLUME ULTRASONIC NEBULIZER	32	A			C			N
A7010	CORRUGATED TUBING, DISPOSABLE, USED WITH LARGE VOLUME NEBULIZER, 100 FEET	32	A			C			N
A7011	CORRUGATED TUBING, NON-DISPOSABLE, USED WITH LARGE VOLUME NEBULIZER, 10 FEET	46	A			C			N
A7012	WATER COLLECTION DEVICE, USED WITH LARGE VOLUME NEBULIZER	32	A			C			N

HCPCS	Long Description	PII	MPI	Statute	X-Ref	Coverage	ASC Pay Grp	ASC Pay Grp Eff Date	Action Code
A7013	FILTER, DISPOSABLE, USED WITH AEROSOL COMPRESSOR	32	A			C			N
A7014	FILTER, NONDISPOSABLE, USED WITH AEROSOL COMPRESSOR OR ULTRASONIC GENERATOR	32	A			C			N
A7015	AEROSOL MASK, USED WITH DME NEBULIZER	32	A			C			N
A7016	DOME AND MOUTHPIECE, USED WITH SMALL VOLUME ULTRASONIC NEBULIZER	32	A			C			N
A7017	NEBULIZER, DURABLE, GLASS OR AUTOCLAVABLE PLASTIC, BOTTLE TYPE, NOT USED WITH OXYGEN	32	A			D			N
A7018	WATER, DISTILLED, USED WITH LARGE VOLUME NEBULIZER, 1000 ML	32	A			C			N
A7019	SALINE SOLUTION, PER 10 ML, METERED DOSE DISPENSER, FOR USE WITH INHALATION DRUGS	34	A			C			D
A7020	STERILE WATER OR STERILE SALINE, 1000 ML, USED WITH LARGE VOLUME NEBULIZER	34	A			C			D
A7025	HIGH FREQUENCY CHEST WALL OSCILLATION SYSTEM VEST, REPLACEMENT FOR USE WITH PATIENT OWNED EQUIPMENT, EACH	32	A			C			N
A7026	HIGH FREQUENCY CHEST WALL OSCILLATION SYSTEM HOSE, REPLACEMENT FOR USE WITH PATIENT OWNED EQUIPMENT, EACH	32	A			C			N
A7030	FULL FACE MASK USED WITH POSITIVE AIRWAY PRESSURE DEVICE, EACH	32	A			C			N
A7031	FACE MASK INTERFACE, REPLACEMENT FOR FULL FACE MASK, EACH	32	A			C			N
A7032	REPLACEMENT CUSHION FOR NASAL APPLICATION DEVICE, EACH	32	A			C			N
A7033	REPLACEMENT PILLOWS FOR NASAL APPLICATION DEVICE, PAIR	32	A			C			N
A7034	NASAL INTERFACE (MASK OR CANNULA TYPE) USED WITH POSITIVE AIRWAY PRESSURE DEVICE, WITH OR WITHOUT HEAD STRAP	32	A			C			N
A7035	HEADGEAR USED WITH POSITIVE AIRWAY PRESSURE DEVICE	32	A			C			N
A7036	CHINSTRAP USED WITH POSITIVE AIRWAY PRESSURE DEVICE	32	A			C			N
A7037	TUBING USED WITH POSITIVE AIRWAY PRESSURE DEVICE	32	A			C			N
A7038	FILTER, DISPOSABLE, USED WITH POSITIVE AIRWAY PRESSURE DEVICE	32	A			C			N
A7039	FILTER, NON DISPOSABLE, USED WITH POSITIVE AIRWAY PRESSURE DEVICE	32	A			C			N
A7042	IMPLANTED PLEURAL CATHETER, EACH	38	A			C			N
A7043	VACUUM DRAINAGE BOTTLE AND TUBING FOR USE WITH IMPLANTED CATHETER	38	A			C			N
A7044	ORAL INTERFACE USED WITH POSITIVE AIRWAY PRESSURE DEVICE, EACH	32	A			C			N
A7046	WATER CHAMBER FOR HUMIDIFIER, USED WITH POSITIVE AIRWAY PRESSURE DEVICE, REPLACEMENT, EACH	32	A			D			A
A7501	TRACHEOSTOMA VALVE, INCLUDING DIAPHRAGM, EACH	37	A			D			N

HCPCS	Long Description	PTI	MPI	Statute	X-Refl	Coverage	ASC Pay Grp	ASC Pay Grp Eff Date	Action Code
A7502	REPLACEMENT DIAPHRAGM/FACEPLATE FOR TRACHEOSTOMA VALVE, EACH	37	A			D			N
A7503	FILTER HOLDER OR FILTER CAP, REUSABLE, FOR USE IN A TRACHEOSTOMA HEAT AND MOISTURE EXCHANGE SYSTEM, EACH	37	A			D			N
A7504	FILTER FOR USE IN A TRACHEOSTOMA HEAT AND MOISTURE EXCHANGE SYSTEM, EACH	37	A			D			N
A7505	HOUSING, REUSABLE WITHOUT ADHESIVE, FOR USE IN A HEAT AND MOISTURE EXCHANGE SYSTEM AND/OR WITH A TRACHEOSTOMA VALVE, EACH	37	A			D			N
A7506	ADHESIVE DISC FOR USE IN A HEAT AND MOISTURE EXCHANGE SYSTEM AND/OR WITH TRACHEOSTOMA VALVE, ANY TYPE EACH	37	A			D			N
A7507	FILTER HOLDER AND INTEGRATED FILTER WITHOUT ADHESIVE, FOR USE IN A TRACHEOSTOMA HEAT AND MOISTURE EXCHANGE SYSTEM, EACH	37	A			D			N
A7508	HOUSING AND INTEGRATED ADHESIVE, FOR USE IN A TRACHEOSTOMA HEAT AND MOISTURE EXCHANGE SYSTEM AND/OR WITH A TRACHEOSTOMA VALVE, EACH	37	A			D			N
A7509	FILTER HOLDER AND INTEGRATED FILTER HOUSING, AND ADHESIVE, FOR USE AS A TRACHEOSTOMA HEAT AND MOISTURE EXCHANGE SYSTEM, EACH	37	A			D			N
A7520	TRACHEOSTOMY/LARYNGECTOMY TUBE, NON-CUFFED, POLYVINYLCHLORIDE (PVC), SILICONE OR EQUAL, EACH	37	A			C			A
A7521	TRACHEOSTOMY/LARYNGECTOMY TUBE, CUFFED, POLYVINYLCHLORIDE (PVC), SILICONE OR EQUAL, EACH	37	A			C			A
A7522	TRACHEOSTOMY/LARYNGECTOMY TUBE, STAINLESS STEEL OR EQUAL (STERILIZABLE AND REUSABLE), EACH	37	A			C			A
A7523	TRACHEOSTOMY SHOWER PROTECTOR, EACH	37	A			C			A
A7524	TRACHEOSTOMA STENT/STUD/BUTTON, EACH	37	A			C			A
A7525	TRACHEOSTOMY MASK, EACH	37	A			C			A
A7526	TRACHEOSTOMY TUBE COLLAR/HOLDER, EACH	37	A			C			A
A9150	NON-PRESCRIPTION DRUGS	57	A			D			N
A9160	NON-COVERED SVC. BY PODIATRIST	00	9	1861.R3		S			N
A9170	NON-COVERED SVC. BY CHIROPRACTOR	00	9	1861.R5		S			N
A9190	PERSONAL COMFORT ITEM	00	9	1862.A6		S			N
A9270	NON-COVERED ITEM OR SERVICE	00	9			M			N
A9280	ALERT OR ALARM DEVICE, NOT OTHERWISE CLASSIFIED	00	9	1861		S			A
A9300	EXERCISE EQUIPMENT	00	9			M			N
A9500	SUPPLY OF RADIOPHARMACEUTICAL DIAGNOSTIC IMAGING AGENT, TECHNETIUM TC 99M SESTAMIBI, PER DOSE	57	A			D			N
A9502	SUPPLY OF RADIOPHARMACEUTICAL DIAGNOSTIC IMAGING AGENT, TECHNETIUM TC 99M TETROFOSMIN, PER UNIT DOSE	57	A			D			N
A9503	SUPPLY OF RADIOPHARMACEUTICAL DIAGNOSTIC IMAGING AGENT, TECHNETIUM TC 99M, MEDRONATE, UP TO 30 MCI	57	A			D			N
A9504	SUPPLY OF RADIOPHARMACEUTICAL DIAGNOSTIC IMAGING AGENT, TECHNETIUM TC 99M APCITIDE	57	A			C			N

HCPCS	Long Description	PII	MPI	Statute	X-Reff	Coverage	ASC Pay Grp	ASC Pay Grp Eff Date	Action Code
A9505	SUPPLY OF RADIOPHARMACEUTICAL DIAGNOSTIC IMAGING AGENT, THALLOUS CHLORIDE TL	57	A			D			N
A9507	SUPPLY OF RADIOPHARMACEUTICAL DIAGNOSTIC IMAGING AGENT, INDIUM IN 111 CAPROMAB PENDETIDE, PER DOSE	57	A			D			N
A9508	SUPPLY OF RADIOPHARMACEUTICAL DIAGNOSTIC IMAGING AGENT, IOBENGUANE SULFATE I-131, PER 0.5 MCI	51	A			D			N
A9510	SUPPLY OF RADIOPHARMACEUTICAL DIAGNOSTIC IMAGING AGENT, TECHNETIUM TC99M DISOFENIN, PER VIAL	51	A			D			N
A9511	SUPPLY OF RADIOPHARMACEUTICAL DIAGNOSTIC IMAGING AGENT, TECHNETIUM TC 99M, DEPREOTIDE, PER MCI	57	A			C			N
A9512	SUPPLY OF RADIOPHARMACEUTICAL DIAGNOSTIC IMAGING AGENT, TECHNETIUM TC-99M PERTECHNETATE, PER MCI	57	A			C			N
A9513	SUPPLY OF RADIOPHARMACEUTICAL DIAGNOSTIC IMAGING AGENT, TECHNETIUM TC-99M MEBROFENIN, PER MCI	57	A			C			N
A9514	SUPPLY OF RADIOPHARMACEUTICAL DIAGNOSTIC IMAGING AGENT, TECHNETIUM TC-99M PYROPHOSPHATE, PER MCI	57	A			C			N
A9515	SUPPLY OF RADIOPHARMACEUTICAL DIAGNOSTIC IMAGING AGENT, TECHNETIUM TC-99M PENTETATE, PER MCI	57	A			C			N
A9516	SUPPLY OF RADIOPHARMACEUTICAL DIAGNOSTIC IMAGING AGENT, I-123 SODIUM IODIDE CAPSULE, PER 100 UCI	57	A			C			N
A9517	SUPPLY OF RADIOPHARMACEUTICAL THERAPEUTIC IMAGING AGENT, I-131 SODIUM IODIDE CAPSULE, PER MCI	57	A			C			S
A9518	SUPPLY OF RADIOPHARMACEUTICAL THERAPEUTIC IMAGING AGENT, I-131 SODIUM IODIDE SOLUTION, PER UCI	57	A		A9530	C			D
A9519	SUPPLY OF RADIOPHARMACEUTICAL DIAGNOSTIC IMAGING AGENT, TECHNETIUM TC-99M MACROAGGREGATED ALBUMIN, PER MCI	57	A			C			N
A9520	SUPPLY OF RADIOPHARMACEUTICAL DIAGNOSTIC IMAGING AGENT, TECHNETIUM TC-99M SULFUR COLLOID, PER MCI	57	A			C			N
A9521	SUPPLY OF RADIOPHARMACEUTICAL DIAGNOSTIC IMAGING AGENT, TECHNETIUM TC-99M EXAMETAZINE, PER DOSE	57	A			C			N
A9522	SUPPLY OF RADIOPHARMACEUTICAL DIAGNOSTIC IMAGING AGENT, INDIUM-111 IBRITUMOMAB TIUXETAN, PER MCI	51	A			D			N
A9523	SUPPLY OF RADIOPHARMACEUTICAL THERAPEUTIC IMAGING AGENT, YTTRIUM 90 IBRITUMOMAB TIUXETAN, PER MCI	51	A			D			N
A9524	SUPPLY OF RADIOPHARMACEUTICAL DIAGNOSTIC IMAGING AGENT, IODINATED I-131 SERUM ALBUMIN, 5 MICROCURIES	57	A			D			N
A9525	SUPPLY OF LOW OR ISO-OSMOLAR CONTRAST MATERIAL, 10 MG OF IODINE	51	A			D			A
A9526	SUPPLY OF RADIOPHARMACEUTICAL DIAGNOSTIC IMAGING AGENT, AMMONIA N-13, PER DOSE	53	A			D			A
A9528	SUPPLY OF RADIOPHARMACEUTICAL DIAGNOSTIC AGENT, I-131 SODIUM IODIDE CAPSULE, PER MILLICURIE	57	A			C			A
A9529	SUPPLY OF RADIOPHARMACEUTICAL DIAGNOSTIC AGENT, I-131 SODIUM IODIDE SOLUTION, PER MILLICURIE	57	A			C			A
A9530	SUPPLY OF RADIOPHARMACEUTICAL THERAPEUTIC AGENT, I-131 SODIUM IODIDE SOLUTION, PER MILLICURIE	57	A			C			A
A9531	SUPPLY OF RADIOPHARMACEUTICAL DIAGNOSTIC AGENT, I-131 SODIUM IODIDE, PER MICROCURIE (UP TO 100 MICROCURIES)	57	A			C			A

HCPCS	Long Description	PTI	MPI	Statute	X-Reff	Coverage	ASC Pay Grp	ASC Pay Grp Eff Date	Action Code
A9532	SUPPLY OF RADIOPHARMACEUTICAL THERAPEUTIC AGENT, IODINATED I-125, SERUM ALBUMIN, 5 MICROCURIES	57	A			C			A
A9533	SUPPLY OF RADIOPHARMACEUTICAL DIAGNOSTIC IMAGING AGENT, I-131 TOSITUMOMAB, PER MILLICURIE	57	A			C			A
A9534	SUPPLY OF RADIOPHARMACEUTICAL THERAPEUTIC IMAGING AGENT, I-131 TOSITUMOMAB, PER MILLICURIE	57	A			C			A
A9600	SUPPLY OF THERAPEUTIC RADIOPHARMACEUTICAL, STRONTIUM-89 CHLORIDE, PER MCI	57	A			C			N
A9605	SUPPLY OF THERAPEUTIC RADIOPHARMACEUTICAL, SAMARIUM SM 153 LEXIDRONAMM, 50 MCI	57	A			C			N
A9699	SUPPLY OF RADIOPHARMACEUTICAL THERAPEUTIC IMAGING AGENT, NOT OTHERWISE CLASSIFIED	57	A			C			N
A9700	SUPPLY OF INJECTABLE CONTRAST MATERIAL FOR USE IN ECHOCARDIOGRAPHY, PER STUDY	57	A			D			N
A9900	MISCELLANEOUS DME SUPPLY, ACCESSORY, AND/OR SERVICE COMPONENT OF ANOTHER HCPCS CODE	46	A			C			N
A9901	DME DELIVERY, SET UP, AND/OR DISPENSING SERVICE COMPONENT OF ANOTHER HCPCS CODE	46	A			C			N
A9999	MISCELLANEOUS DME SUPPLY OR ACCESSORY, NOT OTHERWISE SPECIFIED	46	A			C			A
B4034	ENTERAL FEEDING SUPPLY KIT; SYRINGE, PER DAY	39	A			D			N
B4035	ENTERAL FEEDING SUPPLY KIT; PUMP FED, PER DAY	39	A			D			N
B4036	ENTERAL FEEDING SUPPLY KIT; GRAVITY FED, PER DAY	39	A			D			N
B4081	NASOGASTRIC TUBING WITH STYLET	39	A			D			N
B4082	NASOGASTRIC TUBING WITHOUT STYLET	39	A			D			N
B4083	STOMACH TUBE - LEVINE TYPE	39	A			D			N
B4084	GASTROSTOMY/JEJUNOSTOMY TUBING	39	A			D			N
B4085	GASTROSTOMY TUBE, SILICONE WITH SLIDING RING, EACH	39	A			C			N
B4086	GASTROSTOMY / JEJUNOSTOMY TUBE, ANY MATERIAL, ANY TYPE, (STANDARD OR LOW PROFILE), EACH	39	A			C			N
B4100	FOOD THICKENER, ADMINISTERED ORALLY, PER OUNCE	00	9			I			N
B4150	ENTERAL FORMULAE; CATEGORY I; SEMI-SYNTHETIC INTACT PROTEIN/PROTEIN ISOLATES, ADMINISTERED THROUGH AN ENTERAL FEEDING TUBE, 100 CALORIES = 1 UNIT	39	A			D			N
B4151	ENTERAL FORMULAE; CATEGORY I; NATURAL INTACT PROTEIN/PROTEIN ISOLATES, ADMINISTERED THROUGH AN ENTERAL FEEDING TUBE, 100 CALORIES = 1 UNIT	39	A			D			N
B4152	ENTERAL FORMULAE; CATEGORY II; INTACT PROTEIN/PROTEIN ISOLATES (CALORICALLY DENSE), ADMINISTERED THROUGH AN ENTERAL FEEDING TUBE, 100 CALORIES = 1 UNIT	39	A			D			N
B4153	ENTERAL FORMULAE; CATEGORY III; HYDROLIZED PROTEIN/AMINO ACIDS, ADMINISTERED THROUGH AN ENTERAL FEEDING TUBE, 100 CALORIES = 1 UNIT	39	A			D			N
B4154	ENTERAL FORMULAE; CATEGORY IV; DEFINED FORMULA FOR SPECIAL METABOLIC NEED, ADMINISTERED THROUGH AN ENTERAL FEEDING TUBE, 100 CALORIES = 1 UNIT	39	A			D			N

HCPCS	Long Description	PII	MPI	Statute	X-Ref	Coverage	ASC Pay Grp	ASC Pay Grp Eff Date	Action Code
B4155	ENTERAL FORMULAE; CATEGORY V; MODULAR COMPONENTS, ADMINISTERED THROUGH AN ENTERAL FEEDING TUBE, 100 CALORIES = 1 UNIT	39	A			D			N
B4156	ENTERAL FORMULAE; CATEGORY VI; STANDARDIZED NUTRIENTS, ADMINISTERED THROUGH AN ENTERAL FEEDING TUBE, 100 CALORIES = 1 UNIT	39	A			D			N
B4164	PARENTERAL NUTRITION SOLUTION: CARBOHYDRATES (DEXTROSE), 50% OR LESS (500 ML = 1 UNIT) - HOMEMIX	39	A			D			N
B4168	PARENTERAL NUTRITION SOLUTION; AMINO ACID, 3.5%, (500 ML = 1 UNIT) - HOMEMIX	39	A			D			N
B4172	PARENTERAL NUTRITION SOLUTION; AMINO ACID, 5.5% THROUGH 7%, (500 ML = 1 UNIT) - - HOMEMIX	39	A			D			N
B4176	PARENTERAL NUTRITION SOLUTION; AMINO ACID, 7% THROUGH 8.5%, (500 ML = 1 UNIT) - - HOMEMIX	39	A			D			N
B4178	PARENTERAL NUTRITION SOLUTION: AMINO ACID, GREATER THAN 8.5% (500 ML = 1 UNIT) - HOMEMIX	39	A			D			N
B4180	PARENTERAL NUTRITION SOLUTION; CARBOHYDRATES (DEXTROSE), GREATER THAN 50% (500 ML=1 UNIT) - HOMEMIX	39	A			D			N
B4184	PARENTERAL NUTRITION SOLUTION; LIPIDS, 10% WITH ADMINISTRATION SET (500 ML = 1 UNIT)	39	A			D			N
B4186	PARENTERAL NUTRITION SOLUTION, LIPIDS, 20% WITH ADMINISTRATION SET (500 ML = 1 UNIT)	39	A			D			N
B4189	PARENTERAL NUTRITION SOLUTION; COMPOUNDED AMINO ACID AND CARBOHYDRATES WITH ELECTROLYTES, TRACE ELEMENTS, AND VITAMINS, INCLUDING PREPARATION, ANY STRENGTH, 10 TO 51 GRAMS OF PROTEIN - PREMIX	39	A			D			N
B4193	PARENTERAL NUTRITION SOLUTION; COMPOUNDED AMINO ACID AND CARBOHYDRATES WITH ELECTROLYTES, TRACE ELEMENTS, AND VITAMINS, INCLUDING PREPARATION, ANY STRENGTH, 52 TO 73 GRAMS OF PROTEIN - PREMIX	39	A			D			N
B4197	PARENTERAL NUTRITION SOLUTION; COMPOUNDED AMINO ACID AND CARBOHYDRATES WITH ELECTROLYTES, TRACE ELEMENTS AND VITAMINS, INCLUDING PREPARATION, ANY STRENGTH, 74 TO 100 GRAMS OF PROTEIN - PREMIX	39	A			D			N
B4199	PARENTERAL NUTRITION SOLUTION; COMPOUNDED AMINO ACID AND CARBOHYDRATES WITH ELECTROLYTES, TRACE ELEMENTS AND VITAMINS, INCLUDING PREPARATION, ANY STRENGTH, OVER 100 GRAMS OF PROTEIN - PREMIX	39	A			D			N
B4216	PARENTERAL NUTRITION; ADDITIVES (VITAMINS, TRACE ELEMENTS, HEPARIN, ELECTROLYTES) HOMEMIX PER DAY	39	A			D			N
B4220	PARENTERAL NUTRITION SUPPLY KIT; PREMIX, PER DAY	39	A			D			N
B4222	PARENTERAL NUTRITION SUPPLY KIT; HOME MIX, PER DAY	39	A			D			N
B4224	PARENTERAL NUTRITION ADMINISTRATION KIT, PER DAY	39	A			D			N
B5000	PARENTERAL NUTRITION SOLUTION: COMPOUNDED AMINO ACID AND CARBOHYDRATES WITH ELECTROLYTES, TRACE ELEMENTS, AND VITAMINS, INCLUDING PREPARATION, ANY STRENGTH, RENAL - AMIROSYN RF, NEPHRAMINE, RENAMINE - PREMIX	39	A			D			N
B5100	PARENTERAL NUTRITION SOLUTION: COMPOUNDED AMINO ACID AND CARBOHYDRATES WITH ELECTROLYTES, TRACE ELEMENTS, AND VITAMINS, INCLUDING PREPARATION, ANY STRENGTH, HEPATIC - FREAMINE HBC, HEPATAMINE - PREMIX	39	A			D			N
B5200	PARENTERAL NUTRITION SOLUTION: COMPOUNDED AMINO ACID AND CARBOHYDRATES WITH ELECTROLYTES, TRACE ELEMENTS, AND VITAMINS, INCLUDING PREPARATION, ANY STRENGTH, STRESS - BRANCH CHAIN AMINO ACIDS - PREMIX	39	A			D			N
B9000	ENTERAL NUTRITION INFUSION PUMP - WITHOUT ALARM	39	A			D			N

HCPCS	Long Description	PTI	MPI	Statute	X-Ref1	Coverage	ASC Pay Grp	ASC Pay Grp Eff Date	Action Code
B9002	ENTERAL NUTRITION INFUSION PUMP - WITH ALARM	39	A			D			N
B9004	PARENTERAL NUTRITION INFUSION PUMP, PORTABLE	39	A			D			N
B9006	PARENTERAL NUTRITION INFUSION PUMP, STATIONARY	39	A			D			N
B9998	NOC FOR ENTERAL SUPPLIES	57	A			D			N
B9999	NOC FOR PARENTERAL SUPPLIES	57	A			D			N
C1000	CLOSURE, ARTERIAL VASCULAR DEVICE, PERCLOSE CLOSER ARTERIAL VASCULAR CLOSURE DEVICE, PROSTAR ARTERIAL VASCULAR CLOSURE DEVICE, CLOSER S ARTERIAL VASCULAR DEVICE	53	A	1833(T)		D			N
C1001	CATHETER, DIAGNOSTIC ULTRASOUND, ACUNAV DIAGNOSTIC ULTRASOUND CATHETER	53	A	1833(T)		D			N
C1003	CATHETER, LIVEWIRE TC ABLATION CATHETER 402132, 402133, 402134, 402135, 402136, 402137, 402145, 402146, 402147, 402148, 402149, 402150, 402151, 402152, 402153, 402154, 402155, 402156, 7 FR CSM LIVEWIRE EP CATHETER (MODEL 401935), 5FR DECAPOLAR (MODELS 401938, 401939, 401940, 401941), LIVEWIRE TC COMPASS ABLATION CATHETER (MODELS 402205, 402006, 402207, 402208)	53	A	1833(t)		D			N
C1004	FAST-CATH, SWARTZ, SAFL, CSTA, SEPT, RAMP GUIDING INTRODUCER	53	A	1833(t)		D			N
C1005	INTRAOCULAR LENS, SENSAR SOFT ACRYLIC ULTRAVIOLET LIGHT ABSORBING POSTERIOR CHAMBER INTRAOCULAR LENS	53	A	1833(T)		D			N
C1006	INTRAOCULAR LENS, ARRAY MULTIFOCAL SILICONE POSTERIOR CHAMBER INTRAOCULAR LENS	53	A	1833(T)		D			N
C1007	PROSTHESIS, PENILE, AMS 700 PENILE PROSTHESIS, AMS AMBICOR PENILE PROSTHESIS, DURA II PENILE PROSTHESIS, AMS MALLEABLE 650 PENILE PROSTHESIS. NOTE: ONLY THE AMS AMBICOR PENILE PROSTHESIS IS EFFECTIVE OCTOBER 1, 2000.	53	A	1833(T)		D			N
C1008	STENT, UROLUME, COOK HARRISON FETAL BLADDER STENT	53	A	1833(T)		D			N
C1009	PLASMA, CRYOPRECIPITATE REDUCED, EACH UNIT	53	A	1833(T)		D			N
C1010	WHOLE BLOOD OR RED BLOOD CELLS, LEUKOREDUCED, CMV NEGATIVE, EACH UNIT	53	A	1833(T)		D			D
C1011	PLATELET, HLA-MATCHED LEUKOREDUCED, APHERESIS/PHERESIS, EACH UNIT	53	A	1833(T)		D			D
C1012	PLATELET CONCENTRATE, LEUKOREDUCED, IRRADIATED, EACH UNIT	53	A	1833(T)	P9033	D			N
C1013	PLATELET CONCENTRATE, LEUKOREDUCED, EACH UNIT	53	A	1833(T)	P9031	D			N
C1014	PLATELET, LEUKOREDUCED, APHERESIS/PHERESIS, EACH UNIT	53	A	1833(T)	P9035	D			N
C1015	PLATELETS, PHERESIS, LEUKOCYTE-REDUCED, CMV NEGATIVE, IRRADIATED, EACH UNIT	53	A	1833(t)		D			D
C1016	WHOLE BLOOD OR RED BLOOD CELLS, LEUKOREDUCED, FROZEN, DEGLYCEROL, WASHED, EACH UNIT	53	A	1833(T)		D			D

HCPCS	Long Description	PII	MPI	Statute	X-Ref	Coverage	ASC Pay Grp	ASC Pay Grp Eff Date	Action Code
C1017	PLATELET, LEUKOREDUCED, CMV-NEGATIVE, APHERESIS/PHERESIS, EACH UNIT	53	A	1833(T)		D			D
C1018	WHOLE BLOOD, LEUKOREDUCED, IRRADIATED, EACH UNIT	53	A	1833(T)		D			D
C1019	PLATELET, LEUKOREDUCED, IRRADIATED, APHERESIS/PHERESIS, EACH UNIT	53	A	1833(T)		D			N
C1020	RED BLOOD CELLS, FROZEN/DEGLYCEROLIZED/WASHED, LEUKOCYTE-REDUCED, IRRADIATED, EACH UNIT	53	A	1833(T)		D			D
C1021	RED BLOOD CELLS, LEUKOCYTE-REDUCED, CMV NEGATIVE, IRRADIATED, EACH UNIT	53	A	1833(T)		D			D
C1022	PLASMA, FROZEN WITHIN 24 HOURS OF COLLECTION, EACH UNIT	53	A	1833(T)		D			D
C1024	QUINOPRISTIN/DALFOPRISTIN, 10ML, SYNERCID IV	53	A	1833(T)		D			N
C1025	CATHETER, MARINR CS CATHETER	53	A	1833(T)		D			N
C1026	CATHETER ABLATION, RF PERFORMR, 5F RF MARINR	53	A	1833(T)		D			N
C1027	STENT, CORONARY, MAGIC WALLSTENT EXTRA SHORT OR SHORT CORONARY SELF-EXPANDING STENT WITH DELIVERY SYSTEM, RADIUS 14MM SELF EXPANDING STENT WITH OVER THE WIRE DELIVERY SYSTEM	53	A	1833(T)		D			N
C1028	SLING FIXATION SYSTEM FOR TREATMENT OF STRESS URINARY INCONTINENCE, PRECISION TWIST TRANSVAGINAL ANCHOR SYSTEM, PRECISION TACK TRANSVAGINAL ANCHOR SYSTEM, VESICA PRESS-IN ANCHOR SYSTEM, CAPIO CL (TVB/S) TRANSVAGINAL SUTURING DEVICE	53	A	1833(T)		D			N
C1029	CATHETER, BALLOON DILATATION, CONTROLLED RADIAL EXPANSION (CRE) BALLOON DILATATION CATHETER WIRE GUIDED AND FIXED WIRE, QUANTUM DILATION BALLOON, MS CLASSIQUE BALLOON DILATION CATHETER	53	A	1833(T)		D			N
C1030	CATHETER, BALLOON DILATATION, MARSHAL, BLUE MAX 20, ULTRA-THIN DIAMOND, ULTRA-THIN BALLOON DILATATION CATHETER, ULTRA-THIN ST BALLOON DILATATION CATHETER, ULTRA-THIN BALLOON DILATATION CATHETER WITH GLIDEX HYDROPHILIC COATED BALLOON, ULTRA-THIN ST BALLOON DILATATION CATHETER WITH GLIDEX HYDROPHILIC COATED BALLOON	53	A	1833(T)		D			N
C1031	ELECTRODE, NEEDLE, ABLATION, MR COMPATIBLE LEVEEN, MODIFIED LEVEEN NEEDLE ELECTRODE	53	A	1833(T)		D			N
C1033	CATHETER, IMAGING, SONICATH ULTRA MODEL 37-410 ULTRASOUND IMAGING CATHETER, SONICATH ULTRA 9 MHZ ULTRASOUND IMAGING CATHETER	53	A	1833(T)		D			N
C1034	CATHETER, CORONARY ANGIOPLASTY, SURPASS SUPERFUSION CATHETER, LONG 30 SURPASS SUPERFUSION CATHETER	53	A	1833(T)		D			N
C1035	CATHETER, INTRACARDIAC ECHOCARDIOGRAPHY, ULTRA ICE 6F, 12.5 MHZ CATHETER (WITH DISPOSABLE SHEATH), ULTRA ICE 9F, 9 MHZ CATHETER (WITH DISPOSABLE SHEATH)	53	A	1833(t)		D			N
C1036	PORT/RESERVOIR, VENOUS ACCESS DEVICE, VAXCEL IMPLANTABLE VASCULAR ACCESS SYSTEM, R PORT PREMIER VASCULAR ACCESS SYSTEM (MODEL 45-100), BARD PORT IMPLANTED PORT, BARD ROSENBLATT LUMEN PORT, BARD ULTRA LOW PROFILE PORT, BARDPORT TITANIUM IMPLANTED PORT, BARDPORT X-PORT IMPLANTED PORT, BARDPORT M.R.I. DUAL IMPLANTED PORT, BARDPORT M.R.I. HARD-BASE IMPLANTED PORT	53	A	1833(T)		D			N

HCPCS	Long Description	PTI	MPI	Statute	X-Ref	Coverage	ASC Pay Grp	ASC Pay Grp Eff Date	Action Code
C1037	CATHETER, VAXCEL CHRONIC DIALYSIS CATHETER, MEDCOMP BIO FLEX TESIO CATHETER, MEDCOMP SILICONE TESIO CATHETER, MEDCOMP HEMO-CATH LONG TERM SILICONE CATHETER, BARD NIAGARA DUAL LUMEN CATHETER, BARD OPTI-FLOW DUAL LUMEN CATHETER, MEDCOMP ASH SPLIT CATHETER	53	A	1833(T)		D			N
C1038	CATHETER, IMAGING, ULTRACROSS 2.9F 30MHZ CORONARY IMAGING CATHETER, ULTRACROSS 3.2F MHZ CORONARY IMAGING CATHETER	53	A	1833(t)		D			N
C1039	STENT, TRACHEOBRONCHIAL, WALLSTENT TRACHEOBRONCHIAL ENDOPROSTHESIS (COVERED), WALLSTENT TRACHEOBRONCHIAL ENDOPROSTHESIS WITH PERMALUME COVERING AND UNISTEP PLUS DELIVERY SYSTEM, WALLSTENT RP TRACHEOBRONCHIAL ENDOPROSTHESIS WITH UNISTEP PLUS DELIVERY SYSTEM NOTE: ONLY THE WALLSTENT RP TRACHEOBRONCHIAL ENDOPROSTHESIS WITH UNISTEP PLUS DELIVERY SYSTEM IS EFFECTIVE OCTOBER 1, 2000. THE WALLSTENT TRACHEOBRONCHIAL WAS EFFECTIVE AUGUST 1, 2000.	53	A	1833(T)		D			N
C1040	STENT, SELF-EXPANDABLE FOR CREATION OF INTRAHEPATIC SHUNTS, WALLSTENT TRANSJUGULAR INTRAHEPATIC PORTOSYSTEMIC SHUNT (TIPS) WITH UNISTEP PLUS DELIVERY SYSTEM (40/42/60/68MM IN LENGTH), WALLSTENT RP ENDOPROSTHESIS WITH UNISTEP PLUS DELIVERY SYSTEM (42/68MM IN LENGTH) NOTE: ONLY THE WALLSTENT RP TIPS ENDOPROSTHESIS WITH UNISTEP PLUS DELIVERY SYSTEM IS EFFECTIVE OCTOBER 1, 2000. THE WALLSTENT TIPS ENDOPROSTHESIS WITH UNISTEP PLUS DELIVERY SYSTEM WAS EFFECTIVE AUGUST 1, 2000.	53	A	1833(T)		D			N
C1042	STENT, BILIARY, WALLSTENT BILIARY ENDOPROSTHESIS WITH UNISTEP PLUS DELIVERY SYSTEM, WALLSTENT BILIARY ENDOPROSTHESIS WITH UNISTEP DELIVERY SYSTEM (BILIARY STENT AND CATHETER), WALLSTENT RP BILIARY ENDOPROSTHESIS WITH UNISTEP PLUS DELIVERY SYSTEM, ULTRAFLEX DIAMOND BILIARY STENT SYSTEM, NEW MICROVASIVE BILIARY STENT AND DELIVERY SYSTEM NOTE: ONLY THE WALLSTENT RP BILIARY ENDOPROSTHESIS WITH UNISTEP PLUS DELIVERY SYSTEM IS EFFECTIVE OCTOBER 1, 2000. THE WALLSTENT, ULTRAFLEX DIAMOND, NEW MICROVASIVE BILIARY STENT SYSTEMS WERE EFFECTIVE AUGUST 1, 2000.	53	A	1833(T)		D			N
C1043	ATHERECTOMY SYSTEM, CORONARY, ROTABLATOR ROTALINK ATHERECTOMY CATHETER AND BURR, ROTABLATOR ROTALINK ROTATIONAL ATHERECTOMY SYSTEM ADVANCER AND GUIDE WIRE, ATHEROCATH-GTO ATHERECTOMY CATHETER, INTERVENTIONAL TECHNOLOGIES TRANSLUMINAL EXTRACTION CORONARY (TEC) ATHERECTOMY SYSTEM	53	A	1833(T)		D			N
C1045	SUPPLY OF RADIOPHARMACEUTICAL DIAGNOSTIC IMAGING AGENT, I-131 MIBG [IOBENGUANE SULFATE I-131], PER 0.5 MCI	53	A	1833(T)		D			N
C1047	CATHETER, DIAGNOSTIC, NAVI-STAR DIAGNOSTIC DEFLECTABLE TIP CATHETER, NOGA-STAR DIAGNOSTIC DEFLECTABLE TIP CATHETER	53	A	1833(T)		D			N
C1048	GENERATOR, BIPOLAR PULSE, CYBERONICS NEUROCYBERNETIC PROSTHESIS GENERATOR	53	A	1833(T)		D			N
C1050	PROTEIN A IMMUNOADSORPTION, PROSORBA COLUMN	53	A	1833(T)		D			N
C1051	CATHETER, THROMBECTOMY, OASIS THROMBECTOMY CATHETER, FOGARTY ADHERENT CLOT CATHETER (4 FR, 5 FR, 6 FR), 6 FR THROMBEX PMT CATHETER (60CM, 120CM)	53	A	1833(t)		D			N
C1053	CATHETER, DIAGNOSTIC, ENSITE 3000 CATHETER	53	A	1833(T)		D			N
C1054	CATHETER, THROMBECTOMY, HYDROLYSER 6F MECHANICAL THROMBECTOMY CATHETER, HYDROLYSER 7F MECHANICAL THROMBECTOMY CATHETER	53	A	1833(t)		D			N
C1055	CATHETER, TRANSESOPHAGEAL 210 ATRIAL PACING CATHETER, TRANSESOPHAGEAL 210-S ATRIAL PACING CATHETER, FLEX-EZ BALLOON DILATOR, EZ RESOLUTION BALLOON DILATOR (MODELS 3802, 3804, 3806)	53	A	1833(t)		D			N
C1056	CATHETER, GYNECARE THERMACHOICE II CATHETER, COOK INTRAUTERINE INSEMINATION CATHETER, COOK JANSEN-ANDERSON INSEMINATION SET, COOK OB/GYN SUPRAPUBIC BALLOONS, COOK UROLOGICAL OBRIEN SUPRAPUBIC ACCESS SET, COOK UROLOGICAL SUPRAPUBIC BALLOONS, PRODUCT HEALTH INDUCT BREAST MICROCATHETER, COOK CHORIONIC VILLUS SAMPLING SET	53	A	1833(t)		D			N
C1057	TISSUE MARKER, 11-GAUGE MICROMARK II TISSUE MARKER	53	A	1833(T)		D			N

HCPCS	Long Description	PII	MPI	Statute	X-Ref1	Coverage	ASC Pay Grp	ASC Pay Grp Eff Date	Action Code
C1058	SUPPLY OF RADIOPHARMACEUTICAL DIAGNOSTIC IMAGING AGENT, TECHNETIUM TC 99M OXIDRONATE, PER VIAL	53	A	1833(T)	Q3009	D			N
C1059	AUTOLOGOUS CULTURED CHONDROCYTES, IMPLANTATION, CARTICEL	53	A	1833(T)		D			N
C1060	STENT, CORONARY, ACS MULTI-LINK TRISTAR CORONARY STENT SYSTEM AND DELIVERY SYSTEM, ACS MULTI-LINK ULTRA CORONARY STENT SYSTEM NOTE: ACS MULTI-LINK ULTRA IS EFFECTIVE 01/01/01. ACS MULTI-LINK TRISTAR WAS EFFECTIVE 08/01/00	53	A	1833(T)		D			N
C1061	CATHETER, CORONARY GUIDE, ACS VIKING GUIDING CATHETER, CARDIMA VUEPORT BALLOON OCCLUSION GUIDING CATHETER, MERIT MEDICAL SYSTEMS PERFORMA VESSEL SIZING CATHETER, MERIT MEDICAL SYSTEMS PEDIATRIC/ADULT PIGTAIL CATHETER	53	A	1833(T)		D			N
C1063	LEAD, DEFIBRILLATOR, ENDOTAK ENDURANCE EZ, ENDOTAK ENDURANCE RX, ENDOTAK ENDURANCE 0134, 0135, 0136 NOTE: ENDOTAK ENDURANCE IS EFFECTIVE 01/01/01. ENDOTAK ENDURANCE EZ AND RX WERE EFFECTIVE 08/01/00.	53	A	1833(T)		D			N
C1064	SUPPLY OF RADIOPHARMACUTICAL THERAPEUTIC IMAGING AGENT, SODIUM IODIDE I-131, CAPSULE, EACH ADDITIONAL MCI	53	A	1833(T)		D			N
C1065	SUPPLY OF RADIOPHARMACUETICAL THERAPEUTIC IMAGING AGENT, SODIUM IODIDE I-131, SOLUTION, EACH ADDITIONAL MCI	53	A	1833(T)		D			N
C1066	SUPPLY OF RADIOPHARMACEUTICAL DIAGNOSTIC IMAGING AGENT, INDIUM 111 SATUMOMAB PENDETIDE, PER VIAL	53	A	1833(T)	A4642	D			N
C1067	STENT, BILIARY, MEGALINK BILIARY STENT, PALMAZ BALLOON EXPANDABLE STENT AND DELIVERY SYSTEM, SPIRAL Z BILIARY METAL EXPANDABLE STENT, ZA BILIARY METAL EXPANDABLE STENT, WALLSTENT TRANSHEPATIC BILIARY ENDOPROSTHESIS	53	A	1833(T)		D			N
C1068	PACEMAKER, DUAL CHAMBER, PULSAR DDD, UNITY VDDR (MODEL 292-07)	53	A	1833(T)		D			N
C1069	PACEMAKER, DUAL CHAMBER, DISCOVERY DR	53	A	1833(T)		D			N
C1071	PACEMAKER, SINGLE CHAMBER, PULSAR MAX SR, PULSAR SR, VIGOR SSI	53	A	1833(T)		D			N
C1072	CATHETER, BALLOON DILATATION, CORONARY, RX ESPRIT, RX GEMINI, RX SOLARIS, OTW PHOTON, OTW SOLARIS	53	A	1833(T)		D			N
C1073	MORCELLATOR, LAPAROSCOPIC, GYNECARE X-TRACT LAPARASCOPIC MORCELLATOR	53	A	1833(T)		D			N
C1074	CATHETER, PERIPHERAL DILATATION, RX VIATRAC 14 PERIPHERAL DILATATION CATHETER, OTW VIATRAC 18 PERIPHERAL DILATATION CATHETER	53	A	1833(T)		D			N
C1075	LEAD, PACEMAKER, SELUTE PICOTIP, SELUTE, SWEET PICOTIP RX, SWEET TIP RX, FINELINE, FINELINE EZ, THINLINE, THINLINE EZ	53	A	1833(T)		D			N
C1076	DEFIBRILLATOR, SINGLE CHAMBER, AUTOMATIC, IMPLANTABLE, VENTAK MINI IV, VENTAK MINI IV+ (MODELS 1793, 1796), VENTAK MINI III HE, VENTAK MINI III HE+ (MODELS 1788, 1789), VENTAK MINI III, VENTAK MINI III + (MODELS 1783, 1786) NOTE: ONLY THE VENTAK MINI IV+, VENTAK MINI III HE+ AND VENTAK MINI III+ ARE EFFECTIVE 01/01/01. VENTAK MINI IV, VENTAK MINI III HE, AND VENTAK MINI III WERE EFFECTIVE 08/01/00	53	A	1833(T)		D			N
C1077	DEFIBRILLATOR, SINGLE CHAMBER, AUTOMATIC, IMPLANTABLE, VENTAK PRIZM VR, VENTAK VR	53	A	1833(T)		D			N
C1078	DEFIBRILLATOR, DUAL CHAMBER, AUTOMATIC, IMPLANTABLE, VENTAK PRIZM, VENTAK AV III DR	53	A	1833(T)		D			N
C1079	SUPPLY OF RADIOPHARMACEUTICAL DIAGNOSTIC IMAGING AGENT, CYANOCOBALAMIN CO 57/58, PER 0.5 MICROCURIE	53	A	1833(T)		D			N
C1084	DENILEUKIN DIFTITOX, 300 MCG, ONTAK IV	51	A	1833(T)		D			N
C1086	TEMOZOLOMIDE, 5 MG, TEMODAR	51	A	1833(T)		D			N
C1087	SUPPLY OF RADIOPHARMACEUTICAL DIAGNOSTIC IMAGING AGENT, SODIUM IODIDE 1-123 PER 100 MICROCURIES	53	A	1833(T)		D			N
C1088	LASER OPTIC TREATMENT SYSTEM, INDIGO LASEROPTIC TREATMENT SYSTEM	53	A	1833(T)		D			T

HCPCS	Long Description	PII	MPI	Statute	X-Ref1	Coverage	ASC Pay Grp	ASC Pay Grp Eff Date	Action Code
C1089	SUPPLY OF RADIOPHARMACEUTICAL DIAGNOSTIC IMAGING AGENT, CYANOCOBALAMIN CO 57, 0.5 MCI, CAPSULE	53	A	1833(T)		D			N
C1090	SUPPLY OF RADIOPHARMACEUTICAL DIAGNOSTIC IMAGING AGENT, INDIUM IN 111 CHLORIDE, PER MCI	53	A	1833(T)		D			N
C1091	SUPPLY OF RADIOPHARMACEUTICAL DIAGNOSTIC IMAGING AGENT, INDIUM 111 OXYQUINOLINE, PER 0.5 MILLICURIE	53	A	1833(T)		D			N
C1092	SUPPLY OF RADIOPHARMACEUTICAL DIAGNOSTIC IMAGING AGENT, INDIUM 111 PENTETATE, PER 0.5 MILLICURIE	53	A	1833(T)		D			N
C1094	SUPPLY OF RADIOPHARMACEUTICAL DIAGNOSTIC IMAGING AGENT, TECHNETIUM TC 99M ALBUMIN AGGREGATED, PER 1.0 MILLICURIE	53	A	1833(T)		D			N
C1095	SUPPLY OF RADIOPHARMACEUTICAL DIAGNOSTIC IMAGING AGENT, TECHNETIUM TC 99M DEPREOTIDE, PER VIAL	53	A	1833(T)		D			N
C1096	SUPPLY OF RADIOPHARMACEUTICAL DIAGNOSTIC IMAGING AGENT, TECHNETIUM TC 99M EXAMETAZIME, PER DOSE	53	A	1833(T)		D			N
C1097	SUPPLY OF RADIOPHARMACEUTICAL DIAGNOSTIC IMAGING AGENT, TECHNETIUM TC 99M MEBROFENIN, PER VIAL	53	A	1833(T)		D			N
C1098	SUPPLY OF RADIOPHARMACEUTICAL DIAGNOSTIC IMAGING AGENT, TECHNETIUM TC 99M PENTETATE, PER VIAL	53	A	1833(T)		D			N
C1099	SUPPLY OF RADIOPHARMACEUTICAL DIAGNOSTIC IMAGING AGENT, TECHNETIUM TC 99M PYROPHOSPHATE, PER VIAL	53	A	1833(T)		D			N
C1100	GUIDE WIRE, PERCUTANEOUS TRANSLUMINAL CORONARY ANGIOPLASTY, MEDTRONIC AVE GT1 GUIDE WIRE, MEDTRONIC AVE GT2 FUSION GUIDE WIRE, INTERVENTIONAL TECHNOLOGIES TRACKWIRE, INTERVENTIONAL TECHNOLOGIES TRACKWIRE SUPPORT, INTERVENTIONAL TECHNOLOGIES TRACKWIRE EXTRA SUPPORT	53	A	1833(T)		D			N
C1101	CATHETER, PERCUTANEOUS TRANSLUMINAL CORONARY ANGIOPLASTY GUIDE, MEDTRONIC AVE 5F, 6F, 7F, 8F, 9F ZUMA GUIDE CATHETER, MEDTRONIC AVE Z2 5F, 6F, 7F, 8F, 9F ZUMA GUIDE CATHETER, MEDTRONIC AVE VECTOR GUIDE CATHETER, MEDTRONIC AVE VECTOR X GUIDE CATHETER. NOTE: ONLY THE MEDTRONIC AVE Z2 ZUMA GUIDE CATHETERS ARE EFFECTIVE OCTOBER 1, 2000. THE MEDTRONIC AVE ZUMA GUIDE CATHETERS WERE EFFECTIVE AUGUST 1, 2000.	53	A	1833(T)		D			N
C1102	GENERATOR, PULSE, NEUROSTIMULATOR, MEDTRONIC SYNERGY NEUROSTIMULATOR GENERATOR AND EXTENSION	53	A	1833(T)		D			N
C1103	DEFIBRILLATOR, IMPLANTABLE, MICRO JEWEL, MICRO JEWEL II	53	A	1833(T)		D			N
C1104	CATHETER, ABLATION, RF CONDUCTR MC 4MM, RF CONDUCTR MC 5MM (MODELS 6042, 7544) NOTE: RF CONDUCTR MC 5MM IS EFFECTIVE 01/01/01. RF CONDUCTR MC 4MM WAS EFFECTIVE 08/01/00. CATHETER, ABLATION, RF CONDUCTR MC--EXT (WITH STIFFER TIP) 07864447, 078754447	53	A	1833(T)		D			N
C1105	PACEMAKER, DUAL CHAMBER, SIGMA 300 VDD	53	A	1833(T)		D			N
C1106	NEUROSTIMULATOR, PATIENT PROGRAMMER, SYNERGY EZ PATIENT PROGRAMMER	53	A	1833(T)		D			N
C1107	CATHETER, DIAGNOSTIC, ELECTROPHYSIOLOGY, TORQR, SOLOIST, DYNAMIC XT DECAPOLAR CATHETER	53	A	1833(T)		D			N

HCPCS	Long Description	PTI	MPI	Statute	X-Ref	Coverage	ASC Pay Grp	ASC Pay Grp Eff Date	Action Code
C1109	ANCHOR, IMPLANTABLE, MITEK GII ANCHOR, MITEK KNOTLESS, MITEK TACIT, MITEK ROTATOR CUFF, MITEK GLS, MITEK MINI, MITEK FASTIN, MITEK SUPER, MITEK PANALOK, MITEK MICRO, MITEK PANALOK RC, MITEK FASTIN RC, INNOVASIVE ROC EZ, INNOVASIVE MINIROC, INNOVASIVE BIOROC, INNOVASIVE ROC XS, INNOVASIVE CONTACK, BIOMET 3.5MM CORTICAL SCREW, BIOMET 4.5MM CORTICAL SCREW (FULLY THREADED), BIOMET 6.5MM CANCELLOUS LAG SCREW (32MM THREAD LENGTH), BIOMET 6.5MM CANNULATED CANCELLOUS SCREW (20MM THREAD LENGTH)	53	A	1833(T)		D			N
C1110	CATHETER, DIAGNOSTIC, ELECTROPHYSIOLOGY, STABLE MAPPER	53	A	1833(T)		D			N
C1111	STENT GRAFT SYSTEM, ANEURX AORTO-UNI-ILIAC-STENT GRAFT SYSTEM	53	A	1833(T)		D			N
C1112	STENT GRAFT SYSTEM, ANEURX STENT GRAFT SYSTEM	53	A	1833(T)		D			N
C1113	STENT GRAFT SYSTEM, TALENT ENDOLUMINAL SPRING STENT GRAFT SYSTEM	53	A	1833(T)		D			N
C1114	STENT GRAFT SYSTEM, TALENT SPRING STENT GRAFT SYSTEM	53	A	1833(T)		D			N
C1115	LEAD, PACEMAKER, 5038S, 5038, 5038L, 2188 CORONARY SINUS LEAD, 4057M, 4058M, 4557M, 4558M, 5058, 6416 PACEMAKER LEAD, INNOMEDICA SUTURELESS MYOCARDIAL (MODELS 4045, 4046, 4047, 4058), UNIPASS (MODELS 425-02, 425-04, 425-06)	53	A	1833(T)		D			N
C1116	LEAD, PACEMAKER, CAPSURE SP NOVUS, CAPSURE SP, CAPSURE, EXCELLENCE +, S+, PS+, CAPSURE Z NOVUS, CAPSURE Z, IMPULSE	53	A	1833(T)		D			N
C1117	ENDOGRAFT SYSTEM, ANCURE ENDOGRAFT DELIVERY SYSTEM	53	A	1833(t)		D			N
C1118	PACEMAKER, DUAL CHAMBER, SIGMA 300 DR, LEGACY II DR, LEGACY II S	53	A	1833(T)		D			N
C1119	LEAD, DEFIBRILLATOR, SPRINT 6932, SPRINT 6943	53	A	1833(T)		D			N
C1120	LEAD, DEFIBRILLATOR, SPRINT 6942, SPRINT 6945	53	A	1833(T)		D			N
C1121	DEFIBRILLATOR, IMPLANTABLE, GEM	53	A	1833(T)		D			N
C1122	SUPPLY OF RADIOPHARMACEUTICAL DIAGNOSTIC IMAGING AGENT, TECHNETIUM TC 99M ARCITUMOMAB, PER VIAL	53	A	1833(T)		D			N
C1123	DEFIBRILLATOR, IMPLANTABLE, GEM II VR, GEM III VR (MODEL 7231)	53	A	1833(T)		D			N
C1124	LEAD, NEUROSTIMULATOR, KIT, INTERSTIM TEST STIMULATION LEAD KIT	53	A	1833(T)		D			N
C1125	PACEMAKER, SINGLE CHAMBER, KAPPA 400 SR, TOPAZ II SR, TOPAZ3/TOPAZ SR (MODEL 540)	53	A	1833(T)		D			N
C1126	PACEMAKER, DUAL CHAMBER, KAPPA 700 DR (ALL MODELS), CLARITY DR (MODELS 860, 862, 865), DIAMOND 3/DIAMOND DR (MODEL 840)	53	A	1833(T)		D			N
C1127	PACEMAKER, SINGLE CHAMBER, KAPPA 700 SR, CLARITY SR (MODELS 560, 562, 565)	53	A	1833(T)		D			N
C1128	PACEMAKER, DUAL CHAMBER, KAPPA 700 D, RUBY II D, RUBY 3/RUBY 3 D (MODEL 740), VITA 2 DR (MODEL 830)	53	A	1833(T)		D			N

HCPCS	Long Description	PTI	MPI	Statute	X-Ref1	Coverage	ASC Pay Grp	ASC Pay Grp Eff Date	Action Code
C1129	PACEMAKER, KAPPA 700 VDD	53	A	1833(T)		D			N
C1130	PACEMAKER, DUAL CHAMBER, SIGMA 200 D, LEGACY II D	53	A	1833(T)		D			N
C1131	PACEMAKER, DUAL CHAMBER, SIGMA 200 DR	53	A	1833(T)		D			N
C1132	PACEMAKER, SINGLE CHAMBER, SIGMA 200 SR, LEGACY II SR	53	A	1833(T)		D			N
C1133	PACEMAKER, SINGLE CHAMBER, SIGMA 300 SR, VITA SR, VITA 2 SR (MODEL 530)	53	A	1833(T)		D			N
C1134	PACEMAKER, DUAL CHAMBER, SIGMA 300 D	53	A	1833(T)		D			N
C1135	PACEMAKER, DUAL CHAMBER, RATE-RESPONSIVE, ENTITY DR 5326L, ENTITY DR 5326R, ENTITY DR 5326 NOTE: ONLY THE ENTITY DR 5326 IS EFFECTIVE 01/01/01. ENTITY DR 5326L AND 5326R WERE EFFECTIVE 08/01/00.	53	A	1833(t)		D			N
C1136	PACEMAKER, DUAL CHAMBER, RATE-RESPONSIVE, AFFINITY DR 5330L, AFFINITY DR 5330R, AFFINITY DR 5330 NOTE: ONLY THE AFFINITY DR 5330 IS EFFECTIVE 01/01/01. AFFINITY DR 5330L AND 5330R WERE EFFECTIVE 08/01/00.	53	A	1833(t)		D			N
C1137	SEPTAL DEFECT IMPLANT SYSTEM, CARDIOSEAL SEPTAL OCCLUSION SYSTEM, CARDIOSEAL OCCLUDER DELIVERY CATHETER, AGA MEDICAL AMPLATZER PFO OCCLUDER	53	A	1833(T)		D			N
C1143	PACEMAKER, DUAL CHAMBER, ADDVENT 2060BL, PARAGON III (MODELS 2314L, 2315 M/S)	53	A	1833(T)		D			N
C1144	PACEMAKER, SINGLE CHAMBER, RATE-RESPONSIVE, AFFINITY SR 5130, AFFINITY SR 5130L, AFFINITY SR 5130R, INTEGRITY SR 5142, INTEGRITY U SR 5136. NOTE: ONLY THE AFFINITY SR 5130 IS EFFECTIVE 01/01/01. AFFINITY SR 5130L, AFFINITY SR 5130R, AND INTEGRITY SR 5142 WERE EFFECTIVE 08/01/00.	53	A	1833(T)		D			N
C1145	VASCULAR CLOSURE DEVICE, ANGIO-SEAL 6 FRENCH VASCULAR CLOSURE DEVICE (MODEL 610091), ANGIO-SEAL 8 FRENCH VASCULAR CLOSURE DEVICE (610089, 610097), ANGIO-SEAL 6 FR EV VASCULAR CLOSURE DEVICE, ANGIO-SEAL 8 FR EV VASCULAR CLOSURE DEVICE (MODELS 610099, 610101). NOTE: MODEL 610097 IS EFFECTIVE 01/01/01. MODELS 610091 AND 610089 WERE EFFECTIVE 08/01/00	53	A	1833(T)		D			N
C1146	ENDOTRACHEAL TUBE, VETT TRACHEOBRONCHIAL TUBE	53	A	1833(T)		D			N
C1147	LEAD, PACEMAKER, AV PLUS DX 1368/52, AV PLUS DX 1368/58, AV PLUS DX 1368/65 NOTE: THE AV PLUS DX 1368/65 IS EFFECTIVE 01/01/01. MODELS 1368/52 AND 1368/58 WERE EFFECTIVE 08/01/00.	53	A	1833(T)		D			N
C1148	DEFIBRILLATOR, SINGLE CHAMBER, IMPLANTABLE, CONTOUR MD V-175, CONTOUR MD V-175A, CONTOUR MD V-175AC, CONTOUR MD V-175B, CONTOUR MD V-175C, CONTOUR MD V-175D, CONTOUR II (MODELS V-185AC, V-185B, V-185C)	53	A	1833(T)		D			N
C1149	PACEMAKER, DUAL CHAMBER, NON-RATE RESPONSIVE, ENTITY DC 5226R, ENTITY DC 5226 NOTE: MODEL 5226 IS EFFECTIVE 01/01/01. MODEL 5226R WAS EFFECTIVE 08/01/00.	53	A	1833(T)		D			N
C1151	LEAD, PACEMAKER, PASSIVE PLUS DX 1343K/46, PASSIVE PLUS DX 1343K/52, PASSIVE PLUS DX 1345K/52, PASSIVE PLUS DX 1345K/58, PASSIVE PLUS DX 1336T/52, PASSIVE PLUS DX 1336T/58, PASSIVE PLUS DX 1342T/46, PASSIVE PLUS DX 1342T/52, PASSIVE PLUS DX 1346T/52, PASSIVE PLUS DX 1346T/58, PASSIVE PLUS TIN (MODEL 1242T)	53	A	1833(T)		D			N
C1152	ACCESS SYSTEM, DIALYSIS, LIFESITE ACCESS SYSTEM	53	A	1833(T)		D			N
C1153	PACEMAKER, SINGLE CHAMBER, REGENCY SC+ 2402L	53	A	1833(T)		D			N
C1154	LEAD, DEFIBRILLATOR, SPL SP01, SP02, SPL SP04, 6721L, 6721M, 6721S, 6939 OVAL PATCH LEAD, CAPSURE 4965, DP-3238, ENDOTAK DSP, TRANSVENE 6933, TRANSVENE 6937	53	A	1833(T)		D			N
C1155	REPLIFORM TISSUE REGENERATION MATRIX, PER 8 SQUARE CENTIMETERS	53	A	1833(T)		D			N

HCPCS	Long Description	PII	MPI	Statute	X-Ref	Coverage	ASC Pay Grp	ASC Pay Grp Eff Date	Action Code
C1156	PACEMAKER, SINGLE CHAMBER, AFFINITY SR 5131M/S, TEMPO VR 1102, TRILOGY SR+ 2260L, TRILOGY SR+ 2264L, SOLUS II (MODELS 2006L, 2007 M/S)	53	A	1833(T)		D			N
C1157	PACEMAKER, DUAL CHAMBER, TRILOGY DC+2318L, SYNCHRONY III (MODELS 2028L, 2029 M/S)	53	A	1833(T)		D			N
C1158	LEAD, DEFIBRILLATOR, TVL SV01, TVL SV02, TVL SV04	53	A	1833(T)		D			N
C1159	LEAD, DEFIBRILLATOR, TVL RV02, TVL RV06, TVL RV07	53	A	1833(T)		D			N
C1160	LEAD, DEFIBRILLATOR, TVL-ADX 1559/65	53	A	1833(T)		D			N
C1161	LEAD, PACEMAKER, TENDRIL DX 1388K/46, TENDRIL DX 1388K/52, TENDRIL DX 1388K/58, TENDRIL DX 1388T/46, TENDRIL DX 1388T/52, TENDRIL DX 1388T/58, TENDRIL DX 1388T/85, TENDRIL DX 1388T/100, TENDRIL DX 1388TC/46, TENDRIL DX 1388TC/52, TENDRIL DX 1388T/58	53	A	1833(T)		D			N
C1162	PACEMAKER, DUAL-CHAMBER, AFFINITY DR 5331 M/S, TEMPO DR 2102, TRILOGY DR+ 2360L, TRILOGY DR+ 2364L	53	A	1833(T)		D			N
C1163	LEAD, PACEMAKER, TENDRIL SDX 1488T/46, TENDRIL SDX 1488T/52, TENDRIL SDX 1488T/58, TENDRIL SDX 1488TC/46, TENDRIL SDX 1488TC/52, TENDRIL SDX 1488TC/58	53	A	1833(T)		D			N
C1164	BRACHYTHERAPY SEED, I-125 SEED	53	A	1833(T)		D			N
C1166	INJECTION, CYTARABINE LIPOSOME, PER 10 MG	53	A	1833(T)		D			D
C1167	INJECTION, EPIRUBICIN HYDROCHLORIDE, 2 MG	53	A	1833(T)		D			D
C1170	BIOPSY DEVICE, BREAST, ABBI DEVICE	53	A	1833(T)		D			N
C1171	SITE MARKER DEVICE, DISPOSABLE, AUTO SUTURE SITE MARKER DEVICE	53	A	1833(T)		D			N
C1172	BALLOON, TISSUE DISSECTOR, SPACEMAKER TISSUE DISSECTION BALLOON, SPACEMAKER 1000CC HERNIA BALLOON DISSECTOR NOTE: THE HERNIA BALLOON DISSECTOR IS EFFECTIVE 01/01/01. THE SPACEMAKER TISSUE DISSECTION BALLOON IS EFFECTIVE 08/01/00	53	A	1833(T)		D			N
C1173	STENT, CORONARY, S540 OVER-THE-WIRE CORONARY STENT SYSTEM, S670 WITH DISCRETE TECHNOLOGY OVER-THE-WIRE CORONARY STENT SYSTEM, S670 WITH DISCRETE TECHNOLOGY RAPID EXCHANGE CORONARY STENT SYSTEM	53	A	1833(T)		D			N
C1174	NEEDLE, BRACHYTHERAPY, BARD BRACHYSTAR BRACHYTHERAPY NEEDLE	53	A	1833(T)		D			N
C1175	BIOPSY DEVICE, MIBB DEVICE	53	A	1833(t)		D			N
C1176	BIOPSY DEVICE, MAMMOTOME HH HAND-HELD PROBE WITH SMARTVAC VACUUM SYSTEM	53	A	1833(t)		D			N
C1177	BIOPSY DEVICE, 11-GAUGE MAMMOTOME PROBE WITH VACUUM CANNISTER	53	A	1833(t)		D			N
C1178	INJECTION, BUSULFAN, PER 6 MG	51	A	1833(T)		D			T
C1179	BIOPSY DEVICE, 14-GAUGE MAMMOTOME PROBE WITH VACUUM CANNISTER	53	A	1833(t)		D			N
C1180	PACEMAKER, SINGLE CHAMBER, VIGOR SR	53	A	1833(t)		D			N
C1181	PACEMAKER, SINGLE CHAMBER, MERIDIAN SSI	53	A	1833(t)		D			N
C1182	PACEMAKER, SINGLE CHAMBER, PULSAR SSI	53	A	1833(t)		D			N

HCPCS	Long Description	PH	MPI	Statute	X-Ref1	Coverage	ASC Pay Grp	ASC Pay Grp Eff Date	Action Code
C1183	PACEMAKER, SINGLE CHAMBER, JADE II S, SIGMA 300 S, JADE 3/JADE 3S (MODEL 340)	53	A	1833(t)		D			N
C1184	PACEMAKER, SINGLE CHAMBER, SIGMA 200 S, SIGMA 100 S	53	A	1833(t)		D			N
C1188	SUPPLY OF RADIOPHARMACEUTICAL THERAPEUTIC IMAGING AGENT, SODIUM IODIDE I-131, CAPSULE, PER INITIAL 1-5 MCI	53	A	1833(T)		D			N
C1200	SUPPLY OF RADIOPHARMACEUTICAL DIAGNOSTIC IMAGING AGENT, TECHNETIUM TC 99M SODIUM GLUCOHEPTONATE, PER VIAL	53	A	1833(T)		D			N
C1201	SUPPLY OF RADIOPHARMACEUTICAL DIAGNOSTIC IMAGING AGENT, TECHNETIUM TC 99M SUCCIMER, PER VIAL	53	A	1833(T)		D			N
C1202	SUPPLY OF RADIOPHARMACEUTICAL DIAGNOSTIC IMAGING AGENT, TECHNETIUM TC 99M SULFUR COLLOID, PER DOSE	53	A	1833(T)		D			N
C1203	INJECTION, VISUDYNE (VERTEPORFIN)	53	A	1833(T)		D			N
C1205	SUPPLY OF RADIOPHARMACEUTICAL DIAGNOSTIC IMAGING AGENT, TECHNETIUM TC 99M DISOFENIN, PER VIAL	53	A	1833(T)		D			N
C1207	OCTREOTIDE ACETATE, 1 MG	53	A	1833(T)		D			D
C1300	HYPERBARIC OXYGEN UNDER PRESSURE, FULL BODY CHAMBER, PER 30 MINUTE INTERVAL	53	A	1833(T)		D			T
C1302	LEAD, DEFIBRILLATOR, TVL SQ01	53	A	1833(T)		D			N
C1303	LEAD, DEFIBRILLATOR, CAPSURE FIX 6940, CAPSURE FIX 4068-110	53	A	1833(t)		D			N
C1304	CATHETER, IMAGING, SONICATH ULTRA MODEL 37-416 ULTRASOUND IMAGING CATHETER, SONICATH ULTRA MODEL 37-418 ULTRASOUND IMAGING CATHETER	53	A	1833(T)		D			N
C1305	APLIGRAF, PER 44 SQUARE CENTIMETERS	53	A	1833(T)		D			T
C1306	LEAD, NEUROSTIMULATOR, CYBERONICS NEUROCYBERNETIC PROSTHESIS LEAD, OCTAD LEAD 3898-33/389861, ON-POINT MODEL 3987, PISCES-QUAD PLUS MODEL 3888, RESUME TL MODEL 3986, PISCES-QUAD MODEL 3487A, RESUME II MODEL 3587A, SYMMIX LEAD 3982	53	A	1833(T)		D			N
C1311	PACEMAKER, DUAL CHAMBER, TRILOGY DR+/DAO	53	A	1833(T)		D			N
C1312	STENT, CORONARY, MAGIC WALLSTENT MINI CORONARY SELF EXPANDING STENT WITH DELIVERY SYSTEM	53	A	1833(T)		D			N
C1313	STENT, CORONARY, MAGIC WALLSTENT MEDIUM CORONARY SELF EXPANDING STENT WITH DELIVERY SYSTEM, RADIUS 31MM SELF EXPANDING STNET WITH OVER THE WIRE DELIVERY SYSTEM	53	A	1833(T)		D			N
C1314	STENT, CORONARY, MAGIC WALLSTENT LONG CORONARY SELF EXPANDING STENT WITH DELIVERY SYSTEM	53	A	1833(T)		D			N
C1315	PACEMAKER, DUAL CHAMBER, VIGOR DR, MERIDIAN DR, VIGOR DDD, VISTA DDD	53	A	1833(T)		D			N
C1316	PACEMAKER, DUAL CHAMBER, MERIDIAN DDD	53	A	1833(T)		D			N
C1317	PACEMAKER, SINGLE CHAMBER, DISCOVERY SR	53	A	1833(T)		D			N
C1318	PACEMAKER, SINGLE CHAMBER, MERIDIAN SR	53	A	1833(T)		D			N

HCPCS	Long Description	PTI	MPI	Statute	X-Ref	Coverage	ASC Pay Grp	ASC Pay Grp Eff Date	Action Code
C1319	STENT, ENTERAL, WALLSTENT ENTERAL ENDOPROSTHESIS AND UNISTEP DELIVERY SYSTEM (60MM IN LENGTH), ENTERAL WALLSTENT ENDOPROSTHESIS AND UNISTEP PLUS DELIVERY SYSTEM/SINGLE-USE COLONIC AND DUODENAL ENDOPROSTHESIS WITH UNISTEP PLUS DELIVERY SYSTEM (60MM IN LENGTH), ESOPHAGEAL Z METAL EXPANDABLE STENT WITH DUA ANTI-REFLUX VALVE, ESOPHAGEAL Z METAL EXPANDABLE STENT WITH UNCOATED FLANGES, ULTRAFLEX ESOPHAGEAL STENT SYSTEM, WALLSTENT ESOPHAGEAL PROSTHESIS (DOUBLE), WALLSTENT ESOPHAGEAL PROSTHESIS WITH DELIVERY SYSTEM, WILSON-COOK ESOPHAGEAL Z METAL EXPANDABLE STENT, BARD MEMOTHERM ESOPHAGEAL STENT. NOTE: ONLY THE ENTERAL WALSLTENT ENDOPROSTHESIS AND UNISTEP PLUS DELIVERY SYSTEM IS EFFECTIVE OCTOBER 1, 2000. THE WALLSTENT ENTERAL ENDOPROSTHESIS AND UNISTEP DELIVERY SYSTEM WAS EFFECTIVE AUGUST 1, 2000.	53	A	1833(T)		D			N
C1320	STENT, ILIAC, WALLSTENT ILIAC ENDOPROSTHESIS WITH UNISTEP PLUS DELIVERY SYSTEM, WALLSTENT RP ILIAC ENDOPROSTHESIS WITH UNISTEP PLUS DELIVERY SYSTEM NOTE: ONLY THE WALLSTENT RP ILIAC ENDOPROSTHESIS WITH UNISTEP PLUS DELIVERY SYSTEM IS EFFECTIVE OCTOBER 1, 2000. THE WALLSTENT ILIAC ENDOPROSTHESIS WITH UNISTEP PLUS DELIVERY SYSTEM WAS EFFECTIVE AUGUST 1, 2000.	53	A	1833(T)		D			N
C1321	ELECTRODE, DISPOSABLE, PALATE SOMNOPLASTY COAGULATING ELECTRODE, BASE OF TONGUE SOMNOPLASTY COAGULATING ELECTRODE	53	A	1833(t)		D			N
C1322	ELECTRODE, DISPOSABLE, TURBINATE SOMNOPLASTY COAGULATING ELECTRODE	53	A	1833(t)		D			N
C1323	ELECTRODE, DISPOSABLE, VAPR ELECTRODE, VAPR T THERMAL ELECTRODE	53	A	1833(t)		D			N
C1324	ELECTRODE, DISPOSABLE, LIGASURE DISPOSABLE ELECTRODE	53	A	1833(T)		D			N
C1325	BRACHYTHERAPY SEED, PALLADIUM-103 SEED	53	A	1833(T)		D			N
C1326	CATHETER, THROMBECTOMY, ANGIOJET RHEOLYTIC THROMBECTOMY CATHETER	53	A	1833(T)		D			N
C1328	EXTERNAL TRANSMITTER, NEUROSTIMULATION SYSTEM, ANS RENEW SPINAL CORD STIMULATOR SYSTEM	53	A	1833(T)		D			N
C1329	ELECTRODE, DISPOSABLE, GYNECARE VERSAPOINT RESECTOSCOPIC SYSTEM BIPOLAR ELECTRODE	53	A	1833(t)		D			N
C1333	STENT, BILIARY, PALMAZ CORINTHIAN TRANSHEPATIC BILIARY STENT AND DELIVERY SYSTEM, COOK OASIS ONE ACTION STENT INTRODUCTORY SYSTEM, COOK Z STENT GIANTURCO-ROSCH BILIARY DESIGN, CORDIS PALMAZ XL TRANSHEPATIC BILIARY STENT, LARGE PALMAZ BALLOON EXPANDABLE STENT WITH DELIVERY SYSTEM	53	A	1833(T)		D			N
C1334	STENT, CORONARY, PALMAZ-SCHATZ CROWN STENT, MINI-CROWN STENT, CROSSFLEX LC STENT, COOK GIANTURCO-ROUBIN FLEX-STENT CORONARY STENT	53	A	1833(T)		D			N
C1335	MESH, HERNIA, PROLENE POLYPROPYLENE HERNIA SYSTEM, PROLENE SOFT MESH (POLYPROPYLENE), TRELEX NATURAL MESH	53	A	1833(T)		D			N
C1336	INFUSION PUMP, IMPLANTABLE, NON-PROGRAMMABLE, CONSTANT FLOW IMPLANTABLE PUMP WITH BOLUS SAFETY VALVE MODEL 3000, MODEL 3000-16 (16ML), MODEL 3000-50 (50ML) NOTE: CONSTANT FLOW IMPLANTABLE PUMP MODEL 3000 WAS EFFECTIVE AUGUST 1, 2000. MODELS 3000-16 AND 3000-50 ARE EFFECTIVE OCTOBER 1, 2000	53	A	1833(T)		D			N
C1337	INFUSION PUMP, IMPLANTABLE, NON-PROGRAMMABLE, ISOMED INFUSION PUMP MODEL 8472-20, 8472-35, 8472-60	53	A	1833(t)		D			N
C1348	SUPPLY OF RADIOPHARMACEUTICAL THERAPEUTIC IMAGING AGENT, SODIUM IODIDE I-131, SOLUTION, PER INITIAL 1-6 MCI	53	A	1833(T)		D			N
C1350	BRACHYTHERAPY, PER SOURCE, PROSTASEED I-125	53	A	1833(T)		D			N
C1351	LEAD, PACEMAKER, CAPSUREFIX, SUREFIX, PIROUET +, S+	53	A	1833(T)		D			N
C1352	DEFIBRILLATOR, DUAL CHAMBER, IMPLANTABLE, GEM II DR	53	A	1833(T)		D			N

HCPCS	Long Description	PI	MPI	Statute	X-Refl	Coverage	ASC Pay Grp	ASC Pay Grp Eff Date	Action Code
C1353	NEUROSTIMULATOR, IMPLANTABLE, ITREL II/SOLETRA IMPLANTABLE NEUROSTIMULATOR AND EXTENSION, ITREL III IMPLANTABLE NEUROSTIMULATOR AND EXTENSION, INTERSTIM NEUROSTIMULATOR (IMPLANTABLE) AND EXTENSION, NEUROCONTROL STIM SYSTEM	53	A	1833(T)		D			N
C1354	PACEMAKER, DUAL CHAMBER, KAPPA 400 DR, DIAMOND II 820 DR	53	A	1833(T)		D			N
C1355	PACEMAKER, DUAL CHAMBER, KAPPA 600 DR, VITA DR	53	A	1833(T)		D			N
C1356	DEFIBRILLATOR, SINGLE CHAMBER, IMPLANTABLE, PROFILE MD V-186HV3	53	A	1833(T)		D			N
C1357	DEFIBRILLATOR, SINGLE CHAMBER, IMPLANTABLE, ANGSTROM MD V-190HV3	53	A	1833(T)		D			N
C1358	PACEMAKER, DUAL CHAMBER, NON-RATE RESPONSIVE, AFFINITY DC 5230R, AFFINITY DC 5230 NOTE: MODEL 5230 IS EFFECTIVE 01/01/01. MODEL 5230R WAS EFFECTIVE 08/01/00.	53	A	1833(T)		D			N
C1359	PACEMAKER, DUAL CHAMBER, PULSAR DR, PULSAR MAX DR	53	A	1833(T)		D			N
C1360	OCULAR PHOTODYNAMIC THERAPY	53	A	1833(T)		D			N
C1361	RECORDER, CARDIAC EVENT, IMPLANTABLE, REVEAL, REVEAL PLUS	53	A	1833(T)		D			N
C1362	STENT, BILIARY, RX HERCULINK 14 BILIARY STENT, OTW MEGALINK SDS BILIARY STENT	53	A	1833(T)		D			N
C1363	DEFIBRILLATOR, IMPLANTABLE, DUAL CHAMBER, GEM DR, GEM III DR (MODEL 7275)	53	A	1833(t)		D			N
C1364	DEFIBRILLATOR, DUAL CHAMBER, PHOTON DR V-230HV3	53	A	1833(t)		D			N
C1365	GUIDE WIRE, PERIPHERAL, HI-TORQUE SPARTACORE 14 GUIDE WIRE, HI-TORQUE MEMCORE FIRM 14 GUIDE WIRE, HI-TORQUE STEELCORE 18 GUIDE WIRE, HI-TORQUE STEELCORE 18 LT GUIDE WIRE, HI-TORQUE SUPRA CORE 35 GUIDE WIRE, DOC WIRE, HI-TORQUE EXTRA BALANCE, HI-TORQUE EXTRA SPORT, HI-TORQUE EXTRA SUPPORT, HI-TORQUE FLOPPY II, HI-TORQUE INTERMEDIATE, HI-TORQUE STANDARD, HI-TORQUE TRAVERSE, TAD II GUIDE WIRE SYSTEM (145CM, 200CM, 260CM, 300CM), TAD GUIDE WIRE SYSTEM (145CM), WHOLEY HI-TORQUE MODIFIED J GUIDE WIRE SYSTEM (145CM, 175CM, 260CM, 300CM), WHOLEY HI-TORQUE FLOPPY GUIDE WIRE SYSTEM (145CM, 175CM, 260CM), WHOLEY HI-TORQUE STANDARD GUIDE WIRE SYSTEM (145CM, 300CM), LOC GUIDE WIRE EXTENSION (115CM), HOBBS MEDICAL FLEX-EX GUIDE WIRE (MODELS 3406, 3408, 3410, 3412, 3413). NOTE: ONLY THE HI-TORQUE STEELCORE 18 LT GUIDE WIRE IS EFFECTIVE OCTOBER 1, 2000. THE OTHER GUIDE WIRES	53	A	1833(t)		D			N
C1366	GUIDE WIRE, PERCUTANEOUS TRANSLUMINAL CORONARY ANGIOPLASTY, HI-TORQUE IRON MAN, HI-TORQUE BALANCE MIDDLEWEIGHT, HI-TORQUE ALL STAR, HI-TORQUE BALANCE HEAVYWEIGHT, HI-TORQUE BALANCE TREK	53	A	1833(t)		D			N
C1367	GUIDE WIRE, PERCUTANEOUS TRANSLUMINAL CORONARY ANGIOPLASTY, HI-TORQUE CROSS IT, HI-TORQUE CROSS-IT 100XT, HI-TORQUE CROSS-IT 200XT, HI-TORQUE CROSS-IT 300XT, HI-TORQUE WIGGLE	53	A	1833(t)		D			N
C1368	INFUSION SYSTEM, ON-Q PAIN MANAGEMENT SYSTEM, ON-Q SOAKER PAIN MANAGEMENT SYSTEM, AND PAINBUSTER PAIN MANAGEMENT SYSTEM NOTE: THE ON-Q PAIN MANAGEMENT SYSTEM, ON-Q SOAKER PAIN MANAGEMENT SYSTEM, AND PAINBUSTER PAIN MANAGEMENT SYSTEM ARE EFFECTIVE AUGUST 1, 2000	53	A	1833(t)		D			N
C1369	INTERNAL RECEIVER, NEUROSTIMULATION SYSTEM, ANS RENEW SPINAL CORD STIMULATOR SYSTEM, MEDTRONIC MATTRIX RECEIVER/TRANSMITTER	53	A	1833(t)		D			N
C1370	SINGLE USE DEVICE FOR TREATMENT OF FEMALE STRESS URINARY INCONTINENCE, TENSION-GREE VAGINAL TAPE SINGLE USE DEVICE	53	A	1833(t)		D			N

HCPCS	Long Description	PII	MPI	Statute	X-Refl	Coverage	ASC Pay Grp	ASC Pay Grp Eff Date	Action Code
C1371	STENT, BILIARY, SYMPHONY NITINOL STENT TRANSHEPATIC BILIARY SYSTEM, NIR BILIARY STENT SYSTEM	53	A	1833(t)		D			N
C1372	STENT, BILIARY, SMART CORDIS NITINOL STENT AND DELIVERY SYSTEM, CORDIS SMART .018 NITINOL TRANSHEPATIC BILIARY STENT	53	A	1833(t)		D			N
C1375	STENT, CORONARY, NIR ON RANGER STENT DELIVERY SYSTEM, NIR W/SOX STENT SYSTEM, NIR PRIMO PREMOUNTED STENT SYSTEM	53	A	1833(t)		D			N
C1376	LEAD, NEUROSTIMULATOR, ANS RENEW SPINAL CORD STIMULATION SYSTEM LEAD (WITH OR WITHOUT EXTENSION)	53	A	1833(t)		D			N
C1377	LEAD, NEUROSTIMULATOR, SPECIFY 3988 LEAD	53	A	1833(t)		D			N
C1378	LEAD, NEUROSTIMULATOR, INERSTIM THERAPY 3080 LEAD, INTERSTIM THERAPY 3886 LEAD	53	A	1833(t)		D			N
C1379	LEAD, NEUROSTIMULATOR, PISCES-QUAD COMPACT 3887 LEAD	53	A	1833(t)		D			N
C1420	ANCHOR SYSTEM, STAPLETAC2 BONE ANCHOR SYSTEM WITH DERMIS, STAPLETAC2 BONE ANCHOR SYSTEM WITH DERMIS, BIOSORB FX SYSTEM	53	A	1833(T)		D			N
C1421	ANCHOR SYSTEM, STAPLETAC2 BONE ANCHOR SYSTEM WITHOUT DERMIS	53	A	1833(T)		D			N
C1450	ORTHOSPHERE SPHERICAL INTERPOSITIONAL ARTHROPLASTY	53	A	1833(T)		D			N
C1451	ORTHOSPHERE SPHERICAL INTERPOSITIONAL ARTHROPLASTY KIT	53	A	1833(T)		D			N
C1500	ATHERECTOMY SYSTEM, PERIPHERAL, ROTABLATOR ROTATIONAL ANGIOPLASTY SYSTEM WITH ROTALINK EXCHANGEABLE CATHETER, ADVANCER, AND GUIDE WIRE	53	A	1833(t)		D			N
C1531	STENT, COLORECTAL, BARD MEMOTHERM COLORECTAL STENT MODEL S30R060	53	A	1833(t)		D			N
C1700	NEEDLE, BRACHYTHERAPY, AUTHENTIC MICK TP BRACHYTHERAPY NEEDLE, COOK UROLOGICAL BRACHYTHERAPY NEEDLE	53	A	1833(t)		D			N
C1701	NEEDLE, BRACHYTHERAPY, MEDTEC MT-BT-5201-25 BRACHYTHERAPY NEEDLE, AVID MEDICAL METAL HUB PRE-LOAD STYLE BRACHYTHERAPY SEEDING INSERTION NEEDLE, MICK STYLE BRACHYTHERAPY SEEDING INSERTION NEEDLE	53	A	1833(t)		D			N
C1702	NEEDLE, BRACHYTHERAPY, WWMT BRACHYTHERAPY NEEDLE, NUCLETRON PANCREAS FLEXIBLE BRACHYTHERAPY NEEDLE	53	A	1833(t)		D			N
C1703	NEEDLE, BRACHYTHERAPY, MENTOR PROSTATE BRACHYTHERAPY NEEDLE	53	A	1833(t)		D			N
C1704	NEEDLE, BRACHYTHERAPY, MEDTEC MT-BT-5001-25, MT-BT-5051-25	53	A	1833(t)		D			N
C1705	NEEDLE, BRACHYTHERAPY, BEST FLEXI NEEDLE BRACHYTHERAPY SEED IMPLANTATION (13G, 14G, 15G, 16G, 17G, 18G), BEST INDUSTRIES PROSTATE BRACHYTHERAPY NEEDLE, NYCOMED AMERSHAM MICK APPLICATOR STYLE BRACHYTHERAPY NEEDLE, NYCOMED AMERSHAM BRACHYTHERAPY NEEDLE	53	A	1833(t)		D			N
C1706	NEEDLE, BRACHYTHERAPY, INDIGO PROSTATE SEEDING NEEDLE	53	A	1833(T)		D			N
C1707	NEEDLE, BRACHYTHERAPY, VARISOURCE INTERSTITIAL IMPLANT NEEDLE	53	A	1833(T)		D			N
C1708	NEEDLE, BRACHYTHERAPY, UROMED PROSTATE SEEDING NEEDLE	53	A	1833(T)		D			N
C1709	NEEDLE, BRACHYTHERAPY, REMINGTON MEDICAL BRACHYTHERAPY NEEDLE	53	A	1833(T)		D			N
C1710	NEEDLE, BRACHYTHERAPY, US BIOPSY PROSTATE SEEDING NEEDLE	53	A	1833(T)		D			N

HCPCS	Long Description	PII	MPI	Statute	X-Ref	Coverage	ASC Pay Grp	ASC Pay Grp Eff Date	Action Code
C1711	NEEDLE, BRACHYTHERAPY, MD TECH P.S.S. PROSTATE SEEDING SET (NEEDLE)	53	A	1833(T)		D			N
C1712	NEEDLE, BRACHYTHERAPY, IMAGYN MEDICAL TECHNOLOGIES ISOSTAR PROSTATE BRACHYTHERAPY NEEDLE	53	A	1833(T)		D			N
C1713	ANCHOR/SCREW FOR OPPOSING BONE-TO-BONE OR SOFT TISSUE-TO-BONE (IMPLANTABLE)	53	A	1833(T)		D			N
C1714	CATHETER, TRANSLUMINAL ATHERECTOMY, DIRECTIONAL	53	A	1833(T)		D			N
C1715	BRACHYTHERAPY NEEDLE	53	A	1833(T)		D			N
C1716	BRACHYTHERAPY SOURCE, GOLD 198	53	A	1833(T)		D			C
C1717	BRACHYTHERAPY SEED, HIGH DOSE RATE IRIDIUM 192	53	A	1833(T)		D			D
C1718	BRACHYTHERAPY SOURCE, IODINE 125	53	A	1833(T)		D			C
C1719	BRACHYTHERAPY SOURCE, NON-HIGH DOSE RATE IRIDIUM 192	53	A	1833(T)		D			C
C1720	BRACHYTHERAPY SOURCE, PALLADIUM 103	53	A	1833(T)		D			C
C1721	CARDIOVERTER-DEFIBRILLATOR, DUAL CHAMBER (IMPLANTABLE)	53	A	1833(T)		D			N
C1722	CARDIOVERTER-DEFIBRILLATOR, SINGLE CHAMBER (IMPLANTABLE)	53	A	1833(T)		D			N
C1723	CATHETER, ABLATION, NON-CARDIAC	53	A	1833(T)		D			N
C1724	CATHETER, TRANSLUMINAL ATHERECTOMY, ROTATIONAL	53	A	1833(T)		D			N
C1725	CATHETER, TRANSLUMINAL ANGIOPLASTY, NON-LASER (MAY INCLUDE GUIDANCE, INFUSION/PERFUSION CAPABILITY)	53	A	1833(T)		D			N
C1726	CATHETER, BALLOON DILATATION, NON-VASCULAR	53	A	1833(T)		D			N
C1727	CATHETER, BALLOON TISSUE DISSECTOR, NON-VASCULAR (INSERTABLE)	53	A	1833(T)		D			N
C1728	CATHETER, BRACHYTHERAPY SEED ADMINISTRATION	53	A	1833(T)		D			N
C1729	CATHETER, DRAINAGE	53	A	1833(T)		D			N
C1730	CATHETER, ELECTROPHYSIOLOGY, DIAGNOSTIC, OTHER THAN 3D MAPPING (19 OR FEWER ELECTRODES)	53	A	1833(T)		D			N
C1731	CATHETER, ELECTROPHYSIOLOGY, DIAGNOSTIC, OTHER THAN 3D MAPPING (20 OR MORE ELECTRODES)	53	A	1833(T)		D			N
C1732	CATHETER, ELECTROPHYSIOLOGY, DIAGNOSTIC/ABLATION, 3D OR VECTOR MAPPING	53	A	1833(T)		D			N
C1733	CATHETER, ELECTROPHYSIOLOGY, DIAGNOSTIC/ABLATION, OTHER THAN 3D OR VECTOR MAPPING, OTHER THAN COOL-TIP	53	A	1833(T)		D			N
C1750	CATHETER, HEMODIALYSIS, LONG-TERM	53	A	1833(T)		D			N
C1751	CATHETER, INFUSION, INSERTED PERIPHERALLY, CENTRALLY OR MIDLINE (OTHER THAN HEMODIALYSIS)	53	A	1833(T)		D			N
C1752	CATHETER, HEMODIALYSIS, SHORT-TERM	53	A	1833(T)		D			N

HCPCS	Long Description	PII	MPI	Statute	X-Ref	Coverage	ASC Pay Grp	ASC Pay Grp Eff Date	Action Code
C1753	CATHETER, INTRAVASCULAR ULTRASOUND	53	A	1833(T)		D			N
C1754	CATHETER, INTRADISCAL	53	A	1833(T)		D			N
C1755	CATHETER, INTRASPINAL	53	A	1833(T)		D			N
C1756	CATHETER, PACING, TRANSESOPHAGEAL	53	A	1833(T)		D			N
C1757	CATHETER, THROMBECTOMY/EMBOLECTOMY	53	A	1833(T)		D			N
C1758	CATHETER, URETERAL	53	A	1833(T)		D			N
C1759	CATHETER, INTRACARDIAC ECHOCARDIOGRAPHY	53	A	1833(T)		D			N
C1760	CLOSURE DEVICE, VASCULAR (IMPLANTABLE/INSERTABLE)	53	A	1833(T)		D			N
C1762	CONNECTIVE TISSUE, HUMAN (INCLUDES FASCIA LATA)	53	A	1833(T)		D			N
C1763	CONNECTIVE TISSUE, NON-HUMAN (INCLUDES SYNTHETIC)	53	A	1833(T)		D			N
C1764	EVENT RECORDER, CARDIAC (IMPLANTABLE)	53	A	1833(T)		D			N
C1765	ADHESION BARRIER	53	A	1833(T)		D			N
C1766	INTRODUCER/SHEATH, GUIDING, INTRACARDIAC ELECTROPHYSIOLOGICAL, STEERABLE, OTHER THAN PEEL-AWAY	53	A	1833(T)		D			N
C1767	GENERATOR, NEUROSTIMULATOR (IMPLANTABLE)	53	A	1833(T)		D			N
C1768	GRAFT, VASCULAR	53	A	1833(T)		D			N
C1769	GUIDE WIRE	53	A	1833(T)		D			N
C1770	IMAGING COIL, MAGNETIC RESONANCE (INSERTABLE)	53	A	1833(T)		D			N
C1771	REPAIR DEVICE, URINARY, INCONTINENCE, WITH SLING GRAFT	53	A	1833(T)		D			N
C1772	INFUSION PUMP, PROGRAMMABLE (IMPLANTABLE)	53	A	1833(T)		D			N
C1773	RETRIEVAL DEVICE, INSERTABLE (USED TO RETRIEVE FRACTURED MEDICAL DEVICES)	53	A	1833(T)		D			N
C1774	INJECTION, DARBEPOETIN ALFA (FOR NON ESRD USE), PER 1 MCG	53	A	1833(T)		D			D
C1775	SUPPLY OF RADIOPHARMACEUTICAL DIAGNOSTIC IMAGING AGENT, FLUORODEOXYGLUCOSE F18 (2-DEOXY-2-[18F]FLUORO-D-GLUCOSE), PER DOSE (4-40 MCI/ML)	53	A	1833(T)		D			T
C1776	JOINT DEVICE (IMPLANTABLE)	53	A	1833(T)		D			N
C1777	LEAD, CARDIOVERTER-DEFIBRILLATOR, ENDOCARDIAL SINGLE COIL (IMPLANTABLE)	53	A	1833(T)		D			N
C1778	LEAD, NEUROSTIMULATOR (IMPLANTABLE)	53	A	1833(T)		D			N
C1779	LEAD, PACEMAKER, TRANSVENOUS VDD SINGLE PASS	53	A	1833(T)		D			N
C1780	LENS, INTRAOCULAR (NEW TECHNOLOGY)	53	A	1833(T)		D			N
C1781	MESH (IMPLANTABLE)	53	A	1833(T)		D			N
C1782	MORCELLATOR	53	A	1833(T)		D			N

HCPCS	Long Description	PI1	MPI	Statute	X-Refl	Coverage	ASC Pay Grp	ASC Pay Grp Eff Date	Action Code
C1783	OCULAR IMPLANT, AQUEOUS DRAINAGE ASSIST DEVICE	53	A	1833(T)		D			N
C1784	OCULAR DEVICE, INTRAOPERATIVE, DETACHED RETINA	53	A	1833(T)		D			N
C1785	PACEMAKER, DUAL CHAMBER, RATE-RESPONSIVE (IMPLANTABLE)	53	A	1833(T)		D			N
C1786	PACEMAKER, SINGLE CHAMBER, RATE-RESPONSIVE (IMPLANTABLE)	53	A	1833(T)		D			N
C1787	PATIENT PROGRAMMER, NEUROSTIMULATOR	53	A	1833(T)		D			N
C1788	PORT, INDWELLING (IMPLANTABLE)	53	A	1833(T)		D			N
C1789	PROSTHESIS, BREAST (IMPLANTABLE)	53	A	1833(T)		D			N
C1790	BRACHYTHERAPY SEED, NUCLETRON IRIDIUM 192 HDR, MDS NORDION THERASPHERE (YTTRIUM-90) BRACHYTHERAPY SEED, MDS NORDION GAMMA MED IRIDIUM-192 HDR BRACHYTHERAPY SEED	53	A	1833(T)		D			N
C1791	BRACHYTHERAPY SEED, NYCOMED AMERSHAM I-125 (ONCOSEED, RAPID STRAND)	53	A	1833(T)		D			N
C1792	BRACHYTHERAPY SEED, UROMED SYMMETRA I-125	53	A	1833(T)		D			N
C1793	BRACHYTHERAPY SEED, BARD INTERSOURCE-103 PALLADIUM SEED 1031L, 1031C, INTERNATIONAL BRACHYTHERAPY INTERSOURCE-103 (PALLADIUM 103)	53	A	1833(T)		D			N
C1794	BRACHYTHERAPY SEED, BARD ISOSEED 103 PALLADIUM SEED PD3S111L, PD3S111P	53	A	1833(T)		D			N
C1795	BRACHYTHERAPY SEED, BARD BRACHYSOURCE-125 IODINE SEED 1251L, 1251C, INTERNATIONAL BRACHYTHERAPY INTERSOURCE-125	53	A	1833(t)		D			N
C1796	BRACHYTHERAPY SEED, SOURCE TECH MEDICAL I-125 SEED MODEL STM 1251	53	A	1833(T)		D			N
C1797	BRACHYTHERAPY SEED, DRAXIMAGE I-125 SEED MODEL LS-1	53	A	1833(T)		D			N
C1798	BRACHYTHERAPY SEED, SYNCOR I-125 PHARMASEED MODEL BT-125-1	53	A	1833(T)		D			N
C1799	BRACHYTHERAPY SEED, I-PLANT IODINE 125 MODEL 3500	53	A	1833(T)		D			N
C1800	BRACHYTHERAPY SEED, MENTOR PDGOLD PD-103	53	A	1833(t)		D			N
C1801	BRACHYTHERAPY SEED, MENTOR IOGOLD I-125	53	A	1833(t)		D			N
C1802	BRACHYTHERAPY SEED, BEST IRIDIUM 192, BEST DUMMY RIBBON BRACHYTHERAPY SEED	53	A	1833(t)		D			N
C1802	(MODEL 3 DR, 4 DR SERIES)								
C1803	BRACHYTHERAPY SEED, BEST INDUSTRIES IODINE 125	53	A	1833(t)		D			N
C1804	BRACHYTHERAPY SEED, BEST INDUSTRIES PALLADIUM 103	53	A	1833(t)		D			N
C1805	BRACHYTHERAPY SEED, IMAGYN ISOSTAR IODINE-125 INTERSTITIAL BRACHYTHERAPY SEED	53	A	1833(t)		D			N
C1806	BRACHYTHERAPY SEED, BEST INDUSTRIES GOLD 198	53	A	1833(t)		D			N
C1810	CATHETER, BALLOON DILATATION, D114S OVER-THE-WIRE BALLOON DILATATION CATHETER	53	A	1833(t)		D			N

HCPCS	Long Description	PII	MPI	Statute	X-Refl	Coverage	ASC Pay Grp	ASC Pay Grp Eff Date	Action Code
C1811	ANCHOR, SURGICAL DYNAMICS ANCHORSEW, SURGICAL DYNAMICS S.D. SORB EZ TAC, 'SURGICAL DYNAMICS S.D. SORB SUTURE ANCHOR 2.0MM, SURGICAL DYNAMICS S.D. SORB 'SUTURE ANCHOR 3.0MM, BIOMET BONE MULCH SCREW, BIOMET WASHERLOC SCREW AND WASHERLOC WASHER, WRIGHT MEDICAL TECHNOLOGY HAMMERTOE IMPLANT (SWANSON TYPE) WEIL DESIGN, WRIGHT MEDICAL TECHNOLOGY SWANSON TITANIUM GREAT TOE IMPLANT, WRIGHT MEDICAL TECHNOLOGY STA - PEG (SUBTALAR ARTHROSIS IMPLANT - SMITH DESIGN), WRIGHT MEDICAL TECHNOLOGY SPIN SNAP-OFF SCREW, WRIGHT MEDICAL TECHNOLOGY BOLD CANNULATED TITANIUM COMPRESSION SCREW, WRIGHT MEDICAL 'TECHNOLOGY I.C.O.S. IDEAL COMPRESSION SCREW, WRIGHT MEDICAL TECHNOLOGY SWANSON FINGER JOINT IMPLANT WITH GROMMETS, WRIGHT MEDICAL TECHNOLOGY SWANSON BASAL 'THUMB IMPLANT, WRIGHT MEDICAL TECHNOLOGY SWANSON TITANIUM CARPAL SCAPHOID 'IMPLANT, WRIGHT MEDICAL TECHNOLOGY SWANSON TRAPEZIUM IMPLANT, BIOMET BECTON COLLES' FRACTURE PLATE, BIOMET REPICCI II UNICONDYLAR KNEE SYTEM, WRIGHT MEDICAL TECHNOLOGY OSTEOSET BONE GRAFT SUBSTITUTE (5CC, 10CC, 20CC, 50CC), WRIGHT MEDICAL	53	A	1833(t)		D			N
C1812	ANCHOR, OBL 2.0MM MINI TAC ACHOR, OBL 2.8MM HS ANCHOR, OBL 2.8MM S ANCHOR, OBL '3.5MM TI ANCHOR, OBL RC5 ANCHOR, OBL PRC5 ANCHOR, ARTHREX ANTERIOR CRUCIATE LIGAMENT (ACL) AVULSION LAG SCREW WITH SHEATH, ARTHREX CHRONDRAL DART, ARTHREX 'BIO-ABSORBABLE CORKSCREW, ARTHREX BIO-FASTAK SUTURE ANCHOR, ARTHREX HEADED BIO-ABSORBABLE CORKSCREW, ARTHREX BIO-INTERFERENCE SCREW, ARTHREX CANNULATED INTERFERENCE SCREW, ARTHREX SUTURE ANCHOR SCREW, ARTHREX FASTAK SUTURE ANCHOR, ARTHREX PARACHUTE CORKSCREW ANCHOR, ARTHREX TISSUETAK, BIONX BANKART TACK PLLA 'IMPLANT, BIONX CANNULATED SMARTSCREW PLLA IMPLANT, BIONX CONTOUR LABRAL NAIL PLLA IMPLANT, BIONX SMARTNAIL PLLA IMPLANT, BIONX SMARTSCREW PLLA IMPLANT, BIONX SMARTPIN PLLA AND PGA IMPLANT, BIONX WEDGE PLA IMPLANT, BIONX BIOCUFF PLA 'IMPLANT, BIONX MENISCUS ARROW PLA IMPLANT, BIONX SMARTSCREW ACL INTERFERENCE SCREW PLA IMPLANT, DEPUY NEUFLEX PIP FINGER, MEDTRONIC XOMED EPIDISC OTOLOGIC LAMINA (MODEL 14-17000)	53	A	1833(T)		D			N
C1813	PROSTHESIS, PENILE, INFLATABLE	53	A	1833(T)		D			N
C1814	RETINAL TAMPONADE DEVICE, SILICONE OIL	53	A	1833t		D			A
C1815	PROSTHESIS, URINARY SPHINCTER (IMPLANTABLE)	53	A	1833(T)		D			N
C1816	RECEIVER AND/OR TRANSMITTER, NEUROSTIMULATOR (IMPLANTABLE)	53	A	1833(T)		D			N
C1817	SEPTAL DEFECT IMPLANT SYSTEM, INTRACARDIAC	53	A	1833(T)		D			N
C1818	INTEGRATED KERATOPROSTHESIS	53	A	1833T		D			A
C1850	REPLIFORM TISSUE REGENERATION MATRIX, PER 14 OR 21 SQUARE CENTIMETERS	53	A	1833(t)		D			N
C1851	REPLIFORM TISSUE REGENERATION MATRIX, PER 24 OR 28 SQUARE CENTIMETERS	53	A	1833(t)		D			N
C1852	TRANSCYTE, PER 247 SQUARE CENTIMETERS	53	A	1833(t)		D			N
C1853	SUSPEND TUTOPLAST PROCESSED FASCIA LATA, PER 8 OR 14 SQUARE CENTIMETERS	53	A	1833(T)		D			N
C1854	SUSPEND TUTOPLAST PROCESSED FASCIA LATA, PER 24 OR 28 SQUARE CENTIMETERS	53	A	1833(t)		D			N
C1855	SUSPEND TUTOPLAST PROCESSED FASCIA LATA, PER 36 SQUARE CENTIMETERS	53	A	1833(t)		D			N
C1856	SUSPEND TUTOPLAST PROCESSED FASCIA LATA, PER 48 SQUARE CENTIMETERS	53	A	1833(t)		D			N
C1857	SUSPEND TUTOPLAST PROCESSED FASCIA LATA, PER 84 SQUARE CENTIMETERS	53	A	1833(t)		D			N
C1858	DURADERM ACELLULAR ALLOGRAFT, PER 8 OR 14 SQUARE CENTIMETERS	53	A	1833(t)		D			N

HCPCS	Long Description	PII	MPI	Statute	X-Refl	Coverage	ASC Pay Grp	ASC Pay Grp Eff Date	Action Code
C1859	DURADERM ACELLULAR ALLOGRAFT, PER 21, 24, OR 28 SQUARE CENTIMETERS	53	A	1833(t)		D			N
C1860	DURADERM ACELLULAR ALLOGRAFT, PER 48 SQUARE CENTIMETERS	53	A	1833(t)		D			N
C1861	DURADERM ACELLULAR ALLOGRAFT, PER 36 SQUARE CENTIMETERS	53	A	1833(t)		D			N
C1862	DURADERM ACELLULAR ALLOGRAFT, PER 72 SQUARE CENTIMETERS	53	A	1833(t)		D			N
C1863	DURADERM ACELLULAR ALLOGRAFT, PER 84 SQUARE CENTIMETERS	53	A	1833(t)		D			N
C1864	BARD SPERMA TEX MESH, PER 13.44 SQUARE CENTIMETERS	53	A	1833(t)		D			N
C1865	BARD FASLATA ALLOGRAFT TISSUE, PER 8 OR 14 SQUARE CENTIMETERS	53	A	1833(t)		D			N
C1866	BARD FASLATA ALLOGRAFT TISSUE, PER 24 OR 28 SQUARE CENTIMETERS	53	A	1833(T)		D			N
C1867	BARD FASLATA ALLOGRAFT TISSUE, PER 36 OR 48 SQUARE CENTIMETERS	53	A	1833(t)		D			N
C1868	BARD FASLATA ALLOGRAFT TISSUE, PER 96 SQUARE CENTIMETERS	53	A	1833(t)		D			N
C1869	GORE THYROPLASTY DEVICE, PER 8, 12, 30, OR 37.5 SQUARE CENTIMETERS (0.6MM)	53	A	1833(t)		D			N
C1870	DERMMATRIX SURGICAL MESH, PER 16 SQUARE CENTIMETERS	53	A	1833(T)		D			N
C1871	DERMMATRIX SURGICAL MESH, PER 32 OR 64 SQUARE CENTIMETERS	53	A	1833(T)		D			N
C1872	DERMAGRAFT, PER 37.5 SQUARE CENTIMETERS	53	A	1833(T)		D			N
C1873	BARD 3DMAX MESH, MEDIUM OR LARGE SIZE	53	A	1833(T)		D			N
C1874	STENT, COATED/COVERED, WITH DELIVERY SYSTEM	53	A	1833(T)		D			N
C1875	STENT, COATED/COVERED, WITHOUT DELIVERY SYSTEM	53	A	1833(T)		D			N
C1876	STENT, NON-COATED/NON-COVERED, WITH DELIVERY SYSTEM	53	A	1833(T)		D			N
C1877	STENT, NON-COATED/NON-COVERED, WITHOUT DELIVERY SYSTEM	53	A	1833(T)		D			N
C1878	MATERIAL FOR VOCAL CORD MEDIALIZATION, SYNTHETIC (IMPLANTABLE)	53	A	1833(T)		D			N
C1879	TISSUE MARKER (IMPLANTABLE)	53	A	1833(T)		D			N
C1880	VENA CAVA FILTER	53	A	1833(T)		D			N
C1881	DIALYSIS ACCESS SYSTEM (IMPLANTABLE)	53	A	1833(T)		D			N
C1882	CARDIOVERTER-DEFIBRILLATOR, OTHER THAN SINGLE OR DUAL CHAMBER (IMPLANTABLE)	53	A	1833(T)		D			N
C1883	ADAPTOR/EXTENSION, PACING LEAD OR NEUROSTIMULATOR LEAD (IMPLANTABLE)	53	A	1833(T)		D			N
C1884	EMBOLIZATION PROTECTIVE SYSTEM	53	A	1833T		D			A
C1885	CATHETER, TRANSLUMINAL ANGIOPLASTY, LASER	53	A	1833(T)		D			N
C1887	CATHETER, GUIDING (MAY INCLUDE INFUSION/PERFUSION CAPABILITY)	53	A	1833(T)		D			N

HCPCS	Long Description	PII	MPI	Statute	X-Ref	Coverage	ASC Pay Grp	ASC Pay Grp Eff Date	Action Code
C1888	CATHETER, ABLATION, NON-CARDIAC, ENDOVASCULAR (IMPLANTABLE)	53	A	1833(T)		D			N
C1891	INFUSION PUMP, NON-PROGRAMMABLE, PERMANENT (IMPLANTABLE)	53	A	1833(T)		D			N
C1892	INTRODUCER/SHEATH, GUIDING, INTRACARDIAC ELECTROPHYSIOLOGICAL, FIXED-CURVE, PEEL-AWAY	53	A	1833(T)		D			N
C1893	INTRODUCER/SHEATH, GUIDING, INTRACARDIAC ELECTROPHYSIOLOGICAL, FIXED-CURVE, OTHER THAN PEEL-AWAY	53	A	1833(T)		D			N
C1894	INTRODUCER/SHEATH, OTHE THAN GUIDING, INTRACARDIAC ELECTROPHYSIOLOGICAL, NON-LASER	53	A	1833(T)		D			N
C1895	LEAD, CARDIOVERTER-DEFIBRILLATOR, ENDOCARDIAL DUAL COIL (IMPLANTABLE)	53	A	1833(T)		D			N
C1896	LEAD, CARDIOVERTER-DEFIBRILLATOR, OTHER THAN ENDOCARDIAL SINGLE OR DUAL COIL (IMPLANTABLE)	53	A	1833(T)		D			N
C1897	LEAD, NEUROSTIMULATOR TEST KIT (IMPLANTABLE)	53	A	1833(T)		D			N
C1898	LEAD, PACEMAKER, OTHER THAN TRANSVENOUS VDD SINGLE PASS	53	A	1833(T)		D			N
C1899	LEAD, PACEMAKER/CARDIOVERTER-DEFIBRILLATOR COMBINATION (IMPLANTABLE)	53	A	1833(T)		D			N
C1900	LEAD, LEFT VENTRICULAR CORONARY VENOUS SYSTEM	53	A	1833(T)		D			N
C1929	CATHETER, MAVERICK MONORAIL PTCA CATHETER, MAVERICK OVER-THE-WIRE PTCA CATHETER	53	A	1833(T)		D			N
C1930	CATHETER, PERCUTANEOUS TRANSLUMINAL CORONARY ANGIOPLASTY, COYOTE DILATATION CATHETER 20MM/30MM/40MM	53	A	1833(t)		D			N
C1931	CATHETER, TALON BALLOON DILATATION CATHETER	53	A	1833(t)		D			N
C1932	CATHETER, SCIMED REMEDY CORONARY BALLOON DILATATION INFUSION CATHETER (20MM), DISPATCH CORONARY INFUSION CATHETER, ULTRA FUSE 4MM, ULTRA FUSE 8MM, ULTRA FUSE-X, ANGIODYNAMICS PULSE SPRAY INFUSION CATHETER, ANGIODYNAMICS UNIFUSE INFUSION CATHETER, CORDIS COMMODORE TEMPORARY OCCLUSION BALLOON CATHETER, CORDIS RAPIDTRANSIT INFUSION CATHETER, CORDIS REGATTA FLOW GUIDED INFUSION CATHETER, CORDIS PROWLER PLUS MICROCATHETER, CORDIS PROWLER SMALL PROFILE INFUSION MICROCATHETER, CORDIS PLUS MICROCATHETER, CORDIS MASSTRANSIT MAX ID MICROCATHETER, CORDIS TRANSIT MICROCATHETER, MERIT MEDICAL SYSTEMS MISTIQUE INFUSION CATHETER	53	A	1833(t)		D			N
C1933	CATHETER, OPTI-PLAST CENTURION 5.5F PTA CATHETER (SHAFT LENGTH 50 CM TO 120 CM), OPTI-PLAST XL 5.5F PTA CATHETER (SHAFT LENGTH 75 CM TO 120 CM), OPTI-PLAST PTA CATHETER (5.5 FR), TRU TRAC 5FR PERCUTANEOUS TRANSLUMINAL ANGIOPLASTY BALLOON DILATATION CATHETER, OPTIPLAST XT 5 FR PERCUTANEOUS TRANSLUMINAL ANGIOPLASTY CATHETER (VARIOUS SIZES)	53	A	1833(t)		D			N
C1934	CATHETER, ULTRAVERSE 3.5F BALLOON DILATATION CATHETER, INTERVENTIONAL TECHNOLOGIES CUTTING BALLOON	53	A	1833(t)		D			N
C1935	CATHETER, WORKHORSE PTA BALLOON CATHETER	53	A	1833(t)		D			N
C1936	CATHETER, UROMAX ULTRA HIGH PRESSURE BALLOON DILATATION CATHETER WITH HYDROPLUS COATING, URETHRAMAX HIGH PRESSURE URETHRAL BALLOON DILATATION CATHETER, CARSON ZERO TIP BALLOON DILATATION CATHETERS WITH HYDROPLUS COATING, PASSPORT BALLOON ON A WIRE DILATATION CATHETERS WITH HYDROPLUS COATING, TANDEM THIN-SHAFT TRANSURETEROSCOPIC BALLOON DILATATION CATHETER WITH HYDROPLUS COATING, TRILOGY LOW PROFILE BALLOON DILATATION CATHETERS WITH HYDROPLUS COATING, URETERAL DILATORS WITH HYDROPLUS COATING AND PROCEDURAL SHEATH, AMPLATZ RENAL DILATOR SET	53	A	1833(t)		D			N

HCPCS	Long Description	PII	MPI	Statute	X-Refll	Coverage	ASC Pay Grp	ASC Pay Grp Eff Date	Action Code
C1937	CATHETER, SYNERGY BALLOON DILATATION CATHETER, EXPLORER ST (6 FR), EXPLORER 360 JR., EXPLORER 360, EXPLORER ST, SYMMETRY SMALL VESSEL BALLOON DILATATION CATHETER WITH GLIDEX HYDROPHILIC COATING, SYMMETRY STIFF SHAFT SMALL VESSEL BALLOON DILATATION CATHETER WITH GLIDEX HYDROPHILIC COATING, XXL LARGE BALLOON DILATATION CATHETER	53	A	1833(t)		D			N
C1938	CATHETER, BARD UROFORCE BALLOON DILATATION CATHETER, COOK UROLOGICAL URODYNAMIC CATHETER	53	A	1833(t)		D			N
C1939	CATHETER, NINJA PTCA DILATATION CATHETER, RAPTOR PTCA DILATATION CATHETER, NC RAPTOR PTCA DILATATION CATHETER, CHARGER PTCA DILATATION CATHETER, TITAN PTCA DILATATION CATHETER, TITAN MEGA PTCA DILATATION CATHETER NOTE: ONLY THE NC RAPTOR, CHARGER, TITAN, AND TITAN MEGA PTCA DILATATION CATHETERS ARE EFFECTIVE 01/01/01. THE NINJA AND RAPTOR PTCA DILATATION CATHETERS WERE EFFECTIVE 10/01/00	53	A	1833(t)		D			N
C1940	CATHETER, CORDIS POWERFLEX EXTREME PTA BALLOON CATHETER, CORDIS POWERFLEX PLUS PTA BALLOON CATHETER, CORDIS OPTA LP PTA BALLOON CATHETER, CORDIS OPTA 5 PTA BALLOON CATHETER, CORDIS POWERFLEX P3 PTA BALLOON CATHETER	53	A	1833(t)		D			N
C1941	CATHETER, JUPITER PTA BALLOON DILATATION CATHETER, CORDIS OPTA PROPTA DILATATION CATHETER, CORDIS SLALOM PTA DILATATION CATHETER	53	A	1833(t)		D			N
C1942	CATHETER, CORDIS MAXI LD PTA BALLOON CATHETER	53	A	1833(t)		D			N
C1943	CATHETER, RX CROSSSAIL CORONARY DILATATION CATHETER, OTW OPENSAIL CORONARY DILATATION CATHETER	53	A	1833(t)		D			N
C1944	CATHETER, RAPID EXCHANGE SINGLE-USE BILIARY BALLOON DILATATION CATHETER, MAXFORCE SINGLE-USE BILIARY BALLOON DILATATION CATHETER	53	A	1833(T)		D			N
C1945	CATHETER, CORDIS SAVVY PTA DILATATION CATHETER	53	A	1833(T)		D			N
C1946	CATHETER, R1S RAPID EXCHANGE PRE-DILATATION BALLOON CATHETER	53	A	1833(T)		D			N
C1947	CATHETER, GAZELLE BALLOON DILATATION CATHETER	53	A	1833(T)		D			N
C1948	CATHETER, PURSUIT BALLOON ANGIOPLASTY CATHETER, COOK ACCENT BALLOON ANGIOPLASTY CATHETER	53	A	1833(T)		D			N
C1949	CATHETER, ENDOSONICS ORACLE MEGASONICS FIVE-64 F/X PTCA CATHETER	53	A	1833(T)		D			N
C1979	CATHETER, ENDOSONICS VISIONS PV 8.2F INTRAVASCULAR ULTRASOUND IMAGING CATHETER, ENDOSONICS AVANAR F/X INTRAVASCULAR ULTRASOUND IMAGING CATHETER	53	A	1833(T)		D			N
C1980	CATHETER, ATLANTIS SR CORONARY IMAGING CATHETER	53	A	1833(T)		D			N
C1981	CATHETER ,CORONARY ANGIOPLASTY BALLOON, ADANTE, BONNIE, BONNIE 15MM, BONNIE MONORAIL 30MM OR 40MM, BONNIE SLIDING RAIL, BYPASS SPEEDY, CHUBBY, CHUBBY SLIDING RAIL, COYOTE 20MM, COYOTE 9/15/25MM, MAXXUM, NC RANGER, NC RANGER 9MM, RANGER 20MM, LONG RANGER 30MM OR 40MM, NC RANGER 16/18MM, NC RANGER 22/25/30MM, NC BIG RANGER, QUANTUM RANGER, QUANTUM RANGER 1/4 SIZES, QUANTUM RANGER 9/16/18MM, QUANTUM RANGER 22/30MM, QUANTUM RANGER 25MM, RANGER LP 20/30/40, VIVA/LONG VIVA, ACE - 1CM, ACE - 2CM, ACE GRAFT, LONG ACE, PIVOT COBRA (10, 14, 18, 30, 40MM IN LENGTHS) NOTE: ONLY THE BONNIE MONORAIL 30MM OR 40MM, LONG RANGER 30MM OR 40MM, AND RANGER 20MM ARE EFFECTIVE 01/01/01. THE OTHER CATHETERS WERE EFFECTIVE 08/01/00.	53	A	1833(t)		D			N
C2000	CATHETER, ORBITER ST STEERABLE ELECTRODE CATHETER	53	A	1833(t)		D			N
C2001	CATHETER, CONSTELLATION DIAGNOSTIC CATHETER	53	A	1833(t)		D			N
C2002	CATHETER, IRVINE INQUIRY STEERABLE ELECTROPHYSIOLOGY 5F CATHETER, LIVEWIRE STEERABLE ELECTROPHYSIOLOGY CATHETER, LIVEWIRE EP CATHETER, 7 FR DUO-DECAPOLAR (MODEL 401932), MARINR RF MARINR MC	53	A	1833(t)		D			N

HCPCS	Long Description	PTI	MPI	Statute	X-Ref	Coverage	ASC Pay Grp	ASC Pay Grp Eff Date	Action Code
C2003	CATHETER, IRVINE INQUIRY STEERABLE ELECTROPHYSIOLOGY 6F CATHETER	53	A	1833(t)		D			N
C2004	CATHETER, ELECTROPHYSIOLOGY, BIOSENSE WEBSTER DEFLECTABLE TIP ELECTROPHYSIOLOGY CATHETER	53	A	1833(t)		D			N
C2005	CATHETER, ELECTROPHYSIOLOGY, EP DEFLECTABLE TIP CATHETER (HEXAPOLAR SMALL ANATOMY MODELS ONLY)	53	A	1833(t)		D			N
C2006	CATHETER, ELECTROPHYSIOLOGY, EP DEFLECTABLE TIP CATHETER (DECAPOLAR SMALL ANATOMY MODELS ONLY)	53	A	1833(t)		D			N
C2007	CATHETER, ELECTROPHYSIOLOGY, IRVINE LUMA-CATH 6F FIXED CURVE ELECTROPHYSIOLOGY CATHETER, IBI-1000 INQUIRY FIXED CURVE EP CATHETER (5 FR), IBI-1000 INQUIRY FIXED CURVE EP CATHETER (6 FR, BIPOLAR), IBI-1000 INQUIRY FIXED CURVE EP CATHETER (6 FR, DECAPOLAR), IBI-1000 INQUIRY FIXED CURVE EP CATHETER (6 FR, OCTAPOLAR), IBI-1000 INQUIRY FIXED CURVE EP CATHETER (6 FR, QUADRAPOLAR), SANTORO FIXED CURVE CATHETER, ISMUS CATH DEFLECTABLE 20-POLE CATHETER/CRISTA CATH II DEFLECTABLE 20-POLE CATHETER	53	A	1833(t)		D			N
C2008	CATHETER, ELECTROPHYSIOLOGY, IRVINE LUMA-CATH 7F STEERABLE ELECTROPHYSIOLOGY CATHETER MODEL 81910, MODEL 81912, MODEL 81915	53	A	1833(T)		D			N
C2009	CATHETER, ELECTROPHYSIOLOGY, IRVINE LUMA-CATH 7F STEERABLE ELECTROPHYSIOLOGY CATHETER MODEL 81920	53	A	1833(T)		D			N
C2010	CATHETER, DIAGNOSTIC, ELECTROPHYSIOLOGY, RESPONSE FIXED CURVE CATHETER, SUPREME FIXED CURVE CATHETER, TORQR CS, BIOSENSE WEBSTER FIXED CURVE DIAGNOSTIC ELECTROPHYSIOLOGY CATHETER	53	A	1833(t)		D			N
C2011	CATHETER, ELECTROPHYSIOLOGY, DEFLECTABLE TIP CATHETER (QUADRAPOLAR SMALL ANATOMY MODELS ONLY)	53	A	1833(t)		D			N
C2012	CATHETER, ABLATION, BIOSENSE WEBSTER CELSIUS BRAIDED TIP ABLATION CATHETER, BIOSENSE WEBSTER CELSIUS 5MM TEMPERATURE ABLATION CATHETER, BIOSENSE WEBSTER CELSIUS TEMPERATURE SENSING DIAGNOSTIC/ABLATION TIP CATHETER, BIOSENSE WEBSTER CELSIUS LONG REACH ABLATION CATHETER NOTE: ONLY THE CELSIUS LONG REACH ABLAITON CATHETER IS EFFECTIVE 01/01/01. THE OTHER ABLATION CATHETERS WERE EFFECTIVE 10/01/00.	53	A	1833(t)		D			N
C2013	CATHETER, ABLATION, BIOSENSE WEBSTER CELSIUS LARGE DOME ABLATION CATHETER	53	A	1833(t)		D			N
C2014	CATHETER, ABLATION, BIOSENSE WEBSTER CELSIUS II ASYMMETRICAL ABLATION CATHETER	53	A	1833(t)		D			N
C2015	CATHETER, ABLATION, BIOSENSE WEBSTER CELSIUS II SYMMETRICAL ABLATION CATHETER	53	A	1833(t)		D			N
C2016	CATHETER, ABLATION, NAVI-STAR DS DIAGNOSTIC/ABLATION CATHETER, NAVI-STAR THERMO-COOL TEMPERATURE DIAGNOSTIC/ABLATION CATHETER	53	A	1833(t)		D			N
C2017	CATHETER, ABLATION, NAVI-STAR DIAGNOSTIC/ABLATION DEFLECTABLE TIP CATHETER	53	A	1833(t)		D			N
C2018	CATHETER, ABLATION, POLARIS T ABLATION CATHETER, MECA ABLATION CATHETER, STEEROCATH-A, STEEROCATH-T, POLARIS LE (7 FR), POLARIS DX	53	A	1833(t)		D			N
C2019	CATHETER, EP MEDSYSTEMS DEFLECTABLE ELECTROPHYSIOLOGY CATHETER, EP MEDSYSTEMS NON-DEFLECTABLE PLATINUM ELECTROPHYSIOLOGY CATHETER, CARDIMA NAVIPORT DEFLECTABLE TIP GUIDING CATHETER, CARDIMA VENAPORT GUIDING CATHETER	53	A	1833(t)		D			N
C2020	CATHETER, ABLATION, BLAZER II XP, BLAZER II 6F, BLAZER II HIGH TORQUE DISTAL (HTD), BLAZER II (7 FR)	53	A	1833(t)		D			N
C2021	CATHETER, EP MEDSYSTEMS SILVERFLEX ELECTROPHYSIOLOGY CATHETER, NON-DEFLECTABLE	53	A	1833(t)		D			N
C2022	CATHETER, ABLATION, CARDIAC PATHWAYS CHILLI COOLED ABLATION CATHETER MODELS 41422, 41442, 45422, 45442, 43422, 43442	53	A	1833(T)		D			N
C2023	CATHETER, ABLATION, CARDIAC PATHWAYS CHILLI COOLED ABLATION CATHETER, STANDARD CURVE 3005 OR LARGE CURVE 3006	53	A	1833(T)		D			N

HCPCS	Long Description	PI	MPI	Statute	X-Ref	Coverage	ASC Pay Grp	ASC Pay Grp Eff Date	Action Code
C2100	CATHETER, ELECTROPHYSIOLOGY, CARDIAC PATHWAYS CS REFERENCE CATHETER, BOSTON SCIENTIFIC SPECIAL PROCEDURE STEERO DX OCTA, BOSTON SCIENTIFIC MAP PACING CATHETER	53	A	1833(T)		D			N
C2101	CATHETER, ELECTROPHYSIOLOGY, CARDIAC PATHWAYS RV REFERENCE CATHETER, BOSTON SCIENTIFIC EPT-DX STEERABLE	53	A	1833(T)		D			N
C2102	CATHETER, ELECTROPHYSIOLOGY, CARDIAC PATHWAYS 7F RADII CATHETER	53	A	1833(T)		D			N
C2103	CATHETER, ELECTROPHYSIOLOGY, CARDIAC PATHWAYS 7F RADII CATHETER WITH TRACKING, BOSTON SCIENTIFIC VALVE MAPPER STEERODX	53	A	1833(T)		D			N
C2104	CATHETER, ELECTROPHYSIOLOGY, LASSO DEFLECTABLE CIRCULAR TIP MAPPING CATHETER, CARDIMA TRACER OVER-THE-WIRE MAPPING MICROCATHETER, CARDIMA PATHFINDER MICROCATHETER, CARDIMA REVELATION MICROCATHETER	53	A	1833(T)		D			N
C2151	CATHETER, VERIPATH PERIPHERAL GUIDING CATHETER	53	A	1833(t)		D			N
C2152	CATHETER, CORDIS 5F, 6F, 7F, 8F, 9F, 10F VISTA BRITE TIP GUIDING CATHETER, CORDIS 0.056 VISTA BRITE TIP GUIDING CATHETER (5 FR), CORDIS VISTA BRITE TIP IG INTRODUCER GUIDING CATHETER (7 FR), CORDIS VISTA BRITE TIP IG INTRODUCER GUIDING CATHETER (8 FR), CORDIS VISTA BRITE TIP SUPRA-AORTIC GUIDING CATHETER (8 FR), CORDIS VISTA BRITE TIP SUPRA-AORTIC GUIDING CATHETER (9 FR), CORDIS ENVOY LARGE LUMEN GUIDING CATHETER (5 FR), CORDIS ENVOY LARGE LUMEN GUIDING CATHETER (6 FR)	53	A	1833(T)		D			N
C2153	CATHETER, ELECTROPHYSIOLOGY, BARD VIKING FIXED CURVE CATHETER (BIPOLAR, QUADRAPOLAR, AND ASP MODELS ONLY)	53	A	1833(T)		D			N
C2200	CATHETER, ARROW-TREROTOLA PERCUTANEOUS THROMBOLYTIC DEVICE CATHETER CATHETER, VARISOURCE STANDARD CATHETER, NUCLETRON NASOPHARYNGEAL BRACHYTHERAPY CATHETER	53	A	1833(t)		D			N
C2597	CLINICATH PERIPHERALLY INSERTED MIDLINE CATHETER (PICC) DUAL-LUMEN POLYFLOW POLYURETHANE CATHETER 18G (INCLUDES CATHETER AND INTRODUCER), CLINICATH PERIPHERALLY INSERTED CENTRAL CATHETER (PICC) DUAL-LUMEN POLYFLOW POLYURETHANE 16G/18G (INCLUDES CATHETER AND INTRODUCER), CLINICATH PERIPHERALLY INSERTED CENTRAL CATHETER (PICC) SINGLE-LUMEN POLYFLOW POLYURETHANE 16G (INCLUDES CATHETER AND INTRODUCER), BD FIRST MIDCATH CATHETER (3 FR, 4 FR, 5 FR, 20CM/4 'FR, 20CM/5 FR), DUAL LUMEN SILICONE MIDLINE CATHETER, DUAL LUMEN SILICONE MIDLINE CATHETER (5 FR/5FR, 20 CM), BDL SINGLE-LUMEN POLYURETHANE PICC, BDL SINGLE-LUMEN POLYURETHANE MIDLINE CATHETER (CATHETER AND INTRODUCER ONLY), BARD PER-Q-CATH, BARD PER-Q-CATH PLUS, BARD RADPICC, BARD GROSHONG PERIPHERALLY INSERTED CENTRAL CATHETER (PICC), ETHICON ENDO-SURGERY 18G/20G SINGLE LUMEN BIOVUE MIDLINE CATHETER STARTER SET (CATHETER AND INTRODUCER ONLY), ETHICON ENDO-SURGERY 18G DUAL LUMEN BIOVUE MIDLINE CATHETER STARTER SET (CATHETER AND INTRODUCER ONLY)	53	A	1833(t)		D			N
C2598	CATHETER, CLINICATH PERIPHERALLY INSERTED CENTRAL CATHETER (PICC) SINGLE-LUMEN 'POLYFLOW POLYURETHANE CATHETER 18G/20G/24G (CATHETER AND INTRODUCER), CLINICATH 'PERIPHERALLY INSERTED MIDLINE CATHETER (PICC) SINGLE-LUMEN POLYFLOW 'POLYURETHANE CATHETER 20G/24G (CATHETER AND INTRODUCER), BD FIRST PICC 'CATHETER, 5FR DUAL LUMEN SILICONE PICC (CATHETER AND INTRODUCER ONLY), BDL '16G/18G/20G DUAL LUMEN CATH CATHETER (CATHETER AND INTRODUCER ONLY)	53	A	1833(t)		D			N
C2599	CLINICATH PERIPHERALLY INSERTED CENTRAL CATHETER (PICC) SINGLE-LUMEN POLYFLOW POLYURETHANE CATHETER 16G/18G/19G (INCLUDES CATHETER AND INTRODUCER), BD FIRST PICC CATHETER, 1.9 FR, 2.8 FR, 3 FR, 4 FR, 5 FR SINGLE-LUMEN SILICONE PICC (CATHETER AND INTRODUCER ONLY), BOSTON SCIENTIFIC VAXCEL PERIPHERALLY INSERTED CENTRAL CATHETER (PICC), COOK PERIPHERALLY INSERTED CENTRAL VENOUS CATHETER, ETHICON ENDO-SURGERY 18G/20G/24G SINGLE LUMEN BIOVUE PERIPHERALLY INSERTED CENTRAL CATHETER STARTER SET (CATHETER AND INTRODUCER ONLY), ETHICON ENDO-SURGERY 16G/18G DUAL LUMEN BIOVUE PERIPHERALLY INSERTED CENTRAL CATHETER STARTER SET (CATHETER AND INTRODUCER ONLY)	53	A	1833(t)		D			N
C2600	CATHETER, GOLD PROBE SINGLE-USE ELECTROHEMOSTASIS CATHETER	53	A	1833(t)		D			N

HCPCS	Long Description	PTI	MPI	Statute	X-Ref	Coverage	ASC Pay Grp	ASC Pay Grp Eff Date	Action Code
C2601	CATHETER, BARD DUAL LUMEN URETERAL CATHETER, COOK UROLOGICAL URETERAL DILATATION BALLOON, FLEXIMA URETERAL CATHETER, AXXCESS URETERAL CATHETER (6 FR), C-FLEX URETERAL CATHETER, BOSTON SCIENTIFIC DUAL LUMEN URETERAL CATHETER	53	A	1833(t)		D			N
C2602	CATHETER, SPECTRANETICS 1.4/1.7MM VITESSE CONCENTRIC LASER CATHETER, SPECTRANETICS 0.9 MM VITESSE C CONCENTRIC LASER CATHETER (MODEL 110-003)	53	A	1833(t)		D			N
C2603	CATHETER, SPECTRANETICS 2.0MM VITESSE COS CONCENTRIC LASER CATHETER	53	A	1833(t)		D			N
C2604	CATHETER, SPECTRANETICS 2.0MM VITESSE E ECCENTRIC LASER CATHETER	53	A	1833(t)		D			N
C2605	CATHETER, SPECTRANETICS EXTREME LASER CATHETER, SPECTRANETICS EXTREME 0.9MM CORONARY ANGIOPLASTY CATHETER (MODEL 110-001)	53	A	1833(t)		D			N
C2606	CATHETER, ORATEC SPINECATH XL INTRADISCAL CATHETER	53	A	1833(t)		D			N
C2607	CATHETER, ORATEC SPINECATH INTRADISCAL CATHETER	53	A	1833(t)		D			N
C2608	CATHETER, SCIMED 6F WISEGUIDE GUIDE CATHETER, CYBER GUIDE CATHETER, MERIT MEDICAL SYSTEMS TRAX INTERVENTIONAL GUIDE CATHETER (7 FR), MERIT MEDICAL SYSTEMS TRAX CAVERN INTERVENTIONAL GUIDE CATHETER (8 FR), MIGHTY MAX GUIDE CATHETER (7 FR), TRIGUIDE-FLEX GUIDE CATHETER (10 FR)	53	A	1833(T)		D			N
C2609	CATHETER, FLEXIMA BILIARY DRAINAGE CATHETER WITH LOCKING PIGTAIL, FLEXIMA BILIARY DRAINAGE CATHETER WITH TWIST LOC HUB, FLEXIMA BILARY DRAINAGE CATHETERS WITH TEMP TIP	53	A	1833(t)		D			N
C2610	CATHETER, ARROW FLEX TIP PLUS INTRASPINAL CATHETER KIT	53	A	1833(T)		D			N
C2611	CATHETER, MEDTRONIC PS MEDICAL ALGOLINE INTRASPINAL CATHETER SYSTEM/KIT 81102, 81192	53	A	1833(T)		D			N
C2612	CATHETER, MEDTRONIC INDURA INTRASPINAL CATHETER, MYELOTEC VIDEO GUIDED CATHETER, EBI VUECATH STEERABLE SPINAL CATHETER, SYNCHROMED VASCULAR CATHETER (MODELS 8702, 8700A, 8700V)	53	A	1833(T)		D			N
C2614	PROBE, PERCUTANEOUS LUMBAR DISCECTOMY	53	A	1833(T)		D			N
C2615	SEALANT, PULMONARY, LIQUID	53	A	1833(T)		D			N
C2616	BRACHYTHERAPY SOURCE, YTTRIUM-90	53	A	1833(T)		D			C
C2617	STENT, NON-CORONARY, TEMPORARY, WITHOUT DELIVERY SYSTEM	53	A	1833(T)		D			N
C2618	PROBE, CRYOABLATION	53	A	1833(T)		D			N
C2619	PACEMAKER, DUAL CHAMBER, NON RATE-RESPONSIVE (IMPLANTABLE)	53	A	1833(T)		D			N
C2620	PACEMAKER, SINGLE CHAMBER, NON RATE-RESPONSIVE (IMPLANTABE)	53	A	1833(T)		D			N
C2621	PACEMAKER, OTHER THAN SINGLE OR DUAL CHAMBER (IMPLANTABLE)	53	A	1833(T)		D			N
C2622	PROSTHESIS, PENILE, NON-INFLATABLE	53	A	1833(T)		D			N
C2625	STENT, NON-CORONARY, TEMPORARY, WITH DELIVERY SYSTEM	53	A	1833(T)		D			N
C2626	INFUSION PUMP, NON-PROGRAMMABLE, TEMPORARY (IMPLANTABLE)	53	A	1833(T)		D			N
C2627	CATHETER, SUPRAPUBIC/CYSTOSCOPIC	53	A	1833(T)		D			N
C2628	CATHETER, OCCLUSION	53	A	1833(T)		D			N

HCPCS	Long Description	PH	MPI	Statute	X-Reff	Coverage	ASC Pay Grp	ASC Pay Grp Eff Date	Action Code
C2629	INTRODUCER/SHEATH, OTHER THAN GUIDING, INTRACARDIAC ELECTROPHYSIOLOGICAL, LASER	53	A	1833(T)		D			N
C2630	CATHETER, ELECTROPHYSIOLOGY, DIAGNOSTIC/ABLATION, OTHER THAN 3D OR VECTOR MAPPING, COOL-TIP	53	A	1833(T)		D			N
C2631	REPAIR DEVICE, URINARY, INCONTINENCE, WITHOUT SLING GRAFT	53	A	1833(T)		D			N
C2632	BRACHYTHERAPY SOLUTION, IODINE-125, PER MCI	53	A	1833(T)		D			N
C2676	CATHETER, RESPONSE CV CATHETER	53	A	1833(T)		D			N
C2700	DEFIBRILLATOR, SINGLE CHAMBER, IMPLANTABLE, MYCROPHYLAX PLUS	53	A	1833(T)		D			N
C2701	DEFIBRILLATOR, SINGLE CHAMBER, IMPLANTABLE, PHYLAX XM	53	A	1833(T)		D			N
C2702	DEFIBRILLATOR, SINGLE CHAMBER, IMPLANTABLE, VENTAK PRIZM 2 VR 1860	53	A	1833(T)		D			N
C2703	DEFIBRILLATOR, SINGLE CHAMBER, IMPLANTABLE, VENTAK PRIZM VR HE 1857, 1858	53	A	1833(T)		D			N
C2704	DEFIBRILLATOR, SINGLE CHAMBER, IMPLANTABLE, VENTAK MINI IV+ 1793, 1796	53	A	1833(T)		D			N
C2801	DEFIBRILLATOR, DUAL CHAMBER, IMPLANTABLE, ELA MEDICAL DEFENDER IV DR MODEL 612	53	A	1833(t)		D			N
C2802	DEFIBRILLATOR, DUAL CHAMBER, IMPLANTABLE, PHYLAX AV	53	A	1833(t)		D			N
C2803	DEFIBRILLATOR, DUAL CHAMBER, IMPLANTABLE, VENTAK PRIZM DR HE MODELS 1853, 1858, BIOTRONIK TACHOS DR	53	A	1833(T)		D			N
C2804	DEFIBRILLATOR, DUAL CHAMBER, IMPLANTABLE, VENTAK PRIZM 2 DR 1861	53	A	1833(T)		D			N
C2805	DEFIBRILLATOR, DUAL CHAMBER, IMPLANTABLE, JEWEL AF 7250	53	A	1833(T)		D			N
C2806	DEFIBRILLATOR, IMPLANTABLE, GEM VR 7227	53	A	1833(T)		D			N
C2807	DEFIBRILLATOR, IMPLANTABLE, CONTAK CD 1823	53	A	1833(T)		D			N
C2808	DEFIBRILLATOR, IMPLANTABLE, CONTAK TR 1241	53	A	1833(T)		D			N
C3001	LEAD, DEFIBRILLATOR, IMPLANTABLE, KAINOX SL, KAINOX RV	53	A	1833(t)		D			N
C3002	LEAD, DEFIBRILLATOR, IMPLANTABLE, EASYTRAK 4510, 4511, 4512, 4513	53	A	1833(T)		D			N
C3003	LEAD, DEFIBRILLATOR, IMPLANTABLE, ENDOTAK SQ ARRAY XP (MODEL 0085), ENDOTAK SQ ARRAY (MODELS 0048, 0049), ENDOTAK SQ PATCH (MODELS 0047, 0063) ENDOTAK RELIANCE (MODELS 0147, 0148, 0149, S-0127, S-0128, S-0129)	53	A	1833(T)		D			N
C3004	LEAD, DEFIBRILLATOR, IMPLANTABLE, INTERVENE 497-23, 497-24	53	A	1833(T)		D			N
C3400	PROSTHESIS, BREAST, MENTOR SALINE-FILLED CONTOUR PROFILE, MENTOR SILTEX SPECTRUM MAMMARY PROSTHESIS, MENTOR SILTEX GEL-FILLED MAMMARY PROSTHESIS, SMOOTH-SURFACE GEL-FILLED MAMMARY PROSTHESIS, MCGHAN BIODIMENSIONAL ANATOMICAL TISSUE EXPANDER SALINE-FILLED (BIOSPAN TEXTURED, STYLE 133, 133FV, 133MV, 133LV), MENTOR TISSUE EXPANDER, MENTOR CONTOUR PROFILE TISSUE EXPANDER, MENTOR SILTEX BECKER EXPANDER/MAMMARY PROSTHESIS	53	A	1833(t)		D			N
C3401	PROSTHESIS, BREAST, MENTOR SALINE-FILLED SPECTRUM, MCGHAN BIOCURVE ROUND, BIOCELL TEXTURED, SALINE-FILLED MODERATE PROFILE (STYLE 168), MCGHAN BIOCURVE ROUND, SMOOTH SALINE-FILLED MODERATE PROFILE (STYLE 68), MCGHAN BIODIMENSIONAL BIOCURVE SHAPED (BIOCELL TEXTURED FULL HEIGHT, SALINE FILLED, STYLE 163), MCGHAN BREAST IMPLANT SMOOTH SILICONE-FILLED INTRASHIEL BARRIER (MODERATE PROFILE, ROUND, STYLE 110), MCGHAN BIOCELL TEXTURED SILICONE-FILLED INTRASHIEL BARRIER (STANDARD PROFILE, ROUND, STYLE 40)	53	A	1833(t)		D			N
C3500	PROSTHESIS, PENILE, MENTOR ALPHA I INFLATABLE PENILE PROSTHESIS, MENTOR ALPHA I NARROW-BASE INFLATABLE PENILE PROSTHESIS, MENTOR ACU-FORM MALLEABLE PENILE PROSTHESIS, MENTOR MALLEABLE PENILE PROSTHESIS NOTE: THE MENTOR ALPHA I NARROW-BASE INFLATABLE PENILE PROSTHESIS IS EFFECTIVE OCT 1, 2000. THE MENTOR ALPHA I INFLATABLE PENILE PROSTHESIS WAS EFFECTIVE AUG 1, 2000	53	A	1833(t)		D			N

HCPCS	Long Description	PII	MPI	Statute	X-Ref	Coverage	ASC Pay Grp	ASC Pay Grp Eff Date	Action Code
C3510	PROSTHESIS, AMS SPHINCTER 800 URINARY PROSTHESIS	53	A	1833(T)		D			N
C3551	GUIDE WIRE, PERCUTANEOUS TRANSLUMINAL CORONARY ANGIOPLASTY, CHOICE, LUGE, PATRIOT, PT GRAPHIX INTERMEDIATE, TROOPER, MAILMAN 182/300 CM, GLIDEWIRE GOLD GUIDEWIRE, PLATINUM PLUS GUIDEWIRE, PLATINUM PLUS GUIDEWIRE WITH GLIDEX HYDROPHILIC COATING, JAGWIRE SINGLE-USE HIGH PERFORMANCE GUIDE WIRE, MERIT MEDICAL SYSTEMS EXTENDER GUIDEWIRE, MERIT MEDICAL SYSTEMS TOMCAT PTCA GUIDEWIRE, PLATINUM PLUS GUIDEWIRE (0.014 AND 0.018 IN DIAMETERS)	53	A	1833(t)		D			N
C3552	GUIDE WIRE, HI-TORQUE WHISPER, ZEBRA SINGLE-USE EXCHANGE GUIDEWIRE	53	A	1833(T)		D			N
C3553	GUIDE WIRE, CORDIS STABILIZER MARKER WIRE STEERABLE GUIDEWIRE, CORDIS WIZDOM 'MARKER WIRE STEERABLE GUIDEWIRE, CORDIS ATW MARKER WIRE STEERABLE GUIDEWIRE, CORDIS SHINOBI STEERABLE GUIDEWIRE, CORDIS ATW STEERABLE GUIDEWIRE, CORDIS CINCH QR STEERABLE GUIDEWIRE EXTENSION, CORDIS STOR Q GUIDEWIRE, CORDIS ESSENCE STEERABLE GUIDEWIRE, CORDIS INSTINCT STEERABLE GUIDEWIRE, CORDIS AGILITY 10 HYDROPHILIC STEERABLE GUIDEWIRE, CORDIS AGILITY 14 HYDROPHILIC STEERABLE 'GUIDEWIRE, CORDIS STABILIZER BALANCED PERFORMANCE GUIDEWIRE, CORDIS STABILIZER PLUS STEERABLE GUIDEWIRE, CORDIS SHINOBI PLUS STEERABLE GUIDEWIRE (MODELS '547-214, 547-214X), CORDIS STABILIZER XS STEERABLE GUIDEWIRE (MODELS 527-914, '527-914J, 527-914X, 527-914Y), CORDIS SV GUIDEWIRE--5CM DISTAL TAPER 'CONFIGURATION (MODELS 503-558, 503-558X), 8CM DISTAL TAPER CONFIGURATION (MODELS 503-658, 503-658X), 14CM DISTAL TAPER CONFIGURATION (MODELS 503-758, '503-758X), CORDIS WISDOM ST STEERABLE GUIDEWIRE (MODELS 537-114, 537-114J, '537-	53	A	1833(T)		D			N
C3554	GUIDE WIRE, JINDO TAPERED PERIPHERAL GUIDEWIRE	53	A	1833(T)		D			N
C3555	GUIDE WIRE, WHOLEY HI-TORQUE PLUS GUIDE WIRE SYSTEM, 145CM, 190CM, 300CM	53	A	1833(T)		D			N
C3556	GUIDE WIRE, ENDOSONICS CARDIOMETRICS WAVEWIRE PRESSURE GUIDE WIRE, CARDIOMETRICS FLOWIRE DOPPLER GUIDE WIRE	53	A	1833(T)		D			N
C3557	GUIDEWIRE, HYTEK GUIDEWIRE, BIOTRONIK GALEO HYDRO GUIDE WIRE, MICROVENA ULTRA SELECT NITINOL GUIDEWIRE, WILSON-COOK AXCESS 21 WIRE GUIDE, WILSON-COOK ROADRUNNER EXTRA SUPPORT WIRE GUIDE, WILSON-COOK TRACER WIRE GUIDE, WILSON-COOK TRACER HYBRID WIRE GUIDE, WILSON-COOK TRACER METRO WIRE GUIDE, WILSON-COOK PROTECTOR WIRE GUIDES	53	A	1833(T)		D			N
C3800	INFUSION PUMP, IMPLANTABLE, PROGRAMMABLE, SYNCHROMED EL INFUSION PUMP, SYNCHROMED INFUSION PUMP	53	A	1833(T)		D			N
C3801	INFUSION PUMP, ARROW/MICROJECT PCA SYSTEM	53	A	1833(T)		D			N
C3851	INTRAOCULAR LENS, STAAR ELASTIC ULTRAVIOLET-ABSORBING SILICONE POSTERIOR CHAMBER INTRAOCULAR LENS WITH TORIC OPTIC MODEL AA-4203T, MODEL AA-4203TF, MODEL AA-4203TL	53	A	1833(t)		D			N
C4000	PACEMAKER, SINGLE CHAMBER, ELA MEDICAL OPUS G MODEL 4621, 4624	53	A	1833(t)		D			N
C4001	PACEMAKER, SINGLE CHAMBER, ELA MEDICAL OPUS S MODEL 4121, 4124	53	A	1833(t)		D			N
C4002	PACEMAKER, SINGLE CHAMBER, ELA MEDICAL TALENT MODEL 113	53	A	1833(t)		D			N
C4003	PACEMAKER, SINGLE CHAMBER, KAIROS SR	53	A	1833(t)		D			N
C4004	PACEMAKER, SINGLE CHAMBER, ACTROS SR+, ACTROS SR-B+	53	A	1833(t)		D			N
C4005	PACEMAKER, SINGLE CHAMBER, PHILOS SR, PHILOS SR-B	53	A	1833(T)		D			N
C4006	PACEMAKER, SINGLE CHAMBER, PULSAR MAX II SR 1180, 1181	53	A	1833(T)		D			N

HCPCS	Long Description	PII	MPI	Statute	X-Reff	Coverage	ASC Pay Grp	ASC Pay Grp Eff Date	Action Code
C4007	PACEMAKER, SINGLE CHAMBER, MARATHON SR 291-09, 292-09R, 292-09X	53	A	1833(T)		D			N
C4008	PACEMAKER, SINGLE CHAMBER, DISCOVERY II SSI 481	53	A	1833(T)		D			N
C4009	PACEMAKER, SINGLE CHAMBER, DISCOVERY II SR 1184, 1185, 1186, 1187	53	A	1833(T)		D			N
C4300	PACEMAKER, DUAL CHAMBER, INTEGRITY AFX DR MODEL 5342, INTEGRITY U DR 5336	53	A	1833(t)		D			N
C4301	PACEMAKER, DUAL CHAMBER, INTEGRITY AFX DR MODEL 5346	53	A	1833(t)		D			N
C4302	PACEMAKER, DUAL CHAMBER, AFFINITY VDR 5430	53	A	1833(t)		D			N
C4303	PACEMAKER, DUAL CHAMBER, ELA BRIO MODEL 112 PACEMAKER SYSTEM	53	A	1833(t)		D			N
C4304	PACEMAKER, DUAL CHAMBER, ELA MEDICAL BRIO MODEL 212, TALENT MODEL 213, TALENT MODEL 223	53	A	1833(t)		D			N
C4305	PACEMAKER, DUAL CHAMBER, ELA MEDICAL BRIO MODEL 222	53	A	1833(t)		D			N
C4306	PACEMAKER, DUAL CHAMBER, ELA MEDICAL BRIO MODEL 220	53	A	1833(t)		D			N
C4307	PACEMAKER, DUAL CHAMBER, KAIROS DR	53	A	1833(t)		D			N
C4308	PACEMAKER, DUAL CHAMBER, INOS 2, INOS 2+	53	A	1833(t)		D			N
C4309	PACEMAKER, DUAL CHAMBER, ACTROS DR+, ACTROS D+, ACTROS DR-A+, ACTROS SLR+	53	A	1833(t)		D			N
C4310	PACEMAKER, DUAL CHAMBER, ACTROS DR-B+	53	A	1833(t)		D			N
C4311	PACEMAKER, DUAL CHAMBER, PHILOS DR, PHILOS DR-B, PHILOS SLR	53	A	1833(t)		D			N
C4312	PACEMAKER, DUAL CHAMBER, PULSAR MAX II DR 1280	53	A	1833(T)		D			N
C4313	PACEMAKER, DUAL CHAMBER, MARATHON DR 293-09, 294-09, 294-09R, 294-10	53	A	1833(T)		D			N
C4314	PACEMAKER, DUAL CHAMBER, MOMENTUM DR 294-23	53	A	1833(T)		D			N
C4315	PACEMAKER, DUAL CHAMBER, SELECTION AFM 902 SLC 902C	53	A	1833(T)		D			N
C4316	PACEMAKER, DUAL CHAMBER, DISCOVERY II DR 1283, 1284, 1285, 1286	53	A	1833(T)		D			N
C4317	PACEMAKER, DUAL CHAMBER, DISCOVERY II DDD 981	53	A	1833(T)		D			N
C4600	LEAD, PACEMAKER, SYNOX, POLYROX, ELOX, RETROX, SL-BP, ELC, PR-B PERMANENT 'IMPLANTABLE PACING LEAD (MODELS PR 44 B, PR 48 B, PR 52 B, PR 58 B), PR-S 'PERMANENT IMPLANTABLE PACING LEAD (MODELS PR 44 S, PR 48 S, PR 52 S, PR 58 S), 'PY-PSBV PERMANENT IMPLANTABLE PACING LEAD (MODELS PY 44 PSBV, PY 48 PSBV, PY 52 'PSBV, PY 58 PSBV), PY-PV PERMANENT IMPLANTABLE PACING LEAD (MODELS PY 48 PV, PY '52 PV, PY 58 PV), ZY-PBV PERMANENT IMPLANTABLE PACING LEAD (MODELS ZY 52 PBV, 'ZY 58 PBV), ZY-PJBV PERMANENT IMPLANTABLE PACING LEAD (MODELS ZY 48 PJBV, ZY 52 'PJBV, ZY-PJUSBV PERMANENT IMPLANTABLE PACING LEAD (MODELS ZY 44 PJUSBV, ZY 48 'PJUSBV, ZY 52 PJUSBV) ZY-PJUV PERMANENT IMPLANTABLE PACING LEAD (MODELS ZY 48 'PJUV, ZY 52 PJUV), ZY-PJV PERMANENT IMPLANTABLE PACING LEAD (MODELS ZY 48 PJV, 'ZY 52 PJV), ZY PUSBV PERMANENT IMPLANTABLE PACING LEAD (MODELS ZY 52 PUSBV, ZY '58 PUSBV), ZY-PUV PERMANENT IMPLANTABLE PACING LEAD (MODELS ZY 52 PUV, ZY 58 'PUV), ZY-PV PERMANENT IMPLANTABLE PACING LEAD (MODELS ZY 52 PV, ZY 58 PV)	53	A	1833(t)		D			N
C4601	LEAD, PACEMAKER, AESCULA LV 1055K	53	A	1833(T)		D			N
C4602	LEAD, PACEMAKER, TENDRIL SDX 1488K/46, TENDRIL SDX 1488K/52, TENDRIL SDX '1488K/58	53	A	1833(T)		D			N

HCPCS	Long Description	PTI	MPI	Statute	X-Refl	Coverage	ASC Pay Grp	ASC Pay Grp Eff Date	Action Code
C4603	LEAD, PACEMAKER, OSCOR PR 4015, 4016, 4017, 4018, FLEXION 4015, 4016, 4017, '4018, ELA MEDICAL STELA PACING LEAD (MODELS BJ44, BJ45), ELA MEDICAL STELID II 'PACING LEAD (MODEL BTFR26D), ELA MEDICAL STELIX PACING LEAD (MODEL BR45D), 'HT-PB PERMANENT IMPLANTABLE PACING LEAD (MODELS HT 48 PB, HT 52 PB, HT 58 PB), 'OSCOR PY (MODELS 4439, 4440, 4441), OSCOR ZY (MODELS 4036, 4037, 4038, 4039, '4042, 4056, 4057), RT-TJV PERMANENT IMPLANTABLE PACING LEAD (MODELS RT 48 TJV, 'RT 52 TJV), RT-TV PERMANENT IMPLANTABLE PACING LEAD (MODELS RT 52 TV, RT 58 'TV), RU-TBV PERMANENT IMPLANTABLE PACING LEAD (MODELS RU 52 TBV, RU 58 TBV, RU '70 TBV), RU-TJSBV PERMANENT IMPLANTABLE PACING LEAD (MODELS RU 44 TJSBV, RU 48 'TJSBV, RU 52 TJSBV), RU-TJV PERMANENT IMPLANTABLE PACING LEAD (MODELS RU 48 'TJV, RU 52 TJV), RU-TSBV PERMANENT IMPLANTABLE PACING LEAD (MODELS RU 52 TSBV, 'RU 58 TSBV, RU 70 TSBV), RU-TV PERMANENT IMPLANTABLE PACING LEAD (MODELS RU 52 'TV, RU 58 TV)	53	A	1833(T)		D			N
C4604	LEAD, PACEMAKER, CRYSTALLINE ACTFIX ICF09, CAPSUREFIX NOVUS 5076	53	A	1833(T)		D			N
C4605	LEAD, PACEMAKER, CAPSURE EPI 4968	53	A	1833(T)		D			N
C4606	LEAD, PACEMAKER, FLEXTEND 4080, 4081, 4082	53	A	1833(T)		D			N
C4607	LEAD, PACEMAKER, FINELINE II 4452, 4453, 4454, 4455, 4477, 4478, FINELINE II EZ '4463, 4464, 4465, 4466, 4467, 4468, THINLINE II 430-25, 430-35, 432-35, 'THINLINE II EZ 438-25, 438-35, FINELINE II EZ STEROL (MODELS 4469, 4470, '4471, 4472, 4473, 4474), FINELINE II STEROX (MODELS 4456, 4457, 4459, 4479, '4480) THINLINE II EZ STEROX (MODELS 438-25S, 438-35S), THINLINE II STEROX '(MODELS 430-25S, 430-35S, 432-35S)	53	A	1833(T)		D			N
C5000	STENT, BILIARY, BX VELOCITY WITH HEPACOAT ON RAPTOR STENT SYSTEM (28 OR 33MM IN 'LENGTH)	53	A	1833(T)		D			N
C5001	STENT, BILIARY, BARD MEMOTHERM-FLEX BILIARY STENT (SMALL/MEDIUM DIAMETER)	53	A	1833(t)		D			N
C5002	STENT, BILIARY, BARD MEMOTHERM-FLEX BILIARY STENT, LARGE DIAMETER	53	A	1833(t)		D			N
C5003	STENT, BILIARY, BARD MEMOTHERM-FLEX BILIARY STENT, X-LARGE DIAMETER	53	A	1833(t)		D			N
C5004	STENT, BILIARY, CORDIS PALMAZ CORINTHIAN IQ TRANSHEPATIC BILIARY STENT	53	A	1833(t)		D			N
C5005	STENT, BILIARY, CORDIS PALMAZ CORINTHIAN IQ TRANSHEPATIC BILIARY STENT AND 'DELIVERY SYSTEM	53	A	1833(t)		D			N
C5006	STENT, BILIARY, CORDIS MEDIUM PALMAZ TRANSHEPATIC BILIARY STENT AND DELIVERY 'SYSTEM	53	A	1833(t)		D			N
C5007	STENT, BILIARY, CORDIS PALMAZ XL TRANSHEPATIC BILIARY STENT (40MM LENGTH)	53	A	1833(t)		D			N
C5008	STENT, BILIARY, CORDIS PALMAZ XL TRANSHEPATIC BILIARY STENT (50MM LENGTH)	53	A	1833(t)		D			N
C5009	STENT, BILIARY, BILIARY VISTAFLEX STENT	53	A	1833(t)		D			N
C5010	STENT, BILIARY, RAPID EXCHANGE SINGLE-USE BILIARY STENT SYSTEM	53	A	1833(t)		D			N
C5011	STENT, BILIARY, INTRASTENT, INTRASTENT LP,, WILSON-COOK ST2 SOEHENDRA TANNENBAUM	53	A	1833(t)		D			N
C5012	STENT, BILIARY, INTRASTENT DOUBLESTRUT LD, INTRASTENT DOUBLE STRUT PARA MOUNT 'BILIARY STENT, OLYMPUS DOUBLE LAYER BILIARY STENT	53	A	1833(t)		D			N
C5013	STENT, BILIARY, INTRASTENT DOUBLESTRUT, INTRASTENT DOUBLESTRUT XS	53	A	1833(t)		D			N
C5014	STENT, BILIARY, MEDTRONIC AVE BRIDGE STENT SYSTEM--BILIARY INDICATION (10MM, '17MM, 28MM)	53	A	1833(t)		D			N

HCPCS	Long Description	PH	MPI	Statute	X-Refl	Coverage	ASC Pay Grp	ASC Pay Grp Eff Date	Action Code
C5015	STENT, BILIARY, MEDTRONIC AVE BRIDGE STENT SYSTEM--BILIARY INDICATION (40-60MM, '80-100MM), MEDTRONIC AVE BRIDGE X3 BILIARY STENT SYSTEM (17MM)	53	A	1833(T)		D			N
C5016	STENT, BILIARY, WALLSTENT SINGLE-USE COVERED BILIARY ENDOPROSTHESIS WITH 'UNISTEP PLUS DELIVERY SYSTEM, GORE BILIARY ENDOPROSTHESIS	53	A	1833(t)		D			N
C5017	STENT, BILIARY, WALLSTENT RP BILIARY ENDOPROSTHESIS WITH UNISTEP PLUS DELIVERY 'SYSTEM (20/40/42/60/68 MM IN LENGTH)	53	A	1833(T)		D			N
C5018	STENT, BILIARY, WALLSTENT RP BILIARY ENDOPROSTHESIS WITH UNISTEP PLUS DELIVERY 'SYSTEM (80/94 MM IN LENGTH)	53	A	1833(t)		D			N
C5019	STENT, BILIARY, FLEXIMA SINGLE-USE BILIARY STENT SYSTEM	53	A	1833(T)		D			N
C5020	STENT, BILIARY, CORDIS SMART NITINOL STENT TRANSHEPATIC BILIARY SYSTEM (20MM 'IN LENGTH)	53	A	1833(T)		D			N
C5021	STENT, BILIARY, CORDIS SMART NITINOL STENT TRANSHEPATIC BILIARY SYSTEM (40 OR '60MM IN LENGTH)	53	A	1833(T)		D			N
C5022	STENT, BILIARY, CORDIS SMART NITINOL STENT TRANSHEPATIC BILIARY SYSTEM (80MM IN 'LENGTH)	53	A	1833(T)		D			N
C5023	STENT, BILIARY, BX VELOCITY TRANSHEPATIC BILIARY STENT AND DELIVERY SYSTEM (8 'OR 13MM IN LENGTH)	53	A	1833(T)		D			N
C5024	STENT, BILIARY, BX VELOCITY TRANSHEPATIC BILIARY STENT AND DELIVERY SYSTEM '(18MM IN LENGTH)	53	A	1833(T)		D			N
C5025	STENT, BILIARY, BX VELOCITY TRANSHEPATIC BILIARY STENT AND DELIVERY SYSTEM '(23MM IN LENGTH)	53	A	1833(T)		D			N
C5026	STENT, BILIARY, BX VELOCITY TRANSHEPATIC BILIARY STENT AND DELIVERY SYSTEM (28 '0R 33MM IN LENGTH)	53	A	1833(T)		D			N
C5027	STENT, BILIARY, BX VELOCITY WITH HEPACOAT ON RAPTOR STENT SYSTEM (8 OR 13MM IN 'LENGTH), BX VELOCITY E.5/5.0 BALLOON EXPANDABLE STENT WITH RAPTOR OVER-THE-WIRE 'DELIVERY SYSTEM	53	A	1833(T)		D			N
C5028	STENT, BILIARY, BX VELOCITY WITH HEPACOAT ON RAPTOR STENT SYSTEM (18MM IN 'LENGTH)	53	A	1833(T)		D			N
C5029	STENT, BILIARY, BX VELOCITY WITH HEPACOAT ON RAPTOR STENT SYSTEM (23MM IN 'LENGTH)	53	A	1833(T)		D			N
C5030	STENT, CORONARY, S660 DISCRETE TECHNOLOGY OVER-THE-WIRE CORONARY STENT SYSTEM '(9MM, 12MM), S660 WITH DISCRETE TECHNOLOGY RAPID EXCHANGE CORONARY STENT 'SYSTEM (9MM, 12MM), BIODIVYSIO AS PC COATED CORONARY STENT DELIVERY SYSTEM (11 'MM)	53	A	1833(t)		D			N
C5031	STENT, CORONARY, S660 DISCRETE TECHNOLOGY OVER-THE-WIRE CORONARY STENT SYSTEM '(15MM, 18MM), S660 WITH DISCRETE TECHNOLOGY RAPID EXCHANGE CORONARY STENT 'SYSTEM (15MM, 18MM), BIODIVYSIO AS PC COATED CORONARY STENT DELIVERY SYSTEM (15 'MM)	53	A	1833(t)		D			N
C5032	STENT, CORONARY, S660 DISCRETE TECHNOLOGY OVER-THE-WIRE CORONARY STENT SYSTEM '24MM, 30MM S660 WITH DISCRETE TECHNOLOGY RAPID EXCHANGE CORONARY STENT SYSTEM '24MM, 30MM	53	A	1833(t)		D			N
C5033	STENT, CORONARY, NIROYAL ADVANCE PREMOUNTED STENT SYSTEM (9MM), TENAX-XR STENT 'AND DELIVERY SYSTEM	53	A	1833(t)		D			N
C5034	STENT, CORONARY, NIROYAL ADVANCE PREMOUNTED STENT SYSTEM (12MM/15MM)	53	A	1833(t)		D			N
C5035	STENT, CORONARY, NIROYAL ADVANCE PREMOUNTED STENT SYSTEM (18MM)	53	A	1833(t)		D			N
C5036	STENT, CORONARY, NIROYAL ADVANCE PREMOUNTED STENT SYSTEM (25MM)	53	A	1833(t)		D			N
C5037	STENT, CORONARY, NIROYAL ADVANCE PREMOUNTED STENT SYSTEM (31MM)	53	A	1833(t)		D			N
C5038	STENT, CORONARY, BX VELOCITY BALLOON-EXPANDABLE STENT WITH RAPTOR OVER-THE-WIRE 'DELIVERY SYSTEM	53	A	1833(t)		D			N
C5039	STENT, PERIPHERAL, INTRACOIL PERIPHERAL STENT (40MM STENT LENGTH), DYNALINK 'PERIPHERAL SELF-EXPANDING STENT SYSTEM	53	A	1833(T)		D			N

HCPCS	Long Description	PTI	MPI	Statute	X-Refl	Coverage	ASC Pay Grp	ASC Pay Grp Eff Date	Action Code
C5040	STENT, PERIPHERAL, INTRACOIL PERIPHERAL STENT (60MM STENT LENGTH)	53	A	1833(T)		D			N
C5041	STENT, CORONARY, MEDTRONIC BESTENT 2 OVER-THE-WIRE CORONARY STENT SYSTEM (24MM, '30MM), MEDTRONIC BESTENT 2 RAPID EXCHANGE CORONARY STENT SYSTEM (24MM, 30MM)	53	A	1833(t)		D			N
C5042	STENT, CORONARY, MEDTRONIC BESTENT 2 OVER-THE-WIRE CORONARY STENT SYSTEM '(18MM), MEDTRONIC BESTENT 2 RAPID EXCHANGE (18MM)	53	A	1833(T)		D			N
C5043	STENT, CORONARY, MEDTRONIC BESTENT 2 OVER-THE-WIRE CORONARY STENT SYSTEM '(15MM), MEDTRONIC BESTENT 2 RAPID EXCHANGE (15MM)	53	A	1833(t)		D			N
C5044	STENT, CORONARY, MEDTRONIC BESTENT 2 OVER-THE-WIRE CORONARY STENT SYSTEM (9MM, '12MM), MEDTRONIC BESTENT 2 RAPID EXCHANGE CORONARY STENT SYSTEM (9MM, 12MM)	53	A	1833(t)		D			N
C5045	STENT, CORONARY, MULTILINK TETRA CORONARY STENT SYSTEM	53	A	1833(t)		D			N
C5046	STENT, CORONARY, RADIUS 20MM SELF EXPANDING STENT WITH OVER THE WIRE DELIVERY 'SYSTEM	53	A	1833(t)		D			N
C5047	STENT, CORONARY, NIROYAL ELITE PREMOUNTED STENT SYSTEM 15MM, 25MM, OR 31MM	53	A	1833(T)		D			N
C5048	STENT, CORONARY, GR II CORONARY STENT	53	A	1833(T)		D			N
C5130	STENT, COLON, WILSON-COOK COLONIC Z-STENT	53	A	1833(t)		D			N
C5131	STENT, COLORECTAL, BARD MEMOTHERM COLORECTAL STENT MODEL S30R060	53	A	1833(T)		D			N
C5132	STENT, COLORECTAL, BARD MEMOTHERM COLORECTAL STENT MODEL S30R080	53	A	1833(T)		D			N
C5133	STENT, COLORECTAL, BARD MEMOTHERM COLORECTAL STENT MODEL S30R100	53	A	1833(t)		D			N
C5134	STENT, ENTERAL, WALLSTENT ENTERAL ENDOPROSTHESIS AND UNISTEP DELIVERY SYSTEM '(90MM IN LENGTH), ENTERAL WALLSTENT ENDOPROSTHESIS WITH UNISTEP PLUS DELIVERY 'SYSTEM (90MM IN LENGTH) NOTE: ONLY THE ENTERAL WALLSTENT ENDOPROSTHESIS WITH 'UNISTEP PLUS DELIVERY SYSTEM IS EFFECTIVE OCTOBER 1, 2000. THE WALLSTENT 'ENTERAL AND UNISTEP DELIVERY SYSTEM WAS EFFECTIVE AUGUST 1, 2000	53	A	1833(t)		D			N
C5279	STENT, URETERAL, BOSTON SCIENTIFIC CONTOUR SOFT PERCUFLEX STENT WITH HYDROPLUS 'COATING (BRAIDED), CONTOUR SOFT PERCUFLEX STENT WITH HYDROPLUS COATING, CONTOUR 'VL VARIABLE LENGTH PERCUFLEX STENT WITH HYDROPLUS COATING, PERCUFLEX PLUS STENT 'WITH HYDROPLUS COATING, PERCUFLEX STENT (BRAIDED), CONTOUR CLOSED SOFT 'PERCUFLEX STENT WITH HYDROPLUS COATING, CONTOUR INJECTION SOFT PERCUFLEX STENT 'WITH HYDROPLUS COATING, SOFT PERCUFLEX STENT, PERCUFLEX TAIL PLUS TAPERED 'URETERAL STENT, CONTOUR POLARIS URETERAL STENT WITH HYDROPLUS COATING, MARDIS 'FIRM STENT WITH HYDROPLUS COATING, MARDIS SOFT STENT WITH HYDROPLUS COATING, 'MARDIS SOFT VARIABLE LENGTH STENT WITH HYDROPLUS COATING, NOTTINGHAM ONE-STEP 'TAPERED DILATORS WITH HYDROPLUS COATING, STRETCH VL VARIABLE LENGTH FLEXIMA 'STENT WITH HYDROPLUS COATING, PERCUFLEX URINARY DIVERSION STENT NOTE: THE 'CONTOUR CLOSED SOFT PERCUFLEX STENT, CONOUR INJECTION SOFT PERCUFLEX STENT, 'SOFT PERCUFLEX, AND PERCUFLEX TAIL PLUS TAPERED URETERAL STENT ARE EFFECTIVE '01/01/01. THE OTHER URETERAL STENTS WERE EFFECTIVE 10/01/00	53	A	1833(T)		D			N

HCPCS	Long Description	PII	MPI	Statute	X-Ref	Coverage	ASC Pay Grp	ASC Pay Grp Eff Date	Action Code
C5280	STENT, URETERAL, BARD INLAY DOUBLE PIGTAIL URETERAL STENT, COOK KLEIN RECTAL 'TAMPONADE BALLOON, COOK UROLOGICAL CYSTOSTOMY CATHETER, COOK UROLOGICAL 'URETERAL DILATOR SET, COOK UROLOGICAL FASCIAL DILATOR SET, CIRCON SURGITEK 'CLASSIC DOUBLE PIGTAIL URETERAL STENT, CIRCON SURGITEK CLASSIC DOUBLE PIGTAIL 'HYDROPHILIC COATED URETERAL STENT, CIRCON SURGITEK QUADRACOIL URETERAL STENT, 'CIRCON SURGITEK DOUBLE J II URETERAL STENT, CIRCON SURGITEK LITHOSTENT URETERAL 'STENT, CIRCON SURGITEK SOFT-CURL URETERAL STENT, COOK UROLOGICAL LSE DOUBLE 'PIGTAIL URETERAL STENT, COOK UROLOGICAL LSE MULTI LENGTH URETERAL STENT, COOK 'UROLOGICAL MULTI LENGTH URETERAL STENT, COOK UROLOGICAL DOUBLE PIGTAIL URETERAL 'STENT, COOK UROLOGICAL DOUBLE PIGTAIL URETERAL STENT WITH AQ (HYDROPHILIC) 'COATING, COOK UROLOGICAL MAZER ANTEGRADE DOUBLE PIGTAIL URETERAL STENT SET	53	A	1833(t)		D			N
C5281	STENT, TRACHEOBRONCHIAL, WALLGRAFT TRACHEOBRONCHIAL ENDOPROSTHESIS WITH UNISTEP 'DELIVERY SYSTEM (70MM IN LENGTH)	53	A	1833(t)		D			N
C5282	STENT, TRACHEOBRONCHIAL, WALLGRAFT TRACHEOBRONCHIAL ENDOPROSTHESIS WITH UNISTEP 'DELIVERY SYSTEM (20MM, 30MM, 50MM IN LENGTH)	53	A	1833(t)		D			N
C5283	STENT, SELF-EXPANDABLE FOR CREATION OF INTRAHEPATIC SHUNTS, WALLSTENT TRANSJUGULAR INTRAHEPATIC PROTOSYSTEMIC SHUNT (TIPS) WITH UNISTEP PLUS DELIVERY SYSTEM (90/94MM IN LENGTH), WALLSTENT RP TIPS ENDOPROSTHESIS WITH UNISTEP PLUS DELIVERY SYSTEM (94MM IN LENGTH) NOTE: ONLY THE WALLSTENT RP TIPS ENDOPROSTHESIS WITH UNISTEP PLUS DELIVERY SYSTEM IS EFFECTIVE OCTOBER 1, 2000. THE WALLSTENT TIPS WITH UNISTEP PLUST DELIVERY SYSTEM WAS EFFECTIVE AUGUST 1, 2000	53	A	1833(t)		D			N
C5284	STENT, TRACHEOBRONCHIAL, ULTRAFLEX TRACHEOBRONCHIAL ENDOPROSTHESIS (COVERED AND NON-COVERED)	53	A	1833(t)		D			N
C5600	VASCULAR CLOSURE DEVICE, VASOSEAL ES (EXTRAVASCULAR SECURITY) DEVICE	53	A	1833(t)		D			N
C5601	VASCULAR CLOSURE DEVICE, VASCULAR SOLUTIONS DUETT SEALING DEVICE 1000	53	A	1833(T)		D			N
C6001	MESH, HERNIA, BARD COMPOSIX MESH, PER 8 OR 21 INCHES, ATRIUM HERNIA/SURGICAL MESH, BARD COMPOSIX E/X MESH, BARD KUGEL HERNIA PATCH (LARGE CIRCLE, 12 CM X 12 CM), BARD KUGEL HERNIA PATCH (SMALL CIRCLE, 8 CM X 8 CM), BARD KUGEL HERNIA PATCH (LARGE OVAL, 14 CM X 18 CM), BARD KUGEL HERNIA PATCH (MEDIUM OVAL, 11 CM X 14 CM), BARD KUGEL HERNIA PATCH (SMALL OVAL, 8 CM X 12 CM), BARD MESH PERFIX PLUG, BARD VISILEX MESH (3 IN X 6 IN), BARD VISILEX MESH (4.5 IN X 6 IN)	53	A	1833(t)		D			N
C6002	MESH, HERNIA, BARD COMPOSIX MESH, PER 32 INCHES	53	A	1833(T)		D			N
C6003	MESH, HERNIA, BARD COMPOSIX MESH, PER 48 INCHES	53	A	1833(t)		D			N
C6004	MESH, HERNIA, BARD COMPOSIX MESH, PER 80 INCHES	53	A	1833(T)		D			N
C6005	MESH, HERNIA, BARD COMPOSIX MESH, PER 140 INCHES	53	A	1833(t)		D			N
C6006	MESH, HERNIA, BARD COMPOSIX MESH, PER 144 INCHES	53	A	1833(t)		D			N
C6012	PELVICOL ACELLULAR COLLAGEN MATRIX, PER 8 OR 14 QUARE CENTIMETERS, CONTIGEN BARD COLLAGEN IMPLANT (CONTIGEN IMPLANT)	53	A	1833(t)		D			N
C6013	PELVICOL ACELLULAR COLLAGEN MATRIX, PER 21, 24, OR 28 SQUARE CENTIMETERS	53	A	1833(t)		D			N
C6014	PELVICOL ACELLULAR COLLAGEN MATRIX, PER 40 SQUARE CENTIMETERS	53	A	1833(t)		D			N
C6015	PELVICOL ACELLULAR COLLAGEN MATRIX, PER 48 SQUARE CENTIMETERS	53	A	1833(t)		D			N
C6016	PELVICOL ACELLULAR COLLAGEN MATRIX, PER 96 SQUARE CENTIMETERS	53	A	1833(T)		D			N

HCPCS	Long Description	PII	MPI	Statute	X-Ref	Coverage	ASC Pay Grp	ASC Pay Grp Eff Date	Action Code
C6017	GORE-TEX DUALMESH BIOMATERIAL, PER 75 OR 96 SQUARE CENTIMETERS (1MM THICK)	53	A	1833(t)		D			N
C6018	GORE-TEX DUALMESH BIOMATERIAL, PER 150 SQUARE CENTIMETERS OVAL SHAPED (1MM THICK)	53	A	1833(t)		D			N
C6019	GORE-TEX DUALMESH BIOMATERIAL, PER 285 SQUARE CENTIMETERS OVAL SHAPED (1MM THICK)	53	A	1833(t)		D			N
C6020	GORE-TEX DUALMESH BIOMATERIAL, PER 432 SQUARE CENTIMETERS (1MM THICK)	53	A	1833(t)		D			N
C6021	GORE-TEX DUALMESH BIOMATERIAL, PER 600 SQUARE CENTIMETERS (1MM THICK)	53	A	1833(t)		D			N
C6022	GORE-TEX DUALMESH BIOMATERIAL, PER 884 SQUARE CENTIMETERS (1MM THICK)	53	A	1833(t)		D			N
C6023	GORE-TEX DUALMESH PLUS BIOMATERIAL, PER 75 OR 96 SQUARE CENTIMETERS (1MM THICK)	53	A	1833(t)		D			N
C6024	GORE-TEX DUALMESH PLUS BIOMATERIAL, PER 150 SQUARE CENTIMETERS OVAL SHAPED (1MM THICK)	53	A	1833(t)		D			N
C6025	GORE-TEX DUALMESH PLUS BIOMATERIAL, PER 285 SQUARE CENTIMETERS OVAL SHAPED (1MM THICK)	53	A	1833(t)		D			N
C6026	GORE-TEX DUALMESH PLUS BIOMATERIAL, PER 432 SQUARE CENTIMETERS (1MM THICK)	53	A	1833(t)		D			N
C6027	GORE-TEX DUALMESHPLUS BIOMATERIAL, PER 600 SQUARE CENTIMETERS (1MM THICK)	53	A	1833(t)		D			N
C6028	GORE-TEX DUALMESH PLUS BIOMATERIAL, PER 884 SQUARE CENTIMETERS OVAL SHAPED (1MM THICK)	53	A	1833(t)		D			N
C6029	GORE-TEX DUALMESH PLUS BIOMATERIAL, PER 150 SQUARE CENTIMETERS OVAL SHAPED (2MM THICK)	53	A	1833(t)		D			N
C6030	GORE-TEX DUALMESH PLUS BIOMATERIAL, PER 285 SQUARE CENTIMETERS OVAL SHAPED (2MM THICK)	53	A	1833(t)		D			N
C6031	GORE-TEX DUALMESH PLUS BIOMATERIAL, PER 432 SQUARE CENTIMETERS (2MM THICK)	53	A	1833(t)		D			N
C6032	GORE-TEX DUALMESH PLUS BIOMATERIAL, PER 600 SQUARE CENTIMETERS (2MM THICK)	53	A	1833(t)		D			N
C6033	GORE-TEX DUALMESH PLUS BIOMATERIAL, PER 884 SQUARE CENTIMETERS (2MM THICK)	53	A	1833(t)		D			N
C6034	BARD RECONIX EPTFE RECONSTRUCTION PATCH 150 SQUARE CENTIMETERS (2MM THICK)	53	A	1833(t)		D			N
C6035	BARD RECONIX EPTFE RECONSTRUCTION PATCH 150 SQUARE CENTIMETERS (1MM THICK), 75 SQUARE CENTIMETERS (2MM THICK)	53	A	1833(t)		D			N

HCPCS	Long Description	PH	MPI	Statute	X-Refl	Coverage	ASC Pay Grp	ASC Pay Grp Eff Date	Action Code
C6036	BARD RECONIX EPTFE RECONSTRUCTION PATCH 50/75 SQUARE CENTIMETERS (1MM THICK), 50 SQUARE CENTIMETERS (2MM THICK)	53	A	1833(t)		D			N
C6037	BARD RECONIX EPTFE RECONSTRUCTION PATCH 300 SQUARE CENTIMETERS (1 MM THICK)	53	A	1833(t)		D			N
C6038	BARD RECONIX EPTFE RECONSTRUCTION PATCH 600 SQUARE CENTIMETERS (1MM THICK), 300 SQUARE CENTIMETERS (2MM THICK)	53	A	1833(t)		D			N
C6039	BARD RECONIX EPTFE RECONSTRUCTION PATCH 884 SQUARE CENTIMETERS OVAL SHAPED (1MM THICK)	53	A	1833(t)		D			N
C6040	BARD RECONIX EPTFE RECONSTRUCTION PATCH 600 SQUARE CENTIMETERS (2MM THICK)	53	A	1833(T)		D			N
C6041	BARD RECONIX EPTFE RECONSTRUCTION PATCH 884 SQUARE CENTIMETERS OVAL SHAPED (2MM THICK)	53	A	1833(t)		D			N
C6050	SLING FIXATION SYSTEM FOR TREATMENT OF STRESS URINARY INCONTINENCE, FEMALE IN-FAST SLING FIXATION SYSTEM WITH ELECTRIC INSERTER WITH SLING MATERIAL, FEMALE IN-FAST SLING FIXATION SYSTEM WITH ELECTRIC INSERTER WITHOUT SLING MATERIAL, ADVANCED UROSCIENCE ACYST	53	A	1833(t)		D			N
C6051	DEPUY ORTHOTECH RESTORE, STRATASIS URETHRAL SLING, 20/40 CM	53	A	1833(t)		D			N
C6052	STRATASIS URETHRAL SLING, 60 CM	53	A	1833(t)		D			N
C6053	SURGISIS SOFT TISSUE GRAFT, PER 70CM, 105CM, OR 140CM	53	A	1833(T)		D			N
C6054	SURGISIS ENHANCED STRENGTH SOFT TISSUE GRAFT, PER 4.2CM, 20CM, 28CM OR 40CM	53	A	1833(T)		D			N
C6055	SURGISIS ENHANCED STRENGTH SOFT TISSUE GRAFT, PER 52.5CM, 60CM, OR 70CM	53	A	1833(T)		D			N
C6056	SURGISIS ENHANCED STRENGTH SOFT TISSUE GRAFT, PER 105CM, 140CM	53	A	1833(T)		D			N
C6057	SURGISIS HERNIA GRAFT, PER 195CM	53	A	1833(T)		D			N
C6058	SUGIPRO HERNIA MATE PLUG, MEDIUM OR LARGE	53	A	1833(T)		D			N
C6080	SLING FIXATION SYSTEM FOR TREATMENT OF STRESS URINARY INCONTINENCE, MALE STRAIGHT-IN FIXATION SYSTEM WITH ELECTRIC INSERTER WITH SLING MATERIAL AND DISPOSABLE PRESSURE SENSOR, MALE STRAIGHT-IN FIXATION SYSTEM WITH ELECTRIC INSERTER WITHOUT SLING MATERIAL AND DISPOSABLE PRESSURE SENSOR	53	A	1833(t)		D			N
C6200	VASCULAR GRAFT, EXXCEL SOFT EPTFE VASCULAR GRAFT, EXXCEL EPTFE VASCULAR GRAFT (6MM OR GREATER IN DIAMETER), B. BRAUN VENA TECH LGM VENA CAVA FILTER (DUAL APPROACH--MODEL #31328, JUGULAR APPROACH--MODEL #31326, FEMORAL APPROACH--MODEL #31327), CORDIS TRAPEASE PERMANENT VENA CAVA FILTER, STAINLESS STEEL GREEN FIELD VENA CAVA FILTER WITH 12 FR INTRODUCER SYSTEM	53	A	1833(T)		D			N
C6201	VASCULAR GRAFT, IMPRA VENAFLO VASCULAR GRAFT WITH CARBON (STRAIGHT GRAFT, 10CM OR 20CM IN LENGTH), ATRIUM HYBRID PTFE VASCULAR GRAFT	53	A	1833(T)		D			N
C6202	VASCULAR GRAFT, IMPRA VENAFLO VASCULAR GRAFT WITH CARBON, STRAIGHT GRAFT 30CM OR 40CM IN LENGTH	53	A	1833(T)		D			N
C6203	VASCULAR GRAFT, IMPRA VENAFLO VASCULAR GRAFT WITH CARBON, STRAIGHT GRAFT (50CM IN LENGTH) OR CENTERFLEX VENAFLO STEPPED GRAFT (45CM IN LENGTH)	53	A	1833(T)		D			N
C6204	VASCULAR GRAFT, IMPRA VENAFLO VASCULAR GRAFT WITH CARBON, STEPPED GRAFT 20CM, 25CM, 30CM, 35CM, 40CM, OR 45CM IN LENGTH	53	A	1833(T)		D			N
C6205	VASCULAR GRAFT, IMPRA CARBOFLO VASCULAR GRAFT (STRAIGHT GRAFT, 10CM IN LENGTH), ATRIUM ADVANTA PTFE VASCULAR GRAFT	53	A	1833(T)		D			N
C6206	VASCULAR GRAFT, IMPRA CARBOFLO VASCULAR GRAFT, STRAIGHT GRAFT 20CM IN LENGTH	53	A	1833(T)		D			N

HCPCS	Long Description	PTT	MPI	Statute	X-Ref1	Coverage	ASC Pay Grp	ASC Pay Grp Eff Date	Action Code
C6207	VASCULAR GRAFT, IMPRA CARBOFLO VASCULAR GRAFT, STRAIGHT GRAFT 30CM, 35CM OR 40CM IN LENGTH	53	A	1833(T)		D			N
C6208	VASCULAR GRAFT, IMPRA CARBOFLO VASCULAR GRAFT, STRAIGHT GRAFT (50CM IN LENGTH), ACCESS TAPERED GRAFT (40CM IN LENGTH), OR STEPPED GRAFT (45 OR 50CM IN LENGTH)	53	A	1833(T)		D			N
C6209	VASCULAR GRAFT, IMPRA CARBOFLO VASCULAR GRAFT, CENTERFLEX STRAIGHT GRAFT (40CM OR 50CM IN LENGTH) OR CENTERFLEX STEPPED GRAFT (40CM, 45CM, OR 50CM IN LENGTH)	53	A	1833(T)		D			N
C6210	EXXCEL EPTFE VASCULAR GRAFT (LESS THAN 6MM IN DIAMETER), HEMASHIELD WOVEN DOUBLE VELOUR FABRIC, HEMASHIELD FINESSE ULTRA-THIN, KNITTED CARDIOVASCULAR PATCH	53	A	1833(T)		D			N
C6300	STENT GRAFT SYSTEM, VANGUARD III BIFURCATED ENDOVASCULAR AORTIC GRAFT	53	A	1833(T)		D			N
C6500	SHEATH, GUIDING, PREFACE BRAIDED GUIDING SHEAT (ANTERIOR CURVE, MULTIPURPOSE CURVE, POSTERIOR CURVE)	53	A	1833(t)		D			N
C6501	SHEATH, SOFT-TIP SHEATHS	53	A	1833(t)		D			N
C6502	SHEATH, ELECTROPHYSIOLOGY, PERRY EXCHANGE DILATOR	53	A	1833(T)		D			N
C6525	SPECTRANETICS LASER SHEATH 12F 500-001, 14F 500-012, 16F 500-013	53	A	1833(T)		D			N
C6600	PROBE, MICROVASIVE SWISS F/G LITHOCLAST FLEXIBLE PROBE .89MM, MICROVASIVE SWISS F/G LITHOCLAST FLEXIBLE PROBE II .89MM	53	A	1833(t)		D			N
C6650	INTRODUCER, GUIDING, FAST-CATH TWO-PIECE GUIDING INTRODUCER (MODELS 406869, 406892, 406893, 406904), ACCUSTICK II WITH RO MARKER INTRODUCER SYSTEM, COOK EXTRA LARGE CHECK-FLO INTRODUCER, COOK KELLER-TIMMERMANS INTRODUCER, FAST-CATH HEMOSTASIS INTRODUCER, MAXIMUM HEMOSTASIS INTRODUCER, FAST-CATH DUO SL1 GUIDING INTRODUCER FAST-CATH DUO SL2 GUIDING INTRODUCER	53	A	1833(T)		D			N
C6651	INTRODUCER, GUIDING, SEAL-AWAY CS GUIDING INTRODUCER 407508, 407510	53	A	1833(T)		D			N
C6652	INTRODUCER, BARD SAFETY EXCALIBUR INTRODUCER, BARD RADSTIC MICROINTRODUCER, BARD UNIVERSAL MICROINTRODUCER	53	A	1833(T)		D			N
C6700	SYNTHETIC ABSORBABLE SEALANT, FOCAL SEAL-L, PERFLUORON (PER 2ML VIAL, 5ML VIAL OR 7ML VIAL)	53	A	1833(T)		D			N
C8099	SPECTRANETICS LEAD LOCKING DEVICE (MODELS 518-018, 518-019, 518-020), OSCOR C/VS PERMANENT IMPLANTABLE PACING LEAD ADAPTOR (MODELS C/VS-10, C/VS-40), OSCOR M/VS PERMANENT IMPLANTABLE PACING LEAD ADAPTOR (MODELS M/VS-10, M/VS-40), OSCOR VS/M PERMANENT IMPLANTABLE PACING LEAD ADAPTOR (MODEL VS/M-10), OSCOR VV PERMANENT IMPLANTABLE PACING LEAD EXTENSION (MODELS VV-10, VV-40)	53	A	1833(T)		D			N
C8100	ADHESION BARRIER, ADCON-L	53	A	1833(t)		D			N
C8102	SURGI-VISION ESOPHAGEAL STYLET INTERNAL COIL	53	A	1833(T)		D			N
C8103	CAPIO SUTURE CAPTURING DEVICE, STANDARD OR OPEN ACCESS	53	A	1833(T)		D			N
C8500	CATHETER, ATHERECTOMY, ATHEROCATH-GTO ATHERECTOMY CATHETER	53	A	1833(t)		D			N
C8501	PACEMAKER, SINGLE CHAMBER, VIGOR SSI	53	A	1833(t)		D			N
C8502	CATHETER, DIAGNOSTIC, ELECTROPHYSIOLOGY, LIVEWIRE STEERABLE ELECTROPHYSIOLOGY CATHETER	53	A	1833(t)		D			N
C8503	CATHETER, SYNCHROMED VASCULAR CATHETER MODEL 8702	53	A	1833(t)		D			N
C8504	CLOSURE DEVICE, VASOSEAL VASCULAR HEMOSTASIS DEVICE	53	A	1833(t)		D			N

HCPCS	Long Description	PTI	MPI	Statute	X-Refl	Coverage	ASC Pay Grp	ASC Pay Grp Eff Date	Action Code
C8505	INFUSION PUMP, IMPLANTABLE, PROGRAMMABLE, SYNCHROMED INFUSION PUMP	53	A	1833(t)(b)		D			N
C8506	LEAD, PACEMAKER, 4057M, 4058M, 4557M, 4558M,5058	53	A	1833(t)		D			N
C8507	LEAD, PACEMAKER,6721L, 6721M, 6721S, 6939 OVAL PATCH LEAD	53	A	1833(t)		D			N
C8508	LEAD, DEFIBRILLATOR, CAPSURE 4965	53	A	1833(t)		D			N
C8509	LEAD, DEFIBRILLATOR, TRANSVENE 6933, TRANSVENE 6937	53	A	1833(t)		D			N
C8510	LEAD, DEFIBRILLATOR, DP-3238	53	A	1833(T)		D			N
C8511	LEAD, DEFIBRILLATOR, ENDOTAK DSP	53	A	1833(t)		D			N
C8512	LEAD, NEUROSTIMULATION, ON-POINT MODEL 3987, PISCES-QUAD PLUS MODEL 3888, RESUME TL MODEL 3986	53	A	1833(t)		D			N
C8513	LEAD, NEUROSTIMULATION, PISCES-QUAD MODEL 3487A, RESUME II MODEL 3587A	53	A	1833(t)		D			N
C8514	PROSTHESIS, PENILE, DURA II PENILE PROSTHESIS	53	A	1833(t)		D			N
C8515	PROSTHESIS, PENILE, MENTOR ALPHA I NARROW-BASE INFLATABLE PENILE PROSTHESIS	53	A			D			N
C8516	PROSTHESIS, PENILE, MENTOR ACU-FORM MALLEABLE PENILE PROSTHESIS, MENTOR	53	A	1833(t)		D			N
C8516	MALLEABLE PENILE PROSTHESIS								
C8517	PROSTHESIS, PENILE, AMBICOR PENILE PROSTHESIS	53	A	1833(t)(b)		D			N
C8518	PACEMAKER, DUAL CHAMBER, VIGOR DDD	53	A	1833(t)		D			N
C8519	PACEMAKER, DUAL CHAMBER, VISTA DDD	53	A	1833(t)		D			N
C8520	PACEMAKER, SINGLE CHAMBER, LEGACY II S	53	A	1833(t)		D			N
C8521	RECEIVER/TRANSMITTER, NEUROSTIMULATOR, MEDTRONIC MATTRIX	53	A	1833(t)		D			N
C8522	STENT, BILIARY, PALMAZ BALLOON EXPANDABLE STENT	53	A	1833(t)		D			N
C8523	STENT, BILIARY, WALLSTENT TRANSHEPATIC BILIARY ENDOPROSTHESIS	53	A	1833(t)		D			N
C8524	STENT, ESOPHAGEAL, WALLSTENT ESOPHAGEAL PROSTHESIS	53	A	1833(t)		D			N
C8525	STENT, ESOPHAGEAL, WALLSTENT ESOPHAGEAL PROSTHESIS (DOUBLE)	53	A	1833(t)		D			N
C8526	OPTIPLAST XT 5F PERCUTANEOUS TRANSLUMINAL ANGIOPLASTY CATHETER (VARIOUS SIZES)	53	A	1833(t)		D			N
C8528	MS CLASSIQUE BALLOON DILATATION CATHETER	53	A	1833(t)		D			N
C8529	ISMUS CATH DEFLECTABLE 20-POLE CATHETER/CRISTA CATH II DEFLECTABLE 20-POLE CATHETER	53	A	1833(t)		D			N
C8530	MENTOR SILTEX GEL-FILLED MAMMARY PROSTHESIS, SMOOTH-SURFACE GEL-FILLED MAMMARY PROSTHESIS	53	A	1833(t)		D			N
C8531	WILSON-COOK ESOPHAGEAL Z METAL EXPANDABLE STENT	53	A	1833(t)		D			N
C8532	STENT, ESOPHAGEAL, ULTRAFLEX ESOPHAGEAL STENT SYSTEM	53	A	1833(t)		D			N

HCPCS	Long Description	PI1	MPI	Statute	X-Refl	Coverage	ASC Pay Grp	ASC Pay Grp Eff Date	Action Code
C8533	CATHETER, SYNCHROMED VASCULAR CATHETER MODEL 8700A, MODEL 8700V	53	A	1833(t)		D			N
C8534	PROSTHESIS, PENILE, AMS MALLEABLE 650 PENILE PROSTHESIS	53	A	1833(t)		D			N
C8535	STENT, BILIARY, SPIRAL Z BILIARY METAL EXPANDABLE STENT, ZA BILIARY METAL EXPANDABLE STENT	53	A	1833(T)		D			N
C8536	STENT, ESOPHAGEAL, ESOPHAGEAL Z METAL EXPANDABLE STENT WITH DUA ANTI-REFLUX VALVE, ESOPHAGEAL Z METAL EXPANDABLE STENT WITH UNCOATED FLANGES	53	A	1833(T)		D			N
C8539	WILSON-COOK QUANTUM DILATATION BALLOON	53	A	1833(T)		D			N
C8540	FLEX-EZ (ESOPHAGEAL) BALLOON DILATOR 3302, 3304, 3306	53	A	1833(T)		D			N
C8541	CARSON ZERO TIP BALLOON DILATATION CATHETERS WITH HYDROPLUS COATING KIT, PASSPORT BALLOON ON A WIRE DILATATION CATHETERS WITH HYDROPLUS COATING KIT	53	A	1833(T)		D			N
C8542	URETHRAMAX HIGH PRESSURE URETHRAL BALLOON DILATATION CATHETER/KIT	53	A	1833(T)		D			N
C8543	AMPLATZ RENAL DILATOR SET	53	A	1833(T)		D			N
C8550	CATHETER, LIVEWIRE EP CATHETER, 7F CSM 401935, 5F DECAPOLAR 401938, 401939, 401940, 401941	53	A	1833(T)		D			N
C8551	CATHETER, LIVEWIRE EP CATHETER, 7F DUO-DECAPOLAR 401932	53	A	1833(T)		D			N
C8552	CATHETER, SANTURO FIXED CURVE CATHETER	53	A	1833(T)		D			N
C8597	GUIDE WIRE, CORDIS WISDOM ST STEERABLE GUIDEWIRE 537-114, 537-114J, 537-114X, 537-114Y	53	A	1833(T)		D			N
C8598	GUIDE WIRE, CORDIS SV GUIDEWIRE 5CM DISTAL TAPER CONFIGURATION (MODELS 503-558, 503-558X), 8CM DISTAL TAPER CONFIGURATION (MODELS 503-658, 503-658X), 14CM DISTAL TAPER CONFIGURATION (MODELS 503-758, 503-758X)	53	A	1833(T)		D			N
C8599	GUIDE WIRE, CORDIS STABILIZER XS STEERABLE GUIDEWIRE 527-914, 527-914J, 527-914X, 527-914Y	53	A	1833(T)		D			N
C8600	GUIDE WIRE, CORDIS SHINOBI PLUS STEERABLE GUIDEWIRE 547-214, 547-214X	53	A	1833(T)		D			N
C8650	INTRODUCER, COOK EXTRA LARGE CHECK-FLO INTRODUCER	53	A	1833(T)		D			N
C8724	LEAD, NEUROSTIMULATION, OCTAD LEAD 3898-33/389861	53	A	1833(T)		D			N
C8725	LEAD, NEUROSTIMULATION, SYMMIX LEAD 3982	53	A	1833(T)		D			N
C8748	LEAD, DEFIBRILLATOR, ENDOTAK SQ PATCH 0047, 0063	53	A	1833(T)		D			N
C8749	LEAD, DEFIBRILLATOR, ENDOTAK SQ ARRAY 0048, 0049	53	A	1833(T)		D			N
C8750	PACEMAKER, DUAL CHAMBER, UNITY VDDR 292-07	53	A	1833(T)		D			N
C8775	LEAD, PACEMAKER, 2188 CORONARY SINUS LEAD	53	A	1833(T)		D			N
C8776	LEAD, PACEMAKER, INNOMEDICA SUTURELESS MYOCARDIAL 4045, 4058, 4046, 4047	53	A	1833(T)		D			N
C8777	LEAD, PACEMAKER, UNIPASS 425-02, 425-04, 425-06	53	A	1833(T)		D			N
C8800	STENT, BILIARY, LARGE PALMAZ BALLOON EXPANDABLE STENT WITH DELIVERY SYSTEM	53	A	1833(T)		D			N
C8801	STENT, BILIARY, COOK Z STENT GIANTURCO-ROSCH BILIARY DESIGN	53	A	1833(T)		D			N
C8802	STENT, BILIARY, COOK OASIS ONE ACTION STENT INTRODUCTORY SYSTEM	53	A	1833(T)		D			N
C8830	STENT, CORONARY, COOK GIANTURCO-ROUBIN FLEX-STENT CORONARY STENT	53	A	1833(T)		D			N
C8890	PERFLUORON, PER 2ML	53	A	1833(T)		D			N

HCPCS	Long Description	PTI	MPI	Statute	X-Refl	Coverage	ASC Pay Grp	ASC Pay Grp Eff Date	Action Code
C8891	PERFLUORON, PER 5ML VIAL OR 7ML VIAL	53	A	1833(T)		D			N
C8900	MAGNETIC RESONANCE ANGIOGRAPHY WITH CONTRAST, ABDOMEN	53	A	1833(t)(2)		D			N
C8901	MAGNETIC RESONANCE ANGIOGRAPHY WITHOUT CONTRAST, ABDOMEN	53	A	1833(t)(2)		D			N
C8902	MAGNETIC RESONANCE ANGIOGRAPHY WITHOUT CONTRAST FOLLOWED BY WITH CONTRAST, ABDOMEN	53	A	1833(t)(2)		D			N
C8903	MAGNETIC RESONANCE IMAGING WITH CONTRAST, BREAST; UNILATERAL	53	A	1833(t)(2)		D			N
C8904	MAGNETIC RESONANCE IMAGING WITHOUT CONTRAST, BREAST; UNILATERAL	53	A	1833(t)(2)		D			N
C8905	MAGNETIC RESONANCE IMAGING WITHOUT CONTRAST FOLLOWED BY WITH CONTRAST, BREAST; UNILATERAL	53	A	1833(t)(2)		D			N
C8906	MAGNETIC RESONANCE IMAGING WITH CONTRAST, BREAST; BILATERAL	53	A	1833(t)(2)		D			N
C8907	MAGNETIC RESONANCE IMAGING WITHOUT CONTRAST, BREAST; BILATERAL	53	A	1833(t)(2)		D			N
C8908	MAGNETIC RESONANCE IMAGING WITHOUT CONTRAST FOLLOWED BY WITH CONTRAST, BREAST; BILATERAL	53	A	1833(t)(2)		D			N
C8909	MAGNETIC RESONANCE ANGIOGRAPHY WITH CONTRAST, CHEST (EXCLUDING MYOCARDIUM)	53	A	1833(t)(2)		D			N
C8910	MAGNETIC RESONANCE ANGIOGRAPHY WITHOUT CONTRAST, CHEST (EXCLUDING MYOCARDIUM)	53	A	1833(t)(2)		D			N
C8911	MAGNETIC RESONANCE ANGIOGRAPHY WITHOUT CONTRAST FOLLOWED BY WITH CONTRAST, CHEST (EXCLUDING MYOCARDIUM)	53	A	1833(t)(2)		D			N
C8912	MAGNETIC RESONANCE ANGIOGRAPHY WITH CONTRAST, LOWER EXTREMITY	53	A	1833(t)(2)		D			N
C8913	MAGNETIC RESONANCE ANGIOGRAPHY WITHOUT CONTRAST, LOWER EXTREMITY	53	A	1833(t)(2)		D			N
C8914	MAGNETIC RESONANCE ANGIOGRAPHY WITHOUT CONTRAST FOLLOWED BY WITH CONTRAST, LOWER EXTREMITY	53	A	1833(t)(2)		D			N
C8918	MAGNETIC RESONANCE ANGIOGRAPHY WITH CONTRAST, PELVIS	53	A	430 BIPA		D			A
C8919	MAGNETIC RESONANCE ANGIOGRAPHY WITHOUT CONTRAST, PELVIS	53	A	430 BIPA		D			A
C8920	MAGNETIC RESONANCE ANGIOGRAPHY WITHOUT CONTRAST FOLLOWED BY WITH CONTRAST, PELVIS	53	A	430 BIPA		D			A
C9000	INJECTION, SODIUM CHROMATE CR51, PER 0.25 MCI	53	A	1833(t)		D			N
C9001	LINEZOLID INJECTION, PER 200MG	53	A	1833(t)		D			N
C9002	TENECTEPLASE, PER 50MG/VIAL	53	A	1833(t)		D			N
C9003	PALIVIZUMAB-RSV-IGM, PER 50 MG	53	A	1833(t)		D			N
C9004	INJECTION, GEMTUZUMAB OZOGAMICIN, PER 5 MG	53	A	1833(T)		D			N
C9005	INJECTION, RETEPLASE, 18.8 MG (ONE SINGLE-USE VIAL)	53	A	1833(t)		D			N
C9006	INJECTION, TACROLIMUS, PER 5 MG (1 AMP)	53	A	1833(t)		D			N
C9007	BACLOFEN INTRATHECAL SCREENING KIT (1 AMP)	53	A	1833(t)		D			N
C9008	BACLOFEN INTRATHECAL REFILL KIT, PER 500 MCG	53	A	1833(t)		D			N
C9009	BACLOFEN INTRATHECAL REFILL KIT, PER 2000 MCG	53	A	1833(t)		D			N
C9010	BACLOFEN INTRATHECAL REFILL KIT, PER 4000 MCG	53	A	1833(T)		D			D

HCPCS	Long Description	PTI	MPI	Statute	X-Refl	Coverage	ASC Pay Grp	ASC Pay Grp Eff Date	Action Code
C9011	INJECTION, CAFFEINE CITRATE, PER 1ML	53	A	1833(T)		D			N
C9012	INJECTION, ARSENIC TRIOXIDE, PER 1 MG/KG	53	A	1833(T)		D			N
C9013	SUPPLY OF CO 57 COBALTOUS CHLORIDE, RADIOPHARMACEUTICAL DIAGNOSTIC IMAGING AGENT	53	A	1833(t)		D			N
C9017	LOMUSTINE, 10 MG	53	A	1833(T)		D			N
C9018	BOTULINUM TOXIN TYPE B, PER 100 UNITS	53	A	1833(T)		D			N
C9019	INJECTION, CASPOFUNGIN ACETATE, 5 MG	53	A	1833(T)	J0637	D			N
C9020	SIROLIMUS TABLET, 1 MG	53	A	1833(T)	J7520	D			N
C9100	SUPPLY OF RADIOPHARMACEUTICAL DIAGNOSTIC IMAGING AGENT, IODINATED I-131 ALBUMIN, PER MCI	53	A	1833(t)		D			N
C9102	SUPPLY OF RADIOPHARMACEUTICAL DIAGNOSTIC IMAGING AGENT, 51 SODIUM CHROMATE, PER 50 MCI	53	A	1833(t)		D			N
C9103	SUPPLY OF RADIOPHARMACEUTICAL DIAGNOSTIC IMAGING AGENT, SODIUM IOTHALAMATE I-125 INJECTION, PER 10 UCI	53	A	1833(t)		D			N
C9104	ANTI-THYMOCYTE GLOBULIN, PER 25 MG	53	A	1833(t)		D			N
C9105	INJECTION, HEPATITIS B IMMUNE GLOBULIN, PER 1 ML	53	A	1833(t)		D			N
C9106	SIROLIMUS, PER 1 MG/ML	53	A	1833(t)		D			N
C9107	INJECTION, TINZAPARIN SODIUM, PER 2ML VIAL	53	A	1833(T)		D			N
C9108	INJECTION, THYROTROPIN ALPHA, 1.1 MG	53	A	1833(T)	J3240	D			N
C9109	INJECTION, TIROFIBAN HYDROCHLORIDE, 6.25 MG	53	A	1833(T)		D			N
C9110	INJECTION, ALEMTUZUMAB, PER 10 MG/ ML	53	A	1833(T)	J9010	D			N
C9111	INJECTION, BIVALIRUDIN, 250 MG PER VIAL	53	A	1833(t)		D			D
C9112	INJECTION, PERFLUTREN LIPID MICROSPHERE, PER 2 ML VIAL	53	A	1833(t)		D			T
C9113	INJECTION, PANTOPRAZOLE SODIUM, PER VIAL	53	A	1833(T)		D			N
C9114	INJECTION, NESIRITIDE, PER 1.5 MG VIAL	53	A	1833(T)	J2324	D			N
C9115	INJECTION, ZOLEDRONIC ACID, PER 2 MG	53	A	1833(T)	J3487	D			N
C9116	INJECTION, ERTAPENEM SODIUM, PER 1 GRAM VIAL	53	A	1833(t)		D			D
C9117	INJECTION, YTTRIUM-90 IBRITUMOMAB TIUXETAN, PER MCI	53	A	1833(t)	A9523	D			N
C9118	INJECTION, INDIUM-111 IBRITUMOMAB TIUXETAN, PER MCI	53	A	1833(t)	A9522	D			N
C9119	INJECTION, PEGFILGRASTIM, PER 6 MG SINGLE DOSE VIAL	53	A	1833(t)		D			D
C9120	INJECTION, FULVESTRANT, PER 50 MG	53	A	1833(T)		D			D
C9121	INJECTION, ARGATROBAN, PER 5 MG	53	A	1833(T)		D			N
C9123	TRANSCYTE, PER 247 SQUARE CENTIMETERS	53	A	1833T		D			A

HCPCS	Long Description	PII	MPI	Statute	X-Refl	Coverage	ASC Pay Grp	ASC Pay Grp Eff Date	Action Code
C9200	ORCEL, PER 36 SQUARE CENTIMETERS	53	A	1833(T)		D			N
C9201	DERMAGRAFT, PER 37.5 SQUARE CENTIMETERS	53	A	1833(T)		D			N
C9202	INJECTION, SUSPENSION OF MICROSPHERES OF HUMAN SERUM ALBUMIN WITH OCTAFLUOROPROPANE, PER 3 ML	53	A	1833T		D			A
C9203	INJECTION, PERFLEXANE LIPID MICROSPHERES, PER 10 ML VIAL	53	A	1833T		D			A
C9204	INJECTION, ZIPRASIDONE MESYLATE, PER 20 MG	53	A	1833T		D			D
C9205	INJECTION, OXALIPLATIN, PER 5 MG	53	A	1833T		D			D
C9208	INJECTION, AGALSIDASE BETA, PER 1 MG	53	A	1833T		D			A
C9209	INJECTION, LARONIDASE, PER 2.9 MG	53	A	1833T		D			A
C9500	PLATELETS, IRRADIATED, EACH UNIT	53	A	1833(t)		D			N
C9501	PLATELETS, PHERESIS, EACH UNIT	53	A	1833(t)		D			N
C9502	PLATELETS, PHERESIS, IRRADIATED, EACH UNIT	53	A	1833(t)		D			N
C9503	FRESH FROZEN PLASMA, DONOR RETESTED, EACH UNIT	53	A	1833(t)		D			D
C9504	RED BLOOD CELLS, DEGLYCEROLIZED, EA UNIT	53	A	1883(T)		D			N
C9505	RED BLOOD CELLS, IRRADIATED, EACH UNIT	53	A	1833(T)		D			N
C9506	GRANULOCYTES, PHERESIS, EACH UNIT	53	A	1833(T)		D			N
C9700	WATER INDUCED THERMOTHERAPY	53	A	1833(T)		D			N
C9701	STRETTA SYSTEM	53	A	1833(T)		D			T
C9702	CHECKMATE INTRAVASCULAR BRACHYTHERAPY SYSTEM, NOVOSTE BETA-CATH INTRAVASCULAR BRACHYTHERAPY SYSTEM, GALILEO INTRAVASCULAR RADIOTHERAPY SYSTEM	53	A	1833(T)		D			N
C9703	BARD ENDOSCOPIC SUTURING SYSTEM	53	A	1833(T)		D			T
C9708	PREVIEW TREATMENT PLANNING SOFTWARE	53	A	1833(T)		D			N
C9711	H.E.L.P. APHERESIS SYSTEM	53	A	1833(T)		D			T
D0120	PERIODIC ORAL EVALUATION	00	9	1862A(12)		S			N
D0140	LIMITED ORAL EVALUATION - PROBLEM FOCUSED	00	9	1862A(12)		S			N
D0150	COMPREHENSIVE ORAL EVALUATION - NEW OR ESTABLISHED PATIENT	13	A			D			N
D0160	DETAILED AND EXTENSIVE ORAL EVALUATION - PROBLEM FOCUSED, BY REPORT	00	9	1862A(12)		S			N
D0170	RE-EVALUATION-LIMITED, PROBLEM FOCUSED (ESTABLISHED PATIENT; NOT POST-OPERATIVE VISIT)	00	9	1862a(12)		S			N
D0180	COMPREHENSIVE PERIODONTAL EVALUATION - NEW OR ESTABLISHED PATIENT	00	9	1862a(12)		S			N

HCPCS	Long Description	PTI	MPI	Statute	X-Ref1	Coverage	ASC Pay Grp	ASC Pay Grp Eff Date	Action Code
D0210	INTRAORAL-COMPLETE SERIES (INCLUDING BITEWINGS)	00	9		70320	I			N
D0220	INTRAORAL-PERIAPICAL-FIRST FILM	00	9		70300	I			N
D0230	INTRAORAL-PERIAPICAL-EACH ADDITIONAL FILM	00	9		70310	I			N
D0240	INTRAORAL-0CCLUSAL FILM	13	A			D			N
D0250	EXTRAORAL-FIRST FILM	13	A			D			N
D0260	EXTRAORAL-EACH ADDITIONAL FILM	13	A			D			N
D0270	BITEWING-SINGLE FILM	13	A			D			N
D0272	BITEWINGS-TWO FILMS	13	A			D			N
D0274	BITEWINGS-FOUR FILMS	13	A			D			N
D0277	VERTICAL BITEWINGS - 7 TO 8 FILMS	13	A			D			N
D0290	POSTERIOR-ANTERIOR OR LATERAL SKULL AND FACIAL BONE SURVEY FILM	00	9		70150	I			N
D0310	SIALOGRAPHY	00	9		70390	I			N
D0320	TEMPOROMANDIBULAR JOINT ARTHROGRAM, INCLUDING INJECTION	00	9		70332	I			N
D0321	OTHER TEMPOROMANDIBULAR JOINT FILMS, BY REPORT	00	9		76499	I			N
D0322	TOMOGRAPHIC SURVEY	00	9		CPT	I			N
D0330	PANORAMIC FILM	00	9		70320	I			N
D0340	CEPHALOMETRIC FILM	00	9		70350	I			N
D0350	ORAL/FACIAL IMAGES (INCLUDES INTRA AND EXTRAORAL IMAGES)	00	9			I			N
D0415	BACTERIOLOGIC STUDIES FOR DETERMINATION OF PATHOLOGIC AGENTS	00	9	1862 A(12)	D0410	S			N
D0425	CARIES SUSCEPTIBILITY TESTS	00	9	1862 A(12)	D0420	S			N
D0460	PULP VITALITY TESTS	13	A			D			N
D0470	DIAGNOSTIC CASTS	00	9	1862 a(12)		S			N
D0472	ACCESSION OF TISSUE, GROSS EXAMINATION, PREPARATION AND TRANSMISSION OF WRITTEN REPORT	13	A			D			N
D0473	ACCESSION OF TISSUE, GROSS AND MICROSCOPIC EXAMINATION, PREPARATION AND TRANSMISSION OF WRITTEN REPORT	13	A			D			N
D0474	ACCESSION OF TISSUE, GROSS AND MICROSCOPIC EXAMINATION, INCLUDING ASSESSMENT OF SURGICAL MARGINS FOR PRESENCE OF DISEASE, PREPARATION AND TRANSMISSION OF WRITTEN REPORT	13	A			D			N
D0480	PROCESSING AND INTERPRETATION OF CYTOLOGIC SMEARS, INCLUDING THE PREPARATION AND TRANSMISSION OF WRITTEN REPORT	13	A			D			N
D0501	HISTOPATHOLOGIC EXAMINATIONS	13	A			D			N

HCPCS	Long Description	PH	MPI	Statute	X-Ref	Coverage	ASC Pay Grp	ASC Pay Grp Eff Date	Action Code
D0502	OTHER ORAL PATHOLOGY PROCEDURES, BY REPORT	13	A			D			N
D0999	UNSPECIFIED DIAGNOSTIC PROCEDURE, BY REPORT	13	A			D			N
D1110	PROPHYLAXIS-ADULT	00	9	1862 a(12)		S			N
D1120	PROPHYLAXIS-CHILD	00	9	1862 a(12)		S			N
D1201	TOPICAL APPLICATION OF FLUORIDE (INCLUDING PROPHYLAXIS)-CHILD	00	9	1862 a(12)		S			N
D1203	TOPICAL APPLICATION OF FLUORIDE (PROPHYLAXIS NOT INCLUDED)-CHILD	00	9	1862 a(12)		S			N
D1204	TOPICAL APPLICATION OF FLUORIDE (PROPHYLAXIS NOT INCLUDED)-ADULT	00	9	1862 a(12)		S			N
D1205	TOPICAL APPLICATION OF FLUORIDE (INCLUDING PROPHYLAXIS)-ADULT	00	9	1862 a(12)	D1202	S			N
D1310	NUTRITIONAL COUNSELING FOR THE CONTROL OF DENTAL DISEASE	00	9			M			N
D1320	TOBACCO COUNSELING FOR THE CONTROL AND PREVENTION OF ORAL DISEASE	00	9			M			N
D1330	ORAL HYGIENE INSTRUCTION	00	9			M			N
D1351	SEALANT-PER TOOTH	00	9	1862 a(12)		S			N
D1510	SPACE MAINTAINER-FIXED UNILATERAL	13	A			D			N
D1515	SPACE MAINTAINER-FIXED BILATERAL	13	A			D			N
D1520	SPACE MAINTAINER-REMOVABLE UNILATERAL	13	A			D			N
D1525	SPACE MAINTAINER-REMOVABLE BILATERAL	13	A			D			N
D1550	RECEMENTATION OF SPACE MAINTAINER	13	A			D			N
D2110	AMALGAM-ONE SURFACE, PRIMARY	00	9	1862 a(12)		S			N
D2120	AMALGAM-TWO SURFACES, PRIMARY	00	9	1862 a(12)		S			N
D2130	AMALGAM-THREE SURFACES, PRIMARY	00	9	1862 a(12)		S			N
D2131	AMALGAM-FOUR OR MORE SURFACES, PRIMARY	00	9	1862 a(12)		S			N
D2140	AMALGAM-ONE SURFACE, PRIMARY OR PERMANENT	00	9	1862 a(12)		S			N
D2150	AMALGAM-TWO SURFACES, PRIMARY OR PERMANENT	00	9	1862 a(12)		S			N
D2160	AMALGAM-THREE SURFACES, PRIMARY OR PERMANENT	00	9	1862 a(12)		S			N

HCPCS	Long Description	Pri	MPI	Statute	X-Ref	Coverage	ASC Pay Grp	ASC Pay Grp Eff Date	Action Code
D2161	AMALGAM-FOUR OR MORE SURFACES, PRIMARY OR PERMANENT	00	9	1862 a(12)		S			N
D2330	RESIN-ONE SURFACE, ANTERIOR	00	9	1862 a(12)		S			N
D2331	RESIN-TWO SURFACES, ANTERIOR	00	9	1861 a(12)		S			N
D2332	RESIN-THREE SURFACES, ANTERIOR	00	9	1862 a(12)		S			N
D2335	RESIN-FOUR OR MORE SURFACES OR INVOLVING INCISAL ANGLE (ANTERIOR)	00	9	1862 a(12)		S			N
D2336	COMPOSITE RESIN CROWN-ANTERIOR-PRIMARY	00	9	1862 a(12)		S			N
D2337	RESIN-BASED COMPOSITE CROWN, ANTERIOR-PERMANENT	00	9	1862a(12)		S			N
D2380	RESIN-ONE SURFACE, POSTERIOR-PRIMARY	00	9	1862 a(12)		S			N
D2381	RESIN-TWO SURFACES, POSTERIOR-PRIMARY	00	9	1862 a(12)		S			N
D2382	RESIN-THREE OR MORE SURFACES, POSTERIOR-PRIMARY	00	9	1862 a(12)		S			N
D2385	RESIN-ONE SURFACE, POSTERIOR-PERMANENT	00	9	1862 a(12)		S			N
D2386	RESIN-TWO SURFACES, POSTERIOR-PERMANENT	00	9	1862 a(12)		S			N
D2387	RESIN-THREE OR MORE SURFACES, POSTERIOR-PERMANENT	00	9	1862 a(12)		S			N
D2388	RESIN-BASED COMPOSITE - FOUR OR MORE SURFACES, POSTERIOR PERMANENT	00	9	1862a(12)		S			N
D2390	RESIN-BASED COMPOSITE CROWN, ANTERIOR	00	9	1862a(12)		S			N
D2391	RESIN-BASED COMPOSITE - ONE SURFACE, POSTERIOR	00	9	1862a(12)		S			N
D2392	RESIN-BASED COMPOSITE - TWO SURFACES, POSTERIOR	00	9	1862a(12)		S			N
D2393	RESIN-BASED COMPOSITE - THREE SURFACES, POSTERIOR	00	9	1862a(12)		S			N
D2394	RESIN-BASED COMPOSITE - FOUR OR MORE SURFACES, POSTERIOR	00	9	1862a(12)		S			N
D2410	GOLD FOIL-ONE SURFACE	00	9	1862 a(12)		S			N
D2420	GOLD FOIL-TWO SURFACES	00	9	1862 a(12)		S			N
D2430	GOLD FOIL-THREE SURFACES	00	9	1862 a(12)		S			N
D2510	INLAY-METALLIC-ONE SURFACE	00	9	1862 a(12)		S			N
D2520	INLAY-METALLIC-TWO SURFACES	00	9	1862 a(12)		S			N
D2530	INLAY-METALLIC-THREE OR MORE SURFACES	00	9	1862 a(12)		S			N

HCPCS	Long Description	PTI	MPI	Statute	X-Ref1	Coverage	ASC Pay Grp	ASC Pay Grp Eff Date	Action Code
D2542	ONLAY-METALLIC-TWO SURFACES	00	9	1862a(12)		S			N
D2543	ONLAY - METALLIC - THREE SURFACES	00	9	1862 a(12)		S			N
D2544	ONLAY - METALLIC - FOUR OR MORE SURFACES	00	9	1862 a(12)		S			N
D2610	INLAY-PORCELAIN/CERAMIC-ONE SURFACE	00	9	1862 a(12)		S			N
D2620	INLAY-PORCELAIN/CERAMIC-TWO SURFACES	00	9	1862 a(12)		S			N
D2630	INLAY-PORCELAIN/CERAMIC-THREE OR MORE SURFACES	00	9	1862 a(12)		S			N
D2642	ONLAY - PORCELAIN/CERAMIC - TWO SURFACES	00	9	1862 a(12)		S			N
D2643	ONLAY - PORCELAIN/CERAMIC - THREE SURFACES	00	9	1862 a(12)		S			N
D2644	ONLAY - PORCELAIN/CERAMIC - FOUR OR MORE SURFACES	00	9	1862 a(12)		S			N
D2650	INLAY - RESIN-BASED COMPOSITE - ONE SURFACE	00	9	1862 a(12)		S			N
D2651	INLAY - RESIN-BASED COMPOSITE - TWO SURFACES	00	9	1862 a(12)		S			N
D2652	INLAY - RESIN-BASED COMPOSITE - THREE OR MORE SURFACES	00	9	1862 a(12)		S			N
D2662	ONLAY - RESIN-BASED COMPOSITE - TWO SURFACES	00	9	1862 a(12)		S			N
D2663	ONLAY - RESIN-BASED COMPOSITE - THREE SURFACES	00	9	1862 a(12)		S			N
D2664	ONLAY - - RESIN-BASED COMPOSITE - FOUR OR MORE SURFACES	00	9	1862 a(12)		S			N
D2710	CROWN - RESIN (INDIRECT)	00	9	1862a(12)		S			N
D2720	CROWN-RESIN WITH HIGH NOBLE METAL	00	9	1862a(12)		S			N
D2721	CROWN-RESIN WITH PREDOMINANTLY BASE METAL	00	9	1862a(12)		S			N
D2722	CROWN-RESIN WITH NOBLE METAL	00	9	1862a(12)		S			N
D2740	CROWN-PORCELAIN/CERAMIC SUBSTRATE	00	9	1862a(12)		S			N
D2750	CROWN-PORCELAIN FUSED TO HIGH NOBLE METAL	00	9	1862a(12)		S			N
D2751	CROWN-PROCELAIN FUSED TO PREDOMINANTLY BASE METAL	00	9	1862a(12)		S			N
D2752	CROWN-PORCELAIN FUSED TO NOBLE METAL	00	9	1862a(12)		S			N
D2780	CROWN - 3/4 CAST HIGH NOBLE METAL	00	9	1862a(12)		S			N
D2781	CROWN - 3/4 CAST PREDOMINANTLY BASE METAL	00	9	1862a(12)		S			N

HCPCS	Long Description	PTI	MPI	Statute	X-Ref1	Coverage	ASC Pay Grp	ASC Pay Grp Eff Date	Action Code
D2782	CROWN - 3/4 CAST NOBLE METAL	00	9	1862a(12)		S			N
D2783	CROWN - 3/4 PORCELAIN/CERAMIC	00	9	1862a(12)		S			N
D2790	CROWN-FULL CAST HIGH NOBLE METAL	00	9	1862a(12)		S			N
D2791	CROWN-FULL CAST PREDOMINANTLY BASE METAL	00	9	1862a(12)		S			N
D2792	CROWN-FULL CAST NOBLE METAL	00	9	1862a(12)		S			N
D2799	PROVISIONAL CROWN	00	9	1862a(12)		S			N
D2910	RECEMENT INLAY	00	9	1862a(12)		S			N
D2920	RECEMENT CROWN	00	9	1862a(12)		S			N
D2930	PREFABRICATED STAINLESS STEEL CROWN-PRIMARY TOOTH	00	9	1862a(12)		S			N
D2931	PREFABRICATED STAINLESS STEEL CROWN-PERMANENT TOOTH	00	9	1862a(12)		S			N
D2932	PREFABRICATED RESIN CROWN	00	9	1862a(12)		S			N
D2933	PREFABRICATED STAINLESS STEEL CROWN WITH RESIN WINDOW	00	9	1862a(12)		S			N
D2940	SEDATIVE FILLING	00	9	1862a(12)		S			N
D2950	CORE BUILD-UP, INCLUDING ANY PINS	00	9	1862a(12)		S			N
D2951	PIN RETENTION-PER TOOTH, IN ADDITION TO RESTORATION	00	9	1862a(12)		S			N
D2952	CAST POST AND CORE IN ADDITION TO CROWN	00	9	1862a(12)		S			N
D2953	EACH ADDITIONAL CAST POST - SAME TOOTH	00	9	1862a(12)		S			N
D2954	PREFABRICATED POST AND CORE IN ADDITION TO CROWN	00	9	1862a(12)		S			N
D2955	POST REMOVAL (NOT IN CONJUCTION WITH ENDODONTIC THERAPY)	00	9	1862a(12)		S			N
D2957	EACH ADDITIONAL PREFABRICATED POST - SAME TOOTH	00	9	1862a(12)		S			N
D2960	LABIAL VENEER (LAMINATE)-CHAIRSIDE	00	9	1862a(12)		S			N
D2961	LABIAL VENEER (RESIN LAMINATE)-LABORATORY	00	9	1862a(12)		S			N
D2962	LABIAL VENEER (PORCELAIN LAMINATE)-LABORATORY	00	9	1862a(12)		S			N
D2970	TEMPORARY (FRACTURED TOOTH)	13	A			D			N
D2980	CROWN REPAIR, BY REPORT	00	9	1862a(12)		S			N
D2999	UNSPECIFIED RESTORATIVE PROCEDURE, BY REPORT	13	A			D			N
D3110	PULP CAP-DIRECT (EXCLUDING FINAL RESTORATION)	00	9	1862a(12)		S			N
D3120	PULP CAP-INDIRECT (EXCLUDING FINAL RESTORATION)	00	9	1862a(12)		S			N

HCPCS	Long Description	PI	MPI	Statute	X-Ref1	Coverage	ASC Pay Grp	ASC Pay Grp Eff Date	Action Code
D3220	THERAPEUTIC PULPOTOMY (EXCLUDING FINAL RESTORATION) REMOVAL OF PULP CORONAL TO THE DENTINOCEMENTAL JUNCTION AND APPLICATION OF MEDICAMENT	00	9	1862a(12)		S			N
D3221	PULPAL DEBRIDEMENT, PRIMARY AND PERMANENT TEETH	00	9	1862a(12)		S			N
D3230	PULPAL THERAPY (RESORBABLE FILLING)-ANTERIOR, PRIMARY TOOTH (EXCLUDING FINAL RESTORATION)	00	9	1862a(12)		S			N
D3240	PULPAL THERAPY (RESORBABLE FILLING)-POSTERIOR, PRIMARY TOOTH (EXCLUDING FINAL RESTORATION)	00	9	1862a(12)		S			N
D3310	ANTERIOR (EXCLUDING FINAL RESTORATION)	00	9	1862a(12)		S			N
D3320	BICUSPID (EXCLUDING FINAL RESTORATION)	00	9	1862a(12)		S			N
D3330	MOLAR (EXCLUDING FINAL RESTORATION)	00	9	1862a(12)		S			N
D3331	TREATMENT OF ROOT CANAL OBSTRUCTION; NON-SURGICAL ACCESS	00	9	1862a(12)		S			N
D3332	INCOMPLETE ENDODONTIC THERAPY; INOPERABLE OR FRACTURED TOOTH	00	9	1862a(12)		S			N
D3333	INTERNAL ROOT REPAIR OF PERFORATION DEFECTS	00	9	1862a(12)		S			N
D3346	RETREATMENT OF PREVIOUS ROOT CANAL THERAPY-ANTERIOR	00	9	1862a(12)		S			N
D3347	RETREATMENT OF PREVIOUS ROOT CANAL THERAPY-BICUSPID	00	9	1862a(12)		S			N
D3348	RETREATMENT OF PREVIOUS ROOT CANAL THERAPY-MOLAR	00	9	1862a(12)		S			N
D3351	APEXIFICATION/RECALCIFICATION-INITIAL VISIT (APICAL CLOSURE/CALCIFIC REPAIR OF PERFORATIONS, ROOT RESORPTION, ETC.)	00	9	1862a(12)		S			N
D3352	APEXIFICATION/RECALCIFICATION-INTERIM MEDICATION REPLACEMENT (APICAL CLOSURE/CALCIFIC REPAIR OF PERFORATIONS, ROOT RESORPTION, ETC.)	00	9	1862a(12)		S			N
D3353	APEXIFICATION/RECALCIFICATION-FINAL VISIT (INCLUDES COMPLETED ROOT CANAL THERAPY-APICAL CLOSURE/CALCIFIC REPAIR OF PERFORATIONS, ROOT RESORPTION, ETC.)	00	9	1862a(12)		S			N
D3410	APICOECTOMY/PERIRADICULAR SURGERY-ANTERIOR	00	9	1862a(12)		S			N
D3421	APICOECTOMY/PERIRADICULAR SURGERY-BICUSPID (FIRST ROOT)	00	9	1862a(12)		S			N
D3425	APICOECTOMY/PERIRADICULAR SURGERY-MOLAR (FIRST ROOT).	00	9	1862a(12)		S			N
D3426	APICOECTOMY/PERIRADICULAR SURGERY (EACH ADDITIONAL ROOT)	00	9	1862a(12)		S			N
D3430	RETROGRADE FILLING-PER ROOT	00	9	1862a(12)		S			N
D3450	ROOT AMPUTATION-PER ROOT	00	9	1862a(12)		S			N
D3460	ENDODONTIC ENDOSSEOUS IMPLANT	13	A			D			N
D3470	INTENTIONAL REPLANTATION (INCLUDING NECESSARY SPLINTING)	00	9	1862a(12)		S			N
D3910	SURGICAL PROCEDURE FOR ISOLATION OF TOOTH WITH RUBBER DAM	00	9	1862a(12)		S			N
D3920	HEMISECTION (INCLUDING ANY ROOT REMOVAL), NOT INCLUDING ROOT CANAL THERAPY	00	9	1862a(12)		S			N
D3950	CANAL PREPARATION AND FITTING OF PREFORMED DOWEL OR POST	00	9	1862a(12)		S			N
D3999	UNSPECIFIED ENDODONTIC PROCEDURE, BY REPORT	13	A			D			N
D4210	GINGIVECTOMY OR GINGIVOPLASTY - FOUR OR MORE CONTIGUOUS TEETH OR BOUNDED TEETH SPACES, PER QUADRANT	00	9		41820	I			N

HCPCS	Long Description	PH	MPI	Statute	X-Ref	Coverage	ASC Pay Grp	ASC Pay Grp Eff Date	Action Code
D4211	GINGIVECTOMY OR GINGIVOPLASTY - ONE TO THREE TEETH, PER QUADRANT	00	9		CPT	I			N
D4220	GINGIVAL CURETTAGE, SURGICAL, PER QUADRANT, BY REPORT	00	9	1862a(12)		S			N
D4240	GINGIVAL FLAP PROCEDURE, INCLUDING ROOT PLANING - FOUR OR MORE CONTIGUOUS TEETH OR BOUNDED TEETH SPACES, PER QUADRANT	00	9	1862a(12)		S			N
D4241	GINGIVAL FLAP PROCEDURE, INCLUDING ROOT PLANING - ONE TO THREE TEETH, PER QUADRANT	00	9	1862a(12)		S			N
D4245	APICALLY POSITIONED FLAP	00	9	1862a(12)		S			N
D4249	CLINICAL CROWN LENGTHENING-HARD TISSUE	00	9	1862a(12)		S			N
D4260	OSSEOUS SURGERY (INCLUDING FLAP ENTRY AND CLOSURE) - FOUR OR MORE CONTIGUOUS TEETH OR BOUNDED TEETH SPACES, PER QUADRANT	13	A			D			N
D4261	OSSEOUS SURGERY (INCLUDING FLAP ENTRY AND CLOSURE) - ONE TO THREE TEETH, PER QUADRANT	00	9	1862a(12)		S			N
D4263	BONE REPLACEMENT GRAFT - FIRST SITE IN QUADRANT	13	A			D			N
D4264	BONE REPLACEMENT GRAFT - EACH ADDITIONAL SITE IN QUADRANT	13	A			D			N
D4265	BIOLOGIC MATERIALS TO AID IN SOFT AND OSSEOUS TISSUE REGENERATION	00	9	1862a(12)		S			N
D4266	GUIDED TISSUE REGENERATION - RESORBABLE BARRIER, PER SITE	00	9	1862a(12)		S			N
D4267	GUIDED TISSUE REGENERATION - NONRESORBABLE BARRIER, PER SITE, (INCLUDES MEMBRANE REMOVAL)	00	9	1862a(12)		S			N
D4268	SURGICAL REVISION PROCEDURE, PER TOOTH	00	9			D			N
D4270	PEDICLE SOFT TISSUE GRAFT PROCEDURE	13	A			D			N
D4271	FREE SOFT TISSUE GRAFT PROCEDURE (INCLUDING DONOR SITE SURGERY)	13	A			D			N
D4273	SUBEPITHELIAL CONNECTIVE TISSUE GRAFT PROCEDURES	13	A			D			N
D4274	DISTAL OR PROXIMAL WEDGE PROCEDURE (WHEN NOT PERFORMED IN CONJUCTION WITH SURGICAL PROCEDURES IN THE SAME ANATOMICAL AREA)	00	9	1862a(12)		S			N
D4275	SOFT TISSUE ALLOGRAFT	00	9	1862a(12)		S			N
D4276	COMBINED CONNECTIVE TISSUE AND DOUBLE PEDICLE GRAFT	00	9	1862a(12)		S			N
D4320	PROVISIONAL SPLINTING-INTRACORONAL	00	9	1862a(12)		S			N
D4321	PROVISIONAL SPLINTING-EXTRACORONAL	00	9	1862a(12)		S			N
D4341	PERIODONTAL SCALING AND ROOT PLANING - FOUR OR MORE CONTIGUOUS TEETH OR BOUNDED TEETH SPACES, PER QUADRANT	00	9	1862a(12)		S			N
D4342	PERIODONTAL SCALING AND ROOT PLANING - ONE TO THREE TEETH, PER QUADRANT	00	9	1862a(12)		S			N
D4355	FULL MOUTH DEBRIDEMENT TO ENABLE COMPREHENSIVE EVALUATION AND DIAGNOSIS	13	A			D			N

HCPCS	Long Description	PII	MPI	Statute	X-Refl	Coverage	ASC Pay Grp	ASC Pay Grp Eff Date	Action Code
D4381	LOCALIZED DELIVERY OF CHEMOTHERAPEUTIC AGENTS VIA A CONTROLLED RELEASE VEHICLE INTO DISEASED CREVICULAR TISSUE, PER TOOTH, BY REPORT	13	A			D			N
D4910	PERIODONTAL MAINTENANCE	00	9	1862a(12)		S			N
D5640	REPLACE BROKEN TEETH-PER TOOTH	00	9	1862a(12)		S			N
D5650	ADD TOOTH TO EXISTING PARTIAL DENTURE	00	9	1862a(12)		S			N
D5660	ADD CLASP TO EXISTING PARTIAL DENTURE	00	9	1862a(12)		S			N
D5670	REPLACE ALL TEETH AND ACRYLIC ON CAST METAL FRAMEWORK (MAXILLARY)	00	9	1862a(12)		S			N
D5671	REPLACE ALL TEETH AND ACRYLIC ON CAST METAL FRAMEWORK (MANDIBULAR)	00	9	1862a(12)		S			N
D5710	REBASE COMPLETE MAXILLARY DENTURE	00	9	1862a(12)		S			N
D5711	REBASE COMPLETE MANDIBULAR DENTURE	00	9	1862a(12)		S			N
D5720	REBASE MAXILLARY PARTIAL DENTURE	00	9	1862a(12)		S			N
D5721	REBASE MANDIBULAR PARTIAL DENTURE	00	9	1862a(12)		S			N
D5730	RELINE COMPLETE MAXILLARY DENTURE (CHAIRSIDE)	00	9	1862a(12)		S			N
D5731	RELINE LOWER COMPLETE MANDIBULAR DENTURE (CHAIRSIDE)	00	9	1862a(12)		S			N
D5740	RELINE MAXILLARY PARTIAL DENTURE (CHAIRSIDE)	00	9	1862a(12)		S			N
D5741	RELINE MANDIBULAR PARTIAL DENTURE (CHAIRSIDE)	00	9	1862a(12)		S			N
D5750	RELINE COMPLETE MAXILLARY DENTURE (LABORATORY)	00	9	1862a(12)		S			N
D5751	RELINE COMPLETE MANDIBULAR DENTURE (LABORATORY)	00	9	1862a(12)		S			N
D5760	RELINE MAXILLARY PARTIAL DENTURE (LABORATORY)	00	9	1862a(12)		S			N
D5761	RELINE MANDIBULAR PARTIAL DENTURE (LABORATORY)	13	9	1862a(12)		S			N
D5810	INTERIM COMPLETE DENTURE (MAXILLARY)	00	9	1862a(12)		S			N
D5811	INTERIM COMPLETE DENTURE (MANDIBULAR)	00	9	1862a(12)		S			N
D5820	INTERIM PARTIAL DENTURE (MAXILLARY)	00	9	1862a(12)		S			N
D5821	INTERIM PARTIAL DENTURE (MANDIBULAR)	00	9	1862a(12)		S			N
D5850	TISSUE CONDITIONING, MAXILLARY	00	9	1862a(12)		S			N
D5851	TISSUE CONDITIONING, MANDIBULAR	00	9	1862a(12)		S			N
D5860	OVERDENTURE-COMPLETE, BY REPORT	00	9	1862a(12)		S			N

HCPCS	Long Description	PTI	MPI	Statute	X-Ref	Coverage	ASC Pay Grp	ASC Pay Grp Eff Date	Action Code
D5861	OVERDENTURE-PARTIAL, BY REPORT	00	9	1862a(12)		S			N
D5862	PRECISION ATTACHMENT, BY REPORT	00	9	1862a(12)		S			N
D5867	REPLACEMENT OF REPLACEABLE PART OF SEMI-PRECISION OR PRECISION ATTACHMENT (MALE OR FEMALE COMPONENT)	00	9	1862a(12)		S			N
D5875	MODIFICATION OF REMOVABLE PROSTHESIS FOLLOWING IMPLANT SURGERY	00	9	1862a(12)		S			N
D5899	UNSPECIFIED REMOVABLE PROSTHODONTIC PROCEDURE, BY REPORT	00	9	1862a(12)		S			N
D5911	FACIAL MOULAGE (SECTIONAL)	13	A			D			N
D5912	FACIAL MOULAGE (COMPLETE)	13	A			D			N
D5913	NASAL PROSTHESIS	00	9		21087	I			N
D5914	AURICULAR PROSTHESIS	00	9		21086	I			N
D5915	ORBITAL PROSTHESIS	00	9		L8611	I			N
D5916	OCULAR PROSTHESIS	00	9		CPT, V2623, V2629	I			N
D5919	FACIAL PROSTHESIS	00	9		21088	I			N
D5922	NASAL SEPTAL PROSTHESIS	00	9		30220	I			N
D5923	OCULAR PROSTHESIS, INTERIM	00	9		92330	I			N
D5924	CRANIAL PROSTHESIS	00	9		62143	I			N
D5925	FACIAL AUGMENTATION IMPLANT PROSTHESIS	00	9		21208	I			N
D5926	NASAL PROSTHESIS, REPLACEMENT	00	9		21087	I			N
D5927	AURICULAR PROSTHESIS, REPLACEMENT	00	9		21086	I			N
D5928	ORBITAL PROSTHESIS, REPLACEMENT	00	9		67550	I			N
D5929	FACIAL PROSTHESIS, REPLACEMENT	00	9		21088	I			N
D5931	OBTURATOR PROSTHESIS, SURGICAL	00	9		21079	I			N
D5932	OBTURATOR PROSTHESIS, DEFINITIVE	00	9		21080	I			N
D5933	OBTURATOR PROSTHESIS, MODIFICATION	00	9		21080	I			N
D5934	MANDIBULAR RESECTION PROSTHESIS WITH GUIDE FLANGE	00	9		21081	I			N
D5935	MANDIBULAR RESECTION PROSTHESIS WITHOUT GUIDE FLANGE	00	9		21081	I			N
D5936	OBTURATOR/PROSTHESIS, INTERIM	00	9		21079	I			N
D5937	TRISMUS APPLIANCE (NOT FOR TM TREATMENT)	00	9			I			N
D5951	FEEDING AID	13	A			D			N
D5952	SPEECH AID PROSTHESIS, PEDIATRIC	00	9		21084	I			N
D5953	SPEECH AID PROSTHESIS, ADULT	00	9		21084	I			N

HCPCS	Long Description	PTI	MPI	Statute	X-Ref1	Coverage	ASC Pay Grp	ASC Pay Grp Eff Date	Action Code
D5954	PALATAL AUGMENTATION PROSTHESIS	00	9		21082	I			N
D5955	PALATAL LIFT PROSTHESIS, DEFINITIVE	00	9		21083	I			N
D5958	PALATAL LIFT PROSTHESIS, INTERIM	00	9		21083	I			N
D5959	PALATAL LIFT PROSTHESIS, MODIFICATION	00	9		21083	I			N
D5960	SPEECH AID PROSTHESIS, MODIFICATION	00	9		21084	I			N
D5982	SURGICAL STENT	00	9		21085	I			N
D5983	RADIATION CARRIER	13	A			D			N
D5984	RADIATION SHIELD	13	A			D			N
D5985	RADIATION CONE LOCATOR	13	A			D			N
D5986	FLUORIDE GEL CARRIER	00	9	1862a(12)		S			N
D5987	COMMISSURE SPLINT	13	A			D			N
D5988	SURGICAL SPLINT	13	A		CPT	I			N
D5999	UNSPECIFIED MAXILLOFACIAL PROSTHESIS, BY REPORT	00	9		CPT	I			N
D6010	SURGICAL PLACEMENT OF IMPLANT BODY: ENDOSTEAL IMPLANT	00	9		21248	I			N
D6020	ABUTMENT PLACEMENT OR SUBSTITUTION: ENDOSTEAL IMPLANT	00	9		21248	I			N
D6040	SURGICAL PLACEMENT: EPOSTEAL IMPLANT	00	9		21245	I			N
D6050	SURGICAL PLACEMENT: TRANSOSTEAL IMPLANT	00	9		21244	I			N
D6053	IMPLANT/ABUTMENT SUPPORTED REMOVABLE DENTURE FOR COMPLETELY EDENTULOUS ARCH	00	9			M			N
D6054	IMPLANT/ABUTMENT SUPPORTED REMOVABLE DENTURE FOR PARTIALLY EDENTULOUS ARCH	00	9			M			N
D6055	DENTAL IMPLANT SUPPORTED CONNECTING BAR	00	9			I			N
D6056	PREFABRICATED ABUTMENT	00	9			M			N
D6057	CUSTOM ABUTMENT	00	9			M			N
D6058	ABUTMENT SUPPORTED PORCELAIN/CERAMIC CROWN	00	9			M			N
D6059	ABUTMENT SUPPORTED PORCELAIN FUSED TO METAL CROWN (HIGH NOBLE METAL)	00	9			M			N
D6060	ABUTMENT SUPPORTED PORCELAIN FUSED TO METAL CROWN (PREDOMINANTLY BASE METAL)	00	9			M			N
D6061	ABUTMENT SUPPORTED PORCELAIN FUSED TO METAL CROWN (NOBLE METAL)	00	9			M			N
D6062	ABUTMENT SUPPORTED CAST METAL CROWN (HIGH NOBLE METAL)	00	9			M			N
D6063	ABUTMENT SUPPORTED CAST METAL CROWN (PREDOMINANTLY BASE METAL)	00	9			M			N
D6064	ABUTMENT SUPPORTED CAST METAL CROWN (NOBLE METAL)	00	9			M			N

HCPCS	Long Description	PII	MPI	Statute	X-Ref1	Coverage	ASC Pay Grp	ASC Pay Grp Eff Date	Action Code
D6065	IMPLANT SUPPORTED PORCELAIN/CERAMIC CROWN	00	9			M			N
D6066	IMPLANT SUPPORTED PORCELAIN FUSED TO METAL CROWN (TITANIUM, TITANIUM ALLOY, HIGH NOBLE METAL)	00	9			M			N
D6067	IMPLANT SUPPORTED METAL CROWN (TITANIUM, TITANIUM ALLOY, HIGH NOBLE METAL)	00	9			M			N
D6068	ABUTMENT SUPPORTED RETAINER FOR PORCELAIN/CERAMIC FPD	00	9			M			N
D6069	ABUTMENT SUPPORTED RETAINER FOR PORCELAIN FUSED TO METAL FPD (HIGH NOBLE METAL)	00	9			M			N
D6070	ABUTMENT SUPPORTED RETAINER FOR PORCELAIN FUSED TO METAL FPD (PREDOMINANTLY BASE METAL)	00	9			M			N
D6071	ABUTMENT SUPPORTED RETAINER FOR PORCELAIN FUSED TO METAL FPD (NOBLE METAL)	00	9			M			N
D6072	ABUTMENT SUPPORTED RETAINER FOR CAST METAL FPD (HIGH NOBLE METAL)	00	9			M			N
D6073	ABUTMENT SUPPORTED RETAINER FOR CAST METAL FPD (PREDOMINANTLY BASE METAL)	00	9			M			N
D6074	ABUTMENT SUPPORTED RETAINER FOR CAST METAL FPD (NOBLE METAL)	00	9			M			N
D6075	IMPLANT SUPPORTED RETAINER FOR CERAMIC FPD	00	9			M			N
D6076	IMPLANT SUPPORTED RETAINER FOR PORCELAIN FUSED TO METAL FPD (TITANIUM, TITANIUM ALLOY, OR HIGH NOBLE METAL)	00	9			M			N
D6077	IMPLANT SUPPORTED RETAINER FOR CAST METAL FPD (TITANIUM, TITANIUM ALLOY, OR HIGH NOBLE METAL)	00	9			M			N
D6078	IMPLANT/ABUTMENT SUPPORTED FIXED DENTURE FOR COMPLETELY EDENTULOUS ARCH	00	9			M			N
D6079	IMPLANT/ABUTMENT SUPPORTED FIXED DENTURE FOR PARTIALLY EDENTULOUS ARCH	00	9			M			N
D6080	IMPLANT MAINTENANCE PROCEDURES, INCLUDING: REMOVAL OF PROSTHESIS, CLEANSING OF PROSTHESIS AND ABUTMEN REINSERTION OF PROSTHESIS	00	9			I			N
D6090	REPAIR IMPLANTSUPPORTED PROSTHESIS BY REPORT	00	9		21299	I			N
D6095	REPAIR IMPLANT ABUTMENT, BY REPORT	00	9		21299	I			N
D6100	IMPLANT REMOVAL, BY REPORT	00	9		21299	I			N
D6199	UNSPECIFIED IMPLANT PROCEDURE, BY REPORT	00	9		21299	I			N
D6210	PONTIC-CAST HIGH NOBLE METAL	00	9	1862a(12)		S			N
D6211	PONTIC-CAST PREDOMINANTLY BASE METAL	00	9	1862a(12)		S			N
D6212	PONTIC-CAST NOBLE METAL	00	9	1862a(12)		S			N
D6240	PONTIC-PORCELAIN FUSED TO HIGH NOBLE METAL	00	9	1862a(12)		S			N
D6241	PONTIC-PORCELAIN FUSED TO PREDOMINANTLY BASE METAL	00	9	1862a(12)		S			N

HCPCS	Long Description	PH	MPI	Statute	X-Ref1	Coverage	ASC Pay Grp	ASC Pay Grp Eff Date	Action Code
D6242	PONTIC-PORCELAIN FUSED TO NOBLE METAL	00	9	1862a(12)		S			N
D6245	PONTIC - PORCELAIN/CERAMIC	00	9			M			N
D6250	PONTIC-RESIN WITH HIGH NOBLE METAL	00	9	1862a(12)		S			N
D6251	PONTIC-RESIN WITH PREDOMINANTLY BASE METAL	00	9	1862a(12)		S			N
D6252	PONTIC-RESIN WITH NOBLE METAL	00	9	1862a(12)		S			N
D6253	PROVISIONAL PONTIC	00	9	1862a(12)		S			N
D6519	INLAY/ONLAY - PORCELAIN/CERAMIC	00	9			M			N
D6520	INLAY-METALLIC-TWO SURFACES	00	9	1862a(12)		S			N
D6530	INLAY-METALLIC-THREE OR MORE SURFACES	00	9	1862a(12)		S			N
D6543	ONLAY-METALLIC - THREE SURFACES	00	9	1862a(12)		S			N
D6544	ONLAY-METALLIC - FOUR OR MORE SURFACES	00	9	1862a(12)		S			N
D6545	RETAINER-CAST METAL FOR RESIN BONDED FIXED PROSTHESIS	00	9	1862a(12)		S			N
D6548	RETAINER - PORCELAIN/CERAMIC FOR RESIN BONDED FIXED PROSTHESIS	00	9			M			N
D6600	INLAY-PORCELAIN/CERAMIC, TWO SURFACES	00	9			M			N
D6601	INLAY - PORCELAIN/CERAMIC, THREE OR MORE SURFACES	00	9			M			N
D6602	INLAY - CAST HIGH NOBLE METAL, TWO SURFACES	00	9			M			N
D6603	INLAY - CAST HIGH NOBLE METAL, THREE OR MORE SURFACES	00	9			M			N
D6604	INLAY - CAST PREDOMINANTLY BASE METAL, TWO SURFACES	00	9			M			N
D6605	INLAY - CAST PREDOMINANTLY BASE METAL, THREE OR MORE SURFACES	00	9			M			N
D6606	INLAY - CAST NOBLE METAL, TWO SURFACES	00	9			M			N
D6607	INLAY - CAST NOBLE METAL, THREE OR MORE SURFACES	00	9			M			N
D6608	ONLAY - PORCELAIN/CERAMIC, TWO SURFACES	00	9			M			N
D6609	ONLAY - PORCELAIN/CERAMIC, THREE OR MORE SURFACES	00	9			M			N
D6610	ONLAY - CAST HIGH NOBLE METAL, TWO SURFACES	00	9			M			N
D6611	ONLAY - CAST HIGH NOBLE METAL, THREE OR MORE SURFACES	00	9			M			N
D6612	ONLAY - CAST PREDOMINANTLY BASE METAL, TWO SURFACES	00	9			M			N
D6613	ONLAY - CAST PREDOMINANTLY BASE METAL, THREE OR MORE SURFACES	00	9			M			N

HCPCS	Long Description	PII	MPI	Statute	X-Ref	Coverage	ASC Pay Grp	ASC Pay Grp Eff Date	Action Code
D6614	ONLAY - CAST NOBLE METAL, TWO SURFACES	00	9			M			N
D6615	ONLAY - CAST NOBLE METAL, THREE OR MORE SURFACES	00	9			M			N
D6720	CROWN-RESIN WITH HIGH NOBLE METAL	00	9	1862a(12)		S			N
D6721	CROWN-RESIN WITH PREDOMINANTLY BASE METAL	00	9	1862a(12)		S			N
D6722	CROWN-RESIN WITH NOBLE METAL	00	9	1862a(12)		S			N
D6740	CROWN - PORCELAIN/CERAMIC	00	9			M			N
D6750	CROWN-PORCELAIN FUSED TO HIGH NOBLE METAL	00	9	1862a(12)		S			N
D6751	CROWN-PORCELAIN FUSED TO PREDOMINANTLY BASE METAL	00	9	1862a(12)		S			N
D6752	CROWN-PORCELAIN FUSED TO NOBLE METAL	00	9	1862a(12)		S			N
D6780	CROWN-3/4 CAST HIGH NOBLE METAL	00	9	1862a(12)		S			N
D6781	CROWN - 3/4 CAST PREDOMINANTLY BASED METAL	00	9			M			N
D6782	CROWN - 3/4 CAST NOBLE METAL	00	9			M			N
D6783	CROWN - 3/4 PORCELAIN/CERAMIC	00	9			M			N
D6790	CROWN-FULL CAST HIGH NOBLE METAL	00	9	1862a(12)		S			N
D6791	CROWN-FULL CAST PREDOMINANTLY BASE METAL	00	9	1862a(12)		S			N
D6792	CROWN-FULL CAST NOBLE METAL	00	9	1862a(12)		S			N
D6793	PROVISIONAL RETAINER CROWN	00	9	1862a(12)		S			N
D6920	CONNECTOR BAR	13	A			D			N
D6930	RECEMENT BRIDGE	00	9	1862a(12)		S			N
D6940	STRESS BREAKER	00	9	1862a(12)		S			N
D6950	PRECISION ATTACHMENT	00	9	1862a(12)		S			N
D6970	CAST POST AND CORE IN ADDITION TO BRIDGE RETAINER	00	9	1862a(12)		S			N
D6971	CAST POST AS PART OF BRIDGE RETAINER	00	9	1862a(12)		S			N
D6972	PREFABRICATED POST AND CORE IN ADDITION TO BRIDGE RETAINER	00	9	1862a(12)		S			N
D6973	CORE BUILD UP FOR RETAINER, INCLUDING ANY PINS	00	9	1862a(12)		S			N
D6975	COPING-METAL	00	9	1862a(12)		S			N
D6976	EACH ADDITIONAL CAST POST - SAME TOOTH	00	9			M			N

HCPCS	Long Description	PII	MPI	Statute	X-Ref	Coverage	ASC Pay Grp	ASC Pay Grp Eff Date	Action Code
D6977	EACH ADDITIONAL PREFABRICATED POST - SAME TOOTH	00	9			M			N
D6980	BRIDGE REPAIR, BY REPORT	00	9	1862a(12)		S			N
D6985	PEDIATRIC PARTIAL DENTURE, FIXED	00	9	1862a(12)		S			N
D6999	UNSPECIFIED FIXED PROSTHODONTIC PROCEDURE, BY REPORT	00	9	1862a(12)		S			N
D7110	SINGLE TOOTH	13	A			D			N
D7111	CORONAL REMNANTS - DECIDUOUS TOOTH	13	A			D			N
D7120	EACH ADDITIONAL TOOTH	13	A			D			N
D7130	ROOT REMOVAL-EXPOSED ROOTS	13	A			D			N
D7140	EXTRACTION, ERUPTED TOOTH OR EXPOSED ROOT (ELEVATION AND/OR FORCEPS REMOVAL)	13	A			D			N
D7210	SURGICAL REMOVAL OF ERUPTED TOOTH REQUIRING ELEVATION OF MUCOPERIOSTEAL FLAP AND REMOVAL OF BONE AND/OR SECTION OF TOOTH	13	A			D			N
D7220	REMOVAL OF IMPACTED TOOTH-SOFT TISSUE	13	A			D			N
D7230	REMOVAL OF IMPACTED TOOTH-PARTIALLY BONY	13	A			D			N
D7240	REMOVAL OF IMPACTED TOOTH-COMPLETELY BONY	13	A			D			N
D7241	REMOVAL OF IMPACTED TOOTH-COMPLETELY BONY, WITH UNUSUAL SURGICAL COMPLICATIONS	13	A			D			N
D7250	SURGICAL REMOVAL OF RESIDUAL TOOTH ROOTS (CUTTING PROCEDURE)	13	A			D			N
D7260	ORAL ANTRAL FISTULA CLOSURE	13	A			D			N
D7261	PRIMARY CLOSURE OF A SINUS PERFORATION	13	A			D			N
D7270	TOOTH REIMPLANTATION AND/OR STABILIZATION OF ACCIDENTALLY EVULSED OR DISPLACED TOOTH	00	9	1862a(12)		S			N
D7272	TOOTH TRANSPLANTATION (INCLUDES REIMPLANTATION FROM ONE SITE TO ANOTHER AND SPLINTING AND/OR STABILIZATION)	00	9	1862a(12)		S			N
D7280	SURGICAL ACCESS OF AN UNERUPTED TOOTH	00	9	1862a(12)		S			N
D7281	SURGICAL EXPOSURE OF IMPACTED OR UNERUPTED TOOTH TO AID ERUPTION	00	9	1862a(12)		S			N
D7282	MOBILIZATION OF ERUPTED OR MALPOSITIONED TOOTH TO AID ERUPTION	00	9	1862a(12)		S			N
D7285	BIOPSY OF ORAL TISSUE - HARD (BONE, TOOTH)	00	9		20220, 20225, 20240, 20245	I			N
D7286	BIOPSY OF ORAL TISSUE - SOFT (ALL OTHERS)	00	9		40808	I			N
D7287	CYTOLOGY SAMPLE COLLECTION	00	9			I			N

HCPCS	Long Description	PTI	MPI	Statute	X-Ref	Coverage	ASC Pay Grp	ASC Pay Grp Eff Date	Action Code
D7290	SURGICAL REPOSITIONING OF TEETH	00	9	1862a(12)		S			N
D7291	TRANSSEPTAL FIBEROTOMY/SUPRA CRESTAL FIBEROTOMY, BY REPORT	13	A			D			N
D7310	ALVEOLOPLASTY IN CONJUNCTION WITH EXTRACTIONS - PER QUADRANT	00	9		41874	I			N
D7320	ALVEOLOPLASTY NOT IN CONJUNCTION WITH EXTRACTIONS - PER QUADRANT	00	9		41870	I			N
D7340	VESTIBULOPLASTY-RIDGE EXTENSION (SECOND EPITHELIALIZATION)	00	9		40840, 40842, 40844	I			N
D7350	VESTIBULOPLASTY-RIDGE EXTENSION (INCLUDING SOFT TISSUE GRAFTS, MUSCLE RE-ATTACHMENTS, REVISION OF SOFT TISSUE ATTACHMENT, AND MANAGEMENT OF HYPERTROPHIED AND HYPERPLASTIC TISSUE)	00	9		40845	I			N
D7410	EXCISION OF BENIGN LESION UP TO 1.25 CM	00	9		CPT	I			N
D7411	EXCISION OF BENIGN LESION GREATER THAN 1.25 CM	00	9			I			N
D7412	EXCISION OF BENIGN LESION, COMPLICATED	00	9			I			N
D7413	EXCISION OF MALIGNANT LESION UP TO 1.25 CM	00	9			I			N
D7414	EXCISION OF MALIGNANT LESION GREATER THAN 1.25 CM	00	9			I			N
D7415	EXCISION OF MALIGNANT LESION, COMPLICATED	00	9			I			N
D7420	RADICAL EXCISION-LESION DIAMETER GREATER THAN 1.25 CM	00	9		CPT	I			N
D7430	EXCISION OF BENIGN TUMOR-LESION DIAMETER UP TO 1.25 CM	00	9		CPT	I			N
D7431	EXCISION OF BENIGN TUMOR-LESION DIAMETER GREATER THAN 1.25 CM	00	9		CPT	I			N
D7440	EXCISION OF MALIGNANT TUMOR-LESION DIAMETER UP TO 1.25 CM	00	9		CPT	I			N
D7441	EXCISION OF MALIGNANT TUMOR-LESION DIAMETER GREATER THAN 1.25 CM	00	9		CPT	I			N
D7450	REMOVAL OF BENIGN ODONTOGENIC CYST OR TUMOR-LESION DIAMETER UP T0 1.25 CM	00	9		CPT	I			N
D7451	REMOVAL OF BENIGN ODONTOGENIC CYST OR TUMOR-LESION DIAMETER GREATER THAN 1.25 CM	00	9		CPT	I			N
D7460	REMOVAL OF BENIGN NONODONTOGENIC CYST OR TUMOR-LESION DIAMETER UP TO 1.25 CM	00	9		CPT	I			N
D7461	REMOVAL OF BENIGN NONODONTOGENIC CYST OR TUMOR-LESION DIAMETER GREATER THAN 1.25 CM	00	9		CPT	I			N
D7465	DESTRUCTION OF LESION(S) BY PHYSICAL OR CHEMICAL METHODS, BY REPORT	00	9		41850	I			N
D7471	REMOVAL OF LATERAL EXOSTOSIS (MAXILLA OR MANDIBLE)	00	9		21031,2	I			N
D7472	REMOVAL OF TORUS PALATINUS	00	9			I			N

HCPCS	Long Description	PII	MPI	Statute	X-Ref1	Coverage	ASC Pay Grp	ASC Pay Grp Eff Date	Action Code
D7473	REMOVAL OF TORUS MANDIBULARIS	00	9			I			N
D7480	PARTIAL OSTECTOMY (GUTTERING OR SAUCERIZATION)	00	9		21025	I			N
D7485	SURGICAL REDUCTION OF OSSEOUS TUBEROSITY	00	9			I			N
D7490	RADICAL RESECTION OF MANDIBLE WITH BONE GRAFT	00	9		21095	I			N
D7510	INCISION AND DRAINAGE OF ABSCESS-INTRAORAL SOFT TISSUE	00	9		41800	I			N
D7520	INCISION AND DRAINAGE OF ABSCESS-EXTRAORAL SOFT TISSUE	00	9		40800	I			N
D7530	REMOVAL OF FOREIGN BODY FROM MUCOSA, SKIN, OR SUBCUTANEOUS ALVEOLAR TISSUE	00	9		41805,28	I			N
D7540	REMOVAL OF REACTION-PRODUCING FOREIGN BODIES-MUSCULOSKELETAL SYSTEM	00	9		20520,41 800,806	I			N
D7550	PARTIAL OSTECTOMY/SEQUESTRECTOMY FOR REMOVAL OF NON-VITAL BONE	00	9		20999	I			N
D7560	MAXILLARY SINUSOTOMY FOR REMOVAL OF TOOTH FRAGMENT OR FOREIGN BODY	00	9		31020	I			N
D7610	MAXILLA-OPEN REDUCTION (TEETH IMMOBILIZED IF PRESENT)	00	9		CPT	I			N
D7620	MAXILLA-CLOSED REDUCTION (TEETH IMMOBILIZED IF PRESENT)	00	9		CPT	I			N
D7630	MANDIBLE-OPEN REDUCTION (TEETH IMMOBILIZED IF PRESENT)	00	9		CPT	I			N
D7640	MANDIBLE-CLOSED REDUCTION (TEETH IMMOBILIZED IF PRESENT)	00	9		CPT	I			N
D7650	MALAR AND/OR ZYGOMATIC ARCH-OPEN REDUCTION	00	9		CPT	I			N
D7660	MALAR AND/OR ZYGOMATIC ARCH-CLOSED REDUCTION	00	9		CPT	I			N
D7670	ALVEOLUS - CLOSED REDUCTION, MAY INCLUDE STABILIZATION OF TEETH	00	9		CPT	I			N
D7671	ALVEOLUS - OPEN REDUCTION, MAY INCLUDE STABILIZATION OF TEETH	00	9			I			N
D7680	FACIAL BONES-COMPLICATED REDUCTION WITH FIXATION AND MULTIPLE SURGICAL APPROACHES	00	9		CPT	I			N
D7710	MAXILLA-OPEN REDUCTION	00	9		21346	I			N
D7720	MAXILLA-CLOSED REDUCTION	00	9		21345	I			N
D7730	MANDIBLE-OPEN REDUCTION	00	9		21461,2	I			N
D7740	MANDIBLE-CLOSED REDUCTION	00	9		21455	I			N
D7750	MALAR AND/OR ZYGOMATIC ARCH-OPEN REDUCTION	00	9		21360,5	I			N

HCPCS	Long Description	PTI	MPI	Statute	X-Reff	Coverage	ASC Pay Grp	ASC Pay Grp Eff Date	Action Code
D7760	MALAR AND/OR ZYGOMATIC ARCH-CLOSED REDUCTION	00	9		21355	I			N
D7770	ALVEOLUS - OPEN REDUCTION STABILIZATION OF TEETH	00	9		21422	I			N
D7771	ALVEOLUS, CLOSED REDUCTION STABILIZATION OF TEETH	00	9			I			N
D7780	FACIAL BONES-COMPLICATED REDUCTION WITH FIXATION AND MULTIPLE SURGICAL APPROACHES	00	9		21433,5	I			N
D7810	OPEN REDUCTION OF DISLOCATION	00	9		21490	I			N
D7820	CLOSED REDUCTION OF DISLOCATION	00	9		21480	I			N
D7830	MANIPULATION UNDER ANESTHESIA	00	9		00190	I			N
D7840	CONDYLECTOMY	00	9		21050	I			N
D7850	SURGICAL DISCECTOMY; WITH/WITHOUT IMPLANT	00	9		21060	I			N
D7852	DISC REPAIR	00	9		21299	I			N
D7854	SYNOVECTOMY	00	9		21299	I			N
D7856	MYOTOMY	00	9		21299	I			N
D7858	JOINT RECONSTRUCTION	00	9		21242,3	I			N
D7860	ARTHROTOMY	00	9			I			N
D7865	ARTHROPLASTY	00	9		21240	I			N
D7870	ARTHROCENTESIS	00	9		21060	I			N
D7871	NON-ARTHROSCOPIC LYSIS AND LAVAGE	00	9	1862a(12)		S			N
D7872	ARTHROSCOPY-DIAGNOSIS, WITH OR WITHOUT BIOPSY	00	9		29800	I			N
D7873	ARTHROSCOPY-SURGICAL: LAVAGE AND LYSIS OF ADHESIONS	00	9		29804	I			N
D7874	ARTHROSCOPY-SURGICAL: DISC REPOSITIONING AND STABILIZATION	00	9		29804	I			N
D7875	ARTHROSCOPY-SURGICAL: SYNOVECTOMY	00	9		29804	I			N
D7876	ARTHROSCOPY-SURGICAL: DISCECTOMY	00	9		29804	I			N
D7877	ARTHROSCOPY-SURGICAL: DEBRIDEMENT	00	9		29804	I			N
D7880	OCCLUSAL ORTHOTIC APPLIANCE	00	9		21499	I			N
D7899	UNSPECIFIED TMD THERAPY, BY REPORT	00	9		21499	I			N

HCPCS	Long Description	PI	MPI	Statute	X-Ref1	Coverage	ASC Pay Grp	ASC Pay Grp Eff Date	Action Code
D7910	SUTURE OF RECENT SMALL WOUNDS UP TO 5 CM	00	9		12011,3	I			N
D7911	COMPLICATED SUTURE-UP TO 5 CM	00	9		12051,2	I			N
D7912	COMPLICATED SUTURE-GREATER THAN 5 CM	00	9		13132	I			N
D7920	SKIN GRAFT (IDENTIFY DEFECT COVERED, LOCATION, AND TYPE OF GRAFT)	00	9		CPT	I			N
D7940	OSTEOPLASTY-FOR ORTHOGNATHIC DEFORMITIES	13	A			D			N
D7941	OSTEOTOMY - MANDIBULAR RAMI	00	9		21193,5,6	I			N
D7943	OSTEOTOMY - MANDIBULAR RAMI WITH BONE GRAFT; INCLUDES OBTAINING THE GRAFT	00	9		21194	I			N
D7944	OSTEOTOMY-SEGMENTED OR SUBAPICAL-PER SEXTANT OR QUADRANT	00	9		21198, 21206	I			N
D7945	OSTEOTOMY-BODY OF MANDIBLE	00	9		21193-6	I			N
D7946	LEFORT I (MAXILLA-TOTAL)	00	9		21147	I			N
D7947	LEFORT I (MAXILLA-SEGMENTED)	00	9		21145,6	I			N
D7948	LEFORT II OR LEFORT III (OSTEOPLASTY OF FACIAL BONES FOR MIDFACE HYPOPLASIA OR RETRUSION)-WITHOUT BONE GRAFT	00	9		21150	I			N
D7949	LEFORT II OR LEFORT III-WITH BONE GRAFT	00	9		CPT	I			N
D7950	OSSEOUS, OSTEOPERIOSTEAL, OR CARTILAGE GRAFT OF THE MANDIBLE OR FACIAL BONES-AUTOGENOUS OR NONAUTOGENOUS, BY REPORT	00	9		21247	I			N
D7955	REPAIR OF MAXILLOFACIAL SOFT AND HARD TISSUE DEFECT	00	9		21299	I			N
D7960	FRENULECTOMY (FRENECTOMY OR FRENOTOMY)-SEPARATE PROCEDURE	00	9		40819, 41010, 41115	I			N
D7970	EXCISION OF HYPERPLASTIC TISSUE-PER ARCH	00	9		CPT	I			N
D7971	EXCISION OF PERICORONAL GINGIVA	00	9		41821	I			N
D7972	SURGICAL REDUCTION OF FIBROUS TUBEROSITY	00	9			I			N
D7980	SIALOLITHOTOMY	00	9		42330, 42335, 42340	I			N
D7981	EXCISION OF SALIVARY GLAND, BY REPORT	00	9		42408	I			N
D7982	SIALODOCHOPLASTY	00	9		42500	I			N
D7983	CLOSURE OF SALIVARY FISTULA	00	9		42600	I			N
D7990	EMERGENCY TRACHEOTOMY	00	9		31605	I			N
D7991	CORONOIDECTOMY	00	9		21070	I			N

HCPCS	Long Description	PH	MPI	Statute	X-Ref	Coverage	ASC Pay Grp	ASC Pay Grp Eff Date	Action Code
D7995	SYNTHETIC GRAFT-MANDIBLE OR FACIAL BONES, BY REPORT	00	9		21299	I			N
D7996	IMPLANT-MANDIBLE FOR AUGMENTATION PURPOSES (EXCLUDING ALVEOLAR RIDGE), BY REPORT	00	9		21299	I			N
D7997	APPLIANCE REMOVAL (NOT BY DENTIST WHO PLACED APPLIANCE), INCLUDES REMOVAL OF ARCHBAR	00	9	1862a(12)		S			N
D7999	UNSPECIFIED ORAL SURGERY PROCEDURE, BY REPORT	00	9		21299	I			N
D8010	LIMITED ORTHODONTIC TREATMENT OF THE PRIMARY DENTITION	00	9	1862a(12)		S			N
D8020	LIMITED ORTHODONTIC TREATMENT OF THE TRANSITIONAL DENTITION	00	9	1862a(12)		S			N
D8030	LIMITED ORTHODONTIC TREATMENT OF THE ADOLESCENT DENTITION	00	9	1862a(12)		S			N
D8040	LIMITED ORTHODONTIC TREATMENT OF THE ADULT DENTITION	00	9	1862a(12)		S			N
D8050	INTERCEPTIVE ORTHODONTIC TREATMENT OF THE PRIMARY DENTITION	00	9	1862a(12)		S			N
D8060	INTERCEPTIVE ORTHODONTIC TREATMENT OF THE TRANSITIONAL DENTITION	00	9	1862a(12)		S			N
D8070	COMPREHENSIVE ORTHODONTIC TREATMENT OF THE TRANSITIONAL DENTITION	00	9	1862a(12)		S			N
D8080	COMPREHENSIVE ORTHODONTIC TREATMENT OF THE ADOLESCENT DENTITION	00	9	1862a(12)		S			N
D8090	COMPREHENSIVE ORTHODONTIC TREATMENT OF THE ADULT DENTITION	00	9	1862a(12)		S			N
D8210	REMOVABLE APPLIANCE THERAPY	00	9	1862a(12)		S			N
D8220	FIXED APPLIANCE THERAPY	00	9	1862a(12)		S			N
D8660	PRE-ORTHODONTIC VISIT	00	9	1862a(12)		S			N
D8670	PERIODIC ORTHODONTIC TREATMENT VISIT (AS PART OF CONTRACT)	00	9	1862a(12)		S			N
D8680	ORTHODONTIC RETENTION (REMOVAL OF APPLIANCES, CONSTRUCTION AND PLACEMENT OF RETAINER(S))	00	9	1862a(12)		S			N
D8690	ORTHODONTIC TREATMENT (ALTERNATIVE BILLING TO A CONTRACT FEE)	00	9	1862a(12)		S			N
D8691	REPAIR OF ORTHODONTIC APPLIANCE	00	9	1862a(12)		S			N
D8692	REPLACEMENT OF LOST OR BROKEN RETAINER	00	9	1862a(12)		S			N
D8999	UNSPECIFIED ORTHODONTIC PROCEDURE, BY REPORT	00	9	1862a(12)		S			N
D9110	PALLIATIVE (EMERGENCY) TREATMENT OF DENTAL PAIN-MINOR PROCEDURES	13	A			D			N
D9210	LOCAL ANESTHESIA N0T IN CONJUNCTION WITH OPERATIVE OR SURGICAL PROCEDURES	00	9		90784	I			N
D9211	REGIONAL BLOCK ANESTHESIA	00	9		01995	I			N
D9212	TRIGEMINAL DIVISION BLOCK ANESTHESIA	00	9		64400	I			N
D9215	LOCAL ANESTHESIA	00	9		90784	I			N
D9220	DEEP SEDATION/GENERAL ANESTHESIA-FIRST 30 MINUTES	00	9		CPT	I			N
D9221	DEEP SEDATION/GENERAL ANESTHESIA-EACH ADDITIONAL 15 MINUTES	00	9			I			N

HCPCS	Long Description	PH	MPI	Statute	X-Ref	Coverage	ASC Pay Grp	ASC Pay Grp Eff Date	Action Code
D9230	ANALGESIA, ANXIOLYSIS, INHALATION OF NITROUS OXIDE	13	A			D			N
D9241	INTRAVENOUS CONSCIOUS SEDATION/ANALGESIA - FIRST 30 MINUTES	00	9		90784	I			N
D9242	INTRAVENOUS CONSCIOUS SEDATION/ANALGESIA - EACH ADDITIONAL 15 MINUTES	00	9		90784	I			N
D9248	NON-INTRAVENOUS CONSCIOUS SEDATION	00	9			D			N
D9310	CONSULTATION (DIAGNOSTIC SERVICE PROVIDED BY DENTIST OR PHYSICIAN OTHER THAN PRACTITIONER PROVIDING TREATMENT)	00	9		CPT	I			N
D9410	HOUSE/EXTENDED CARE FACILITY CALL	00	9		CPT	I			N
D9420	HOSPITAL CALL	00	9		CPT	I			N
D9430	OFFICE VISIT FOR OBSERVATION (DURING REGULARLY SCHEDULED HOURS) NO OTHER SERVICES PERFORMED	00	9		CPT	I			N
D9440	OFFICE VISIT-AFTER REGULARLY SCHEDULED HOURS	00	9		99050	I			N
D9450	CASE PRESENTATION, DETAILED AND EXTENSIVE TREATMENT PLANNING	00	9			I			N
D9610	THERAPEUTIC DRUG INJECTION, BY REPORT	00	9		90788,84	I			N
D9630	OTHER DRUGS AND/OR MEDICAMENTS, BY REPORT	13	A			D			N
D9910	APPLICATION OF DESENSITIZING MEDICAMENT	00	9	1862a(12)		S			N
D9911	APPLICATION OF DESENSITIZING RESIN FOR CERVICAL AND/OR ROOT SURFACE, PER TOOTH	00	9	1862a(12)		S			N
D9920	BEHAVIOR MANAGEMENT, BY REPORT	00	9	1862a(12)		S			N
D9930	TREATMENT OF COMPLICATIONS (POSTSURGICAL) - UNUSUAL CIRCUMSTANCES, BY REPORT	13	A			D			N
D9940	OCCLUSAL GUARDS, BY REPORT	13	A			D			N
D9941	FABRICATION OF ATHLETIC MOUTHGUARD	00	9	1862a(12)	21089	S			N
D9950	OCCLUSION ANALYSIS-MOUNTED CASE	13	A			D			N
D9951	OCCLUSAL ADJUSTMENT-LIMITED	13	A			D			N
D9952	OCCLUSAL ADJUSTMENT-COMPLETE	13	A			D			N
D9970	ENAMEL MICROABRASION	00	9	1862a(12)		S			N
D9971	ODONTOPLASTY 1 - 2 TEETH; INCLUDES REMOVAL OF ENAMEL PROJECTIONS	00	9	1862a(12)		S			N
D9972	EXTERNAL BLEACHING - PER ARCH	00	9	1862a(12)		S			N
D9973	EXTERNAL BLEACHING - PER TOOTH	00	9	1862a(12)		S			N
D9974	INTERNAL BLEACHING - PER TOOTH	00	9	1862a(12)		S			N
D9999	UNSPECIFIED ADJUNCTIVE PROCEDURE, BY REPORT	00	9		21499	I			N
E0100	CANE, INCLUDES CANES OF ALL MATERIALS, ADJUSTABLE OR FIXED, WITH TIP	32	A			D			N

HCPCS	Long Description	PTI	MPI	Statute	X-Ref	Coverage	ASC Pay Grp	ASC Pay Grp Eff Date	Action Code
E0105	CANE, QUAD OR THREE PRONG, INCLUDES CANES OF ALL MATERIALS, ADJUSTABLE OR FIXED, WITH TIPS	32	A			D			N
E0110	CRUTCHES, FOREARM, INCLUDES CRUTCHES OF VARIOUS MATERIALS, ADJUSTABLE OR FIXED, PAIR, COMPLETE WITH TIPS AND HANDGRIPS	32	A			D			N
E0111	CRUTCH FOREARM, INCLUDES CRUTCHES OF VARIOUS MATERIALS, ADJUSTABLE OR FIXED, EACH, WITH TIP AND HANDGRIPS	32	A			D			N
E0112	CRUTCHES UNDERARM, WOOD, ADJUSTABLE OR FIXED, PAIR, WITH PADS, TIPS AND HANDGRIPS	32	A			D			N
E0113	CRUTCH UNDERARM, WOOD, ADJUSTABLE OR FIXED, EACH, WITH PAD, TIP AND HANDGRIP	32	A			D			N
E0114	CRUTCHES UNDERARM, OTHER THAN WOOD, ADJUSTABLE OR FIXED, PAIR, WITH PADS, TIPS AND HANDGRIPS	32	A			D			N
E0116	CRUTCH UNDERARM, OTHER THAN WOOD, ADJUSTABLE OR FIXED, EACH, WITH PAD, TIP AND HANDGRIP	32	A			D			N
E0117	CRUTCH, UNDERARM, ARTICULATING, SPRING ASSISTED, EACH	32	A			D			N
E0118	CRUTCH SUBSTITUTE, LOWER LEG PLATFORM, WITH OR WITHOUT WHEELS, EACH	00	9			I			A
E0130	WALKER, RIGID (PICKUP), ADJUSTABLE OR FIXED HEIGHT	32	A			D			N
E0135	WALKER, FOLDING (PICKUP), ADJUSTABLE OR FIXED HEIGHT	32	A			D			N
E0140	WALKER, WITH TRUNK SUPPORT, ADJUSTABLE OR FIXED HEIGHT, ANY TYPE	32	A			D			A
E0141	WALKER, RIGID, WHEELED, ADJUSTABLE OR FIXED HEIGHT	32	A			D			C
E0142	RIGID WALKER, WHEELED, WITH SEAT	32	A			D			D
E0143	WALKER, FOLDING, WHEELED, ADJUSTABLE OR FIXED HEIGHT	32	A			D			C
E0144	WALKER, ENCLOSED, FOUR SIDED FRAMED, RIGID OR FOLDING, WHEELED WITH POSTERIOR SEAT	36	A			D			C
E0145	WALKER, WHEELED, WITH SEAT AND CRUTCH ATTACHMENTS	36	A			D			D
E0146	FOLDING WALKER, WHEELED, WITH SEAT	36	A			D			D
E0147	WALKER, HEAVY DUTY, MULTIPLE BRAKING SYSTEM, VARIABLE WHEEL RESISTANCE	32	A			D			C
E0148	WALKER, HEAVY DUTY, WITHOUT WHEELS, RIGID OR FOLDING, ANY TYPE, EACH	32	A			C			N
E0149	WALKER, HEAVY DUTY, WHEELED, RIGID OR FOLDING, ANY TYPE	32	A			C			C
E0153	PLATFORM ATTACHMENT, FOREARM CRUTCH, EACH	32	A			C			N
E0154	PLATFORM ATTACHMENT, WALKER, EACH	32	A			C			N
E0155	WHEEL ATTACHMENT, RIGID PICK-UP WALKER, PER PAIR	32	A			C			N
E0156	SEAT ATTACHMENT, WALKER	32	A			C			N
E0157	CRUTCH ATTACHMENT, WALKER, EACH	32	A			C			N

HCPCS	Long Description	PII	MPI	Statute	X-Reft	Coverage	ASC Pay Grp	ASC Pay Grp Eff Date	Action Code
E0158	LEG EXTENSIONS FOR WALKER, PER SET OF FOUR (4)	32	A			C			N
E0159	BRAKE ATTACHMENT FOR WHEELED WALKER, REPLACEMENT, EACH	32	A			C			N
E0160	SITZ TYPE BATH OR EQUIPMENT, PORTABLE, USED WITH OR WITHOUT COMMODE	32	A			D			N
E0161	SITZ TYPE BATH OR EQUIPMENT, PORTABLE, USED WITH OR WITHOUT COMMODE, WITH FAUCET ATTACHMENT/S	32	A			D			N
E0162	SITZ BATH CHAIR	32	A			D			N
E0163	COMMODE CHAIR, STATIONARY, WITH FIXED ARMS	32	A			D			N
E0164	COMMODE CHAIR, MOBILE, WITH FIXED ARMS	32	A			D			N
E0165	COMMODE CHAIR, STATIONARY, WITH DETACHABLE ARMS	36	A			D			D
E0166	COMMODE CHAIR, MOBILE, WITH DETACHABLE ARMS	36	A			D			N
E0167	PAIL OR PAN FOR USE WITH COMMODE CHAIR	32	A			D			N
E0168	COMMODE CHAIR, EXTRA WIDE AND/OR HEAVY DUTY, STATIONARY OR MOBILE, WITH OR WITHOUT ARMS, ANY TYPE, EACH	32	A			C			N
E0169	COMMODE CHAIR WITH SEAT LIFT MECHANISM	36	A			C			N
E0175	FOOT REST, FOR USE WITH COMMODE CHAIR, EACH	32	A			C			N
E0176	AIR PRESSURE PAD OR CUSHION, NONPOSITIONING	32	A			D			N
E0177	WATER PRESSURE PAD OR CUSHION, NONPOSITIONING	32	A			D			N
E0178	GEL OR GEL-LIKE PRESSURE PAD OR CUSHION, NONPOSITIONING	32	A			D			N
E0179	DRY PRESSURE PAD OR CUSHION, NONPOSITIONING	32	A			D			N
E0180	PRESSURE PAD, ALTERNATING WITH PUMP	36	A			D			N
E0181	PRESSURE PAD, ALTERNATING WITH PUMP, HEAVY DUTY	36	A			D			N
E0182	PUMP FOR ALTERNATING PRESSURE PAD	36	A			D			N
E0184	DRY PRESSURE MATTRESS	32	A			D			N
E0185	GEL OR GEL-LIKE PRESSURE PAD FOR MATTRESS, STANDARD MATTRESS LENGTH AND WIDTH	32	A			D			N
E0186	AIR PRESSURE MATTRESS	36	A			D			N
E0187	WATER PRESSURE MATTRESS	36	A			D			N
E0188	SYNTHETIC SHEEPSKIN PAD	32	A			D			N

HCPCS	Long Description	PII	MPI	Statute	X-Ref	Coverage	ASC Pay Grp	ASC Pay Grp Eff Date	Action Code
E0189	LAMBSWOOL SHEEPSKIN PAD, ANY SIZE	32	A			D			N
E0190	POSITIONING CUSHION/PILLOW/WEDGE, ANY SHAPE OR SIZE	00	9			I			A
E0191	HEEL OR ELBOW PROTECTOR, EACH	32	A			C			N
E0192	LOW PRESSURE AND POSITIONING EQUALIZATION PAD, FOR WHEELCHAIR	32	A			D			N
E0193	POWERED AIR FLOTATION BED (LOW AIR LOSS THERAPY)	36	A			C			N
E0194	AIR FLUIDIZED BED	36	A		Q0049	D			N
E0196	GEL PRESSURE MATTRESS	36	A			D			N
E0197	AIR PRESSURE PAD FOR MATTRESS, STANDARD MATTRESS LENGTH AND WIDTH	32	A			D			N
E0198	WATER PRESSURE PAD FOR MATTRESS, STANDARD MATTRESS LENGTH AND WIDTH	32	A			D			N
E0199	DRY MATRESS PAD FOR MATTRESS, STANDARD MATTRESS LENGTH AND WIDTH	32	A			D			N
E0200	HEAT LAMP, WITHOUT STAND (TABLE MODEL), INCLUDES BULB, OR INFRARED ELEMENT	32	A			D			N
E0202	PHOTOTHERAPY (BILIRUBIN) LIGHT WITH PHOTOMETER	36	A			C			N
E0203	THERAPEUTIC LIGHTBOX, MINIMUM 10,000 LUX, TABLE TOP MODEL	00	9			I			N
E0205	HEAT LAMP, WITH STAND, INCLUDES BULB, OR INFRARED ELEMENT	32	A			D			N
E0210	ELECTRIC HEAT PAD, STANDARD	32	A			D			N
E0215	ELECTRIC HEAT PAD, MOIST	32	A			D			N
E0217	WATER CIRCULATING HEAT PAD WITH PUMP	32	A			D			N
E0218	WATER CIRCULATING COLD PAD WITH PUMP	36	A			D			N
E0220	HOT WATER BOTTLE	32	A			C			N
E0221	INFRARED HEATING PAD SYSTEM	32	A			C			N
E0225	HYDROCOLLATOR UNIT, INCLUDES PADS	32	A			D			N
E0230	ICE CAP OR COLLAR	32	A			C			N
E0231	NON-CONTACT WOUND WARMING DEVICE (TEMPERATURE CONTROL UNIT, AC ADAPTER AND POWER CORD) FOR USE WITH WARMING CARD AND WOUND COVER	00	9			M			N
E0232	WARMING CARD FOR USE WITH THE NON CONTACT WOUND WARMING DEVICE AND NON CONTACT WOUND WARMING WOUND COVER	00	9			M			N
E0235	PARAFFIN BATH UNIT, PORTABLE (SEE MEDICAL SUPPLY CODE A4265 FOR PARAFFIN)	36	A			D			N
E0236	PUMP FOR WATER CIRCULATING PAD	36	A			D			N
E0238	NON-ELECTRIC HEAT PAD, MOIST	32	A			D			N
E0239	HYDROCOLLATOR UNIT, PORTABLE	32	A			D			N
E0240	BATH/SHOWER CHAIR, WITH OR WITHOUT WHEELS, ANY SIZE	00	9			I			A

HCPCS	Long Description	PTI	MPI	Statute	X-Refl	Coverage	ASC Pay Grp	ASC Pay Grp Eff Date	Action Code
E0241	BATH TUB WALL RAIL, EACH	00	9			M			N
E0242	BATH TUB RAIL, FLOOR BASE	00	9			M			N
E0243	TOILET RAIL, EACH	00	9			M			N
E0244	RAISED TOILET SEAT	00	9			M			N
E0245	TUB STOOL OR BENCH	00	9			M			N
E0246	TRANSFER TUB RAIL ATTACHMENT	00	9			C			N
E0247	TRANSFER BENCH FOR TUB OR TOILET WITH OR WITHOUT COMMODE OPENING	00	9			I			A
E0248	TRANSFER BENCH, HEAVY DUTY, FOR TUB OR TOILET WITH OR WITHOUT COMMODE OPENING	00	9			I			A
E0249	PAD FOR WATER CIRCULATING HEAT UNIT	32	A			D			N
E0250	HOSPITAL BED, FIXED HEIGHT, WITH ANY TYPE SIDE RAILS, WITH MATTRESS	36	A			D			N
E0251	HOSPITAL BED, FIXED HEIGHT, WITH ANY TYPE SIDE RAILS, WITHOUT MATTRESS	36	A			D			N
E0255	HOSPITAL BED, VARIABLE HEIGHT, HI-LO, WITH ANY TYPE SIDE RAILS, WITH MATTRESS	36	A			D			N
E0256	HOSPITAL BED, VARIABLE HEIGHT, HI-LO, WITH ANY TYPE SIDE RAILS, WITHOUT MATTRESS	36	A			D			N
E0260	HOSPITAL BED, SEMI-ELECTRIC (HEAD AND FOOT ADJUSTMENT), WITH ANY TYPE SIDE RAILS, WITH MATTRESS	36	A			D			N
E0261	HOSPITAL BED, SEMI-ELECTRIC (HEAD AND FOOT ADJUSTMENT), WITH ANY TYPE SIDE RAILS, WITHOUT MATTRESS	36	A			D			N
E0265	HOSPITAL BED, TOTAL ELECTRIC (HEAD, FOOT AND HEIGHT ADJUSTMENTS), WITH ANY TYPE SIDE RAILS, WITH MATTRESS	36	A			D			N
E0266	HOSPITAL BED, TOTAL ELECTRIC (HEAD, FOOT AND HEIGHT ADJUSTMENTS), WITH ANY TYPE SIDE RAILS, WITHOUT MATTRESS	36	A			D			N
E0270	HOSPITAL BED, INSTITUTIONAL TYPE INCLUDES: OSCILLATING, CIRCULATING AND STRYKER FRAME, WITH MATTRESS	00	9			M			N
E0271	MATTRESS, INNERSPRING	32	A			D			N
E0272	MATTRESS, FOAM RUBBER	32	A			D			N
E0273	BED BOARD	00	9			M			N
E0274	OVER-BED TABLE	00	9			M			N
E0275	BED PAN, STANDARD, METAL OR PLASTIC	32	A			D			N
E0276	BED PAN, FRACTURE, METAL OR PLASTIC	32	A			D			N
E0277	POWERED PRESSURE-REDUCING AIR MATTRESS	36	A			D			N
E0280	BED CRADLE, ANY TYPE	32	A			C			N
E0290	HOSPITAL BED, FIXED HEIGHT, WITHOUT SIDE RAILS, WITH MATTRESS	36	A			D			N
E0291	HOSPITAL BED, FIXED HEIGHT, WITHOUT SIDE RAILS, WITHOUT MATTRESS	36	A			D			N
E0292	HOSPITAL BED, VARIABLE HEIGHT, HI-LO, WITHOUT SIDE RAILS, WITH MATTRESS	36	A			D			N

HCPCS	Long Description	PH	MPI	Statute	X-Reff	Coverage	ASC Pay Grp	ASC Pay Grp Eff Date	Action Code
E0293	HOSPITAL BED, VARIABLE HEIGHT, HI-LO, WITHOUT SIDE RAILS, WITHOUT MATTRESS	36	A			D			N
E0294	HOSPITAL BED, SEMI-ELECTRIC (HEAD AND FOOT ADJUSTMENT), WITHOUT SIDE RAILS, WITH MATTRESS	36	A			D			N
E0295	HOSPITAL BED, SEMI-ELECTRIC (HEAD AND FOOT ADJUSTMENT), WITHOUT SIDE RAILS, WITHOUT MATTRESS	36	A			D			N
E0296	HOSPITAL BED, TOTAL ELECTRIC (HEAD, FOOT AND HEIGHT ADJUSTMENTS), WITHOUT SIDE RAILS, WITH MATTRESS	36	A			D			N
E0297	HOSPITAL BED, TOTAL ELECTRIC (HEAD, FOOT AND HEIGHT ADJUSTMENTS), WITHOUT SIDE RAILS, WITHOUT MATTRESS	36	A			D			N
E0298	HOSPITAL BED, HEAVY DUTY, EXTRA WIDE, WITH ANY TYPE SIDE RAILS, WITH MATTRESS	00	9		K0549	I			N
E0300	PEDIATRIC CRIB, HOSPITAL GRADE, FULLY ENCLOSED	32	A			C			A
E0301	HOSPITAL BED, HEAVY DUTY, EXTRA WIDE, WITH WEIGHT CAPACITY GREATER THAN 350 POUNDS, BUT LESS THAN OR EQUAL TO 600 POUNDS, WITH ANY TYPE SIDE RAILS, WITHOUT MATTRESS	36	A			D			A
E0302	HOSPITAL BED, EXTRA HEAVY DUTY, EXTRA WIDE, WITH WEIGHT CAPACITY GREATER THAN 600 POUNDS, WITH ANY TYPE SIDE RAILS, WITHOUT MATTRESS	36	A			D			A
E0303	HOSPITAL BED, HEAVY DUTY, EXTRA WIDE, WITH WEIGHT CAPACITY GREATER THAN 350 POUNDS, BUT LESS THAN OR EQUAL TO 600 POUNDS, WITH ANY TYPE SIDE RAILS, WITH MATTRESS	36	A			D			A
E0304	HOSPITAL BED, EXTRA HEAVY DUTY, EXTRA WIDE, WITH WEIGHT CAPACITY GREATER THAN 600 POUNDS, WITH ANY TYPE SIDE RAILS, WITH MATTRESS	36	A			D			A
E0305	BED SIDE RAILS, HALF LENGTH	36	A			D			N
E0310	BED SIDE RAILS, FULL LENGTH	32	A			D			N
E0315	BED ACCESSORY: BOARD, TABLE, OR SUPPORT DEVICE, ANY TYPE	00	9			M			N
E0316	SAFETY ENCLOSURE FRAME/CANOPY FOR USE WITH HOSPITAL BED, ANY TYPE	36	A			C			N
E0325	URINAL; MALE, JUG-TYPE, ANY MATERIAL	32	A			D			N
E0326	URINAL; FEMALE, JUG-TYPE, ANY MATERIAL	32	A			D			N
E0350	CONTROL UNIT FOR ELECTRONIC BOWEL IRRIGATION/EVACUATION SYSTEM	57	A			C			N
E0352	DISPOSABLE PACK (WATER RESERVOIR BAG, SPECULUM, VALVING MECHANISM AND COLLECTION BAG/BOX) FOR USE WITH THE ELECTRONIC BOWEL IRRIGATION/EVACUATION SYSTEM	57	A			C			N
E0370	AIR PRESSURE ELEVATOR FOR HEEL	00	9			C			N
E0371	NONPOWERED ADVANCED PRESSURE REDUCING OVERLAY FOR MATTRESS, STANDARD MATTRESS LENGTH AND WIDTH	36	A			C			N
E0372	POWERED AIR OVERLAY FOR MATTRESS, STANDARD MATTRESS LENGTH AND WIDTH	36	A			C			N
E0373	NONPOWERED ADVANCED PRESSURE REDUCING MATTRESS	36	A			C			N
E0424	STATIONARY COMPRESSED GASEOUS OXYGEN SYSTEM, RENTAL; INCLUDES CONTAINER, CONTENTS, REGULATOR, FLOWMETER, HUMIDIFIER, NEBULIZER, CANNULA OR MASK, AND TUBING	33	A			D			N
E0425	STATIONARY COMPRESSED GAS SYSTEM, PURCHASE; INCLUDES REGULATOR, FLOWMETER, HUMIDIFIER, NEBULIZER, CANNULA OR MASK, AND TUBING	00	9			D			N
E0430	PORTABLE GASEOUS OXYGEN SYSTEM, PURCHASE; INCLUDES REGULATOR, FLOWMETER, HUMIDIFIER, CANNULA OR MASK, AND TUBING	00	9			D			N

HCPCS	Long Description	PII	MPI	Statute	X-Ref	Coverage	ASC Pay Grp	ASC Pay Grp Eff Date	Action Code
E0431	PORTABLE GASEOUS OXYGEN SYSTEM, RENTAL; INCLUDES PORTABLE CONTAINER, REGULATOR, FLOWMETER, HUMIDIFIER, CANNULA OR MASK, AND TUBING	33	A			D			N
E0434	PORTABLE LIQUID OXYGEN SYSTEM, RENTAL; INCLUDES PORTABLE CONTAINER, SUPPLY RESERVOIR, HUMIDIFIER, FLOWMETER, REFILL ADAPTOR, CONTENTS GAUGE, CANNULA OR MASK, AND TUBING	33	A			D			N
E0435	PORTABLE LIQUID OXYGEN SYSTEM, PURCHASE; INCLUDES PORTABLE CONTAINER, SUPPLY RESERVOIR, FLOWMETER, HUMIDIFIER, CONTENTS GAUGE, CANNULA OR MASK, TUBING AND REFILL ADAPTOR	00	9			D			N
E0439	STATIONARY LIQUID OXYGEN SYSTEM, RENTAL; INCLUDES CONTAINER, CONTENTS, REGULATOR, FLOWMETER, HUMIDIFIER, NEBULIZER, CANNULA OR MASK, & TUBING	33	A			D			N
E0440	STATIONARY LIQUID OXYGEN SYSTEM, PURCHASE; INCLUDES USE OF RESERVOIR, CONTENTS INDICATOR, REGULATOR, FLOWMETER, HUMIDIFIER, NEBULIZER, CANNULA OR MASK, AND TUBING	00	9			D			N
E0441	OXYGEN CONTENTS, GASEOUS (FOR USE WITH OWNED GASEOUS STATIONARY SYSTEMS OR WHEN BOTH A STATIONARY AND PORTABLE GASEOUS SYSTEM ARE OWNED), 1 MONTHS SUPPLY = 1 UNIT	33	A			D			N
E0442	OXYGEN CONTENTS, LIQUID (FOR USE WITH OWNED LIQUID STATIONARY SYSTEMS OR WHEN BOTH A STATIONARY AND PORTABLE LIQUID SYSTEM ARE OWNED), 1 MONTHS SUPPLY = 1 UNIT	33	A			D			N
E0443	PORTABLE OXYGEN CONTENTS, GASEOUS (FOR USE ONLY WITH PORTABLE GASEOUS SYSTEMS WHEN NO STATIONARY GAS OR LIQUID SYSTEM IS USED), 1 MONTHS SUPPLY = 1 UNIT	33	A			D			N
E0444	PORTABLE OXYGEN CONTENTS, LIQUID (FOR USE ONLY WITH PORTABLE LIQUID SYSTEMS WHEN NO STATIONARY GAS OR LIQUID SYSTEM IS USED), 1 MONTHS SUPPLY = 1 UNIT	33	A			D			N
E0445	OXIMETER DEVICE FOR MEASURING BLOOD OXYGEN LEVELS NON-INVASIVELY	00	9			C			N
E0450	VOLUME VENTILATOR, STATIONARY OR PORTABLE, WITH BACKUP RATE FEATURE, USED WITH INVASIVE INTERFACE (E.G., TRACHEOSTOMY TUBE)	31	A			D			N
E0454	PRESSURE VENTILATOR WITH PRESSURE CONTROL, PRESSURE SUPPORT AND FLOW TRIGGERING FEATURES	31	A			D			N
E0455	OXYGEN TENT, EXCLUDING CROUP OR PEDIATRIC TENTS	33	A			D			N
E0457	CHEST SHELL (CUIRASS)	32	A			C			N
E0459	CHEST WRAP	36	A			C			N
E0460	NEGATIVE PRESSURE VENTILATOR; PORTABLE OR STATIONARY	31	A			D			N
E0461	VOLUME VENTILATOR, STATIONARY OR PORTABLE, WITH BACKUP RATE FEATURE, USED WITH NON-INVASIVE INTERFACE	31	A			D			N
E0462	ROCKING BED WITH OR WITHOUT SIDE RAILS	36	A			C			N
E0470	RESPIRATORY ASSIST DEVICE, BI-LEVEL PRESSURE CAPABILITY, WITHOUT BACKUP RATE FEATURE, USED WITH NONINVASIVE INTERFACE, E.G., NASAL OR FACIAL MASK (INTERMITTENT ASSIST DEVICE WITH CONTINUOUS POSITIVE AIRWAY PRESSURE DEVICE)	36	A			D			A
E0471	RESPIRATORY ASSIST DEVICE, BI-LEVEL PRESSURE CAPABILITY, WITH BACK-UP RATE FEATURE, USED WITH NONINVASIVE INTERFACE, E.G., NASAL OR FACIAL MASK (INTERMITTENT ASSIST DEVICE WITH CONTINUOUS POSITIVE AIRWAY PRESSURE DEVICE)	31	A			D			A
E0472	RESPIRATORY ASSIST DEVICE, BI-LEVEL PRESSURE CAPABILITY, WITH BACKUP RATE FEATURE, USED WITH INVASIVE INTERFACE, E.G., TRACHEOSTOMY TUBE (INTERMITTENT ASSIST DEVICE WITH CONTINUOUS POSITIVE AIRWAY PRESSURE DEVICE)	31	A			D			A
E0480	PERCUSSOR, ELECTRIC OR PNEUMATIC, HOME MODEL	36	A			D			N
E0481	INTRAPULMONARY PERCUSSIVE VENTILATION SYSTEM AND RELATED ACCESSORIES	00	9			M			N
E0482	COUGH STIMULATING DEVICE, ALTERNATING POSITIVE AND NEGATIVE AIRWAY PRESSURE	36	A			C			N

HCPCS	Long Description	PII	MPI	Statute	X-Ref	Coverage	ASC Pay Grp	ASC Pay Grp Eff Date	Action Code
E0483	HIGH FREQUENCY CHEST WALL OSCILLATION AIR-PULSE GENERATOR SYSTEM, (INCLUDES HOSES AND VEST), EACH	36	A			C			N
E0484	OSCILLATORY POSITIVE EXPIRATORY PRESSURE DEVICE, NON-ELECTRIC, ANY TYPE, EACH	32	A			C			N
E0500	IPPB MACHINE, ALL TYPES, WITH BUILT-IN NEBULIZATION; MANUAL OR AUTOMATIC VALVES; INTERNAL OR EXTERNAL POWER SOURCE	31	A			D			N
E0550	HUMIDIFIER, DURABLE FOR EXTENSIVE SUPPLEMENTAL HUMIDIFICATION DURING IPPB TREATMENTS OR OXYGEN DELIVERY	36	A			D			N
E0555	HUMIDIFIER, DURABLE, GLASS OR AUTOCLAVABLE PLASTIC BOTTLE TYPE, FOR USE WITH REGULATOR OR FLOWMETER	33	A			D			N
E0560	HUMIDIFIER, DURABLE FOR SUPPLEMENTAL HUMIDIFICATION DURING IPPB TREATMENT OR OXYGEN DELIVERY	32	A			D			N
E0561	HUMIDIFIER, NON-HEATED, USED WITH POSITIVE AIRWAY PRESSURE DEVICE	32	A			C			A
E0562	HUMIDIFIER, HEATED, USED WITH POSITIVE AIRWAY PRESSURE DEVICE	32	A			C			A
E0565	COMPRESSOR, AIR POWER SOURCE FOR EQUIPMENT WHICH IS NOT SELF-CONTAINED OR CYLINDER DRIVEN	36	A			C			N
E0570	NEBULIZER, WITH COMPRESSOR	36	A			D			N
E0571	AEROSOL COMPRESSOR, BATTERY POWERED, FOR USE WITH SMALL VOLUME NEBULIZER	36	A			D			N
E0572	AEROSOL COMPRESSOR, ADJUSTABLE PRESSURE, LIGHT DUTY FOR INTERMITTENT USE	36	A			C			N
E0574	ULTRASONIC/ELECTRONIC AEROSOL GENERATOR WITH SMALL VOLUME NEBULIZER	36	A			C			N
E0575	NEBULIZER, ULTRASONIC, LARGE VOLUME	31	A			D			N
E0580	NEBULIZER, DURABLE, GLASS OR AUTOCLAVABLE PLASTIC, BOTTLE TYPE, FOR USE WITH REGULATOR OR FLOWMETER	32	A			D			N
E0585	NEBULIZER, WITH COMPRESSOR AND HEATER	36	A			D			N
E0590	DISPENSING FEE COVERED DRUG ADMINISTERED THROUGH DME NEBULIZER	46	A			C			N
E0600	RESPIRATORY SUCTION PUMP, HOME MODEL, PORTABLE OR STATIONARY, ELECTRIC	36	A			D			N
E0601	CONTINUOUS AIRWAY PRESSURE (CPAP) DEVICE	36	A			D			N
E0602	BREAST PUMP, MANUAL, ANY TYPE	32	A			C			N
E0603	BREAST PUMP, ELECTRIC (AC AND/OR DC), ANY TYPE	00	9			C			N
E0604	BREAST PUMP, HEAVY DUTY, HOSPITAL GRADE, PISTON OPERATED, PULSATILE VACUUM SUCTION/RELEASE CYCLES, VACUUM REGULATOR, SUPPLIES, TRANSFORMER, ELECTRIC (AC AND / OR DC)	00	9			C			N
E0605	VAPORIZER, ROOM TYPE	32	A			D			N
E0606	POSTURAL DRAINAGE BOARD	36	A			D			N
E0607	HOME BLOOD GLUCOSE MONITOR	32	A			D			N
E0608	APNEA MONITOR	36	A		E0618	D			N

HCPCS	Long Description	PI	MPI	Statute	X-Ref	Coverage	ASC Pay Grp	ASC Pay Grp Eff Date	Action Code
E0609	BLOOD GLUCOSE MONITOR WITH SPECIAL FEATURES (EG., VOICE SYNTHESIZERS AUTOMATIC TIMERS, ETC.)	32	A			D			N
E0610	PACEMAKER MONITOR, SELF-CONTAINED, (CHECKS BATTERY DEPLETION, INCLUDES AUDIBLE AND VISIBLE CHECK SYSTEMS)	32	A			D			N
E0615	PACEMAKER MONITOR, SELF CONTAINED, CHECKS BATTERY DEPLETION AND OTHER PACEMAKER COMPONENTS, INCLUDES DIGITAL/VISIBLE CHECK SYSTEMS	32	A			D			N
E0616	IMPLANTABLE CARDIAC EVENT RECORDER WITH MEMORY, ACTIVATOR AND PROGRAMMER	32	A			C			N
E0617	EXTERNAL DEFIBRILLATOR WITH INTEGRATED ELECTROCARDIOGRAM ANALYSIS	36	A			C			N
E0618	APNEA MONITOR, WITHOUT RECORDING FEATURE	00	9			C			N
E0619	APNEA MONITOR, WITH RECORDING FEATURE	00	9			C			N
E0620	SKIN PIERCING DEVICE FOR COLLECTION OF CAPILLARY BLOOD, LASER, EACH	32	A			C			N
E0621	SLING OR SEAT, PATIENT LIFT, CANVAS OR NYLON	32	A			D			N
E0625	PATIENT LIFT, KARTOP, BATHROOM OR TOILET	00	9			M			N
E0627	SEAT LIFT MECHANISM INCORPORATED INTO A COMBINATION LIFT-CHAIR MECHANISM	32	A		Q0080	D			N
E0628	SEPARATE SEAT LIFT MECHANISM FOR USE WITH PATIENT OWNED FURNITURE-ELECTRIC	32	A		Q0078	D			N
E0629	SEPARATE SEAT LIFT MECHANISM FOR USE WITH PATIENT OWNED FURNITURE-NON-ELECTRIC	32	A		Q0079	D			N
E0630	PATIENT LIFT, HYDRAULIC, WITH SEAT OR SLING	36	A			D			N
E0635	PATIENT LIFT, ELECTRIC WITH SEAT OR SLING	36	A			D			N
E0636	MULTIPOSITIONAL PATIENT SUPPORT SYSTEM, WITH INTEGRATED LIFT, PATIENT ACCESSIBLE CONTROLS	36	A			C			N
E0637	COMBINATION SIT TO STAND SYSTEM, ANY SIZE, WITH SEAT LIFT FEATURE, WITH OR WITHOUT WHEELS	32	A			C			A
E0638	STANDING FRAME SYSTEM, ANY SIZE, WITH OR WITHOUT WHEELS	32	A			C			A
E0650	PNEUMATIC COMPRESSOR, NON-SEGMENTAL HOME MODEL	32	A			D			N
E0651	PNEUMATIC COMPRESSOR, SEGMENTAL HOME MODEL WITHOUT CALIBRATED GRADIENT PRESSURE	32	A			D			N
E0652	PNEUMATIC COMPRESSOR, SEGMENTAL HOME MODEL WITH CALIBRATED GRADIENT PRESSURE	32	A			D			N
E0655	NON-SEGMENTAL PNEUMATIC APPLIANCE FOR USE WITH PNEUMATIC COMPRESSOR, HALF ARM	32	A			D			N
E0660	NON-SEGMENTAL PNEUMATIC APPLIANCE FOR USE WITH PNEUMATIC COMPRESSOR, FULL LEG	32	A			D			N
E0665	NON-SEGMENTAL PNEUMATIC APPLIANCE FOR USE WITH PNEUMATIC COMPRESSOR, FULL ARM	32	A			D			N
E0666	NON-SEGMENTAL PNEUMATIC APPLIANCE FOR USE WITH PNEUMATIC COMPRESSOR, HALF LEG	32	A			D			N
E0667	SEGMENTAL PNEUMATIC APPLIANCE FOR USE WITH PNEUMATIC COMPRESSOR, FULL LEG	32	A			D			N

HCPCS	Long Description	PI1	MPI	Statute	X-Ref	Coverage	ASC Pay Grp	ASC Pay Grp Eff Date	Action Code
E0668	SEGMENTAL PNEUMATIC APPLIANCE FOR USE WITH PNEUMATIC COMPRESSOR, FULL ARM	32	A			D			N
E0669	SEGMENTAL PNEUMATIC APPLIANCE FOR USE WITH PNEUMATIC COMPRESSOR, HALF LEG	32	A			D			N
E0671	SEGMENTAL GRADIENT PRESSURE PNEUMATIC APPLIANCE, FULL LEG	32	A			D			N
E0672	SEGMENTAL GRADIENT PRESSURE PNEUMATIC APPLIANCE, FULL ARM	32	A			D			N
E0673	SEGMENTAL GRADIENT PRESSURE PNEUMATIC APPLIANCE, HALF LEG	32	A			D			N
E0675	PNEUMATIC COMPRESSION DEVICE, HIGH PRESSURE, RAPID INFLATION/DEFLATION CYCLE,	36	A			C			A
E0690	FOR ARTERIAL INSUFFICIENCY (UNILATERAL OR BILATERAL SYSTEM) ULTRAVIOLET CABINET, APPROPRIATE FOR HOME USE	32	A			D			N
E0691	ULTRAVIOLET LIGHT THERAPY SYSTEM PANEL, INCLUDES BULBS/LAMPS, TIMER AND EYE PROTECTION; TREATMENT AREA 2 SQUARE FEET OR LESS	32	A			C			N
E0692	ULTRAVIOLET LIGHT THERAPY SYSTEM PANEL, INCLUDES BULBS/LAMPS, TIMER AND EYE PROTECTION, 4 FOOT PANEL	32	A			C			N
E0693	ULTRAVIOLET LIGHT THERAPY SYSTEM PANEL, INCLUDES BULBS/LAMPS, TIMER AND EYE PROTECTION, 6 FOOT PANEL	32	A			C			N
E0694	ULTRAVIOLET MULTIDIRECTIONAL LIGHT THERAPY SYSTEM IN 6 FOOT CABINET, INCLUDES BULBS/LAMPS, TIMER AND EYE PROTECTION	32	A			C			N
E0700	SAFETY EQUIPMENT (E.G., BELT, HARNESS OR VEST)	00	9			C			N
E0701	HELMET WITH FACE GUARD AND SOFT INTERFACE MATERIAL, PREFABRICATED	32	A			C			N
E0710	RESTRAINTS, ANY TYPE (BODY, CHEST, WRIST OR ANKLE)	57	A			C			N
E0720	TENS, TWO LEAD, LOCALIZED STIMULATION	32	A			D			N
E0730	TRANSCUTANEOUS ELECTRICAL NERVE STIMULATION DEVICE, FOUR OR MORE LEADS, FOR MULTIPLE NERVE STIMULATION	32	A			D			N
E0731	FORM FITTING CONDUCTIVE GARMENT FOR DELIVERY OF TENS OR NMES (WITH CONDUCTIVE FIBERS SEPARATED FROM THE PATIENTS SKIN BY LAYERS OF FABRIC)	34	A			D			N
E0740	INCONTINENCE TREATMENT SYSTEM, PELVIC FLOOR STIMULATOR, MONITOR, SENSOR AND/OR TRAINER	32	A			D			N
E0744	NEUROMUSCULAR STIMULATOR FOR SCOLIOSIS	36	A			C			N
E0745	NEUROMUSCULAR STIMULATOR, ELECTRONIC SHOCK UNIT	36	A			D			N
E0746	ELECTROMYOGRAPHY (EMG), BIOFEEDBACK DEVICE	52	A			D			N
E0747	OSTEOGENESIS STIMULATOR, ELECTRICAL, NON-INVASIVE, OTHER THAN SPINAL APPLICATIONS	32	A			D			N
E0748	OSTEOGENESIS STIMULATOR, ELECTRICAL, NON-INVASIVE, SPINAL APPLICATIONS	32	A			D			N
E0749	OSTEOGENESIS STIMULATOR, ELECTRICAL, SURGICALLY IMPLANTED	36	A			D			N
E0751	IMPLANTABLE NEUROSTIMULATOR PULSE GENERATOR, OR COMBINATION OF EXTERNAL TRANSMITTER WITH IMPLANTABLE RECEIVER (INCLUDES EXTENSION)	38	A			D			N
E0752	IMPLANTABLE NEUROSTIMULATOR ELECTRODE, EACH	38	A			D			N

HCPCS	Long Description	PH	MPI	Statute	X-Refl	Coverage	ASC Pay Grp	ASC Pay Grp Eff Date	Action Code
E0753	IMPLANTABLE NEUROSTIMULATOR ELECTRODES, PER GROUP OF FOUR	38	A			D			N
E0754	PATIENT PROGRAMMER (EXTERNAL) FOR USE WITH IMPLANTABLE PROGRAMMABLE NEUROSTIMULATOR PULSE GENERATOR	38	A			D			N
E0755	ELECTRONIC SALIVARY REFLEX STIMULATOR (INTRA-ORAL/NON-INVASIVE)	52	A			C			N
E0756	IMPLANTABLE NEUROSTIMULATOR PULSE GENERATOR	38	A			D			N
E0757	IMPLANTABLE NEUROSTIMULATOR RADIOFREQUENCY RECEIVER	38	A			D			N
E0758	RADIOFREQUENCY TRANSMITTER (EXTERNAL) FOR USE WITH IMPLANTABLE NEUROSTIMULATOR RADIOFREQUENCY RECEIVER	38	A			D			N
E0759	RADIOFREQUENCY TRANSMITTER (EXTERNAL) FOR USE WITH IMPLANTABLE SACRAL ROOT NEUROSTIMULATOR RECEIVER FOR BOWEL AND BLADDER MANAGEMENT, REPLACEMENT	38	A			C			N
E0760	OSTOGENESIS STIMULATOR, LOW INTENSITY ULTRASOUND, NON-INVASIVE	32	A			C			N
E0761	NON-THERMAL PULSED HIGH FREQUENCY RADIOWAVES, HIGH PEAK POWER ELECTROMAGNETIC ENERGY TREATMENT DEVICE	00	9			I			N
E0765	FDA APPROVED NERVE STIMULATOR, WITH REPLACEABLE BATTERIES, FOR TREATMENT OF NAUSEA AND VOMITING	32	A			C			N
E0776	IV POLE	32	A			C			N
E0779	AMBULATORY INFUSION PUMP, MECHANICAL, REUSABLE, FOR INFUSION 8 HOURS OR GREATER	36	A			C			N
E0780	AMBULATORY INFUSION PUMP, MECHANICAL, REUSABLE, FOR INFUSION LESS THAN 8 HOURS	32	A			C			N
E0781	AMBULATORY INFUSION PUMP, SINGLE OR MULTIPLE CHANNELS, ELECTRIC OR BATTERY OPERATED, WITH ADMINISTRATIVE EQUIPMENT, WORN BY PATIENT	36	A			D			N
E0782	INFUSION PUMP, IMPLANTABLE, NON-PROGRAMMABLE (INCLUDES ALL COMPONENTS, E.G., PUMP, CATHETER, CONNECTORS, ETC.)	32	A			D			N
E0783	INFUSION PUMP SYSTEM, IMPLANTABLE, PROGRAMMABLE (INCLUDES ALL COMPONENTS, E.G., PUMP, CATHETER, CONNECTORS, ETC.)	32	A			D			N
E0784	EXTERNAL AMBULATORY INFUSION PUMP, INSULIN	36	A			D			N
E0785	IMPLANTABLE INTRASPINAL (EPIDURAL/INTRATHECAL) CATHETER USED WITH IMPLANTABLE INFUSION PUMP, REPLACEMENT	32	A			D			N
E0786	IMPLANTABLE PROGRAMMABLE INFUSION PUMP, REPLACEMENT (EXCLUDES IMPLANTABLE INTRASPINAL CATHETER)	32	A			D			N
E0791	PARENTERAL INFUSION PUMP, STATIONARY, SINGLE OR MULTI-CHANNEL	36	A			D			N
E0830	AMBULATORY TRACTION DEVICE, ALL TYPES, EACH	00	9			D			N
E0840	TRACTION FRAME, ATTACHED TO HEADBOARD, CERVICAL TRACTION	32	A			D			N
E0850	TRACTION STAND, FREE STANDING, CERVICAL TRACTION	32	A			D			N
E0855	CERVICAL TRACTION EQUIPMENT NOT REQUIRING ADDITIONAL STAND OR FRAME	32	A			C			N

HCPCS	Long Description	PII	MPI	Statute	X-Ref1	Coverage	ASC Pay Grp	ASC Pay Grp Eff Date	Action Code
E0860	TRACTION EQUIPMENT, OVERDOOR, CERVICAL	32	A			D			N
E0870	TRACTION FRAME, ATTACHED TO FOOTBOARD, EXTREMITY TRACTION, (E.G. BUCKS)	32	A			D			N
E0880	TRACTION STAND, FREE STANDING, EXTREMITY TRACTION, (E.G., BUCKS)	32	A			D			N
E0890	TRACTION FRAME, ATTACHED TO FOOTBOARD, PELVIC TRACTION	32	A			D			N
E0900	TRACTION STAND, FREE STANDING, PELVIC TRACTION, (E.G., BUCKS)	32	A			D			N
E0910	TRAPEZE BARS, A/K/A PATIENT HELPER, ATTACHED TO BED, WITH GRAB BAR	36	A			D			N
E0920	FRACTURE FRAME, ATTACHED TO BED, INCLUDES WEIGHTS	36	A			D			N
E0930	FRACTURE FRAME, FREE STANDING, INCLUDES WEIGHTS	36	A			D			N
E0935	PASSIVE MOTION EXERCISE DEVICE	31	A			D			N
E0940	TRAPEZE BAR, FREE STANDING, COMPLETE WITH GRAB BAR	36	A			D			N
E0941	GRAVITY ASSISTED TRACTION DEVICE, ANY TYPE	36	A			D			N
E0942	CERVICAL HEAD HARNESS/HALTER	32	A			C			N
E0943	CERVICAL PILLOW	32	A			C			D
E0944	PELVIC BELT/HARNESS/BOOT	32	A			C			N
E0945	EXTREMITY BELT/HARNESS	32	A			C			N
E0946	FRACTURE, FRAME, DUAL WITH CROSS BARS, ATTACHED TO BED, (E.G. BALKEN, 4 POSTER)	36	A			D			N
E0947	FRACTURE FRAME, ATTACHMENTS FOR COMPLEX PELVIC TRACTION	32	A			D			N
E0948	FRACTURE FRAME, ATTACHMENTS FOR COMPLEX CERVICAL TRACTION	32	A			D			N
E0950	WHEELCHAIR ACCESSORY, TRAY, EACH	00	9		K0107	I			C
E0951	HEEL LOOP/HOLDER, WITH OR WITHOUT ANKLE STRAP, EACH	00	9		K0034	C			C
E0952	TOE LOOP/HOLDER, EACH	00	9			I			C
E0953	PNEUMATIC TIRE, EACH	00	9		K0067	I			N
E0954	SEMI-PNEUMATIC CASTER, EACH	00	9		K0075	I			N
E0955	WHEELCHAIR ACCESSORY, HEADREST, CUSHIONED, PREFABRICATED, INCLUDING FIXED MOUNTING HARDWARE, EACH	32	A			C			A
E0956	WHEELCHAIR ACCESSORY, LATERAL TRUNK OR HIP SUPPORT, PREFABRICATED, INCLUDING FIXED MOUNTING HARDWARE, EACH	32	A			C			A
E0957	WHEELCHAIR ACCESSORY, MEDIAL THIGH SUPPORT, PREFABRICATED, INCLUDING FIXED MOUNTING HARDWARE, EACH	32	A			C			A

HCPCS	Long Description	PTI	MPI	Statute	X-Ref1	Coverage	ASC Pay Grp	ASC Pay Grp Eff Date	Action Code
E0958	MANUAL WHEELCHAIR ACCESSORY, ONE-ARM DRIVE ATTACHMENT, EACH	00	9		K0101	C			C
E0959	MANUAL WHEELCHAIR ACCESSORY, ADAPTER FOR AMPUTEE, EACH	00	9		K0100	I			C
E0960	WHEELCHAIR ACCESSORY, SHOULDER HARNESS/STRAPS OR CHEST STRAP, INCLUDING ANY TYPE MOUNTING HARDWARE	32	A			C			A
E0961	MANUAL WHEELCHAIR ACCESSORY, WHEEL LOCK BRAKE EXTENSION (HANDLE), EACH	00	9		K0079	I			C
E0962	1" CUSHION, FOR WHEELCHAIR	32	A			D			N
E0963	2" CUSHION, FOR WHEELCHAIR	32	A			D			N
E0964	3" CUSHION, FOR WHEELCHAIR	32	A			D			N
E0965	4" CUSHION, FOR WHEELCHAIR	32	A			D			N
E0966	MANUAL WHEELCHAIR ACCESSORY, HEADREST EXTENSION, EACH	00	9		K0025	I			C
E0967	MANUAL WHEELCHAIR ACCESSORY, HAND RIM WITH PROJECTIONS, EACH	32	A			D			C
E0968	COMMODE SEAT, WHEELCHAIR	36	A			D			N
E0969	NARROWING DEVICE, WHEELCHAIR	32	A			D			N
E0970	NO.2 FOOTPLATES, EXCEPT FOR ELEVATING LEG REST	00	9		K0037,42	I			N
E0971	ANTI-TIPPING DEVICE WHEELCHAIRS	00	9		K0021	C			N
E0972	WHEELCHAIR ACCESSORY, TRANSFER BOARD OR DEVICE, EACH	00	9		K0103	I			C
E0973	WHEELCHAIR ACCESSORY, ADJUSTABLE HEIGHT, DETACHABLE ARMREST, COMPLETE ASSEMBLY, EACH	00	9			I			C
E0974	MANUAL WHEELCHAIR ACCESSORY, ANTI-ROLLBACK DEVICE, EACH	00	9			I			C
E0975	REINFORCED SEAT UPHOLSTERY, WHEELCHAIR	00	9		E0981	I			D
E0976	REINFORCED BACK, WHEELCHAIR, UPHOLSTERY OR OTHER MATERIAL	00	9		E0982	I			D
E0977	WEDGE CUSHION, WHEELCHAIR	32	A			C			N
E0978	WHEELCHAIR ACCESSORY, SAFETY BELT/PELVIC STRAP, EACH	00	9			I			C
E0979	BELT, SAFETY WITH VELCRO CLOSURE, WHEELCHAIR	00	9		E0978	I			D
E0980	SAFETY VEST, WHEELCHAIR	32	A			C			N
E0981	WHEELCHAIR ACCESSORY, SEAT UPHOLSTERY, REPLACEMENT ONLY, EACH	32	A			C			A
E0982	WHEELCHAIR ACCESSORY, BACK UPHOLSTERY, REPLACEMENT ONLY, EACH	32	A			C			A
E0983	MANUAL WHEELCHAIR ACCESSORY, POWER ADD-ON TO CONVERT MANUAL WHEELCHAIR TO MOTORIZED WHEELCHAIR, JOYSTICK CONTROL	36	A			C			A
E0984	MANUAL WHEELCHAIR ACCESSORY, POWER ADD-ON TO CONVERT MANUAL WHEELCHAIR TO MOTORIZED WHEELCHAIR, TILLER CONTROL	32	A			C			A

HCPCS	Long Description	PTI	MPI	Statute	X-Reff	Coverage	ASC Pay Grp	ASC Pay Grp Eff Date	Action Code
E0985	WHEELCHAIR ACCESSORY, SEAT LIFT MECHANISM	32	A			C			A
E0986	MANUAL WHEELCHAIR ACCESSORY, PUSH-RIM ACTIVATED POWER ASSIST, EACH	32	A			C			A
E0990	WHEELCHAIR ACCESSORY, ELEVATING LEG REST, COMPLETE ASSEMBLY, EACH	00	9		K0048	I			C
E0991	UPHOLSTERY SEAT	00	9		E0981	I			D
E0992	MANUAL WHEELCHAIR ACCESSORY, SOLID SEAT INSERT	32	A		K0030	C			B
E0993	BACK, UPHOLSTERY	00	9		E0982	I			D
E0994	ARM REST, EACH	32	A			D			N
E0995	WHEELCHAIR ACCESSORY, CALF REST/PAD, EACH	00	9		K0049	I			C
E0996	TIRE, SOLID, EACH	00	9		K0066	I			N
E0997	CASTER WITH A FORK	32	A			D			N
E0998	CASTER WITHOUT FORK	32	A			D			N
E0999	PNEUMATIC TIRE WITH WHEEL	32	A			D			N
E1000	TIRE, PNEUMATIC CASTER	00	9		K0074	I			N
E1001	WHEEL, SINGLE	32	A			D			N
E1002	WHEELCHAIR ACCESSORY, POWER SEATING SYSTEM, TILT ONLY	32	A			C			A
E1003	WHEELCHAIR ACCESSORY, POWER SEATING SYSTEM, RECLINE ONLY, WITHOUT SHEAR REDUCTION	32	A			C			A
E1004	WHEELCHAIR ACCESSORY, POWER SEATING SYSTEM, RECLINE ONLY, WITH MECHANICAL SHEAR REDUCTION	32	A			C			A
E1005	WHEELCHAIR ACCESSORY, POWER SEATNG SYSTEM, RECLINE ONLY, WITH POWER SHEAR REDUCTION	32	A			C			A
E1006	WHEELCHAIR ACCESSORY, POWER SEATING SYSTEM, COMBINATION TILT AND RECLINE, WITHOUT SHEAR REDUCTION	32	A			C			A
E1007	WHEELCHAIR ACCESSORY, POWER SEATING SYSTEM, COMBINATION TILT AND RECLINE, WITH MECHANICAL SHEAR REDUCTION	32	A			C			A
E1008	WHEELCHAIR ACCESSORY, POWER SEATING SYSTEM, COMBINATION TILT AND RECLINE, WITH POWER SHEAR REDUCTION	32	A			C			A
E1009	WHEELCHAIR ACCESSORY, ADDITION TO POWER SEATING SYSTEM, MECHANICALLY LINKED LEG ELEVATION SYSTEM, INCLUDING PUSHROD AND LEG REST, EACH	32	A			C			A
E1010	WHEELCHAIR ACCESSORY, ADDITION TO POWER SEATING SYSTEM, POWER LEG ELEVATION SYSTEM, INCLUDING LEG REST, EACH	32	A			C			A
E1011	MODIFICATION TO PEDIATRIC WHEELCHAIR, WIDTH ADJUSTMENT PACKAGE (NOT TO BE DISPENSED WITH INITIAL CHAIR)	32	A			D			N
E1012	INTEGRATED SEATING SYSTEM, PLANAR, FOR PEDIATRIC WHEELCHAIR	32	A			D			N
E1013	INTEGRATED SEATING SYSTEM, CONTOURED, FOR PEDIATRIC WHEELCHAIR	32	A			D			N
E1014	RECLINING BACK, ADDITION TO PEDIATRIC WHEELCHAIR	32	A			D			N

HCPCS	Long Description	PTI	MPI	Statute	X-Ref	Coverage	ASC Pay Grp	ASC Pay Grp Eff Date	Action Code
E1015	SHOCK ABSORBER FOR MANUAL WHEELCHAIR, EACH	32	A			D			N
E1016	SHOCK ABSORBER FOR POWER WHEELCHAIR, EACH	32	A			D			N
E1017	HEAVY DUTY SHOCK ABSORBER FOR HEAVY DUTY OR EXTRA HEAVY DUTY MANUAL WHEELCHAIR, EACH	32	A			D			N
E1018	HEAVY DUTY SHOCK ABSORBER FOR HEAVY DUTY OR EXTRA HEAVY DUTY POWER WHEELCHAIR, EACH	32	A			D			N
E1019	WHEELCHAIR ACCESSORY, POWER SEATING SYSTEM, HEAVY DUTY FEATURE, PATIENT WEIGHT CAPACITY GREATER THAN 250 POUNDS AND LESS THAN OR EQUAL TO 400 POUNDS	32	A			C			A
E1020	RESIDUAL LIMB SUPPORT SYSTEM FOR WHEELCHAIR	32	A			D			N
E1021	WHEELCHAIR ACCESSORY, POWER SEATING SYSTEM, EXTRA HEAVY DUTY FEATURE, WEIGHT CAPACITY GREATER THAN 400 POUNDS	32	A			C			A
E1025	LATERAL THORACIC SUPPORT, NON-CONTOURED, FOR PEDIATRIC WHEELCHAIR, EACH (INCLUDES HARDWARE)	32	A			D			N
E1026	LATERAL THORACIC SUPPORT, CONTOURED, FOR PEDIATRIC WHEELCHAIR, EACH (INCLUDES HARDWARE)	32	A			D			N
E1027	LATERAL/ANTERIOR SUPPORT, FOR PEDIATRIC WHEELCHAIR, EACH (INCLUDES HARDWARE)	32	A			D			N
E1028	WHEELCHAIR ACCESSORY, MANUAL SWINGAWAY, RETRACTABLE OR REMOVABLE MOUNTING HARDWARE FOR JOYSTICK, OTHER CONTROL INTERFACE OR POSITIONING ACCESSORY	32	A			C			A
E1029	WHEELCHAIR ACCESSORY, VENTILATOR TRAY, FIXED	32	A			C			A
E1030	WHEELCHAIR ACCESSORY, VENTILATOR TRAY, GIMBALED	32	A			C			A
E1031	ROLLABOUT CHAIR, ANY AND ALL TYPES WITH CASTORS 5" OR GREATER	36	A			D			N
E1035	MULTI-POSITIONAL PATIENT TRANSFER SYSTEM, WITH INTEGRATED SEAT, OPERATED BY CARE GIVER	36	A			D			N
E1037	TRANSPORT CHAIR, PEDIATRIC SIZE	36	A			D			N
E1038	TRANSPORT CHAIR, ADULT SIZE	36	A			D			N
E1050	FULLY-RECLINING WHEELCHAIR, FIXED FULL LENGTH ARMS, SWING AWAY DETACHABLE ELEVATING LEG RESTS	36	A			D			N
E1060	FULLY-RECLINING WHEELCHAIR, DETACHABLE ARMS, DESK OR FULL LENGTH, SWING AWAY DETACHABLE ELEVATING LEGRESTS	36	A			D			N
E1065	POWER ATTACHMENT (TO CONVERT ANY WHEELCHAIR TO MOTORIZED WHEELCHAIR, E.G., SOLO)	32	A			D			N
E1066	BATTERY CHARGER	00	9		E2366	I			D
E1069	DEEP CYCLE BATTERY	00	9		E2360	I			D
E1070	FULLY-RECLINING WHEELCHAIR, DETACHABLE ARMS (DESK OR FULL LENGTH) SWING AWAY DETACHABLE FOOTREST	36	A			D			N
E1083	HEMI-WHEELCHAIR, FIXED FULL LENGTH ARMS, SWING AWAY DETACHABLE ELEVATING LEG REST	36	A			D			N
E1084	HEMI-WHEELCHAIR, DETACHABLE ARMS DESK OR FULL LENGTH ARMS, SWING AWAY DETACHABLE ELEVATING LEG RESTS	36	A			D			N

HCPCS	Long Description	PH	MPI	Statute	X-Ref1	Coverage	ASC Pay Grp	ASC Pay Grp Eff Date	Action Code
E1085	HEMI-WHEELCHAIR, FIXED FULL LENGTH ARMS, SWING AWAY DETACHABLE FOOT RESTS	00	9		K0002	I			N
E1086	HEMI-WHEELCHAIR DETACHABLE ARMS DESK OR FULL LENGTH, SWING AWAY DETACHABLE FOOTRESTS	00	9		K0002	I			N
E1087	HIGH STRENGTH LIGHTWEIGHT WHEELCHAIR, FIXED FULL LENGTH ARMS, SWING AWAY DETACHABLE ELEVATING LEG RESTS	36	A			D			N
E1088	HIGH STRENGTH LIGHTWEIGHT WHEELCHAIR, DETACHABLE ARMS DESK OR FULL LENGTH, SWING AWAY DETACHABLE ELEVATING LEG RESTS	36	A			D			N
E1089	HIGH STRENGTH LIGHTWEIGHT WHEELCHAIR, FIXED LENGTH ARMS, SWING AWAY DETACHABLE FOOTREST	00	9		K0004	I			N
E1090	HIGH STRENGTH LIGHTWEIGHT WHEELCHAIR, DETACHABLE ARMS DESK OR FULL LENGTH, SWING AWAY DETACHABLE FOOT RESTS	00	9		K0004	I			N
E1091	YOUTH WHEELCHAIR, ANY TYPE	36	A			D			N
E1092	WIDE HEAVY DUTY WHEEL CHAIR, DETACHABLE ARMS (DESK OR FULL LENGTH), SWING AWAY DETACHABLE ELEVATING LEG RESTS	36	A			D			N
E1093	WIDE HEAVY DUTY WHEELCHAIR, DETACHABLE ARMS DESK OR FULL LENGTH ARMS, SWING AWAY DETACHABLE FOOTRESTS	36	A			D			N
E1100	SEMI-RECLINING WHEELCHAIR, FIXED FULL LENGTH ARMS, SWING AWAY DETACHABLE ELEVATING LEG RESTS	36	A			D			N
E1110	SEMI-RECLINING WHEELCHAIR, DETACHABLE ARMS (DESK OR FULL LENGTH) ELEVATING LEG REST	36	A			D			N
E1130	STANDARD WHEELCHAIR, FIXED FULL LENGTH ARMS, FIXED OR SWING AWAY DETACHABLE FOOTRESTS	00	9		K0001	I			N
E1140	WHEELCHAIR, DETACHABLE ARMS, DESK OR FULL LENGTH, SWING AWAY DETACHABLE FOOTRESTS	00	9		K0001	I			N
E1150	WHEELCHAIR, DETACHABLE ARMS, DESK OR FULL LENGTH SWING AWAY DETACHABLE ELEVATING LEGRESTS	36	A			D			N
E1160	WHEELCHAIR, FIXED FULL LENGTH ARMS, SWING AWAY DETACHABLE ELEVATING LEGRESTS	36	A			D			N
E1161	MANUAL ADULT SIZE WHEELCHAIR, INCLUDES TILT IN SPACE	36	A			C			N
E1170	AMPUTEE WHEELCHAIR, FIXED FULL LENGTH ARMS, SWING AWAY DETACHABLE ELEVATING LEGRESTS	36	A			D			N
E1171	AMPUTEE WHEELCHAIR, FIXED FULL LENGTH ARMS, WITHOUT FOOTRESTS OR LEGREST	36	A			D			N
E1172	AMPUTEE WHEELCHAIR, DETACHABLE ARMS (DESK OR FULL LENGTH) WITHOUT FOOTRESTS OR LEGRESTS	36	A			D			N
E1180	AMPUTEE WHEELCHAIR, DETACHABLE ARMS (DESK OR FULL LENGTH) SWING AWAY DETACHABLE FOOTRESTS	36	A			D			N
E1190	AMPUTEE WHEELCHAIR, DETACHABLE ARMS (DESK OR FULL LENGTH) SWING AWAY DETACHABLE ELEVATING LEGRESTS	36	A			D			N
E1195	HEAVY DUTY WHEELCHAIR, FIXED FULL LENGTH ARMS, SWING AWAY DETACHABLE ELEVATING LEGRESTS	36	A			D			N
E1200	AMPUTEE WHEELCHAIR, FIXED FULL LENGTH ARMS, SWING AWAY DETACHABLE FOOTREST	36	A			D			N
E1210	MOTORIZED WHEELCHAIR, FIXED FULL LENGTH ARMS, SWING AWAY DETACHABLE ELEVATING LEG RESTS	36	A			D			N

HCPCS	Long Description	PTI	MPI	Statute	X-Reff	Coverage	ASC Pay Grp	ASC Pay Grp Eff Date	Action Code
E1211	MOTORIZED WHEELCHAIR, DETACHABLE ARMS DESK OR FULL LENGTH SWING AWAY, DETACHABLE ELEVATING LEG REST	36	A			D			N
E1212	MOTORIZED WHEELCHAIR, FIXED FULL LENGTH ARMS, SWING AWAY DETACHABLE FOOT RESTS	00	9		K0010	I			N
E1213	MOTORIZED WHEELCHAIR, DETACHABLE ARMS DESK OR FULL LENGTH, SWING AWAY DETACHABLE FOOT RESTS	00	9		K0010	I			N
E1220	WHEELCHAIR; SPECIALLY SIZED OR CONSTRUCTED, (INDICATE BRAND NAME, MODEL NUMBER, 'IF ANY) AND JUSTIFICATION	45	A			D			N
E1221	WHEELCHAIR WITH FIXED ARM, FOOTRESTS	36	A			D			N
E1222	WHEELCHAIR WITH FIXED ARM, ELEVATING LEGRESTS	36	A			D			N
E1223	WHEELCHAIR WITH DETACHABLE ARMS, FOOTRESTS	36	A			D			N
E1224	WHEELCHAIR WITH DETACHABLE ARMS, ELEVATING LEGRESTS	36	A			D			N
E1225	MANUAL WHEELCHAIR ACCESSORY, SEMI-RECLINING BACK, (RECLINE GREATER THAN 15 DEGREES, BUT LESS THAN 80 DEGREES), EACH	36	A			D			C
E1226	MANUAL WHEELCHAIR ACCESSORY, FULLY RECLINING BACK, EACH	00	9			I			C
E1227	SPECIAL HEIGHT ARMS FOR WHEELCHAIR	32	A			D			N
E1228	SPECIAL BACK HEIGHT FOR WHEELCHAIR	36	A			D			N
E1230	POWER OPERATED VEHICLE (THREE OR FOUR WHEEL NONHIGHWAY) SPECIFY BRAND NAME AND MODEL NUMBER	32	A			D			N
E1231	WHEELCHAIR, PEDIATRIC SIZE, TILT-IN-SPACE, RIGID, ADJUSTABLE, WITH SEATING SYSTEM	36	A			D			N
E1232	WHEELCHAIR, PEDIATRIC SIZE, TILT-IN-SPACE, FOLDING, ADJUSTABLE, WITH SEATING SYSTEM	36	A			D			N
E1233	WHEELCHAIR, PEDIATRIC SIZE, TILT-IN-SPACE, RIGID, ADJUSTABLE, WITHOUT SEATING SYSTEM	36	A			D			N
E1234	WHEELCHAIR, PEDIATRIC SIZE, TILT-IN-SPACE, FOLDING, ADJUSTABLE, WITHOUT SEATING SYSTEM	36	A			D			N
E1235	WHEELCHAIR, PEDIATRIC SIZE, RIGID, ADJUSTABLE, WITH SEATING SYSTEM	36	A			D			N
E1236	WHEELCHAIR, PEDIATRIC SIZE, FOLDING, ADJUSTABLE, WITH SEATING SYSTEM	36	A			D			N
E1237	WHEELCHAIR, PEDIATRIC SIZE, RIGID, ADJUSTABLE, WITHOUT SEATING SYSTEM	36	A			D			N
E1238	WHEELCHAIR, PEDIATRIC SIZE, FOLDING, ADJUSTABLE, WITHOUT SEATING SYSTEM	36	A			D			N
E1240	LIGHTWEIGHT WHEELCHAIR, DETACHABLE ARMS, (DESK OR FULL LENGTH) SWING AWAY DETACHABLE, ELEVATING LEGREST	36	A			D			N
E1250	LIGHTWEIGHT WHEELCHAIR, FIXED FULL LENGTH ARMS, SWING AWAY DETACHABLE FOOTREST	00	9		K0003	I			N
E1260	LIGHTWEIGHT WHEELCHAIR, DETACHABLE ARMS (DESK OR FULL LENGTH) SWING AWAY DETACHABLE FOOTREST	00	9		K0003	I			N

HCPCS	Long Description	PH	MPI	Statute	X-Ref1	Coverage	ASC Pay Grp	ASC Pay Grp Eff Date	Action Code
E1270	LIGHTWEIGHT WHEELCHAIR, FIXED FULL LENGTH ARMS, SWING AWAY DETACHABLE ELEVATING LEGRESTS	36	A			D			N
E1280	HEAVY DUTY WHEELCHAIR, DETACHABLE ARMS (DESK OR FULL LENGTH) ELEVATING LEGRESTS	36	A			D			N
E1285	HEAVY DUTY WHEELCHAIR, FIXED FULL LENGTH ARMS, SWING AWAY DETACHABLE FOOTREST	00	9		K0006	I			N
E1290	HEAVY DUTY WHEELCHAIR, DETACHABLE ARMS (DESK OR FULL LENGTH) SWING AWAY DETACHABLE FOOTREST	00	9		K0006	I			N
E1295	HEAVY DUTY WHEELCHAIR, FIXED FULL LENGTH ARMS, ELEVATING LEGREST	36	A			D			N
E1296	SPECIAL WHEELCHAIR SEAT HEIGHT FROM FLOOR	32	A			D			N
E1297	SPECIAL WHEELCHAIR SEAT DEPTH, BY UPHOLSTERY	32	A			D			N
E1298	SPECIAL WHEELCHAIR SEAT DEPTH AND/OR WIDTH, BY CONSTRUCTION	32	A			D			N
E1300	WHIRLPOOL, PORTABLE (OVERTUB TYPE)	00	9			M			N
E1310	WHIRLPOOL, NON-PORTABLE (BUILT-IN TYPE)	32	A			D			N
E1340	REPAIR OR NONROUTINE SERVICE FOR DURABLE MEDICAL EQUIPMENT REQUIRING THE SKILL OF A TECHNICIAN, LABOR COMPONENT, PER 15 MINUTES	46	A			D			N
E1353	REGULATOR	33	A			D			N
E1355	STAND/RACK	33	A			D			N
E1372	IMMERSION EXTERNAL HEATER FOR NEBULIZER	32	A			D			N
E1375	NEBULIZER PORTABLE WITH SMALL COMPRESSOR, WITH LIMITED FLOW	32	A		E0570	D			N
E1377	OXYGEN CONCENTRATOR, HIGH HUMIDITY SYSTEM EQUIV. TO 244 CU. FT.	33	A			D			N
E1378	OXYGEN CONCENTRATOR, HIGH HUMIDITY SYSTEM EQUIV. TO 488 CU. FT.	33	A			D			N
E1379	OXYGEN CONCENTRATOR, HIGH HUMIDITY SYSTEM EQUIV. TO 732 CU. FT.	33	A			D			N
E1380	OXYGEN CONCENTRATOR, HIGH HUMIDITY SYSTEM EQUIV. TO 976 CU. FT.	33	A			D			N
E1381	OXYGEN CONCENTRATOR, HIGH HUMIDITY SYSTEM EQUIV. TO 1220 CU. FT.	33	A			D			N
E1382	OXYGEN CONCENTRATOR, HIGH HUMIDITY SYSTEM EQUIV. TO 1464 CU. FT.	33	A			D			N
E1383	OXYGEN CONCENTRATOR, HIGH HUMIDITY SYSTEM EQUIV. TO 1708 CU. FT.	33	A			D			N
E1384	OXYGEN CONCENTRATOR, HIGH HUMIDITY SYSTEM EQUIV. TO 1952 CU. FT.	33	A			D			N
E1385	OXYGEN CONCENTRATOR, HIGH HUMIDITY SYSTEM EQUIV. TO OVER 1952 CU. FT.	33	A			D			N

HCPCS	Long Description	PII	MPI	Statute	X-Ref	Coverage	ASC Pay Grp	ASC Pay Grp Eff Date	Action Code
E1390	OXYGEN CONCENTRATOR, SINGLE DELIVERY PORT, CAPABLE OF DELIVERING 85 PERCENT OR GREATER OXYGEN CONCENTRATION AT THE PRESCRIBED FLOW RATE	33	A			D			C
E1391	OXYGEN CONCENTRATOR, DUAL DELIVERY PORT, CAPABLE OF DELIVERING 85 PERCENT OR GREATER OXYGEN CONCENTRATION AT THE PRESCRIBED FLOW RATE, EACH	33	A			D			A
E1399	DURABLE MEDICAL EQUIPMENT, MISCELLANEOUS	46	A			C			N
E1405	OXYGEN AND WATER VAPOR ENRICHING SYSTEM WITH HEATED DELIVERY	33	A			D			N
E1406	OXYGEN AND WATER VAPOR ENRICHING SYSTEM WITHOUT HEATED DELIVERY	33	A			D			N
E1500	CENTRIFUGE, FOR DIALYSIS	52	A			D			N
E1510	KIDNEY, DIALYSATE DELIVERY SYST. KIDNEY MACHINE, PUMP RECIRCULAT- ING, AIR REMOVAL SYST, FLOWRATE METER, POWER OFF, HEATER AND TEMPERATURE CONTROL WITH ALARM, I.V.POLES, PRESSURE GAUGE, CONCENTRATE CONTAINER	52	A			D			N
E1520	HEPARIN INFUSION PUMP FOR HEMODIALYSIS	52	A			D			N
E1530	AIR BUBBLE DETECTOR FOR HEMODIALYSIS, EACH, REPLACEMENT	52	A			D			N
E1540	PRESSURE ALARM FOR HEMODIALYSIS, EACH, REPLACEMENT	52	A			D			N
E1550	BATH CONDUCTIVITY METER FOR HEMODIALYSIS, EACH	52	A			D			N
E1560	BLOOD LEAK DETECTOR FOR HEMODIALYSIS, EACH, REPLACEMENT	52	A			D			N
E1570	ADJUSTABLE CHAIR, FOR ESRD PATIENTS	52	A			D			N
E1575	TRANSDUCER PROTECTORS/FLUID BARRIERS, FOR HEMODIALYSIS, ANY SIZE, PER 10	52	A			D			N
E1580	UNIPUNCTURE CONTROL SYSTEM FOR HEMODIALYSIS	52	A			D			N
E1590	HEMODIALYSIS MACHINE	52	A			D			N
E1592	AUTOMATIC INTERMITTENT PERITONEAL DIALYSIS SYSTEM	52	A			D			N
E1594	CYCLER DIALYSIS MACHINE FOR PERITONEAL DIALYSIS	52	A			D			N
E1600	DELIVERY AND/OR INSTALLATION CHARGES FOR HEMODIALYSIS EQUIPMENT	52	A			D			N
E1610	REVERSE OSMOSIS WATER PURIFICATION SYSTEM, FOR HEMODIALYSIS	52	A			D			N
E1615	DEIONIZER WATER PURIFICATION SYSTEM, FOR HEMODIALYSIS	52	A			D			N
E1620	BLOOD PUMP FOR HEMODIALYSIS, REPLACEMENT	52	A			D			N
E1625	WATER SOFTENING SYSTEM, FOR HEMODIALYSIS	52	A			D			N
E1630	RECIPROCATING PERITONEAL DIALYSIS SYSTEM	52	A			C			N

HCPCS	Long Description	PEI	MPI	Statute	X-Ref1	Coverage	ASC Pay Grp	ASC Pay Grp Eff Date	Action Code
E1632	WEARABLE ARTIFICIAL KIDNEY, EACH	52	A			D			N
E1634	PERITONEAL DIALYSIS CLAMPS, EACH	52	A			D			A
E1635	COMPACT (PORTABLE) TRAVEL HEMODIALYZER SYSTEM	52	A			D			N
E1636	SORBENT CARTRIDGES, FOR HEMODIALYSIS, PER 10	52	A			D			N
E1637	HEMOSTATS, EACH	52	A			D			N
E1638	HEATING PAD, FOR PERITONEAL DIALYSIS, ANY SIZE, EACH	52	A		E0210	D			N
E1639	SCALE, EACH	52	A			D			N
E1640	REPLACEMENT COMPONENTS FOR HEMODIALYSIS AND/OR PERITONEAL DIALYSIS MACHINES THAT ARE OWNED OR BEING PURCHASED BY THE PATIENT	52	A			D			N
E1699	DIALYSIS EQUIPMENT, NOT OTHERWISE SPECIFIED	52	A			D			N
E1700	JAW MOTION REHABILITATION SYSTEM	32	A			C			N
E1701	REPLACEMENT CUSHIONS FOR JAW MOTION REHABILITATION SYSTEM, PKG. OF 6	34	A			C			N
E1702	REPLACEMENT MEASURING SCALES FOR JAW MOTION REHABILITATION SYSTEM, PKG. OF 200	34	A			C			N
E1800	DYNAMIC ADJUSTABLE ELBOW EXTENSION/FLEXION DEVICE, INCLUDES SOFT INTERFACE MATERIAL	36	A			C			N
E1801	BI-DIRECTIONAL STATIC PROGRESSIVE STRETCH ELBOW DEVICE WITH RANGE OF MOTION ADJUSTMENT, INCLUDES CUFFS	36	A			C			N
E1802	DYNAMIC ADJUSTABLE FOREARM PRONATION/SUPINATION DEVICE, INCLUDES SOFT INTERFACE MATERIAL	36	A			C			N
E1805	DYNAMIC ADJUSTABLE WRIST EXTENSION / FLEXION DEVICE, INCLUDES SOFT INTERFACE MATERIAL	36	A			C			N
E1806	BI-DIRECTIONAL STATIC PROGRESSIVE STRETCH WRIST DEVICE WITH RANGE OF MOTION ADJUSTMENT, INCLUDES CUFFS	36	A			C			N
E1810	DYNAMIC ADJUSTABLE KNEE EXTENSION / FLEXION DEVICE, INCLUDES SOFT INTERFACE MATERIAL	36	A			C			N
E1811	BI-DIRECTIONAL STATIC PROGRESSIVE STRETCH KNEE DEVICE WITH RANGE OF MOTION ADJUSTMENT, INCLUDES CUFFS	36	A			C			N
E1815	DYNAMIC ADJUSTABLE ANKLE EXTENSION/FLEXION DEVICE, INCLUDES SOFT INTERFACE MATERIAL	36	A			C			N
E1816	BI-DIRECTIONAL STATIC PROGRESSIVE STRETCH ANKLE DEVICE WITH RANGE OF MOTION ADJUSTMENT, INCLUDES CUFFS	36	A			C			N
E1818	BI-DIRECTIONAL STATIC PROGRESSIVE STRETCH FOREARM PRONATION / SUPINATION DEVICE WITH RANGE OF MOTION ADJUSTMENT, INCLUDES CUFFS	36	A			C			N
E1820	REPLACEMENT SOFT INTERFACE MATERIAL, DYNAMIC ADJUSTABLE EXTENSION/FLEXION DEVICE	32	A			C			N
E1821	REPLACEMENT SOFT INTERFACE MATERIAL/CUFFS FOR BI-DIRECTIONAL STATIC PROGRESSIVE STRETCH DEVICE	32	A			C			N
E1825	DYNAMIC ADJUSTABLE FINGER EXTENSION/FLEXION DEVICE, INCLUDES SOFT INTERFACE MATERIAL	36	A			C			N
E1830	DYNAMIC ADJUSTABLE TOE EXTENSION/FLEXION DEVICE, INCLUDES SOFT INTERFACE MATERIAL	36	A			C			N
E1840	DYNAMIC ADJUSTABLE SHOULDER FLEXION / ABDUCTION / ROTATION DEVICE, INCLUDES SOFT INTERFACE MATERIAL	36	A			C			N

HCPCS	Long Description	PII	MPI	Statute	X-Ref1	Coverage	ASC Pay Grp	ASC Pay Grp Eff Date	Action Code
E1900	SYNTHESIZED SPEECH AUGMENTATIVE COMMUNICATION DEVICE WITH DYNAMIC DISPLAY	00	9			I			N
E1902	COMMUNICATION BOARD, NON-ELECTRONIC AUGMENTATIVE OR ALTERNATIVE COMMUNICATION DEVICE	00	9			C			N
E2000	GASTRIC SUCTION PUMP, HOME MODEL, PORTABLE OR STATIONARY, ELECTRIC	36	A			C			N
E2100	BLOOD GLUCOSE MONITOR WITH INTEGRATED VOICE SYNTHESIZER	32	A			D			N
E2101	BLOOD GLUCOSE MONITOR WITH INTEGRATED LANCING/BLOOD SAMPLE	32	A			D			N
E2120	PULSE GENERATOR SYSTEM FOR TYMPANIC TREATMENT OF INNER EAR ENDOLYMPHATIC FLUID	36	A			C			A
E2201	MANUAL WHEELCHAIR ACCESSORY, NONSTANDARD SEAT FRAME, WIDTH GREATER THAN OR EQUAL TO 20 INCHES AND LESS THAN 24 INCHES	32	A			C			A
E2202	MANUAL WHEELCHAIR ACCESSORY, NONSTANDARD SEAT FRAME WIDTH, 24-27 INCHES	32	A			C			A
E2203	MANUAL WHEELCHAIR ACCESSORY, NONSTANDARD SEAT FRAME DEPTH, 20 TO LESS THAN 22 INCHES	32	A			C			A
E2204	MANUAL WHEELCHAIR ACCESSORY, NONSTANDARD SEAT FRAME DEPTH, 22 TO 25 INCHES	32	A			C			A
E2300	POWER WHEELCHAIR ACCESSORY, POWER SEAT ELEVATION SYSTEM	32	A			C			A
E2301	POWER WHEELCHAIR ACCESSORY, POWER STANDING SYSTEM	32	A			C			A
E2310	POWER WHEELCHAIR ACCESSORY, ELECTRONIC CONNECTION BETWEEN WHEELCHAIR CONTROLLER AND ONE POWER SEATING SYSTEM MOTOR, INCLUDING ALL RELATED ELECTRONICS, INDICATOR FEATURE, MECHANICAL FUNCTION SELECTION SWITCH, AND FIXED MOUNTING HARDWARE	32	A			C			A
E2311	POWER WHEELCHAIR ACCESSORY, ELECTRONIC CONNECTION BETWEEN WHEELCHAIR CONTROLLER AND TWO OR MORE POWER SEATING SYSTEM MOTORS, INCLUDING ALL RELATED ELECTRONICS, INDICATOR FEATURE, MECHANICAL FUNCTION SELECTION SWITCH, AND FIXED MOUNTING HARDWARE	32	A			C			A
E2320	POWER WHEELCHAIR ACCESSORY, HAND OR CHIN CONTROL INTERFACE, REMOTE JOYSTICK OR TOUCHPAD, PROPORTIONAL, INCLUDING ALL RELATED ELECTRONICS, AND FIXED MOUNTING HARDWARE	32	A			C			A
E2321	POWER WHEELCHAIR ACCESSORY, HAND CONTROL INTERFACE, REMOTE JOYSTICK, NONPROPORTIONAL, INCLUDING ALL RELATED ELECTRONICS, MECHANICAL STOP SWITCH, AND FIXED MOUNTING HARDWARE	32	A			C			A
E2322	POWER WHEELCHAIR ACCESSORY, HAND CONTROL INTERFACE, MULTIPLE MECHANICAL SWITCHES, NONPROPORTIONAL, INCLUDING ALL RELATED ELECTRONICS, MECHANICAL STOP SWITCH, AND FIXED MOUNTING HARDWARE	32	A			C			A
E2323	POWER WHEELCHAIR ACCESSORY, SPECIALTY JOYSTICK HANDLE FOR HAND CONTROL INTERFACE, PREFABRICATED	32	A			C			A
E2324	POWER WHEELCHAIR ACCESSORY, CHIN CUP FOR CHIN CONTROL INTERFACE	32	A			C			A
E2325	POWER WHEELCHAIR ACCESSORY, SIP AND PUFF INTERFACE, NONPROPORTIONAL, INCLUDING ALL RELATED ELECTRONICS, MECHANICAL STOP SWITCH, AND MANUAL SWINGAWAY MOUNTING HARDWARE	32	A			C			A
E2326	POWER WHEELCHAIR ACCESSORY, BREATH TUBE KIT FOR SIP AND PUFF INTERFACE	32	A			C			A
E2327	POWER WHEELCHAIR ACCESSORY, HEAD CONTROL INTERFACE, MECHANICAL, PROPORTIONAL, INCLUDING ALL RELATED ELECTRONICS, MECHANICAL DIRECTION CHANGE SWITCH, AND FIXED MOUNTING HARDWARE	32	A			C			A
E2328	POWER WHEELCHAIR ACCESSORY, HEAD CONTROL OR EXTREMITY CONTROL INTERFACE, ELECTRONIC, PROPORTIONAL, INCLUDING ALL RELATED ELECTRONICS AND FIXED MOUNTING HARDWARE	32	A			C			A

HCPCS	Long Description	PII	MPI	Statute	X-Ref	Coverage	ASC Pay Grp	ASC Pay Grp Eff Date	Action Code
E2329	POWER WHEELCHAIR ACCESSORY, HEAD CONTROL INTERFACE, CONTACT SWITCH MECHANISM, NONPROPORTIONAL, INCLUDING ALL RELATED ELECTRONICS, MECHANICAL STOP SWITCH, MECHANICAL DIRECTION CHANGE SWITCH, HEAD ARRAY, AND FIXED MOUNTING HARDWARE	32	A			C			A
E2330	POWER WHEELCHAIR ACCESSORY, HEAD CONTROL INTERFACE, PROXIMITY SWITCH MECHANISM, NONPROPORTIONAL, INCLUDING ALL RELATED ELECTRONICS, MECHANICAL STOP SWITCH, MECHANICAL DIRECTION CHANGE SWITCH, HEAD ARRAY, AND FIXED MOUNTING HARDWARE	32	A			C			A
E2331	POWER WHEELCHAIR ACCESSORY, ATTENDANT CONTROL, PROPORTIONAL, INCLUDING ALL RELATED ELECTRONICS AND FIXED MOUNTING HARDWARE	32	A			C			A
E2340	POWER WHEELCHAIR ACCESSORY, NONSTANDARD SEAT FRAME WIDTH, 20-23 INCHES	32	A			C			A
E2341	POWER WHEELCHAIR ACCESSORY, NONSTANDARD SEAT FRAME WIDTH, 24-27 INCHES	32	A			C			A
E2342	POWER WHEELCHAIR ACCESSORY, NONSTANDARD SEAT FRAME DEPTH, 20 OR 21 INCHES	32	A			C			A
E2343	POWER WHEELCHAIR ACCESSORY, NONSTANDARD SEAT FRAME DEPTH, 22-25 INCHES	32	A			C			A
E2351	POWER WHEELCHAIR ACCESSORY, ELECTRONIC INTERFACE TO OPERATE SPEECH GENERATING DEVICE USING POWER WHEELCHAIR CONTROL INTERFACE	32	A			C			A
E2360	POWER WHEELCHAIR ACCESSORY, 22 NF NON-SEALED LEAD ACID BATTERY, EACH	32	A			C			A
E2361	POWER WHEELCHAIR ACCESSORY, 22NF SEALED LEAD ACID BATTERY, EACH, (E.G. GEL CELL, ABSORBED GLASSMAT)	32	A			C			A
E2362	POWER WHEELCHAIR ACCESSORY, GROUP 24 NON-SEALED LEAD ACID BATTERY, EACH	32	A			C			A
E2363	POWER WHEELCHAIR ACCESSORY, GROUP 24 SEALED LEAD ACID BATTERY, EACH (E.G. GEL CELL, ABSORBED GLASSMAT)	32	A			C			A
E2364	POWER WHEELCHAIR ACCESSORY, U-1 NON-SEALED LEAD ACID BATTERY, EACH	32	A			C			A
E2365	POWER WHEELCHAIR ACCESSORY, U-1 SEALED LEAD ACID BATTERY, EACH (E.G. GEL CELL, ABSORBED GLASSMAT)	32	A			C			A
E2366	POWER WHEELCHAIR ACCESSORY, BATTERY CHARGER, SINGLE MODE, FOR USE WITH ONLY ONE BATTERY TYPE, SEALED OR NON-SEALED, EACH	32	A			C			A
E2367	POWER WHEELCHAIR ACCESSORY, BATTERY CHARGER, DUAL MODE, FOR USE WITH EITHER BATTERY TYPE, SEALED OR NON-SEALED, EACH	32	A			C			A
E2399	POWER WHEELCHAIR ACCESSORY, NOT OTHERWISE CLASSIFIED INTERFACE, INCLUDING ALL RELATED ELECTRONICS AND ANY TYPE MOUNTING HARDWARE	32	A			C			A
E2402	NEGATIVE PRESSURE WOUND THERAPY ELECTRICAL PUMP, STATIONARY OR PORTABLE	36	A			C			A
E2500	SPEECH GENERATING DEVICE, DIGITIZED SPEECH, USING PRE-RECORDED MESSAGES, LESS THAN OR EQUAL TO 8 MINUTES RECORDING TIME	32	A			D			A
E2502	SPEECH GENERATING DEVICE, DIGITIZED SPEECH, USING PRE-RECORDED MESSAGES, GREATER THAN 8 MINUTES BUT LESS THAN OR EQUAL TO 20 MINUTES RECORDING TIME	32	A			D			A
E2504	SPEECH GENERATING DEVICE, DIGITIZED SPEECH, USING PRE-RECORDED MESSAGES, GREATER THAN 20 MINUTES BUT LESS THAN OR EQUAL TO 40 MINUTES RECORDING TIME	32	A			D			A
E2506	SPEECH GENERATING DEVICE, DIGITIZED SPEECH, USING PRE-RECORDED MESSAGES, GREATER THAN 40 MINUTES RECORDING TIME	32	A			D			A

HCPCS	Long Description	PI	MPI	Statute	X-Reff	Coverage	ASC Pay Grp	ASC Pay Grp Eff Date	Action Code
E2508	SPEECH GENERATING DEVICE, SYNTHESIZED SPEECH, REQUIRING MESSAGE FORMULATION BY SPELLING AND ACCESS BY PHYSICAL CONTACT WITH THE DEVICE	32	A			D			A
E2510	SPEECH GENERATING DEVICE, SYNTHESIZED SPEECH, PERMITTING MULTIPLE METHODS OF MESSAGE FORMULATION AND MULTIPLE METHODS OF DEVICE ACCESS	32	A			D			A
E2511	SPEECH GENERATING SOFTWARE PROGRAM, FOR PERSONAL COMPUTER OR PERSONAL DIGITAL ASSISTANT	32	A			D			A
E2512	ACCESSORY FOR SPEECH GENERATING DEVICE, MOUNTING SYSTEM	32	A			D			A
E2599	ACCESSORY FOR SPEECH GENERATING DEVICE, NOT OTHERWISE CLASSIFIED	32	A			D			A
G0001	ROUTINE VENIPUNCTURE FOR COLLECTION OF SPECIMEN(S)	22	A			C			N
G0002	OFFICE PROCEDURE, INSERTION OF TEMPORARY INDWELLING CATHETER, FOLEY TYPE (SEPARATE PROCEDURE)	11	A		51702,3	C			N
G0004	PATIENT DEMAND SINGLE OR MULTIPLE EVENT RECORDING WITH PRE-SYMPTOM MEMORY LOOP AND 24 HOUR ATTENDED MONITORING, PER 30 DAY PERIOD; INCLUDES TRANSMISSION, PHYSICIAN REVIEW AND INTERPRETATION	11	A		93268	D			N
G0005	PATIENT DEMAND SINGLE OR MULTIPLE EVENT RECORDING WITH PRE-SYMPTOM MEMORY LOOP AND 24 HOUR ATTENDED MONITORING, PER 30 DAY PERIOD; RECORDING (INCLUDES HOOK-UP, RECORDING AND DISCONNECTION)	11	A		93270	D			N
G0006	PATIENT DEMAND SINGLE OR MULTIPLE EVENT RECORDING WITH PRE-SYMPTOM MEMORY LOOP AND 24 HOUR ATTENDED MONITORING, PER 30 DAY PERIOD; 24 HOUR ATTENDED MONITORING, RECEIPT OF TRANSMISSIONS, AND ANALYSIS	11	A		93271	D			N
G0007	PATIENT DEMAND SINGLE OR MULTIPLE EVENT RECORDING WITH PRE-SYMPTON MEMORY LOOP AND 24 HOUR ATTENDED MONITORING, PER 30 DAY PERIOD; PHYSICIAN REVIEW AND INTERPRETATION ONLY	11	A		93272	D			N
G0008	ADMINISTRATION OF INFLUENZA VIRUS VACCINE	54	A			C			N
G0009	ADMINISTRATION OF PNEUMOCOCCAL VACCINE	54	A			C			N
G0010	ADMINISTRATION OF HEPATITIS B VACCINE	54	A			C			N
G0015	POST-SYMPTOM TELEPHONIC TRANSMISSION OF ELECTROCARDIOGRAM RHYTHM STRIP(S) AND 24 HOUR ATTENDED MONITORING, PER 30 DAY PERIOD; TRACING ONLY	11	A		93012	D			N
G0016	POST-SYMPTOM TELEPHONIC TRANSMISSION OF ELECTROCARDIOGRAM RHYTHM STRIPS(S) AND 24 HOUR ATTENDED MONITORING, PER 30 DAY PERIOD; PHYSICIAN REVIEW AND INTERPRETATION ONLY	11	A			D			N
G0025	COLLAGEN SKIN TEST KIT	00	9		Q3031	I			D
G0026	FECAL LEUCOCYTE EXAMINATION	21	A			C			N
G0027	SEMEN ANALYSIS; PRESENCE AND/OR MOTILITY OF SPERM EXCLUDING HUHNER	21	A			C			R
G0030	PET MYOCARDIAL PERFUSION IMAGING, (FOLLOWING PREVIOUS PET, G0030 G0047); SINGLE STUDY, REST OR STRESS (EXERCISE AND/OR PHARMACOLOGIC)	11	B			D			N
G0031	PET MYOCARDIAL PERFUSION IMAGING, (FOLLOWING PREVIOUS PET, G0030 G0047); MULTIPLE STUDIES, REST OR STRESS (EXERCISE AND/OR PHARMACOLOGIC)	11	B			D			N
G0032	PET MYOCARDIAL PERFUSION IMAGING, (FOLLOWING REST SPECT, 78464); SINGLE STUDY, REST OR STRESS (EXERCISE AND/OR PHARMACOLOGIC)	11	B			D			N
G0033	PET MYOCARDIAL PERFUSION IMAGING, (FOLLOWING REST SPECT, 78464); MULTIPLE STUDIES, REST OR STRESS (EXERCISE AND/OR PHARMACOLOGIC)	11	B			D			N

HCPCS	Long Description	PET	MPI	Statute	X-Ref	Coverage	ASC Pay Grp	ASC Pay Grp Eff Date	Action Code
G0034	PET MYOCARDIAL PERFUSION IMAGING, (FOLLOWING STRESS SPECT, 78465); SINGLE STUDY, REST OR STRESS (EXERCISE AND/OR PHARMACOLOGIC)	11	B			D			N
G0035	PET MYOCARDIAL PERFUSION IMAGING, (FOLLOWING STRESS SPECT, 78465); MULTIPLE STUDIES, REST OR STRESS (EXERCISE AND/OR PHARMACOLOGIC)	11	B			D			N
G0036	PET MYOCARDIAL PERFUSION IMAGING, (FOLLOWING CORONARY ANGIOGRAPHY, 93510-93529); SINGLE STUDY, REST OR STRESS (EXERCISE AND/OR PHARMACOLOGIC)	11	B			D			N
G0037	PET MYOCARDIAL PERFUSION IMAGING, (FOLLOWING CORONARY ANGIOGRAPHY, 93510-93529); MULTIPLE STUDIES, REST OR STRESS (EXERCISE AND/OR PHARMACOLOGIC)	11	B			D			N
G0038	PET MYOCARDIAL PERFUSION IMAGING, (FOLLOWING STRESS PLANAR MYOCARDIAL PERFUSION, 78460); SINGLE STUDY, REST OR STRESS (EXERCISE AND/OR PHARMACOLOGIC)	11	B			D			N
G0039	PET MYOCARDIAL PERFUSION IMAGING, (FOLLOWING STRESS PLANAR MYOCARDIAL PERFUSION, 78460); MULTIPLE STUDIES, REST OR STRESS (EXERCISE AND/OR PHARMACOLOGIC)	11	B			D			N
G0040	PET MYOCARDIAL PERFUSION IMAGING, (FOLLOWING STRESS ECHOCARDIOGRAM, 93350); SINGLE STUDY, REST OR STRESS (EXERCISE AND/OR PHARMACOLOGIC)	11	B			D			N
G0041	PET MYOCARDIAL PERFUSION IMAGING, (FOLLOWING STRESS ECHOCARDIOGRAM, 93350); MULTIPLE STUDIES, REST OR STRESS (EXERCISE AND/OR PHARMACOLOGIC)	11	B			D			N
G0042	PET MYOCARDIAL PERFUSION IMAGING, (FOLLOWING STRESS NUCLEAR VENTRICULOGRAM, 78481 OR 78483); SINGLE STUDY, REST OR STRESS (EXERCISE AND/OR PHARMACOLOGIC)	11	B			D			N
G0043	PET MYOCARDIAL PERFUSION IMAGING, (FOLLOWING STRESS NUCLEAR VENTRICULOGRAM, 78481 OR 78483); MULTIPLE STUDIES, REST OR STRESS (EXERCISE AND/OR PHARMACOLOGIC)	11	B			D			N
G0044	PET MYOCARDIAL PERFUSION IMAGING, (FOLLOWING REST ECG, 93000); SINGLE STUDY, REST OR STRESS (EXERCISE AND/OR PHARMACOLOGIC)	11	B			D			N
G0045	PET MYOCARDIAL PERFUSION IMAGING, (FOLLOWING REST ECG, 93000); MULTIPLE STUDIES, REST OR STRESS (EXERCISE AND/OR PHARMACOLOGIC)	11	B			D			N
G0046	PET MYOCARDIAL PERFUSION IMAGING, (FOLLOWING STRESS ECG, 93015); SINGLE STUDY, REST OR STRESS (EXERCISE AND/OR PHARMACOLOGIC)	11	B			D			N
G0047	PET MYOCARDIAL PERFUSION IMAGING, (FOLLOWING STRESS ECG, 93015); MULTIPLE STUDIES, REST OR STRESS (EXERCISE AND/OR PHARMACOLOGIC)	11	B			D			N
G0050	MEASUREMENT OF POST-VOIDING RESIDUAL URINE AND/OR BLADDER CAPACITY BY ULTRASOUND	11	A		51798	C			N
G0101	CERVICAL OR VAGINAL CANCER SCREENING; PELVIC AND CLINICAL BREAST EXAMINATION	11	A			D			N
G0102	PROSTATE CANCER SCREENING; DIGITAL RECTAL EXAMINATION	11	A			D			N
G0103	PROSTATE CANCER SCREENING; PROSTATE SPECIFIC ANTIGEN TEST (PSA), TOTAL	21	A			D			N
G0104	COLORECTAL CANCER SCREENING; FLEXIBLE SIGMOIDOSCOPY	11	A			D			N
G0105	COLORECTAL CANCER SCREENING; COLONOSCOPY ON INDIVIDUAL AT HIGH RISK	11	A			D	02	19980101	N
G0106	COLORECTAL CANCER SCREENING; ALTERNATIVE TO G0104, SCREENING SIGMOIDOSCOPY, BARIUM ENEMA	11	A			D			N
G0107	COLORECTAL CANCER SCREENING; FECAL-OCCULT BLOOD TEST, 1-3 SIMULTANEOUS DETERMINATIONS	21	A			D			N
G0108	DIABETES OUTPATIENT SELF-MANAGEMENT TRAINING SERVICES, INDIVIDUAL, PER 30 MINUTES	11	A			C			N
G0109	DIABETES OUTPATIENT SELF-MANAGEMENT TRAINING SERVICES, GROUP SESSION (2 OR MORE), PER 30 MINUTES	11	A			C			N

HCPCS	Long Description	PT	MPI	Statute	X-Ref1	Coverage	ASC Pay Grp	ASC Pay Grp Eff Date	Action Code
G0110	NETT PULM-REHAB; EDUCATION/SKILLS TRAINING, INDIVIDUAL	11	A			G			D
G0111	NETT PULM-REHAB; EDUCATION/SKILLS TRAINING, GROUP	11	A			G			D
G0112	NETT PULM-REHAB; NUTRITIONAL GUIDANCE, INITIAL	11	A			G			D
G0113	NETT PULM-REHAB; NUTRITIONAL GUIDANCE, SUBSEQUENT	11	A			G			D
G0114	NETT PULM-REHAB; PSYCHOSOCIAL CONSULTATION	11	A			G			D
G0115	NETT PULM-REHAB; PSYCHOLOGICAL TESTING	11	A			G			D
G0116	NETT PULM-REHAB; PSYCHOSOCIAL COUNSELLING	11	A			G			D
G0117	GLAUCOMA SCREENING FOR HIGH RISK PATIENTS FURNISHED BY AN OPTOMETRIST OR OPHTHALMOLOGIST	11	A			C			T
G0118	GLAUCOMA SCREENING FOR HIGH RISK PATIENT FURNISHED UNDER THE DIRECT SUPERVISION OF AN OPTOMETRIST OR OPHTHALOMOLOGIST	11	A			C			T
G0120	COLORECTAL CANCER SCREENING; ALTERNATIVE TO G0105, SCREENING COLONOSCOPY, BARIUM ENEMA.	11	A			D			N
G0121	COLORECTAL CANCER SCREENING; COLONOSCOPY ON INDIVIDUAL NOT MEETING CRITERIA FOR HIGH RISK	11	A			D	02	20010701	N
G0122	COLORECTAL CANCER SCREENING; BARIUM ENEMA	00	9			M			N
G0123	SCREENING CYTOPATHOLOGY, CERVICAL OR VAGINAL (ANY REPORTING SYSTEM), COLLECTED IN PRESERVATIVE FLUID, AUTOMATED THIN LAYER PREPARATION, SCREENING BY CYTOTECHNOLOGIST UNDER PHYSICIAN SUPERVISION	21	A			D			N
G0124	SCREENING CYTOPATHOLOGY, CERVICAL OR VAGINAL (ANY REPORTING SYSTEM), COLLECTED IN PRESERVATIVE FLUID, AUTOMATED THIN LAYER PREPARATION, REQUIRING INTERPRETATION BY PHYSICIAN	11	C			D			N
G0125	PET IMAGING REGIONAL OR WHOLE BODY; SINGLE PULMONARY NODULE	11	A			D			N
G0126	PET LUNG IMAGING OF SOLITARY PULMONARY NODULES, USING 2-(FLUORINE-18)-FLUORO-2-DEOXY-D-GLUCOSE (FDG), FOLLOWING CT (71250/71260 OR 71270); INITIAL STAGING OF PATHOLOGICALLY DIAGNOSED NON-SMALL CELL LUNG CANCER	11	A			D			N
G0127	TRIMMING OF DYSTROPHIC NAILS, ANY NUMBER	11	A			D			N
G0128	DIRECT (FACE-TO-FACE WITH PATIENT) SKILLED NURSING SERVICES OF A REGISTERED NURSE PROVIDED IN A COMPREHENSIVE OUTPATIENT REHABILITATION FACILITY, EACH 10 MINUTES BEYOND THE FIRST 5 MINUTES	99	9	1833(a)		D			N
G0129	OCCUPATIONAL THERAPY REQUIRING THE SKILLS OF A QUALIFIED OCCUPATIONAL THERAPIST, FURNISHED AS A COMPONENT OF A PARTIAL HOSPITALIZATION TREATMENT PROGRAM, PER DAY	00	9			C			N
G0130	SINGLE ENERGY X-RAY ABSORPTIOMETRY (SEXA) BONE DENSITY STUDY, ONE OR MORE SITES; APPENDICULAR SKELETON (PERIPHERAL) (EG, RADIUS, WRIST, HEEL)	11	A			D			N
G0131	COMPUTERIZED TOMOGRAPHY BONE MINERAL DENSITY STUDY, ONE OR MORE SITES; AXIAL SKELETON (EG, HIPS, PELVIS, SPINE)	11	A		76070	D			N
G0132	COMPUTERIZED TOMOGRAPHY BONE MINERAL DENSITY STUDY, ONE OR MORE SITES; APPENDICULAR SKELETON (PERIPHERAL) (EG, RADIUS, WRIST, HEEL)	11	A		76071	D			N
G0141	SCREENING CYTOPATHOLOGY SMEARS, CERVICAL OR VAGINAL, PERFORMED BY AUTOMATED SYSTEM, WITH MANUAL RESCREENING, REQUIRING INTERPRETATION BY PHYSICIAN	11	A			C			N

HCPCS	Long Description	PIT	MPI	Statute	X-Ref	Coverage	ASC Pay Grp	ASC Pay Grp Eff Date	Action Code
G0143	SCREENING CYTOPATHOLOGY, CERVICAL OR VAGINAL (ANY REPORTING SYSTEM), COLLECTED IN PRESERVATIVE FLUID, AUTOMATED THIN LAYER PREPARATION, WITH MANUAL SCREENING AND RESCREENING BY CYTOTECHNOLOGIST UNDER PHYSICIAN SUPERVISION	21	A			C			N
G0144	SCREENING CYTOPATHOLOGY, CERVICAL OR VAGINAL (ANY REPORTING SYSTEM), COLLECTED IN PRESERVATIVE FLUID, AUTOMATED THIN LAYER PREPARATION, WITH SCREENING BY AUTOMATED SYSTEM, UNDER PHYSICIAN SUPERVISION	21	A			C			N
G0145	SCREENING CYTOPATHOLOGY, CERVICAL OR VAGINAL (ANY REPORTING SYSTEM), COLLECTED IN PRESERVATIVE FLUID, AUTOMATED THIN LAYER PREPARATION, WITH SCREENING BY AUTOMATED SYSTEM AND MANUAL RESCREENING UNDER PHYSICIAN SUPERVISION	21	A			C			N
G0147	SCREENING CYTOPATHOLOGY SMEARS, CERVICAL OR VAGINAL, PERFORMED BY AUTOMATED SYSTEM UNDER PHYSICIAN SUPERVISION	21	A			C			N
G0148	SCREENING CYTOPATHOLOGY SMEARS, CERVICAL OR VAGINAL, PERFORMED BY AUTOMATED SYSTEM WITH MANUAL RESCREENING	21	A			C			N
G0151	SERVICES OF PHYSICAL THERAPIST IN HOME HEALTH SETTING, EACH 15 MINUTES	00	9			C			N
G0152	SERVICES OF OCCUPATIONAL THERAPIST IN HOME HEALTH SETTING, EACH 15 MINUTES	00	9			C			N
G0153	SERVICES OF SPEECH AND LANGUAGE PATHOLOGIST IN HOME HEALTH SETTING, EACH 15 MINUTES	00	9			C			N
G0154	SERVICES OF SKILLED NURSE IN HOME HEALTH SETTING, EACH 15 MINUTES	00	9			C			N
G0155	SERVICES OF CLINICAL SOCIAL WORKER IN HOME HEALTH SETTING, EACH 15 MINUTES	00	9			C			N
G0156	SERVICES OF HOME HEALTH AIDE IN HOME HEALTH SETTING, EACH 15 MINUTES	00	9			C			N
G0159	PERCUTANEOUS THROMBECTOMY AND/OR REVISION, ARTERIOVENOUS FISTULA, AUTOGENOUS OR NONAUTOGENOUS DIALYSIS GRAFT	00	9			I			N
G0160	CRYOSURGICAL ABLATION OF LOCALIZED PROSTATE CANCER, PRIMARY TREATMENT ONLY (POST OPERATIVE IRRIGATIONS AND ASPIRATION OF SLOUGHING TISSUE INCLUDED)	00	9			I			N
G0161	ULTRASONIC GUIDANCE FOR INTERSTITIAL PLACEMENT OF CRYOSURGICAL PROBES	11	A			D			N
G0163	POSITRON EMISSION TOMOGRAPHY (PET), WHOLE BODY, FOR RECURRENCE OF COLORECTAL METASTATIC CANCER	11	A			D			N
G0164	POSITRON EMISSION TOMOGRAPHY (PET), WHOLE BODY, FOR STAGING AND CHARACTERIZATION OF LYMPHOMA	11	A			D			N
G0165	POSITRON EMISSION TOMOGRAPHY (PET), WHOLE BODY, FOR RECURRENCE OF MELANOMA OR MELANOMA METASTATIC CANCER	11	A			D			N
G0166	EXTERNAL COUNTERPULSATION, PER TREATMENT SESSION	11	A			D			N
G0167	HYPERBARIC OXYGEN TREATMENT NOT REQUIRING PHYSICIAN ATTENDANCE, PER TREATMENT SESSION	11	A			G			D
G0168	WOUND CLOSURE UTILIZING TISSUE ADHESIVE(S) ONLY	00	9			C			N
G0169	REMOVAL OF DEVITALIZED TISSUE, WITHOUT USE OF ANESTHESIA (CONSCIOUS SEDATION, LOCAL, REGIONAL, GENERAL)	11	A			C			N
G0170	APPLICATION OF TISSUE CULTURED SKIN GRAFTS, INCLUDING BILAMINATE SKIN SUBSTITUTES OR NEODERMIS, INCLUDING SITE PREPARATION, INITIAL 25 SO CMS	11	A			C			N
G0171	APPLICATION OF TISSUE CULTURED SKIN GRAFTS, INCLUDING BILAMINATE SKIN SUBSTITUTES OR NEODERMIS, INCLUDING SITE PREPARATION, EACH ADDITIONAL 25 SO CMS	11	A			C			N

HCPCS	Long Description	PII	MPI	Statute	X-Ref	Coverage	ASC Pay Grp	ASC Pay Grp Eff Date	Action Code
G0172	TRAINING AND EDUCATIONAL SERVICES FURNISHED AS A COMPONENT OF A PARTIAL HOSPITALIZATION TREATMENT PROGRAM, PER DAY	00	9		G0177	D			N
G0173	STEREOTACTIC RADIOSURGERY, COMPLETE COURSE OF THERAPY IN ONE SESSION	00	9			D			N
G0174	INTENSITY MODULATED RADIATION THERAPY (IMRT) DELIVERY TO ONE OR MORE TREATMENT AREAS, MULTIPLE COUCH ANGLES/FIELDS/ARC, CUSTOM COLLIMATED PENCIL-BEAMS WITH TREATMENT SETUP AND VERIFICATION IMAGES, COMPLETE COURSE OF THERAPY REQUIRING MORE THAN ONE SESSION, PER SESSION	00	9			G			N
G0175	SCHEDULED INTERDISCIPLINARY TEAM CONFERENCE (MINIMUM OF THREE EXCLUSIVE OF PATIENT CARE NURSING STAFF) WITH PATIENT PRESENT	00	9			C			N
G0176	ACTIVITY THERAPY, SUCH AS MUSIC, DANCE, ART OR PLAY THERAPIES NOT FOR RECREATION, RELATED TO THE CARE AND TREATMENT OF PATIENTS DISABLING MENTAL HEALTH PROBLEMS, PER SESSION (45 MINUTES OR MORE)	00	9			D			N
G0177	TRAINING AND EDUCATIONAL SERVICES RELATED TO THE CARE AND TREATMENT OF PATIENTS DISABLING MENTAL HEALTH PROBLEMS PER SESSION (45 MINUTES OR MORE)	00	9			D			N
G0178	INTENSITY MODULATED RADIATION THERAPY (IMRT) PLAN, INCLUDING DOSE VOLUME HISTOGRAMS FOR TARGET AND CRITICAL STRUCTURE PARTIAL TOLERANCES, INVERSE PLAN OPTIMIZATION PERFORMED FOR HIGHLY CONFORMAL DISTRIBUTIONS, PLAN POSITIONAL ACCURACY AND DOSE VERIFICATION, PER COURSE OF TREATMENT	11	A			G			N
G0179	PHYSICIAN RE-CERTIFICATION FOR MEDICARE-COVERED HOME HEALTH SERVICES UNDER A HOME HEALTH PLAN OF CARE (PATIENT NOT PRESENT), INCLUDING CONTACTS WITH HOME HEALTH AGENCY AND REVIEW OF REPORTS OF PATIENT STATUS REQUIRED BY PHYSICIANS TO AFFIRM THE INITIAL IMPLEMENTATION OF THE PLAN OF CARE THAT MEETS PATIENTS NEEDS, PER RE-CERTIFICATION PERIOD	11	A			C			N
G0180	PHYSICIAN CERTIFICATION FOR MEDICARE-COVERED HOME HEALTH SERVICES UNDER A HOME HEALTH PLAN OF CARE (PATIENT NOT PRESENT), INCLUDING CONTACTS WITH HOME HEALTH AGENCY AND REVIEW OF REPORTS OF PATIENT STATUS REQUIRED BY PHYSICIANS TO AFFIRM THE INITIAL IMPLEMENTATION OF THE PLAN OF CARE THAT MEETS PATIENTS NEEDS, PER CERTIFICATION PERIOD	11	A			C			N
G0181	PHYSICIAN SUPERVISION OF A PATIENT RECEIVING MEDICARE-COVERED SERVICES PROVIDED BY A PARTICIPATING HOME HEALTH AGENCY (PATIENT NOT PRESENT) REQUIRING COMPLEX AND MULTIDISCIPLINARY CARE MODALITIES INVOLVING REGULAR PHYSICIAN DEVELOPMENT AND/OR REVISION OF CARE PLANS, REVIEW OF SUBSEQUENT REPORTS OF PATIENT STATUS, REVIEW OF LABORATORY AND OTHER STUDIES, COMMUNICATION (INCLUDING TELEPHONE CALLS) WITH OTHER HEALTH CARE PROFESSIONALS INVOLVED IN THE PATIENTS CARE, INTEGRATION OF NEW INFORMATION INTO THE MEDICAL TREATMENT PLAN AND/OR ADJUSTMENT OF MEDICAL THERAPY, WITHIN A CALENDAR MONTH, 30 MINUTES OR MORE	11	A			C			N
G0182	PHYSICIAN SUPERVISION OF A PATIENT UNDER A MEDICARE-APPROVED HOSPICE (PATIENT NOT PRESENT) REQUIRING COMPLEX AND MULTIDISCIPLINARY CARE MODALITIES INVOLVING REGULAR PHYSICIAN DEVELOPMENT AND/OR REVISION OF CARE PLANS, REVIEW OF SUBSEQUENT REPORTS OF PATIENT STATUS, REVIEW OF LABORATORY AND OTHER STUDIES, COMMUNICATION (INCLUDING TELEPHONE CALLS) WITH OTHER HEALTH CARE PROFESSIONALS INVOLVED IN THE PATIENTS CARE, INTEGRATION OF NEW INFORMATION INTO THE MEDICAL TREATMENT PLAN AND/OR ADJUSTMENT OF MEDICAL THERAPY, WITHIN A CALENDAR MONTH, 30 MINUTES OR MORE	11	A			C			N
G0184	OCULAR PHOTODYNAMIC THERAPY TREATMENT, SECOND EYE; DESTRUCTION OF LOCALIZED LESION OF CHOROID (INCLUDES INTRAVENOUS INFUSION)	11	A			C			N
G0185	DESTRUCTION OF LOCALIZED LESION OF CHOROID (FOR EXAMPLE, CHOROIDAL NEOVASCULARIZATION); TRANSPUPILLARY THERMOTHERAPY (ONE OR MORE SESSIONS)	00	9		0016T	C			N
G0186	DESTRUCTION OF LOCALIZED LESION OF CHOROID (FOR EXAMPLE, CHOROIDAL NEOVASCULARIZATION); PHOTOCOAGULATION, FEEDER VESSEL TECHNIQUE (ONE OR MORE SESSIONS)	00	9			C			N

HCPCS	Long Description	PII	MPI	Statute	X-Ref	Coverage	ASC Pay Grp	ASC Pay Grp Eff Date	Action Code
G0187	DESTRUCTION OF MACULAR DRUSEN, PHOTOCOAGULATION (ONE OR MORE SESSIONS)	00	9			C			N
G0188	FULL LENGTH RADIOGRAPHY OF LOWER EXTREMITY, WHICH INCLUDES HIP, KNEE AND ANKLE	11	A			C			N
G0190	IMMUNIZATION ADMINISTRATION (INCLUDES PERCUTANEOUS, INTRADERMAL, SUBCUTANEOUS, INTRAMUSCULAR AND JET INJECTIONS; EACH ADDITIONAL VACCINE (SINGLE OR COMBINATION VACCINE/TOXOID)	11	A			C			N
G0191	IMMUNIZATION ADMINISTRATION (INCLUDES PERCUTANEOUS, INTRADERMAL, SUBCUTANEOUS, INTRAMUSCULAR AND JET INJECTIONS); EACH ADDITIONAL VACCINE (SINGLE OR COMBINATION VACCINE/TOXOID) LIST SEPARATELY IN ADDITION TO CODE FOR PRIMARY PROCEDURE	11	A			C			N
G0192	INTRANASAL OR ORAL ADMINISTRATION; ONE VACCINE (SINGLE OR COMBINATION VACCINE/TOXOID)	00	9			M			N
G0193	ENDOSCOPIC STUDY OF SWALLOWING FUNCTION (ALSO FIBEROPTIC ENDOSCOPIC EVALUATION OF SWALLOWING (FEES)	11	A		92612	C			N
G0194	SENSORY TESTING DURING ENDOSCOPIC STUDY OF SWALLOWING (ADD ON CODE) REFERRED TO AS FIBEROPTIC ENDOSCOPIC EVALUATION OF SWALLOWING WITH SENSORY TESTING (FEEST)	11	A		92614	C			N
G0195	CLINICAL EVALUATION OF SWALLOWING FUNCTION (NOT INVOLVING INTERPRETATION OF DYNAMIC RADIOLOGICAL STUDIES OR ENDOSCOPIC STUDY OF SWALLOWING)	11	A		92610	C			N
G0196	EVALUATION OF SWALLOWING INVOLVING SWALLOWING OF RADIO-OPAQUE MATERIALS	11	A		92611	C			N
G0197	EVALUATION OF PATIENT FOR PRESCRIPTION OF SPEECH GENERATING DEVICES	11	A		92607	C			N
G0198	PATIENT ADAPTATION AND TRAINING FOR USE OF SPEECH GENERATING DEVICES	11	A		92609	C			N
G0199	RE-EVALUATION OF PATIENT USING SPEECH GENERATING DEVICES	11	A		92607,8	C			N
G0200	EVALUATION OF PATIENT FOR PRESCRIPTION OF VOICE PROSTHETIC	11	A		92506	C			N
G0201	MODIFICATION OR TRAINING IN USE OF VOICE PROSTHETIC	11	A		92507	C			N
G0202	SCREENING MAMMOGRAPHY, PRODUCING DIRECT DIGITAL IMAGE, BILATERAL, ALL VIEWS	11	A			C			N
G0203	SCREENING MAMMOGRAPHY, FILM PROCESSED TO PRODUCE DIGITAL IMAGES ANALYZED FOR POTENTIAL ABNORMALITIES, BILATERAL, ALL VIEWS	11	A			C			N
G0204	DIAGNOSTIC MAMMOGRAPHY, PRODUCING DIRECT DIGITAL IMAGE, BILATERAL, ALL VIEWS	11	A			C			N
G0205	DIAGNOSTIC MAMMOGRAPHY, FILM PROCESSED TO PRODUCE DIGITAL IMAGE ANALYZED FOR POTENTIAL ABNORMALITIES, BILATERAL, ALL VIEWS	11	A			C			N
G0206	DIAGNOSTIC MAMMOGRAPHY, PRODUCING DIRECT DIGITAL IMAGE, UNILATERAL, ALL VIEWS	11	A			C			N
G0207	DIAGNOSTIC MAMMOGRAPHY, FILM PROCESSED TO PRODUCE DIGITAL IMAGE ANALYZED FOR POTENTIAL ABNORMALITIES, UNILATERAL, ALL VIEWS	11	A			C			N
G0210	PET IMAGING WHOLE BODY; DIAGNOSIS; LUNG CANCER, NON-SMALL CELL	11	A			D			N
G0211	PET IMAGING WHOLE BODY; INITIAL STAGING; LUNG CANCER; NON-SMALL CELL (REPLACES G0126)	11	A			D			N

HCPCS	Long Description	PET	MPI	Statute	X-Refl	Coverage	ASC Pay Grp	ASC Pay Grp Eff Date	Action Code
G0212	PET IMAGING WHOLE BODY; RESTAGING; LUNG CANCER; NON-SMALL	11	A			D			N
G0213	PET IMAGING WHOLE BODY; DIAGNOSIS; COLORECTAL	11	A			D			N
G0214	PET IMAGING WHOLE BODY; INITIAL STAGING; COLORECTAL	11	A			D			N
G0215	PET IMAGING WHOLE BODY; RESTAGING; COLORECTAL CANCER (REPLACES G0163)	11	A			D			N
G0216	PET IMAGING WHOLE BODY; DIAGNOSIS; MELANOMA	11	A			D			N
G0217	PET IMAGING WHOLE BODY; INITIAL STAGING; MELANOMA	11	A			D			N
G0218	PET IMAGING WHOLE BODY; RESTAGING; MELANOMA (REPLACES G0165)	11	A			D			N
G0219	PET IMAGING WHOLE BODY; MELANOMA FOR NON-COVERED INDICATIONS	00	9			M			N
G0220	PET IMAGING WHOLE BODY; DIAGNOSIS; LYMPHOMA	11	A			D			N
G0221	PET IMAGING WHOLE BODY; INITIAL STAGING; LYMPHOMA (REPLACES G0164)	11	A			D			N
G0222	PET IMAGING WHOLE BODY; RESTAGING; LYMPHOMA (REPLACES G0164)	11	A			D			N
G0223	PET IMAGING WHOLE BODY OR REGIONAL; DIAGNOSIS; HEAD AND NECK CANCER; EXCLUDING THYROID AND CNS CANCERS	11	A			D			N
G0224	PET IMAGING WHOLE BODY OR REGIONAL; INITIAL STAGING; HEAD AND NECK CANCER; EXCLUDING THYROID AND CNS CANCERS	11	A			D			N
G0225	PET IMAGING WHOLE BODY OR REGIONAL; RESTAGING; HEAD AND NECK CANCER, EXCLUDING THYROID AND CNS CANCERS	11	A			D			N
G0226	PET IMAGING WHOLE BODY; DIAGNOSIS; ESOPHAGEAL CANCER	11	A			D			N
G0227	PET IMAGING WHOLE BODY; INITIAL STAGING; ESOPHAGEAL CANCER	11	A			D			N
G0228	PET IMAGING WHOLE BODY; RESTAGING; ESOPHAGEAL CANCER	11	A			D			N
G0229	PET IMAGING; METABOLIC BRAIN IMAGING FOR PRE-SURGICAL EVALUATION OF REFRACTORY SEIZURES	11	A			D			N
G0230	PET IMAGING; METABOLIC ASSESSMENT FOR MYOCARDIAL VIABILITY FOLLOWING INCONCLUSIVE SPECT STUDY	11	A			D			N
G0231	PET, WHOLE BODY, FOR RECURRENCE OF COLORECTAL OR COLORECTAL METASTATIC CANCER; GAMMA CAMERAS ONLY	11	A			D			N
G0232	PET, WHOLE BODY, FOR STAGING AND CHARACTERIZATION OF LYMPHOMA; GAMMA CAMERAS ONLY	11	A			D			N
G0233	PET, WHOLE BODY, FOR RECURRENCE OF MELANOMA OR MELANOMA METASTATIC CANCER; GAMMA CAMERAS ONLY	11	A			D			N
G0234	PET, REGIONAL OR WHOLE BODY, FOR SOLITARY PULMONARY NODULE FOLLOWING CT OR FOR INITIAL STAGING OF PATHOLOGICALLY DIAGNOSED NONSMALL CELL LUNG CANCER; GAMMA CAMERAS ONLY	11	A			D			N

HCPCS	Long Description	PT1	MP1	Statute	X-Ref	Coverage	ASC Pay Grp	ASC Pay Grp Eff Date	Action Code
G0236	DIGITIZATION OF FILM RADIOGRAPHIC IMAGES WITH COMPUTER ANALYSIS FOR LESION DETECTION, OR COMPUTER ANALYSIS OF DIGITAL MAMMOGRAM FOR LESION DETECTION, AND FURTHER PHYSICIAN REVIEW FOR INTERPRETATION, DIAGNOSTIC MAMMOGRAPHY (LIST SEPARATELY IN ADDITION TO CODE FOR PRIMARY PROCEDURE)	11	A			C			D
G0237	THERAPEUTIC PROCEDURES TO INCREASE STRENGTH OR ENDURANCE OF RESPIRATORY MUSCLES, FACE TO FACE, ONE ON ONE, EACH 15 MINUTES (INCLUDES MONITORING)	11	A			C			N
G0238	THERAPEUTIC PROCEDURES TO IMPROVE RESPIRATORY FUNCTION, OTHER THAN DESCRIBED BY G0237, ONE ON ONE, FACE TO FACE, PER 15 MINUTES (INCLUDES MONITORING)	11	A			C			N
G0239	THERAPEUTIC PROCEDURES TO IMPROVE RESPIRATORY FUNCTION OR INCREASE STRENGTH OR ENDURANCE OF RESPIRATORY MUSCLES, TWO OR MORE INDIVIDUALS (INCLUDES MONITORING)	11	A			C			N
G0240	CRITICAL CARE SERVICE DELIVERED BY A PHYSICIAN, FACE TO FACE; DURING INTERFACILITY TRANSPORT OF A CRITICALLY ILL OR CRITICALLY INJURED PATIENT; FIRST 30-74 MINUTES OF ACTIVE TRANSPORT	11	A			C			N
G0241	EACH ADDITIONAL 30 MINUTES (LIST SEPARATELY IN ADDITION TO G0240)	11	A			C			N
G0242	MULTI-SOURCE PHOTON STEREOTACTIC RADIOSURGERY (COBALT 60 MULTI-SOURCE CONVERGING BEAMS) PLAN, INCLUDING DOSE VOLUME HISTOGRAMS FOR TARGET AND CRITICAL STRUCTURE TOLERANCES, PLAN OPTIMIZATION PERFORMED FOR HIGHLY CONFORMAL DISTRIBUTIONS, PLAN POSITIONAL ACCURACY AND DOSE VERIFICATION, ALL LESIONS TREATED, PER COURSE OF TREATMENT	00	9			D			N
G0243	MULTI-SOURCE PHOTON STEREOTACTIC RADIOSURGERY, DELIVERY INCLUDING COLLIMATOR CHANGES AND CUSTOM PLUGGING, COMPLETE COURSE OF TREATMENT, ALL LESIONS	00	9			D			N
G0244	OBSERVATION CARE PROVIDED BY A FACILITY TO A PATIENT WITH CHF, CHEST PAIN, OR ASTHMA, MINIMUM EIGHT HOURS, MAXIMUM FORTY EIGHT HOURS	00	9			D			N
G0245	INITIAL PHYSICIAN EVALUATION AND MANAGEMENT OF A DIABETIC PATIENT WITH DIABETIC SENSORY NEUROPATHY RESULTING IN A LOSS OF PROTECTIVE SENSATION (LOPS) WHICH MUST INCLUDE: (1) THE DIAGNOSIS OF LOPS, (2) A PATIENT HISTORY, (3) A PHYSICAL EXAMINATION THAT CONSISTS OF AT LEAST THE FOLLOWING ELEMENTS: (A) VISUAL INSPECTION OF THE FOREFOOT, HINDFOOT AND TOE WEB SPACES, (B)EVALUATION OF A PROTECTIVE SENSATION, (C) EVALUATION OF FOOT STRUCTURE AND BIOMECHANICS, (D) EVALUATION OF VASCULAR STATUS AND SKIN INTEGRITY, AND (E) EVALUATION AND RECOMMENDATION OF FOOTWEAR AND (4) PATIENT EDUCATION	11	A			D			N
G0246	FOLLOW-UP PHYSICIAN EVALUATION AND MANAGEMENT OF A DIABETIC PATIENT WITH DIABETIC SENSORY NEUROPATHY RESULTING IN A LOSS OF PROTECTIVE SENSATION (LOPS) TO INCLUDE AT LEAST THE FOLLOWING: (1) A PATIENT HISTORY, (2) A PHYSICAL EXAMINATION THAT INCLUDES: (A) VISUAL INSPECTION OF THE FOREFOOT, HINDFOOT AND TOE WEB SPACES, (B) EVALUATION OF PROTECTIVE SENSATION, (C) EVALUATION OF FOOT STRUCTURE AND BIOMECHANICS, (D) EVALUATION OF VASCULAR STATUS AND SKIN INTEGRITY, AND (E) EVALUATION AND RECOMMENDATION OF FOOTWEAR, AND (3) PATIENT EDUCATION	11	A			D			N
G0247	ROUTINE FOOT CARE BY A PHYSICIAN OF A DIABETIC PATIENT WITH DIABETIC SENSORY NEUROPATHY RESULTING IN A LOSS OF PROTECTIVE SENSATION (LOPS) TO INCLUDE, THE LOCAL CARE OF SUPERFICIAL WOUNDS (I.E. SUPERFICIAL TO MUSCLE AND FASCIA) AND AT LEAST THE FOLLOWING IF PRESENT: (1) LOCAL CARE OF SUPERFICIAL WOUNDS, (2) DEBRIDEMENT OF CORNS AND CALLUSES, AND (3) TRIMMING AND DEBRIDEMENT OF NAILS	11	A			D			C
G0248	DEMONSTRATION, AT INITIAL USE, OF HOME INR MONITORING FOR PATIENT WITH MECHANICAL HEART VALVE(S) WHO MEETS MEDICARE COVERAGE CRITERIA, UNDER THE DIRECTION OF A PHYSICIAN; INCLUDES: DEMONSTRATING USE AND CARE OF THE INR MONITOR, OBTAINING AT LEAST ONE BLOOD SAMPLE, PROVISION OF INSTRUCTIONS FOR REPORTING HOME INR TEST RESULTS, AND DOCUMENTATION OF PATIENT ABILITY TO PERFORM TESTING	11	A			D			T

HCPCS	Long Description	PH	MPI	Statute	X-Refl	Coverage	ASC Pay Grp	ASC Pay Grp Eff Date	Action Code
G0249	PROVISION OF TEST MATERIALS AND EQUIPMENT FOR HOME INR MONITORING TO PATIENT WITH MECHANICAL HEART VALVE(S) WHO MEETS MEDICARE COVERAGE CRITERIA; INCLUDES PROVISION OF MATERIALS FOR USE IN THE HOME AND REPORTING OF TEST RESULTS TO PHYSICIAN; PER 4 TESTS	11	A			D			T
G0250	PHYSICIAN REVIEW, INTERPRETATION AND PATIENT MANAGEMENT OF HOME INR TESTING FOR A PATIENT WITH MECHANICAL HEART VALVE(S) WHO MEETS OTHER COVERAGE CRITERIA; PER 4 TESTS (DOES NOT REQUIRE FACE-TO-FACE SERVICE)	11	A			D			N
G0251	LINEAR ACCELERATOR BASED STEREOTACTIC RADIOSURGERY, DELIVERY INCLUDING COLLIMATOR CHANGES AND CUSTOM PLUGGING, FRACTIONATED TREATMENT, ALL LESIONS, PER SESSION, MAXIMUM FIVE SESSIONS PER COURSE OF TREATMENT	00	9			D			N
G0252	PET IMAGING, FULL AND PARTIAL-RING PET SCANNERS ONLY, FOR INITIAL DIAGNOSIS OF BREAST CANCER AND/OR SURGICAL PLANNING FOR BREAST CANCER (E.G. INITIAL STAGING OF AXILLARY LYMPH NODES)	00	9			M			N
G0253	PET IMAGING FOR BREAST CANCER, FULL AND PARTIAL-RING PET SCANNERS ONLY, STAGING/RESTAGING OF LOCAL REGIONAL RECURRENCE OR DISTANT METASTASES (I.E., STAGING/RESTAGING AFTER OR PRIOR TO COURSE OF TREATMENT)	11	A			C			N
G0254	PET IMAGING FOR BREAST CANCER, FULL AND PARTIAL- RING PET SCANNERS ONLY, EVALUATION OF RESPONSE TO TREATMENT, PERFORMED DURING COURSE OF TREATMENT	11	A			C			N
G0255	CURRENT PERCEPTION THRESHOLD/SENSORY NERVE CONDUCTION TEST, (SNCT) PER LIMB, ANY NERVE	00	9			M			N
G0256	PROSTATE BRACHYTHERAPY USING PERMANENTLY IMPLANTED PALLADIUM SEEDS, INCLUDING TRANSPERITONEAL PLACEMENT OF NEEDLES OR CATHETERS INTO THE PROSTATE, CYSTOSCOPY AND APPLICATION OF PERMANENT INTERSTITIAL RADIATION SOURCE	00	9			D			N
G0257	UNSCHEDULED OR EMERGENCY DIALYSIS TREATMENT FOR AN ESRD PATIENT IN A HOSPITAL OUTPATIENT DEPARTMENT THAT IS NOT CERTIFIED AS AN ESRD FACILITY	00	9			D			N
G0258	INTRAVENOUS INFUSION DURING SEPARATELY PAYABLE OBSERVATION STAY, PER OBSERVATION STAY (MUST BE REPORTED WITH G0244)	00	9			D			N
G0259	INJECTION PROCEDURE FOR SACROILIAC JOINT; ARTHROGRAPY	00	9			D			N
G0260	INJECTION PROCEDURE FOR SACROILIAC JOINT; PROVISION OF ANESTHETIC, STEROID AND/OR OTHER THERAPEUTIC AGENT AND ARTHROGRAPHY	00	9			D			N
G0261	PROSTATE BRACHYTHERAPY USING PERMANENTLY IMPLANTED IODINE SEEDS, INCLUDING TRANSPERINEAL PLACEMENT OF NEEDLES OR CATHETERS INTO THE PROSTATE, CYSTOSCOPY AND APPLICATION OF PERMANENT INTERSTITIAL RADIATION SOURCE	00	9			D			N
G0262	SMALL INTESTINAL IMAGING; INTRALUMINAL, FROM LIGAMENT OF TREITZ TO THE ILEO CECAL VALVE, INCLUDES PHYSICIAN INTERPRETATION AND REPORT	11	A			G			D
G0263	DIRECT ADMISSION OF PATIENT WITH DIAGNOSIS OF CONGESTIVE HEART FAILURE, CHEST PAIN OR ASTHMA FOR OBSERVATION SERVICES THAT MEET ALL CRITERIA FOR G0244	00	9			D			N
G0264	INITIAL NURSING ASSESSMENT OF PATIENT DIRECTLY ADMITTED TO OBSERVATION WITH DIAGNOSIS OTHER THAN CHF, CHEST PAIN OR ASTHMA OR PATIENT DIRECTLY ADMITTED TO OBSERVATION WITH DIAGNOSIS OF CHF, CHEST PAIN OR ASTHMA WHEN THE OBSERVATION STAY DOES NOT QUALIFY FOR G0244	00	9			D			N
G0265	CRYOPRESERVATION, FREEZING AND STORAGE OF CELLS FOR THERAPEUTIC USE, EACH CELL LINE	13	A			C			N
G0266	THAWING AND EXPANSION OF FROZEN CELLS FOR THERAPEUTIC USE, EACH ALIQUOT	11	A			C			N
G0267	BONE MARROW OR PERIPHERAL STEM CELL HARVEST, MODIFICATION OR TREATMENT TO ELIMINATE CELL TYPE(S) (E.G. T-CELLS, METASTATIC CARCINOMA)	11	A			C			N
G0268	REMOVAL OF IMPACTED CERUMEN (ONE OR BOTH EARS) BY PHYSICIAN ON SAME DATE OF SERVICE AS AUDIOLOGIC FUNCTION TESTING	11	A			C			N

HCPCS	Long Description	PII	MPI	Statute	X-Ref	Coverage	ASC Pay Grp	ASC Pay Grp Eff Date	Action Code
G0269	PLACEMENT OF OCCLUSIVE DEVICE INTO EITHER A VENOUS OR ARTERIAL ACCESS SITE, POST SURGICAL OR INTERVENTIONAL PROCEDURE (E.G. ANGIOSEAL PLUG, VASCULAR PLUG)	00	9			D			N
G0270	MEDICAL NUTRITION THERAPY; REASSESSMENT AND SUBSEQUENT INTERVENTION(S) FOLLOWING SECOND REFERRAL IN SAME YEAR FOR CHANGE IN DIAGNOSIS, MEDICAL CONDITION OR TREATMENT REGIMEN (INCLUDING ADDITIONAL HOURS NEEDED FOR RENAL DISEASE), INDIVIDUAL, FACE TO FACE WITH THE PATIENT, EACH 15 MINUTES	11	A			C			N
G0271	MEDICAL NUTRITION THERAPY, REASSESSMENT AND SUBSEQUENT INTERVENTION(S) FOLLOWING SECOND REFERRAL IN SAME YEAR FOR CHANGE IN DIAGNOSIS, MEDICAL CONDITION, OR TREATMENT REGIMEN (INCLUDING ADDITIONAL HOURS NEEDED FOR RENAL DISEASE), GROUP (2 OR MORE INDIVIDUALS), EACH 30 MINUTES	11	A			C			N
G0272	NASO/ORO GASTRIC TUBE PLACEMENT, REQUIRING PHYSICIANS SKILL AND FLUOROSCOPIC GUIDANCE (INCLUDES FLUOROSCOPY, IMAGE DOCUMENTATION AND REPORT)	11	A			G			D
G0273	RADIOPHARMACEUTICAL BIODISTRIBUTION, SINGLE OR MULTIPLE SCANS ON ONE OR MORE DAYS, PRE-TREATMENT PLANNING FOR RADIOPHARMACEUTICAL THERAPY OF NON-HODGKINS LYMPHOMA, INCLUDES ADMINISTRATION OF RADIOPHARMACEUTICAL (E.G., RADIOLABELED ANTIBODIES)	11	A			G			D
G0274	RADIOPHARMACEUTICAL THERAPY, NON-HODGKINS LYMPHOMA, INCLUDES ADMINISTRATION OF RADIOPHARMACEUTICAL (.E.G. RADIOLABELED ANTIBODIES)	11	A			G			D
G0275	RENAL ARTERY ANGIOGRAPHY (UNILATERAL OR BILATERAL) PERFORMED AT THE TIME OF CARDIAC CATHETERIZATION, INCLUDES CATHETER PLACEMENT, INJECTION OF DYE, FLUSH AORTOGRAM AND RADIOLOGIC SUPERVISION AND INTERPRETATION AND PRODUCTION OF IMAGES (LIST SEPARATELY IN ADDITION TO PRIMARY PROCEDURE)	11	A			C			N
G0278	ILIAC ARTERY ANGIOGRAPHY PERFORMED AT THE SAME TIME OF CARDIAC CATHETERIZATION, INCLUDES CATHETER PLACEMENT, INJECTION OF DYE, RADIOLOGIC SUPERVISION AND INTERPRETATION AND PRODUCTION OF IMAGES (LIST SEPARATELY IN ADDITION TO PRIMARY PROCEDURE)	11	A			C			N
G0279	EXTRACORPOREAL SHOCK WAVE THERAPY; INVOLVING ELBOW EPICONDYLITIS	11	A			C			T
G0280	EXTRACORPOREAL SHOCK WAVE THERAPY; INVOLVING OTHER THAN ELBOW EPICONDYLITIS OR PLANTAR FASCITIS	11	A			C			T
G0281	ELECTRICAL STIMULATION, (UNATTENDED), TO ONE OR MORE AREAS, FOR CHRONIC STAGE III AND STAGE IV PRESSURE ULCERS, ARTERIAL ULCERS, DIABETIC ULCERS, AND VENOUS STATSIS ULCERS NOT DEMONSTRATING MEASURABLE SIGNS OF HEALING AFTER 30 DAYS OF CONVENTIONAL CARE, AS PART OF A THERAPY PLAN OF CARE	11	A			C			N
G0282	ELECTRICAL STIMULATION, (UNATTENDED), TO ONE OR MORE AREAS, FOR WOUND CARE OTHER THAN DESCRIBED IN G0281	00	9			M			N
G0283	ELECTRICAL STIMULATION (UNATTENDED), TO ONE OR MORE AREAS FOR INDICATION(S) OTHER THAN WOUND CARE, AS PART OF A THERAPY PLAN OF CARE	11	A			C			T
G0288	RECONSTRUCTION, COMPUTED TOMOGRAPHIC ANGIOGRAPHY OF AORTA FOR SURGICAL PLANNING FOR VASCULAR SURGERY	11	A			C			N
G0289	ARTHROSCOPY, KNEE, SURGICAL, FOR REMOVAL OF LOOSE BODY, FOREIGN BODY, DEBRIDEMENT/SHAVING OF ARTICULAR CARTILAGE (CHRONDROPLASTY) AT THE TIME OF OTHER SURGICAL KNEE ARTHROSCOPY IN A DIFFERENT COMPARTMENT OF THE SAME KNEE	11	A			C			N
G0290	TRANSCATHETER PLACEMENT OF A DRUG ELUTING INTRACORONARY STENT(S), PERCUTANEOUS, WITH OR WITHOUT OTHER THERAPEUTIC INTERVENTION, ANY METHOD; SINGLE VESSEL	00	9			D			N
G0291	TRANSCATHETER PLACEMENT OF A DRUG ELUTING INTRACORONARY STENT(S), PERCUTANEOUS, WITH OR WITHOUT OTHER THERAPEUTIC INTERVENTION, ANY METHOD; EACH ADDITIONAL VESSEL	00	9			D			N
G0292	ADMINISTRATION(S) OF EXPERIMENTAL DRUG(S) ONLY IN A MEDICARE QUALIFYING CLINICAL TRIAL (INCLUDES ADMINISTRATION FOR CHEMOTHERAPY AND OTHER TYPES OF THERAPY VIA INFUSION AND/OR OTHER THAN INFUSION), PER DAY	00	9			D			N
G0293	NONCOVERED SURGICAL PROCEDURE(S) USING CONSCIOUS SEDATION, REGIONAL, GENERAL OR SPINAL ANESTHESIA IN A MEDICARE QUALIFYING CLINICAL TRIAL, PER DAY	00	9			D			N

HCPCS	Long Description	PH	MPI	Statute	X-Reft	Coverage	ASC Pay Grp	ASC Pay Grp Eff Date	Action Code
G0294	NONCOVERED PROCEDURE(S) USING EITHER NO ANESTHESIA OR LOCAL ANESTHESIA ONLY, IN A MEDICARE QUALIFYING CLINICAL TRIAL, PER DAY	00	9			D			N
G0295	ELECTROMAGNETIC STIMULATION, TO ONE OR MORE AREAS	00	9			M			N
G0296	PET IMAGING, FULL AND PARTIAL RING PET SCANNER ONLY, FOR RESTAGING OF PREVIOUSLY TREATED THYROID CANCER OF FOLLICULAR CELL ORIGIN FOLLOWING NEGATIVE I-131 WHOLE BODY SCAN	13	A			C			A
G0297	INSERTION OF SINGLE CHAMBER PACING CARDIOVERTER DEFIBRILLATOR PULSE GENERATOR	00	9			C			A
G0298	INSERTION OF DUAL CHAMBER PACING CARDIOVERTER DEFIBRILLATOR PULSE GENERATOR	00	9			C			A
G0299	INSERTION OR REPOSITIONING OF ELECTRODE LEAD FOR SINGLE CHAMBER PACING CARDIOVERTER DEFIBRILLATOR AND INSERTION OF PULSE GENERATOR	00	9			C			A
G0300	INSERTION OR REPOSITIONING OF ELECTRODE LEAD(S) FOR DUAL CHAMBER PACING CARDIOVERTER DEFIBRILLATOR AND INSERTION OF PULSE GENERATOR	00	9			C			A
G0302	PRE-OPERATIVE PULMONARY SURGERY SERVICES FOR PREPARATION FOR LVRS, COMPLETE COURSE OF SERVICES, TO INCLUDE A MINIMUM OF 16 DAYS OF SERVICES	00	9			C			A
G0303	PRE-OPERATIVE PULMONARY SURGERY SERVICES FOR PREPARATION FOR LVRS, 10 TO 15 DAYS OF SERVICES	00	9			C			A
G0304	PRE-OPERATIVE PULMONARY SURGERY SERVICES FOR PREPARATION FOR LVRS, 1 TO 9 DAYS SERVICES	00	9			C			A
G0305	POST-DISCHARGE PULMONARY SURGERY SERVICES AFTER LVRS, MINIMUM OF 6 DAYS OF SERVICES	00	9			C			A
G0306	COMPLETE CBC, AUTOMATED (HGB, HCT, RBC, WBC, WITHOUT PLATELET COUNT) AND AUTOMATED WBC DIFFERENTIAL COUNT	00	9			C			A
G0307	COMPLETE (CBC), AUTOMATED (HGB, HCT, RBC, WBC; WITHOUT PLATELET COUNT)	00	9			C			A
G3001	ADMINISTRATION AND SUPPLY OF TOSITUMOMAB, 450 MG	13	A			C			A
G9001	COORDINATED CARE FEE, INITIAL RATE	00	9			D			N
G9002	COORDINATED CARE FEE, MAINTENANCE RATE	00	9			D			N
G9003	COORDINATED CARE FEE, RISK ADJUSTED HIGH, INITIAL	00	9			D			N
G9004	COORDINATED CARE FEE, RISK ADJUSTED LOW, INITIAL	00	9			D			N
G9005	COORDINATED CARE FEE, RISK ADJUSTED MAINTENANCE	00	9			D			N
G9006	COORDINATED CARE FEE, HOME MONITORING	00	9			D			N
G9007	COORDINATED CARE FEE, SCHEDULED TEAM CONFERENCE	00	9			D			N
G9008	COORDINATED CARE FEE, PHYSICIAN COORDINATED CARE OVERSIGHT SERVICES	00	9			D			N
G9009	COORDINATED CARE FEE, RISK ADJUSTED MAINTENANCE, LEVEL 3	00	9			D			N
G9010	COORDINATED CARE FEE, RISK ADJUSTED MAINTENANCE, LEVEL 4	00	9			D			N
G9011	COORDINATED CARE FEE, RISK ADJUSTED MAINTENANCE, LEVEL 5	00	9			D			N
G9012	OTHER SPECIFIED CASE MANAGEMENT SERVICE NOT ELSEWHERE CLASSIFIED	00	9			D			N
G9016	SMOKING CESSATION COUNSELING, INDIVIDUAL, IN THE ABSENCE OF OR IN ADDITION TO ANY OTHER EVALUATION AND MANAGEMENT SERVICE, PER SESSION (6-10 MINUTES) [DEMO PROJECT CODE ONLY]	00	9			M			N

HCPCS	Long Description	Pit	MPI	Statute	X-Ref	Coverage	ASC Pay Grp	ASC Pay Grp Eff Date	Action Code
H0001	ALCOHOL AND/OR DRUG ASSESSMENT	00	9			I			N
H0002	BEHAVIORAL HEALTH SCREENING TO DETERMINE ELIGIBILITY FOR ADMISSION TO TREATMENT PROGRAM	00	9			I			N
H0003	ALCOHOL AND/OR DRUG SCREENING; LABORATORY ANALYSIS OF SPECIMENS FOR PRESENCE OF ALCOHOL AND/OR DRUGS	00	9			I			N
H0004	BEHAVIORAL HEALTH COUNSELING AND THERAPY, PER 15 MINUTES	00	9			I			N
H0005	ALCOHOL AND/OR DRUG SERVICES; GROUP COUNSELING BY A CLINICIAN	00	9			I			N
H0006	ALCOHOL AND/OR DRUG SERVICES; CASE MANAGEMENT	00	9			I			N
H0007	ALCOHOL AND/OR DRUG SERVICES; CRISIS INTERVENTION (OUTPATIENT)	00	9			I			N
H0008	ALCOHOL AND/OR DRUG SERVICES; SUB-ACUTE DETOXIFICATION (HOSPITAL INPATIENT)	00	9			I			N
H0009	ALCOHOL AND/OR DRUG SERVICES; ACUTE DETOXIFICATION (HOSPITAL INPATIENT)	00	9			I			N
H0010	ALCOHOL AND/OR DRUG SERVICES; SUB-ACUTE DETOXIFICATION (RESIDENTIAL ADDICTION PROGRAM INPATIENT)	00	9			I			N
H0011	ALCOHOL AND/OR DRUG SERVICES; ACUTE DETOXIFICATION (RESIDENTIAL ADDICTION PROGRAM INPATIENT)	00	9			I			N
H0012	ALCOHOL AND/OR DRUG SERVICES; SUB-ACUTE DETOXIFICATION (RESIDENTIAL ADDICTION PROGRAM OUTPATIENT)	00	9			I			N
H0013	ALCOHOL AND/OR DRUG SERVICES; ACUTE DETOXIFICATION (RESIDENTIAL ADDICTION PROGRAM OUTPATIENT)	00	9			I			N
H0014	ALCOHOL AND/OR DRUG SERVICES; AMBULATORY DETOXIFICATION	00	9			I			N
H0015	ALCOHOL AND/OR DRUG SERVICES; INTENSIVE OUTPATIENT (TREATMENT PROGRAM THAT OPERATES AT LEAST 3 HOURS/DAY AND AT LEAST 3 DAYS/WEEK AND IS BASED ON AN INDIVIDUALIZED TREATMENT PLAN), INCLUDING ASSESSMENT, COUNSELING; CRISIS INTERVENTION, AND ACTIVITY THERAPIES OR EDUCATION	00	9			I			N
H0016	ALCOHOL AND/OR DRUG SERVICES; MEDICAL/SOMATIC (MEDICAL INTERVENTION IN AMBULATORY SETTING)	00	9			I			N
H0017	BEHAVIORAL HEALTH; RESIDENTIAL (HOSPITAL RESIDENTIAL TREATMENT PROGRAM), WITHOUT ROOM AND BOARD, PER DIEM	00	9			I			N
H0018	BEHAVIORAL HEALTH; SHORT-TERM RESIDENTIAL (NON-HOSPITAL RESIDENTIAL TREATMENT PROGRAM), WITHOUT ROOM AND BOARD, PER DIEM	00	9			I			N
H0019	BEHAVIORAL HEALTH; LONG-TERM RESIDENTIAL (NON-MEDIAL, NON-ACUTE CARE IN A RESIDENTIAL TREATMENT PROGRAM WHERE STAY IS TYPICALLY LONGER THAN 30 DAYS), WITHOUT ROOM AND BOARD, PER DIEM	00	9			I			N
H0020	ALCOHOL AND/OR DRUG SERVICES; METHADONE ADMINISTRATION AND/OR SERVICE (PROVISION OF THE DRUG BY A LICENSED PROGRAM)	00	9			I			N
H0021	ALCOHOL AND/OR DRUG TRAINING SERVICE (FOR STAFF AND PERSONNEL NOT EMPLOYED BY PROVIDERS)	00	9			I			N
H0022	ALCOHOL AND/OR DRUG INTERVENTION SERVICE (PLANNED FACILITATION)	00	9			I			N

HCPCS	Long Description	PII	MPI	Statute	X-Ref	Coverage	ASC Pay Grp	ASC Pay Grp Eff Date	Action Code
H0023	BEHAVIORAL HEALTH OUTREACH SERVICE (PLANNED APPROACH TO REACH A TARGETED POPULATION)	00	9			I			N
H0024	BEHAVIORAL HEALTH PREVENTION INFORMATION DISSEMINATION SERVICE (ONE-WAY DIRECT OR NON-DIRECT CONTACT WITH SERVICE AUDIENCES TO AFFECT KNOWLEDGE AND ATTITUDE)	00	9			I			N
H0025	BEHAVIORAL HEALTH PREVENTION EDUCATION SERVICE (DELIVERY OF SERVICES WITH TARGET POPULATION TO AFFECT KNOWLEDGE, ATTITUDE AND/OR BEHAVIOR)	00	9			I			N
H0026	ALCOHOL AND/OR DRUG PREVENTION PROCESS SERVICE, COMMUNITY-BASED (DELIVERY OF SERVICES TO DEVELOP SKILLS OF IMPACTORS)	00	9			I			N
H0027	ALCOHOL AND/OR DRUG PREVENTION ENVIRONMENTAL SERVICE (BROAD RANGE OF EXTERNAL ACTIVITIES GEARED TOWARD MODIFYING SYSTEMS IN ORDER TO MAINSTREAM PREVENTION THROUGH POLICY AND LAW)	00	9			I			N
H0028	ALCOHOL AND/OR DRUG PREVENTION PROBLEM IDENTIFICATION AND REFERRAL SERVICE (E.G. STUDENT ASSISTANCE AND EMPLOYEE ASSISTANCE PROGRAMS), DOES NOT INCLUDE ASSESSMENT	00	9			I			N
H0029	ALCOHOL AND/OR DRUG PREVENTION ALTERNATIVES SERVICE (SERVICES FOR POPULATIONS THAT EXCLUDE ALCOHOL AND OTHER DRUG USE E.G. ALCOHOL FREE SOCIAL EVENTS)	00	9			I			N
H0030	BEHAVIORAL HEALTH HOTLINE SERVICE	00	9			I			N
H0031	MENTAL HEALTH ASSESSMENT, BY NON-PHYSICIAN	00	9			I			N
H0032	MENTAL HEALTH SERVICE PLAN DEVELOPMENT BY NON-PHYSICIAN	00	9			I			N
H0033	ORAL MEDICATION ADMINISTRATION, DIRECT OBSERVATION	00	9			I			N
H0034	MEDICATION TRAINING AND SUPPORT, PER 15 MINUTES	00	9			I			N
H0035	MENTAL HEALTH PARTIAL HOSPITALIZATION, TREATMENT, LESS THAN 24 HOURS	00	9			I			N
H0036	COMMUNITY PSYCHIATRIC SUPPORTIVE TREATMENT, FACE-TO-FACE, PER 15 MINUTES	00	9			I			N
H0037	COMMUNITY PSYCHIATRIC SUPPORTIVE TREATMENT PROGRAM, PER DIEM	00	9			I			N
H0038	SELF-HELP/PEER SERVICES, PER 15 MINUTES	00	9			I			N
H0039	ASSERTIVE COMMUNITY TREATMENT, FACE-TO-FACE, PER 15 MINUTES	00	9			I			N
H0040	ASSERTIVE COMMUNITY TREATMENT PROGRAM, PER DIEM	00	9			I			N
H0041	FOSTER CARE, CHILD, NON-THERAPEUTIC, PER DIEM	00	9			I			N
H0042	FOSTER CARE, CHILD, NON-THERAPEUTIC, PER MONTH	00	9			I			N
H0043	SUPPORTED HOUSING, PER DIEM	00	9			I			N
H0044	SUPPORTED HOUSING, PER MONTH	00	9			I			N
H0045	RESPITE CARE SERVICES, NOT IN THE HOME, PER DIEM	00	9			I			N
H0046	MENTAL HEALTH SERVICES, NOT OTHERWISE SPECIFIED	00	9			I			N

HCPCS	Long Description	PII	MPI	Statute	X-Ref	Coverage	ASC Pay Grp	ASC Pay Grp Eff Date	Action Code
H0047	ALCOHOL AND/OR OTHER DRUG ABUSE SERVICES, NOT OTHERWISE SPECIFIED	00	9			I			N
H0048	ALCOHOL AND/OR OTHER DRUG TESTING: COLLECTION AND HANDLING ONLY, SPECIMENS OTHER THAN BLOOD	00	9			I			N
H1000	PRENATAL CARE, AT-RISK ASSESSMENT	00	9			I			N
H1001	PRENATAL CARE, AT-RISK ENHANCED SERVICE; ANTEPARTUM MANAGEMENT	00	9			I			N
H1002	PRENATAL CARE, AT RISK ENHANCED SERVICE; CARE COORDINATION	00	9			I			N
H1003	PRENATAL CARE, AT-RISK ENHANCED SERVICE; EDUCATION	00	9			I			N
H1004	PRENATAL CARE, AT-RISK ENHANCED SERVICE; FOLLOW-UP HOME VISIT	00	9			I			N
H1005	PRENATAL CARE, AT-RISK ENHANCED SERVICE PACKAGE (INCLUDES H1001-H1004)	00	9			I			N
H1010	NON-MEDICAL FAMILY PLANNING EDUCATION, PER SESSION	00	9			I			N
H1011	FAMILY ASSESSMENT BY LICENSED BEHAVIORAL HEALTH PROFESSIONAL FOR STATE DEFINED PURPOSES	00	9			I			N
H2000	COMPREHENSIVE MULTIDISCIPLINARY EVALUATION	00	9			I			N
H2001	REHABILITATION PROGRAM, PER 1/2 DAY	00	9			I			N
H2010	COMPREHENSIVE MEDICATION SERVICES, PER 15 MINUTES	00	9			I			A
H2011	CRISIS INTERVENTION SERVICE, PER 15 MINUTES	00	9			I			A
H2012	BEHAVIORAL HEALTH DAY TREATMENT, PER HOUR	00	9			I			A
H2013	PSYCHIATRIC HEALTH FACILITY SERVICE, PER DIEM	00	9			I			A
H2014	SKILLS TRAINING AND DEVELOPMENT, PER 15 MINUTES	00	9			I			A
H2015	COMPREHENSIVE COMMUNITY SUPPORT SERVICES, PER 15 MINUTES	00	9			I			A
H2016	COMPREHENSIVE COMMUNITY SUPPORT SERVICES, PER DIEM	00	9			I			A
H2017	PSYCHOSOCIAL REHABILITATION SERVICES, PER 15 MINUTES	00	9			I			A
H2018	PSYCHOSOCIAL REHABILITATION SERVICES, PER DIEM	00	9			I			A
H2019	THERAPEUTIC BEHAVIORAL SERVICES, PER 15 MINUTES	00	9			I			A
H2020	THERAPEUTIC BEHAVIORAL SERVICES, PER DIEM	00	9			I			A
H2021	COMMUNITY-BASED WRAP-AROUND SERVICES, PER 15 MINUTES	00	9			I			A
H2022	COMMUNITY-BASED WRAP-AROUND SERVICES, PER DIEM	00	9			I			A
H2023	SUPPORTED EMPLOYMENT, PER 15 MINUTES	00	9			I			A

HCPCS	Long Description	PTI	MPI	Statute	X-Ref	Coverage	ASC Pay Grp	ASC Pay Grp Eff Date	Action Code
H2024	SUPPORTED EMPLOYMENT, PER DIEM	00	9			I			A
H2025	ONGOING SUPPORT TO MAINTAIN EMPLOYMENT, PER 15 MINUTES	00	9			I			A
H2026	ONGOING SUPPORT TO MAINTAIN EMPLOYMENT, PER DIEM	00	9			I			A
H2027	PSYCHOEDUCATIONAL SERVICE, PER 15 MINUTES	00	9			I			A
H2028	SEXUAL OFFENDER TREATMENT SERVICE, PER 15 MINUTES	00	9			I			A
H2029	SEXUAL OFFENDER TREATMENT SERVICE, PER DIEM	00	9			I			A
H2030	MENTAL HEALTH CLUBHOUSE SERVICES, PER 15 MINUTES	00	9			I			A
H2031	MENTAL HEALTH CLUBHOUSE SERVICES, PER DIEM	00	9			I			A
H2032	ACTIVITY THERAPY, PER 15 MINUTES	00	9			I			A
H2033	MULTISYSTEMIC THERAPY FOR JUVENILES, PER 15 MINUTES	00	9			I			A
H2034	ALCOHOL AND/OR DRUG ABUSE HALFWAY HOUSE SERVICES, PER DIEM	00	9			I			A
H2035	ALCOHOL AND/OR OTHER DRUG TREATMENT PROGRAM, PER HOUR	00	9			I			A
H2036	ALCOHOL AND/OR OTHER DRUG TREATMENT PROGRAM, PER DIEM	00	9			I			A
H2037	DEVELOPMENTAL DELAY PREVENTION ACTIVITIES, DEPENDENT CHILD OF CLIENT, PER 15 MINUTES	00	9			I			A
J0120	INJECTION, TETRACYCLINE, UP TO 250 MG	51	A			D			N
J0130	INJECTION ABCIXIMAB, 10 MG	51	A			D			N
J0150	INJECTION, ADENOSINE, 6 MG (NOT TO BE USED TO REPORT ANY ADENOSINE PHOSPHATE COMPOUNDS, INSTEAD USE A9270)	51	A			D			N
J0151	INJECTION, ADENOSINE, 90 MG (NOT TO BE USED TO REPORT ANY ADENOSINE PHOSPHATE COMPOUNDS, INSTEAD USE A9270)	51	A		J0152	D			D
J0152	INJECTION, ADENOSINE, 30 MG (NOT TO BE USED TO REPORT ANY ADENOSINE PHOSPHATE COMPOUNDS, INSTEAD USE A9270)	51	A			C			A
J0170	INJECTION, ADRENALIN, EPINEPHRINE, UP TO 1 ML AMPULE	51	A			D			N
J0190	INJECTION, BIPERIDEN LACTATE, PER 5 MG	51	A			D			N
J0200	INJECTION, ALATROFLOXACIN MESYLATE, 100 MG	51	A			D			N
J0205	INJECTION, ALGLUCERASE, PER 10 UNITS	51	A			D			N
J0207	INJECTION, AMIFOSTINE, 500 MG	51	A			D			N
J0210	INJECTION, METHYLDOPATE HCL, UP TO 250 MG	51	A			D			N
J0215	INJECTION, ALEFACEPT, 0.5 MG	51	A			C			A
J0256	INJECTION, ALPHA 1 - PROTEINASE INHIBITOR - HUMAN, 10 MG	51	A			D			N

HCPCS	Long Description	PII	MPI	Statute	X-Ref	Coverage	ASC Pay Grp	ASC Pay Grp Eff Date	Action Code
J0270	INJECTION, ALPROSTADIL, 1.25 MCG (CODE MAY BE USED FOR MEDICARE WHEN DRUG ADMINISTERED UNDER THE DIRECT SUPERVISION OF A PHYSICIAN, NOT FOR USE WHEN DRUG IS SELF ADMINISTERED)	51	A			D			N
J0275	ALPROSTADIL URETHRAL SUPPOSITORY (CODE MAY BE USED FOR MEDICARE WHEN DRUG ADMINISTERED UNDER THE DIRECT SUPERVISION OF A PHYSICIAN, NOT FOR USE WHEN DRUG IS SELF ADMINISTERED)	51	A			D			N
J0280	INJECTION, AMINOPHYLLIN, UP TO 250 MG	51	A			D			N
J0282	INJECTION, AMIODARONE HYDROCHLORIDE, 30 MG	51	A			D			N
J0285	INJECTION, AMPHOTERICIN B, 50 MG	51	A			D			N
J0286	INJECTION, AMPHOTERICIN B, ANY LIPID FORMULATION, 50 MG	51	A			D			N
J0287	INJECTION, AMPHOTERICIN B LIPID COMPLEX, 10 MG	51	A			D			N
J0288	INJECTION, AMPHOTERICIN B CHOLESTERYL SULFATE COMPLEX, 10 MG	51	A			D			N
J0289	INJECTION, AMPHOTERICIN B LIPOSOME, 10 MG	51	A			D			N
J0290	INJECTION, AMPICILLIN SODIUM, 500 MG	51	A			D			N
J0295	INJECTION, AMPICILLIN SODIUM/SULBACTAM SODIUM, PER 1.5 GM	51	A			D			N
J0300	INJECTION, AMOBARBITAL, UP TO 125 MG	51	A			D			N
J0330	INJECTION, SUCCINYLCHOLINE CHLORIDE, UP TO 20 MG	51	A			D			N
J0340	INJECTION, NANDROLONE PHENPROPIONATE, UP TO 50 MG	51	A			D			N
J0350	INJECTION, ANISTREPLASE, PER 30 UNITS	51	A			D			N
J0360	INJECTION, HYDRALAZINE HCL, UP TO 20 MG	51	A			D			N
J0380	INJECTION, METARAMINOL BITARTRATE, PER 10 MG	51	A			D			N
J0390	INJECTION, CHLOROQUINE HYDROCHLORIDE, UP TO 250 MG	51	A			D			N
J0395	INJECTION, ARBUTAMINE HCL, 1 MG	51	A			D			N
J0400	INJECTION, TRIMETHAPHAN CAMSYLATE, UP TO 500 MG	51	A			D			N
J0456	INJECTION, AZITHROMYCIN, 500 MG	51	A			D			N
J0460	INJECTION, ATROPINE SULFATE, UP TO 0.3 MG	51	A			D			N
J0470	INJECTION, DIMERCAPROL, PER 100 MG	51	A			D			N
J0475	INJECTION, BACLOFEN, 10 MG	51	A			D			N
J0476	INJECTION, BACLOFEN, 50 MCG FOR INTRATHECAL TRIAL	51	A			D			N
J0500	INJECTION, DICYCLOMINE HCL, UP TO 20 MG	51	A			D			N
J0510	INJECTION, BENZQUINAMIDE HCL, UP TO 50 MG	51	A			D			N
J0515	INJECTION, BENZTROPINE MESYLATE, PER 1 MG	51	A			D			N

HCPCS	Long Description	PII	MPI	Statute	X-Ref	Coverage	ASC Pay Grp	ASC Pay Grp Eff Date	Action Code
J0520	INJECTION, BETHANECHOL CHLORIDE, MYOTONACHOL OR URECHOLINE, UP TO 5 MG	51	A			D			N
J0530	INJECTION, PENICILLIN G BENZATHINE AND PENICILLIN G PROCAINE, UP TO 600,000 UNITS	51	A			D			N
J0540	INJECTION, PENICILLIN G BENZATHINE AND PENICILLIN G PROCAINE, UP TO 1,200,000 UNITS	51	A			D			N
J0550	INJECTION, PENICILLIN G BENZATHINE AND PENICILLIN G PROCAINE, UP TO 2,400,000 UNITS	51	A			D			N
J0560	INJECTION, PENICILLIN G BENZATHINE, UP TO 600,000 UNITS	51	A			D			N
J0570	INJECTION, PENICILLIN G BENZATHINE, UP TO 1,200,000 UNITS	51	A			D			N
J0580	INJECTION, PENICILLIN G BENZATHINE, UP TO 2,400,000 UNITS	51	A			D			N
J0583	INJECTION, BIVALIRUDIN, 1 MG	51	A			C			A
J0585	BOTULINUM TOXIN TYPE A, PER UNIT	51	A			D			N
J0587	BOTULINUM TOXIN TYPE B, PER 100 UNITS	51	A			D			N
J0590	INJECTION, ETHYLNOREPINEPHRINE HCL, 1 ML	51	A			D			N
J0592	INJECTION, BUPRENORPHINE HYDROCHLORIDE, 0.1 MG	51	A			D			N
J0595	INJECTION, BUTORPHANOL TARTRATE, 1 MG	51	A			C			A
J0600	INJECTION, EDETATE CALCIUM DISODIUM, UP TO 1000 MG	51	A			D			N
J0610	INJECTION, CALCIUM GLUCONATE, PER 10 ML	51	A			D			N
J0620	INJECTION, CALCIUM GLYCEROPHOSPHATE AND CALCIUM LACTATE, PER 10 ML	51	A			D			N
J0630	INJECTION, CALCITONIN SALMON, UP TO 400 UNITS	51	A			D			N
J0635	INJECTION, CALCITRIOL, 1 MCG AMP.	51	A			D			N
J0636	INJECTION, CALCITRIOL, 0.1 MCG	51	A			D			N
J0637	INJECTION, CASPOFUNGIN ACETATE, 5 MG	51	A			C			N
J0640	INJECTION, LEUCOVORIN CALCIUM, PER 50 MG	51	A			D			N
J0670	INJECTION, MEPIVACAINE HYDROCHLORIDE, PER 10 ML	51	A			D			N
J0690	INJECTION, CEFAZOLIN SODIUM, 500 MG	51	A			D			N
J0692	INJECTION, CEFEPIME HYDROCHLORIDE, 500 MG	51	A			C			N
J0694	INJECTION, CEFOXITIN SODIUM, 1 GM	51	A		Q0090	D			N
J0695	INJECTION, CEFONICID SODIUM, 1 GRAM	51	A			D			N
J0696	INJECTION, CEFTRIAXONE SODIUM, PER 250 MG	51	A			D			N
J0697	INJECTION, STERILE CEFUROXIME SODIUM, PER 750 MG	51	A			D			N

HCPCS	Long Description	PII	MPI	Statute	X-Ref1	Coverage	ASC Pay Grp	ASC Pay Grp Eff Date	Action Code
J0698	INJECTION, CEFOTAXIME SODIUM, PER GM	51	A			D			N
J0702	INJECTION, BETAMETHASONE ACETATE AND BETAMETHASONE SODIUM PHOSPHATE, PER 3 MG	51	A			D			N
J0704	INJECTION, BETAMETHASONE SODIUM PHOSPHATE, PER 4 MG	51	A			D			N
J0706	INJECTION, CAFFEINE CITRATE, 5MG	51	A			C			N
J0710	INJECTION, CEPHAPIRIN SODIUM, UP TO 1 GM	51	A			D			N
J0713	INJECTION, CEFTAZIDIME, PER 500 MG	51	A			D			N
J0715	INJECTION, CEFTIZOXIME SODIUM, PER 500 MG	51	A			D			N
J0720	INJECTION, CHLORAMPHENICOL SODIUM SUCCINATE, UP TO 1 GM	51	A			D			N
J0725	INJECTION, CHORIONIC GONADOTROPIN, PER 1,000 USP UNITS	51	A			D			N
J0730	INJECTION, CHLORPHENIRAMINE MALEATE, PER 10 MG	51	A			D			N
J0735	INJECTION, CLONIDINE HYDROCHLORIDE, 1 MG	51	A			D			N
J0740	INJECTION, CIDOFOVIR, 375 MG	51	A			D			N
J0743	INJECTION, CILASTATIN SODIUM; IMIPENEM, PER 250 MG	51	A			D			N
J0744	INJECTION, CIPROFLOXACIN FOR INTRAVENOUS INFUSION, 200 MG	51	A			C			N
J0745	INJECTION, CODEINE PHOSPHATE, PER 30 MG	51	A			D			N
J0760	INJECTION, COLCHICINE, PER 1MG	51	A			D			N
J0770	INJECTION, COLISTIMETHATE SODIUM, UP TO 150 MG	51	A			D			N
J0780	INJECTION, PROCHLORPERAZINE, UP TO 10 MG	51	A			D			N
J0800	INJECTION, CORTICOTROPIN, UP TO 40 UNITS	51	A			D			N
J0810	INJECTION, CORTISONE, UP TO 50 MG	51	A			D			N
J0835	INJECTION, COSYNTROPIN, PER 0.25 MG	51	A			D			N
J0850	INJECTION, CYTOMEGALOVIRUS IMMUNE GLOBULIN INTRAVENOUS (HUMAN), PER VIAL	51	A			D			N
J0880	INJECTION, DARBEPOETIN ALFA, 5 MCG	00	9			I			F
J0895	INJECTION, DEFEROXAMINE MESYLATE, 500 MG	51	A		Q0087	D			N
J0900	INJECTION, TESTOSTERONE ENANTHATE AND ESTRADIOL VALERATE, UP TO 1 CC	51	A			D			N
J0945	INJECTION, BROMPHENIRAMINE MALEATE, PER 10 MG	51	A			D			N
J0970	INJECTION, ESTRADIOL VALERATE, UP TO 40 MG	51	A			D			N

HCPCS	Long Description	PII	MPI	Statute	X-Ref1	Coverage	ASC Pay Grp	ASC Pay Grp Eff Date	Action Code
J1000	INJECTION, DEPO-ESTRADIOL CYPIONATE, UP TO 5 MG	51	A			D			N
J1020	INJECTION, METHYLPREDNISOLONE ACETATE, 20 MG	51	A			D			N
J1030	INJECTION, METHYLPREDNISOLONE ACETATE, 40 MG	51	A			D			N
J1040	INJECTION, METHYLPREDNISOLONE ACETATE, 80 MG	51	A			D			N
J1050	INJECTION, MEDROXYPROGESTERONE ACETATE, 100 MG	51	A			D			N
J1051	INJECTION, MEDROXYPROGESTERONE ACETATE, 50 MG	51	A			D			N
J1055	INJECTION, MEDROXYPROGESTERONE ACETATE FOR CONTRACEPTIVE USE, 150 MG	00	9	1862A1		S			N
J1056	INJECTION, MEDROXYPROGESTERONE ACETATE / ESTRADIOL CYPIONATE, 5MG / 25MG	51	A			C			N
J1060	INJECTION, TESTOSTERONE CYPIONATE AND ESTRADIOL CYPIONATE, UP TO 1 ML	51	A			D			N
J1070	INJECTION, TESTOSTERONE CYPIONATE, UP TO 100 MG	51	A			D			N
J1080	INJECTION, TESTOSTERONE CYPIONATE, 1 CC, 200 MG	51	A			D			N
J1090	INJECTION, TESTOSTERONE CYPIONATE, 1 CC, 50 MG	51	A			D			N
J1094	INJECTION, DEXAMETHASONE ACETATE, 1 MG	51	A			D			N
J1095	INJECTION, DEXAMETHASONE ACETATE, PER 8 MG	51	A			D			N
J1100	INJECTION, DEXAMETHASONE SODIUM PHOSPHATE, 1MG	51	A			D			N
J1110	INJECTION, DIHYDROERGOTAMINE MESYLATE, PER 1 MG	51	A			D			N
J1120	INJECTION, ACETAZOLAMIDE SODIUM, UP TO 500 MG	51	A			D			N
J1160	INJECTION, DIGOXIN, UP TO 0.5 MG	51	A			D			N
J1165	INJECTION, PHENYTOIN SODIUM, PER 50 MG	51	A			D			N
J1170	INJECTION, HYDROMORPHONE, UP TO 4 MG	51	A			D			N
J1180	INJECTION, DYPHYLLINE, UP TO 500 MG	51	A			D			N
J1190	INJECTION, DEXRAZOXANE HYDROCHLORIDE, PER 250 MG	51	A			D			N
J1200	INJECTION, DIPHENHYDRAMINE HCL, UP TO 50 MG	51	A			D			N
J1205	INJECTION, CHLOROTHIAZIDE SODIUM, PER 500 MG	51	A			D			N
J1212	INJECTION, DMSO, DIMETHYL SULFOXIDE, 50%, 50 ML	51	A			D			N
J1230	INJECTION, METHADONE HCL, UP TO 10 MG	51	A			D			N

HCPCS	Long Description	PII	MPI	Statute	X-Ref	Coverage	ASC Pay Grp	ASC Pay Grp Eff Date	Action Code
J1240	INJECTION, DIMENHYDRINATE, UP TO 50 MG	51	A			D			N
J1245	INJECTION, DIPYRIDAMOLE, PER 10 MG	51	A			D			N
J1250	INJECTION, DOBUTAMINE HYDROCHLORIDE, PER 250 MG	51	A			D			N
J1260	INJECTION, DOLASETRON MESYLATE, 10 MG	51	A			D			N
J1270	INJECTION, DOXERCALCIFEROL, 1 MCG	51	A			C			N
J1320	INJECTION, AMITRIPTYLINE HCL, UP TO 20 MG	51	A			D			N
J1325	INJECTION, EPOPROSTENOL, 0.5 MG	51	A			D			N
J1327	INJECTION, EPTIFIBATIDE, 5 MG	51	A			D			N
J1330	INJECTION, ERGONOVINE MALEATE, UP TO 0.2 MG	51	A			D			N
J1335	INJECTION, ERTAPENEM SODIUM, 500 MG	51	A			C			A
J1362	INJECTION, ERYTHROMYCIN GLUCEPTATE, PER 250 MG	51	A			D			N
J1364	INJECTION, ERYTHROMYCIN LACTOBIONATE, PER 500 MG	51	A			D			N
J1380	INJECTION, ESTRADIOL VALERATE, UP TO 10 MG	51	A			D			N
J1390	INJECTION, ESTRADIOL VALERATE, UP TO 20 MG	51	A			D			N
J1410	INJECTION, ESTROGEN CONJUGATED, PER 25 MG	51	A			D			N
J1435	INJECTION, ESTRONE, PER 1 MG	51	A			D			N
J1436	INJECTION, ETIDRONATE DISODIUM, PER 300 MG	51	A			D			N
J1438	INJECTION, ETANERCEPT, 25 MG (CODE MAY BE USED FOR MEDICARE WHEN DRUG ADMINISTERED UNDER THE DIRECT SUPERVISION OF A PHYSICIAN, NOT FOR USE WHEN DRUG IS SELF ADMINISTERED)	51	A			D			N
J1440	INJECTION, FILGRASTIM (G-CSF), 300 MCG	51	A			D			N
J1441	INJECTION, FILGRASTIM (G-CSF), 480 MCG	51	A			D			N
J1450	INJECTION FLUCONAZOLE, 200 MG	51	A			D			N
J1452	INJECTION, FOMIVIRSEN SODIUM, INTRAOCULAR, 1.65 MG	51	A			D			N
J1455	INJECTION, FOSCARNET SODIUM, PER 1000 MG	51	A			D			N
J1460	INJECTION, GAMMA GLOBULIN, INTRAMUSCULAR, 1 CC	51	A			D			N
J1470	INJECTION, GAMMA GLOBULIN, INTRAMUSCULAR, 2 CC	51	A			D			N
J1480	INJECTION, GAMMA GLOBULIN, INTRAMUSCULAR, 3 CC	51	A			D			N
J1490	INJECTION, GAMMA GLOBULIN, INTRAMUSCULAR, 4 CC	51	A			D			N

HCPCS	Long Description	PH	MPI	Statute	X-Reff	Coverage	ASC Pay Grp	ASC Pay Grp Eff Date	Action Code
J1500	INJECTION, GAMMA GLOBULIN, INTRAMUSCULAR, 5 CC	51	A			D			N
J1510	INJECTION, GAMMA GLOBULIN, INTRAMUSCULAR, 6 CC	51	A			D			N
J1520	INJECTION, GAMMA GLOBULIN, INTRAMUSCULAR, 7 CC	51	A			D			N
J1530	INJECTION, GAMMA GLOBULIN, INTRAMUSCULAR, 8 CC	51	A			D			N
J1540	INJECTION, GAMMA GLOBULIN, INTRAMUSCULAR, 9 CC	51	A			D			N
J1550	INJECTION, GAMMA GLOBULIN, INTRAMUSCULAR, 10 CC	51	A			D			N
J1560	INJECTION, GAMMA GLOBULIN, INTRAMUSCULAR, OVER 10 CC	51	A			D			N
J1561	INJECTION, IMMUNE GLOBULIN, INTRAVENOUS, 500 MG	51	A			D			N
J1562	INJECTION, IMMUNE GLOBULIN, INTRAVENOUS, 5 GMS	51	A			D			N
J1563	INJECTION, IMMUNE GLOBULIN, INTRAVENOUS, 1G	51	A			D			N
J1564	INJECTION, IMMUNE GLOBULIN, 10 MG	51	A			D			N
J1565	INJECTION, RESPIRATORY SYNCYTIAL VIRUS IMMUNE GLOBULIN, INTRAVENOUS, 50 MG	51	A			D			N
J1570	INJECTION, GANCICLOVIR SODIUM, 500 MG	51	A			D			N
J1580	INJECTION, GARAMYCIN, GENTAMICIN, UP TO 80 MG	51	A			D			N
J1590	INJECTION, GATIFLOXACIN, 10MG	51	A			C			N
J1595	INJECTION, GLATIRAMER ACETATE, 20 MG	51	A			D			A
J1600	INJECTION, GOLD SODIUM THIOMALATE, UP TO 50 MG	51	A			D			N
J1610	INJECTION, GLUCAGON HYDROCHLORIDE, PER 1 MG	51	A			D			N
J1620	INJECTION, GONADORELIN HYDROCHLORIDE, PER 100 MCG	51	A			D			N
J1626	INJECTION, GRANISETRON HYDROCHLORIDE, 100 MCG	51	A			D			N
J1630	INJECTION, HALOPERIDOL, UP TO 5 MG	51	A			D			N
J1631	INJECTION, HALOPERIDOL DECANOATE, PER 50 MG	51	A			D			N
J1642	INJECTION, HEPARIN SODIUM, (HEPARIN LOCK FLUSH), PER 10 UNITS	51	A			D			N
J1644	INJECTION, HEPARIN SODIUM, PER 1000 UNITS	51	A			D			N
J1645	INJECTION, DALTEPARIN SODIUM, PER 2500 IU	51	A			D			N
J1650	INJECTION, ENOXAPARIN SODIUM, 10 MG	51	A			C			F
J1652	INJECTION, FONDAPARINUX SODIUM, 0.5 MG	51	A			D			N

HCPCS	Long Description	PII	MPI	Statute	X-Ref	Coverage	ASC Pay Grp	ASC Pay Grp Eff Date	Action Code
J1655	INJECTION, TINZAPARIN SODIUM, 1000 IU	46	A			C			N
J1670	INJECTION, TETANUS IMMUNE GLOBULIN, HUMAN, UP TO 250 UNITS	51	A			D			N
J1690	INJECTION, PREDNISOLONE TEBUTATE, UP TO 20 MG	51	A			D			N
J1700	INJECTION, HYDROCORTISONE ACETATE, UP TO 25 MG	51	A			D			N
J1710	INJECTION, HYDROCORTISONE SODIUM PHOSPHATE, UP TO 50 MG	51	A			D			N
J1720	INJECTION, HYDROCORTISONE SODIUM SUCCINATE, UP TO 100 MG	51	A			D			N
J1730	INJECTION, DIAZOXIDE, UP TO 300 MG	51	A			D			N
J1739	INJECTION, HYDROXYPROGESTERONE CAPROATE 125 MG/ML	51	A			D			N
J1741	INJECTION, HYDROXYPROGESTERONE CAPROATE, 250 MG/ML	51	A			D			N
J1742	INJECTION, IBUTILIDE FUMARATE, 1 MG	51	A			D			N
J1745	INJECTION INFLIXIMAB, 10 MG	51	A			D			N
J1750	INJECTION, IRON DEXTRAN, 50 MG	51	A			D			N
J1755	INJECTION, IRON SUCROSE, 20MG	51	A			C			N
J1756	INJECTION, IRON SUCROSE, 1 MG	51	A			C			N
J1785	INJECTION, IMIGLUCERASE, PER UNIT	51	A			D			N
J1790	INJECTION, DROPERIDOL, UP TO 5 MG	51	A			D			N
J1800	INJECTION, PROPRANOLOL HCL, UP TO 1 MG	51	A			D			N
J1810	INJECTION, DROPERIDOL AND FENTANYL CITRATE, UP TO 2 ML AMPULE	51	A			D			N
J1815	INJECTION, INSULIN, PER 5 UNITS	51	A			D			N
J1817	INSULIN FOR ADMINISTRATION THROUGH DME (I.E., INSULIN PUMP) PER 50 UNITS	51	A			C			N
J1820	INJECTION, INSULIN, UP TO 100 UNITS	51	A		J1815	D			N
J1825	INJECTION, INTERFERON BETA-1A, 33 MCG	00	9			I			N
J1830	INJECTION INTERFERON BETA-1B, 0.25 MG (CODE MAY BE USED FOR MEDICARE WHEN DRUG ADMINISTERED UNDER THE DIRECT SUPERVISION OF A PHYSICIAN, NOT FOR USE WHEN DRUG IS SELF ADMINISTERED)	51	A			D			N
J1835	INJECTION, ITRACONAZOLE, 50 MG	51	A			C			N
J1840	INJECTION, KANAMYCIN SULFATE, UP TO 500 MG	51	A			D			N
J1850	INJECTION, KANAMYCIN SULFATE, UP TO 75 MG	51	A			D			N
J1885	INJECTION, KETOROLAC TROMETHAMINE, PER 15 MG	51	A			D			N
J1890	INJECTION, CEPHALOTHIN SODIUM, UP TO 1 GRAM	51	A			D			N

HCPCS	Long Description	PEI	MPI	Statute	X-Refl	Coverage	ASC Pay Grp	ASC Pay Grp Eff Date	Action Code
J1910	INJECTION, KUTAPRESSIN, UP TO 2 ML	51	A			D			D
J1930	INJECTION, PROPIOMAZINE HCL, UP TO 20 MG	51	A			D			N
J1940	INJECTION, FUROSEMIDE, UP TO 20 MG	51	A			D			N
J1950	INJECTION, LEUPROLIDE ACETATE (FOR DEPOT SUSPENSION), PER 3.75 MG	51	A			D			N
J1955	INJECTION, LEVOCARNITINE, PER 1 GM	51	A			D			N
J1956	INJECTION, LEVOFLOXACIN, 250 MG	51	A			D			N
J1960	INJECTION, LEVORPHANOL TARTRATE, UP TO 2 MG	51	A			D			N
J1970	INJECTION, METHOTRIMEPRAZINE, UP TO 20 MG	51	A			D			N
J1980	INJECTION, HYOSCYAMINE SULFATE, UP TO 0.25 MG	51	A			D			N
J1990	INJECTION, CHLORDIAZEPOXIDE HCL, UP TO 100 MG	51	A			D			N
J2000	INJECTION, LIDOCAINE HCL, 50 CC	51	A			D			D
J2001	INJECTION, LIDOCAINE HCL FOR INTRAVENOUS INFUSION, 10 MG	51	A			D			A
J2010	INJECTION, LINCOMYCIN HCL, UP TO 300 MG	51	A			D			N
J2020	INJECTION, LINEZOLID, 200MG	51	A			C			N
J2060	INJECTION, LORAZEPAM, 2 MG	51	A			D			N
J2150	INJECTION, MANNITOL, 25% IN 50 ML	51	A			D			N
J2175	INJECTION, MEPERIDINE HYDROCHLORIDE, PER 100 MG	51	A			D			N
J2180	INJECTION, MEPERIDINE AND PROMETHAZINE HCL, UP TO 50 MG	51	A			D			N
J2185	INJECTION, MEROPENEM, 100 MG	51	A			C			A
J2210	INJECTION, METHYLERGONOVINE MALEATE, UP TO 0.2 MG	51	A			D			N
J2240	INJECTION, METOCURINE IODIDE, UP TO 2 MG	51	A			D			N
J2250	INJECTION, MIDAZOLAM HYDROCHLORIDE, PER 1 MG	51	A			D			N
J2260	INJECTION, MILRINONE LACTATE, 5 MG	51	A			D			N
J2270	INJECTION, MORPHINE SULFATE, UP TO 10 MG	51	A			D			N
J2271	INJECTION, MORPHINE SULFATE, 100MG	51	A			D			N
J2275	INJECTION, MORPHINE SULFATE (PRESERVATIVE-FREE STERILE SOLUTION), PER 10 MG	51	A			D			N
J2280	INJECTION, MOXIFLOXACIN, 100 MG	51	A			C			A
J2300	INJECTION, NALBUPHINE HYDROCHLORIDE, PER 10 MG	51	A			D			N
J2310	INJECTION, NALOXONE HYDROCHLORIDE, PER 1 MG	51	A			D			N

HCPCS	Long Description	PTI	MPI	Statute	X-Ref	Coverage	ASC Pay Grp	ASC Pay Grp Eff Date	Action Code
J2320	INJECTION, NANDROLONE DECANOATE, UP TO 50 MG	51	A			D			N
J2321	INJECTION, NANDROLONE DECANOATE, UP TO 100 MG	51	A			D			N
J2322	INJECTION, NANDROLONE DECANOATE, UP TO 200 MG	51	A			D			N
J2324	INJECTION, NESIRITIDE, 0.5 MG	51	A			D			N
J2330	INJECTION, THIOTHIXENE, UP TO 4 MG	51	A			D			N
J2350	INJECTION, NIACINAMIDE, NIACIN, UP TO 100 MG	51	A			D			N
J2352	INJECTION, OCTREOTIDE ACETATE, 1 MG	51	A			D			D
J2353	INJECTION, OCTREOTIDE, DEPOT FORM FOR INTRAMUSCULAR INJECTION, 1 MG	51	A			C			A
J2354	INJECTION, OCTREOTIDE, NON-DEPOT FORM FOR SUBCUTANEOUS OR INTRAVENOUS INJECTION, 25 MCG	51	A			C			A
J2355	INJECTION, OPRELVEKIN, 5 MG	51	A			D			N
J2360	INJECTION, ORPHENADRINE CITRATE, UP TO 60 MG	51	A			D			N
J2370	INJECTION, PHENYLEPHRINE HCL, UP TO 1 ML	51	A			D			N
J2400	INJECTION, CHLOROPROCAINE HYDROCHLORIDE, PER 30 ML	51	A			D			N
J2405	INJECTION, ONDANSETRON HYDROCHLORIDE, PER 1 MG	51	A			D			N
J2410	INJECTION, OXYMORPHONE HCL, UP TO 1 MG	51	A			D			N
J2430	INJECTION, PAMIDRONATE DISODIUM, PER 30 MG	51	A			D			N
J2440	INJECTION, PAPAVERINE HCL, UP TO 60 MG	51	A			D			N
J2460	INJECTION, OXYTETRACYCLINE HCL, UP TO 50 MG	51	A			D			N
J2480	INJECTION, HYDROCHLORIDES OF OPIUM ALKALOIDS, UP TO 20 MG	51	A			D			N
J2500	INJECTION, PARICALCITOL, 5 MCG	51	A			D			N
J2501	INJECTION, PARICALCITOL, 1 MCG	51	A			D			N
J2505	INJECTION, PEGFILGRASTIM, 6 MG	53	A			C			A
J2510	INJECTION, PENICILLIN G PROCAINE, AQUEOUS, UP TO 600,000 UNITS	51	A			D			N
J2512	INJECTION, PENTAGASTRIN, PER 2 ML	51	A			D			N
J2515	INJECTION, PENTOBARBITAL SODIUM, PER 50 MG	51	A			D			N
J2540	INJECTION, PENICILLIN G POTASSIUM, UP TO 600,000 UNITS	51	A			D			N
J2543	INJECTION, PIPERACILLIN SODIUM/TAZOBACTAM SODIUM, 1 GRAM/0.125 GRAMS (1.125 GRAMS)	51	A			D			N
J2545	PENTAMIDINE ISETHIONATE, INHALATION SOLUTION, PER 300 MG, ADMINISTERED THROUGH A DME	51	A		Q0O77	D			N
J2550	INJECTION, PROMETHAZINE HCL, UP TO 50 MG	51	A			D			N
J2560	INJECTION, PHENOBARBITAL SODIUM, UP TO 120 MG	51	A			D			N

HCPCS	Long Description	PH	MPI	Statute	X-Ref1	Coverage	ASC Pay Grp	ASC Pay Grp Eff Date	Action Code
J2590	INJECTION, OXYTOCIN, UP TO 10 UNITS	51	A			D			N
J2597	INJECTION, DESMOPRESSIN ACETATE, PER 1 MCG	51	A			D			N
J2640	INJECTION, PREDNISOLONE SODIUM PHOSPHATE, TO 20 MG	51	A			D			N
J2650	INJECTION, PREDNISOLONE ACETATE, UP TO 1 ML	51	A			D			N
J2670	INJECTION, TOLAZOLINE HCL, UP TO 25 MG	51	A			D			N
J2675	INJECTION, PROGESTERONE, PER 50 MG	51	A			D			N
J2680	INJECTION, FLUPHENAZINE DECANOATE, UP TO 25 MG	51	A			D			N
J2690	INJECTION, PROCAINAMIDE HCL, UP TO 1 GM	51	A			D			N
J2700	INJECTION, OXACILLIN SODIUM, UP TO 250 MG	51	A			D			N
J2710	INJECTION, NEOSTIGMINE METHYLSULFATE, UP TO 0.5 MG	51	A			D			N
J2720	INJECTION, PROTAMINE SULFATE, PER 10 MG	51	A			D			N
J2725	INJECTION, PROTIRELIN, PER 250 MCG	51	A			D			N
J2730	INJECTION, PRALIDOXIME CHLORIDE, UP TO 1 GM	51	A			D			N
J2760	INJECTION, PHENTOLAMINE MESYLATE, UP TO 5 MG	51	A			D			N
J2765	INJECTION, METOCLOPRAMIDE HCL, UP TO 10 MG	51	A			D			N
J2770	INJECTION, QUINUPRISTIN/DALFOPRISTIN, 500 MG (150/350)	51	A			D			N
J2780	INJECTION, RANITIDINE HYDROCHLORIDE, 25 MG	51	A			D			N
J2783	INJECTION, RASBURICASE, 0.5 MG	51	A			C			A
J2788	INJECTION, RHO D IMMUNE GLOBULIN, HUMAN, MINIDOSE, 50 MCG	51	A			D			N
J2790	INJECTION, RHO D IMMUNE GLOBULIN, HUMAN, FULL DOSE, 300 MCG	51	A			D			N
J2792	INJECTION, RHO D IMMUNE GLOBULIN, INTRAVENOUS, HUMAN, SOLVENT DETERGENT, 100 IU	51	A			D			N
J2795	INJECTION, ROPIVACAINE HYDROCHLORIDE, 1 MG	51	A			C			N
J2800	INJECTION, METHOCARBAMOL, UP TO 10 ML	51	A			D			N
J2810	INJECTION, THEOPHYLLINE, PER 40 MG	51	A			D			N
J2820	INJECTION, SARGRAMOSTIM (GM-CSF), 50 MCG	51	A			D			N
J2860	INJECTION, SECOBARBITAL SODIUM, UP TO 250 MG	51	A			D			N
J2910	INJECTION, AUROTHIOGLUCOSE, UP TO 50 MG	51	A			D			N
J2912	INJECTION, SODIUM CHLORIDE, 0.9%, PER 2 ML	51	A			D			N
J2915	INJECTION, SODIUM FERRIC GLUCONATE COMPLEX IN SUCROSE INJECTION, 62.5 MG	51	A			D			N

HCPCS	Long Description	PIT	MPI	Statute	X-Ref	Coverage	ASC Pay Grp	ASC Pay Grp Eff Date	Action Code
J2916	INJECTION, SODIUM FERRIC GLUCONATE COMPLEX IN SUCROSE INJECTION, 12.5 MG	51	A			D			N
J2920	INJECTION, METHYLPREDNISOLONE SODIUM SUCCINATE, UP TO 40 MG	51	A			D			N
J2930	INJECTION, METHYLPREDNISOLONE SODIUM SUCCINATE, UP TO 125 MG	51	A			D			N
J2940	INJECTION, SOMATREM, 1 MG	51	A	1861s2b		D			N
J2941	INJECTION, SOMATROPIN, 1 MG	51	A	1861s2b		D			N
J2950	INJECTION, PROMAZINE HCL, UP TO 25 MG	51	A			D			N
J2970	INJECTION, METHICILLIN SODIUM, UP TO 1 GM	51	A			D			N
J2993	INJECTION, RETEPLASE, 18.1 MG	51	A			D			N
J2994	INJECTION RETEPLASE, 37.6 MG (TWO SINGLE USE VIALS)	51	A			D			N
J2995	INJECTION, STREPTOKINASE, PER 250,000 IU	51	A			D			N
J2996	INJECTION, ALTEPLASE RECOMBINANT, PER 10 MG	51	A			D			N
J2997	INJECTION, ALTEPLASE RECOMBINANT, 1 MG	51	A			D			N
J3000	INJECTION, STREPTOMYCIN, UP TO 1 GM	51	A			D			N
J3010	INJECTION, FENTANYL CITRATE, 0.1 MG	51	A			D			N
J3030	INJECTION, SUMATRIPTAN SUCCINATE, 6 MG (CODE MAY BE USED FOR MEDICARE WHEN DRUG ADMINISTERED UNDER THE DIRECT SUPERVISION OF A PHYSICIAN, NOT FOR USE WHEN DRUG IS SELF ADMINISTERED)	51	A			D			N
J3070	INJECTION, PENTAZOCINE, 30 MG	51	A			D			N
J3080	INJECTION, CHLORPROTHIXENE, UP TO 50 MG	51	A			D			N
J3100	INJECTION, TENECTEPLASE, 50MG	51	A			C			N
J3105	INJECTION, TERBUTALINE SULFATE, UP TO 1 MG	51	A			D			N
J3120	INJECTION, TESTOSTERONE ENANTHATE, UP TO 100 MG	51	A			D			N
J3130	INJECTION, TESTOSTERONE ENANTHATE, UP TO 200 MG	51	A			D			N
J3140	INJECTION, TESTOSTERONE SUSPENSION, UP TO 50 MG	51	A			D			N
J3150	INJECTION, TESTOSTERONE PROPIONATE, UP TO 100 MG	51	A			D			N
J3230	INJECTION, CHLORPROMAZINE HCL, UP TO 50 MG	51	A			D			N
J3240	INJECTION, THYROTROPIN ALPHA, 0.9 MG, PROVIDED IN 1.1 MG VIAL	51	A			D			N
J3245	INJECTION, TIROFIBAN HYDROCHLORIDE, 12.5 MG	51	A			D			N
J3250	INJECTION, TRIMETHOBENZAMIDE HCL, UP TO 200 MG	51	A			D			N
J3260	INJECTION, TOBRAMYCIN SULFATE, UP TO 80 MG	51	A			D			N
J3265	INJECTION, TORSEMIDE, 10 MG/ML	51	A			D			N

HCPCS	Long Description	PH	MPI	Statute	X-Refl	Coverage	ASC Pay Grp	ASC Pay Grp Eff Date	Action Code
J3270	INJECTION, IMIPRAMINE HCL, UP TO 25 MG	51	A			D			N
J3280	INJECTION, THIETHYLPERAZINE MALEATE, UP TO 10 MG	51	A			D			N
J3301	INJECTION, TRIAMCINOLONE ACETONIDE, PER 10MG	51	A			D			N
J3302	INJECTION, TRIAMCINOLONE DIACETATE, PER 5MG	51	A			D			N
J3303	INJECTION, TRIAMCINOLONE HEXACETONIDE, PER 5MG	51	A			D			N
J3305	INJECTION, TRIMETREXATE GLUCURONATE, PER 25 MG	51	A			D			N
J3310	INJECTION, PERPHENAZINE, UP TO 5 MG	51	A			D			N
J3315	INJECTION, TRIPTORELIN PAMOATE, 3.75 MG	51	A			D			N
J3320	INJECTION, SPECTINOMYCIN DIHYDROCHLORIDE, UP TO 2 GM	51	A			D			N
J3350	INJECTION, UREA, UP TO 40 GM	51	A			D			N
J3360	INJECTION, DIAZEPAM, UP TO 5 MG	51	A			D			N
J3364	INJECTION, UROKINASE, 5000 IU VIAL	51	A			D			N
J3365	INJECTION, IV, UROKINASE, 250,000 I.U. VIAL	51	A		Q0089	D			N
J3370	INJECTION, VANCOMYCIN HCL, 500 MG	51	A			D			N
J3390	INJECTION, METHOXAMINE HCL, UP TO 20 MG	51	A			D			N
J3395	INJECTION, VERTEPORFIN, 15MG	51	A			D			N
J3400	INJECTION, TRIFLUPROMAZINE HCL, UP TO 20 MG	51	A			D			N
J3410	INJECTION, HYDROXYZINE HCL, UP TO 25 MG	51	A			D			N
J3411	INJECTION, THIAMINE HCL, 100 MG	51	A			C			A
J3415	INJECTION, PYRIDOXINE HCL, 100 MG	51	A			C			A
J3420	INJECTION, VITAMIN B-12 CYANOCOBALAMIN, UP TO 1000 MCG	51	A			D			N
J3430	INJECTION, PHYTONADIONE (VITAMIN K), PER 1 MG	51	A			D			N
J3450	INJECTION, MEPHENTERMINE SULFATE, UP TO 30 MG	51	A			D			N
J3465	INJECTION, VORICONAZOLE, 10 MG	51	A			D			A
J3470	INJECTION, HYALURONIDASE, UP TO 150 UNITS	51	A			D			N
J3475	INJECTION, MAGNESIUM SULFATE, PER 500 MG	51	A			D			N
J3480	INJECTION, POTASSIUM CHLORIDE, PER 2 MEQ	51	A			D			N
J3485	INJECTION, ZIDOVUDINE, 10 MG	51	A			D			N
J3486	INJECTION, ZIPRASIDONE MESYLATE, 10 MG	51	A			C			A
J3487	INJECTION, ZOLEDRONIC ACID, 1 MG	51	A			C			N
J3490	UNCLASSIFIED DRUGS	51	A			D			N
J3520	EDETATE DISODIUM, PER 150 MG	00	9			M			N

HCPCS	Long Description	PII	MPI	Statute	X-Ref1	Coverage	ASC Pay Grp	ASC Pay Grp Eff Date	Action Code
J3530	NASAL VACCINE INHALATION	51	A			D			N
J3535	DRUG ADMINISTERED THROUGH A METERED DOSE INHALER	00	9			M			N
J3570	LAETRILE, AMYGDALIN, VITAMIN B17	00	9			M			N
J3590	UNCLASSIFIED BIOLOGICS	51	A			C			N
J7030	INFUSION, NORMAL SALINE SOLUTION , 1000 CC	51	A			D			N
J7040	INFUSION, NORMAL SALINE SOLUTION, STERILE (500 ML=1 UNIT)	51	A			D			N
J7042	5% DEXTROSE/NORMAL SALINE (500 ML = 1 UNIT)	51	A			D			N
J7050	INFUSION, NORMAL SALINE SOLUTION , 250 CC	51	A			D			N
J7051	STERILE SALINE OR WATER, UP TO 5 CC	51	A			D			N
J7060	5% DEXTROSE/WATER (500 ML = 1 UNIT)	51	A			D			N
J7070	INFUSION, D5W, 1000 CC	51	A			D			N
J7100	INFUSION, DEXTRAN 40, 500 ML	51	A			D			N
J7110	INFUSION, DEXTRAN 75, 500 ML	51	A			D			N
J7120	RINGERS LACTATE INFUSION, UP TO 1000 CC	51	A			D			N
J7130	HYPERTONIC SALINE SOLUTION, 50 OR 100 MEQ, 20 CC VIAL	51	A			D			N
J7190	FACTOR VIII (ANTIHEMOPHILIC FACTOR, HUMAN) PER I.U.	51	A			D			N
J7191	FACTOR VIII (ANTIHEMOPHILIC FACTOR (PORCINE)), PER I.U.	51	A			D			N
J7192	FACTOR VIII (ANTIHEMOPHILIC FACTOR, RECOMBINANT) PER I.U.	51	A			D			N
J7193	FACTOR IX (ANTIHEMOPHILIC FACTOR, PURIFIED, NON-RECOMBINANT) PER I.U.	51	A			D			N
J7194	FACTOR IX, COMPLEX, PER I.U.	51	A			D			N
J7195	FACTOR IX (ANTIHEMOPHILIC FACTOR, RECOMBINANT) PER I.U.	51	A			D			N
J7197	ANTITHROMBIN III (HUMAN), PER I.U.	51	A			D			N
J7198	ANTI-INHIBITOR, PER I.U.	51	A			D			N
J7199	HEMOPHILIA CLOTTING FACTOR, NOT OTHERWISE CLASSIFIED	51	A			D			N
J7300	INTRAUTERINE COPPER CONTRACEPTIVE	00	9	1862A1		S			N
J7302	LEVONORGESTREL-RELEASING INTRAUTERINE CONTRACEPTIVE SYSTEM, 52 MG	00	9	1862a1		S			N
J7303	CONTRACEPTIVE SUPPLY, HORMONE CONTAINING VAGINAL RING, EACH	00	9	1862.1		S			A
J7308	AMINOLEVULINIC ACID HCL FOR TOPICAL ADMINISTRATION, 20%, SINGLE UNIT DOSAGE FORM (354 MG)	51	A			C			F
J7310	GANCICLOVIR, 4.5 MG, LONG-ACTING IMPLANT	51	A			D			N
J7315	SODIUM HYALURONATE, 20 MG, FOR INTRA ARTICULAR INJECTION	51	A			C			N

HCPCS	Long Description	PII	MPI	Statute	X-Ref	Coverage	ASC Pay Grp	ASC Pay Grp Eff Date	Action Code
J7316	SODIUM HYALURONATE, 5 MG FOR INTRA-ARTICULAR INJECTION	00	9		J7317	I			N
J7317	SODIUM HYALURONATE, PER 20 TO 25 MG DOSE FOR INTRA-ARTICULAR INJECTION	51	A			C			N
J7320	HYLAN G-F 20, 16 MG, FOR INTRA ARTICULAR INJECTION	51	A			C			N
J7330	AUTOLOGOUS CULTURED CHONDROCYTES, IMPLANT	57	A			C			N
J7340	DERMAL AND EPIDERMAL TISSUE OF HUMAN ORIGIN, WITH OR WITHOUT BIOENGINEERED OR PROCESSED ELEMENTS, WITH METABOLICALLY ACTIVE ELEMENTS, PER SQUARE CENTIMETER	51	A			C			N
J7342	DERMAL TISSUE, OF HUMAN ORIGIN, WITH OR WITHOUT OTHER BIOENGINEERED OR PROCESSED ELEMENTS, WITH METABOLICALLY ACTIVE ELEMENTS, PER SQUARE CENTIMETER	46	A			C			N
J7350	DERMAL TISSUE OF HUMAN ORIGIN, INJECTABLE, WITH OR WITHOUT OTHER BIOENGINEERED OR PROCESSED ELEMENTS, BUT WITHOUT METABOLIZED ACTIVE ELEMENTS, PER 10 MG	51	A			C			N
J7500	AZATHIOPRINE, ORAL, 50 MG	51	A			D			N
J7501	AZATHIOPRINE, PARENTERAL, 100 MG	51	A			D			N
J7502	CYCLOSPORINE, ORAL, 100 MG	57	A			D			N
J7504	LYMPHOCYTE IMMUNE GLOBULIN, ANTITHYMOCYTE GLOBULIN, EQUINE, PARENTERAL, 250 MG	51	A			D			N
J7505	MUROMONAB-CD3, PARENTERAL, 5 MG	51	A			D			N
J7506	PREDNISONE, ORAL, PER 5MG	51	A			D			N
J7507	TACROLIMUS, ORAL, PER 1 MG	51	A			D			N
J7508	TACROLIMUS, ORAL, PER 5 MG	51	A			D			D
J7509	METHYLPREDNISOLONE ORAL, PER 4 MG	51	A			D			N
J7510	PREDNISOLONE ORAL, PER 5 MG	51	A			D			N
J7511	LYMPHOCYTE IMMUNE GLOBULIN, ANTITHYMOCYTE GLOBULIN, RABBIT, PARENTERAL, 25MG	51	A			C			N
J7513	DACLIZUMAB, PARENTERAL, 25 MG	51	A			D			N
J7515	CYCLOSPORINE, ORAL, 25 MG	51	A			C			N
J7516	CYCLOSPORIN, PARENTERAL, 250 MG	51	A			C			N
J7517	MYCOPHENOLATE MOFETIL, ORAL, 250 MG	51	A			C			N
J7520	SIROLIMUS, ORAL, 1 MG	51	A			D			N
J7525	TACROLIMUS, PARENTERAL, 5 MG	51	A			D			N
J7599	IMMUNOSUPPRESSIVE DRUG, NOT OTHERWISE CLASSIFIED	51	A			D			N
J7608	ACETYLCYSTEINE, INHALATION SOLUTION ADMINISTERED THROUGH DME, UNIT DOSE FORM, PER GRAM	51	A			D			N
J7610	ACETYLCYSTEINE, 10%, PER ML, INHALATION SOLUTION ADMINISTERED THROUGH DME	51	A			D			N
J7615	ACETYLCYSTEINE, 20%, PER ML, INHALATION SOLUTION ADMINISTERED THROUGH DME	51	A			D			N

HCPCS	Long Description	PI1	MPI	Statute	X-Ref1	Coverage	ASC Pay Grp	ASC Pay Grp Eff Date	Action Code
J7618	ALBUTEROL, ALL FORMULATIONS INCLUDING SEPARATED ISOMERS, INHALATION SOLUTION ADMINISTERED THROUGH DME, CONCENTRATED FORM, PER 1 MG (ALBUTEROL) OR PER 0.5 MG (LEVALBUTEROL)	51	A			D			N
J7619	ALBUTEROL, ALL FORMULATIONS INCLUDING SEPARATED ISOMERS, INHALATION SOLUTION ADMINISTERED THROUGH DME, UNIT DOSE, PER 1 MG (ALBUTEROL) OR PER 0.5 MG (LEVALBUTEROL)	51	A			D			N
J7620	ALBUTEROL SULFATE, 0.083%, PER ML, INHALATION SOLUTION ADMINISTERED THROUGH DME	51	A			D			N
J7621	ALBUTEROL, ALL FORMULATIONS, INCLUDING SEPARATED ISOMERS, UP TO 5 MG (ALBUTEROL) OR 2.5 MG (LEVOALBUTEROL), AND IPRATROPIUM BROMIDE, UP TO 1 MG, COMPOUNDED INHALATION SOLUTION, ADMINISTERED THROUGH DME	51	A			C			A
J7622	BECLOMETHASONE, INHALATION SOLUTION ADMINISTERED THROUGH DME, UNIT DOSE FORM, PER MILLIGRAM	51	A			C			N
J7624	BETAMETHASONE, INHALATION SOLUTION ADMINISTERED THROUGH DME, UNIT DOSE FORM, PER MILLIGRAM	51	A			C			N
J7625	ALBUTEROL SULFATE, 0.5%, PER ML, INHALATION SOLUTION ADMINISTERED THROUGH DME	51	A			D			N
J7626	BUDESONIDE INHALATION SOLUTION, ADMINISTERED THROUGH DME, UNIT DOSE FORM, 0.25 TO 0.50 MG	51	A			C			N
J7627	BITOLTEROL MESYLATE, 0.2%, PER 10 ML, INHALATION SOLUTION ADMINISTERED THROUGH DME	51	A			C			N
J7628	BITOLTEROL MESYLATE, INHALATION SOLUTION ADMINISTERED THROUGH DME, CONCENTRATED FORM, PER MILLIGRAM	51	A			D			N
J7629	BITOLTEROL MESYLATE, INHALATION SOLUTION ADMINISTERED THROUGH DME, UNIT DOSE FORM, PER MILLIGRAM	51	A			D			N
J7630	CROMOLYN SODIUM, PER 20 MG, INHALATION SOLUTION ADMINISTERED THROUGH DME	51	A			D			N
J7631	CROMOLYN SODIUM, INHALATION SOLUTION ADMINISTERED THROUGH DME, UNIT DOSE FORM, PER 10 MILLIGRAMS	51	A			D			N
J7633	BUDESONIDE, INHALATION SOLUTION ADMINISTERED THROUGH DME, CONCENTRATED FORM, PER 0.25 MILLIGRAM	51	A			C			N
J7635	ATROPINE, INHALATION SOLUTION ADMINISTERED THROUGH DME, CONCENTRATED FORM, PER MILLIGRAM	51	A			D			N
J7636	ATROPINE, INHALATION SOLUTION ADMINISTERED THROUGH DME, UNIT DOSE FORM, PER MILLIGRAM	51	A			D			N
J7637	DEXAMETHASONE, INHALATION SOLUTION ADMINISTERED THROUGH DME, CONCENTRATED FORM, PER MILLIGRAM	51	A			D			N
J7638	DEXAMETHASONE, INHALATION SOLUTION ADMINISTERED THROUGH DME, UNIT DOSE FORM, PER MILLIGRAM	51	A			D			N
J7639	DORNASE ALPHA, INHALATION SOLUTION ADMINISTERED THROUGH DME, UNIT DOSE FORM, PER MILLIGRAM	51	A			D			N
J7640	EPINEPHRINE, 2.25%, PER ML, INHALATION SOLUTION ADMINISTERED THROUGH DME	51	A			D			N
J7641	FLUNISOLIDE, INHALATION SOLUTION ADMINISTERED THROUGH DME, UNIT DOSE, PER MILLIGRAM	51	A			C			N
J7642	GLYCOPYRROLATE, INHALATION SOLUTION ADMINISTERED THROUGH DME, CONCENTRATED FORM, PER MILLIGRAM	51	A			D			N
J7643	GLYCOPYRROLATE, INHALATION SOLUTION ADMINISTERED THROUGH DME, UNIT DOSE FORM, PER MILLIGRAM	51	A			D			N
J7644	IPRATROPIUM BROMIDE, INHALATION SOLUTION ADMINISTERED THROUGH DME, UNIT DOSE FORM, PER MILLIGRAM	51	A			D			N
J7645	IPRATROPIUM BROMIDE 0.02%, PER ML, INHALATION SOLUTION ADMINISTERED THROUGH A DME	51	A			D			N

HCPCS	Long Description	PI	MPI	Statute	X-Ref	Coverage	ASC Pay Grp	ASC Pay Grp Eff Date	Action Code
J7648	ISOETHARINE HCL, INHALATION SOLUTION ADMINISTERED THROUGH DME, CONCENTRATED FORM, PER MILLIGRAM	51	A			D			N
J7649	ISOETHARINE HCL, INHALATION SOLUTION ADMINISTERED THROUGH DME, UNIT DOSE FORM, PER MILLIGRAM	51	A			D			N
J7650	ISOETHARINE HYDROCHLORIDE, 0.1%, PER ML, INHALATION SOLUTION ADMINISTERED THROUGH DME	51	A			D			N
J7651	ISOETHARINE HYDROCHLORIDE, 0.125%, PER ML, INHALATION SOLUTION ADMINISTERED THROUGH DME	51	A			D			N
J7652	ISOETHARINE HYDROCHLORIDE, 0.167%, PER ML, INHALATION SOLUTION ADMINISTERED THROUGH DME	51	A			D			N
J7653	ISOETHARINE HYDROCHLORIDE, 0.2%, PER ML, INHALATION SOLUTION ADMINISTERED THROUGH DME	51	A			D			N
J7654	ISOETHARINE HYDROCHLORIDE, 0.25%, PER ML, INHALATION SOLUTION ADMINISTERED THROUGH DME	51	A			D			N
J7655	ISOETHARINE HYDROCHLORIDE, 1.0%, PER ML, INHALATION SOLUTION ADMINISTERED THROUGH DME	51	A			D			N
J7658	ISOPROTERENOL HCL, INHALATION SOLUTION ADMINISTERED THROUGH DME, CONCENTRATED FORM, PER MILLIGRAM	51	A			D			N
J7659	ISOPROTERENOL HCL, INHALATION SOLUTION ADMINISTERED THROUGH DME, UNIT DOSE FORM, PER MILLIGRAM	51	A			D			N
J7660	ISOPROTERENOL HYDROCHLORIDE, 0.5%, PER ML, INHALATION SOLUTION ADMINISTERED THROUGH DME	51	A			D			N
J7665	ISOPROTERENOL HYDROCHLORIDE, 1.0%, PER ML, INHALATION SOLUTION ADMINISTERED THROUGH DME	51	A			D			N
J7668	METAPROTERENOL SULFATE, INHALATION SOLUTION ADMINISTERED THROUGH DME, CONCENTRATED FORM, PER 10 MILLIGRAMS	51	A			D			N
J7669	METAPROTERENOL SULFATE, INHALATION SOLUTION ADMINISTERED THROUGH DME, UNIT DOSE FORM, PER 10 MILLIGRAMS	51	A			D			N
J7670	METAPROTERENOL SULFATE, 0.4%, PER 2.5 ML, INHALATION SOLUTION ADMINISTERED THROUGH DME THROUGH DME	51	A			D			N
J7672	METAPROTERENOL SULFATE, 0.6%, PER 2.5 ML, INHALATION SOLUTION ADMINISTERED THROUGH DME	51	A			D			N
J7675	METAPROTERENOL SULFATE, 5.0%, PER ML, INHALATION SOLUTION ADMINISTERED THROUGH DME	51	A			D			N
J7680	TERBUTALINE SULFATE, INHALATION SOLUTION ADMINISTERED THROUGH DME, CONCENTRATED FORM, PER MILLIGRAM	51	A			D			N
J7681	TERBUTALINE SULFATE, INHALATION SOLUTION ADMINISTERED THROUGH DME, UNIT DOSE FORM, PER MILLIGRAM	51	A			D			N
J7682	TOBRAMYCIN, UNIT DOSE FORM, 300 MG, INHALATION SOLUTION, ADMINISTERED THROUGH DME	51	A			D			N
J7683	TRIAMCINOLONE, INHALATION SOLUTION ADMINISTERED THROUGH DME, CONCENTRATED FORM, PER MILLIGRAM	51	A			D			N
J7684	TRIAMCINOLONE, INHALATION SOLUTION ADMINISTERED THROUGH DME, UNIT DOSE FORM, PER MILLIGRAM	51	A			D			N
J7699	NOC DRUGS, INHALATION SOLUTION ADMINISTERED THROUGH DME	51	A			D			N
J7799	NOC DRUGS, OTHER THAN INHALATION DRUGS, ADMINISTERED THROUGH DME	51	A			D			N
J8499	PRESCRIPTION DRUG, ORAL, NON CHEMOTHERAPEUTIC, NOS	00	9			M			N
J8510	BUSULFAN; ORAL, 2 MG	51	A			D			N
J8520	CAPECITABINE, ORAL, 150 MG	51	A			D			N
J8521	CAPECITABINE, ORAL, 500 MG	51	A			D			N
J8530	CYCLOPHOSPHAMIDE; ORAL, 25 MG	51	A			D			N
J8560	ETOPOSIDE; ORAL, 50 MG	51	A			D			N
J8600	MELPHALAN; ORAL, 2 MG	51	A			D			N
J8610	METHOTREXATE; ORAL, 2.5 MG	51	A			D			N

HCPCS	Long Description	PTI	MPI	Statute	X-Ref1	Coverage	ASC Pay Grp	ASC Pay Grp Eff Date	Action Code
J8700	TEMOZOLOMIDE, ORAL, 5 MG	51	A			D			N
J8999	PRESCRIPTION DRUG, ORAL, CHEMOTHERAPEUTIC, NOS	51	A			D			N
J9000	DOXORUBICIN HCL, 10 MG	51	A			D			N
J9001	DOXORUBICIN HYDROCHLORIDE, ALL LIPID FORMULATIONS, 10 MG	51	A			D			N
J9010	ALEMTUZUMAB, 10 MG	51	A	1833T		D			N
J9015	ALDESLEUKIN, PER SINGLE USE VIAL	51	A			D			N
J9017	ARSENIC TRIOXIDE, 1MG	51	A			C			N
J9020	ASPARAGINASE, 10,000 UNITS	51	A			D			N
J9031	BCG (INTRAVESICAL) PER INSTILLATION	51	A			D			N
J9040	BLEOMYCIN SULFATE, 15 UNITS	51	A			D			N
J9045	CARBOPLATIN, 50 MG	51	A			D			N
J9050	CARMUSTINE, 100 MG	51	A			D			N
J9060	CISPLATIN, POWDER OR S0LUTION, PER 10 MG	51	A			D			N
J9062	CISPLATIN, 50 MG	51	A			D			N
J9065	INJECTION, CLADRIBINE, PER 1 MG	51	A			D			N
J9070	CYCLOPHOSPHAMIDE, 100 MG	51	A			D			N
J9080	CYCLOPHOSPHAMIDE, 200 MG	51	A			D			N
J9090	CYCLOPHOSPHAMIDE, 500 MG	51	A			D			N
J9091	CYCLOPHOSPHAMIDE, 1.0 GRAM	51	A			D			N
J9092	CYCLOPHOSPHAMIDE, 2.0 GRAM	51	A			D			N
J9093	CYCLOPHOSPHAMIDE, LYOPHILIZED, 100 MG	51	A			D			N
J9094	CYCLOPHOSPHAMIDE, LYOPHILIZED, 200 MG	51	A			D			N
J9095	CYCLOPHOSPHAMIDE, LYOPHILIZED, 500 MG	51	A			D			N
J9096	CYCLOPHOSPHAMIDE, LYOPHILIZED, 1.0 GRAM	51	A			D			N
J9097	CYCLOPHOSPHAMIDE, LYOPHILIZED, 2.0 GRAM	51	A			D			N
J9098	CYTARABINE LIPOSOME, 10 MG	51	A			C			A
J9100	CYTARABINE, 100 MG	51	A			D			N

HCPCS	Long Description	PI	MPI	Statute	X-Ref1	Coverage	ASC Pay Grp	ASC Pay Grp Eff Date	Action Code
J9110	CYTARABINE, 500 MG	51	A			D			N
J9120	DACTINOMYCIN, 0.5 MG	51	A			D			N
J9130	DACARBAZINE, 100 MG	51	A			D			S
J9140	DACARBAZINE, 200 MG	51	A			D			N
J9150	DAUNORUBICIN, 10 MG	51	A			D			N
J9151	DAUNORUBICIN CITRATE, LIPOSOMAL FORMULATION, 10 MG	51	A			D			N
J9160	DENILEUKIN DIFTITOX, 300 MCG	51	A			C			N
J9165	DIETHYLSTILBESTROL DIPHOSPHATE, 250 MG	51	A			D			N
J9170	DOCETAXEL, 20 MG	51	A			D			N
J9178	INJECTION, EPIRUBICIN HCL, 2 MG	51	A			C			A
J9180	EPIRUBICIN HYDROCHLORIDE, 50 MG	51	A			D			D
J9181	ETOPOSIDE, 10 MG	51	A			D			N
J9182	ETOPOSIDE, 100 MG	51	A			D			N
J9185	FLUDARABINE PHOSPHATE, 50 MG	51	A			D			N
J9190	FLUOROURACIL, 500 MG	51	A			D			N
J9200	FLOXURIDINE, 500 MG	51	A			D			N
J9201	GEMCITABINE HCL, 200 MG	51	A			D			N
J9202	GOSERELIN ACETATE IMPLANT, PER 3.6 MG	51	A			D			N
J9206	IRINOTECAN, 20 MG	51	A			D			N
J9208	IFOSFAMIDE, 1 GM	51	A			D			N
J9209	MESNA, 200 MG	51	A			D			N
J9211	IDARUBICIN HYDROCHLORIDE, 5 MG	51	A			D			N
J9212	INJECTION, INTERFERON ALFACON-1, RECOMBINANT, 1 MCG	51	A			D			N
J9213	INTERFERON, ALFA-2A, RECOMBINANT, 3 MILLION UNITS	51	A			D			N
J9214	INTERFERON, ALFA-2B, RECOMBINANT, 1 MILLION UNITS	51	A			D			N
J9215	INTERFERON, ALFA-N3, (HUMAN LEUKOCYTE DERIVED), 250,000 IU	51	A			D			N
J9216	INTERFERON, GAMMA 1-B, 3 MILLION UNITS	51	A			D			N
J9217	LEUPROLIDE ACETATE (FOR DEPOT SUSPENSION), 7.5 MG	51	A			D			N
J9218	LEUPROLIDE ACETATE, PER 1 MG	51	A			D			N
J9219	LEUPROLIDE ACETATE IMPLANT, 65 MG	51	A			D			N
J9230	MECHLORETHAMINE HYDROCHLORIDE, (NITROGEN MUSTARD), 10 MG	51	A			D			N
J9245	INJECTION, MELPHALAN HYDROCHLORIDE, 50 MG	51	A			D			N

HCPCS	Long Description	PH	MPI	Statute	X-Ref	Coverage	ASC Pay Grp	ASC Pay Grp Eff Date	Action Code
J9250	METHOTREXATE SODIUM, 5 MG	51	A			D			N
J9260	METHOTREXATE SODIUM, 50 MG	51	A			D			N
J9263	INJECTION, OXALIPLATIN, 0.5 MG	51	A			C			A
J9265	PACLITAXEL, 30 MG	51	A			D			N
J9266	PEGASPARGASE, PER SINGLE DOSE VIAL	51	A			D			N
J9268	PENTOSTATIN, PER 10 MG	51	A			D			N
J9270	PLICAMYCIN, 2.5 MG	51	A			D			N
J9280	MITOMYCIN, 5 MG	51	A			D			N
J9290	MITOMYCIN, 20 MG	51	A			D			N
J9291	MITOMYCIN, 40 MG	51	A			D			N
J9293	INJECTION, MITOXANTRONE HYDROCHLORIDE, PER 5 MG	51	A			D			N
J9300	GEMTUZUMAB OZOGAMICIN, 5MG	51	A			C			N
J9310	RITUXIMAB, 100 MG	51	A			D			N
J9320	STREPTOZOCIN, 1 GM	51	A			D			N
J9340	THIOTEPA, 15 MG	51	A			D			N
J9350	TOPOTECAN, 4 MG	51	A			D			N
J9355	TRASTUZUMAB, 10 MG	51	A			C			N
J9357	VALRUBICIN, INTRAVESICAL, 200 MG	51	A			D			N
J9360	VINBLASTINE SULFATE, 1 MG	51	A			D			N
J9370	VINCRISTINE SULFATE, 1 MG	51	A			D			N
J9375	VINCRISTINE SULFATE, 2 MG	51	A			D			N
J9380	VINCRISTINE SULFATE, 5 MG	51	A			D			N
J9390	VINORELBINE TARTRATE, PER 10 MG	51	A			D			N
J9395	INJECTION, FULVESTRANT, 25 MG	51	A			C			A
J9600	PORFIMER SODIUM, 75 MG	51	A			D			N
J9999	NOT OTHERWISE CLASSIFIED, ANTINEOPLASTIC DRUGS	51	A			D			N
K0001	STANDARD WHEELCHAIR	36	A			C			N
K0002	STANDARD HEMI (LOW SEAT) WHEELCHAIR	36	A			C			N
K0003	LIGHTWEIGHT WHEELCHAIR	36	A			C			N
K0004	HIGH STRENGTH, LIGHTWEIGHT WHEELCHAIR	36	A			C			N
K0005	ULTRALIGHTWEIGHT WHEELCHAIR	32	A			C			N
K0006	HEAVY DUTY WHEELCHAIR	36	A			C			N

HCPCS	Long Description	PI	MPI	Statute	X-Refl	Coverage	ASC Pay Grp	ASC Pay Grp Eff Date	Action Code
K0007	EXTRA HEAVY DUTY WHEELCHAIR	36	A			C			N
K0008	CUSTOM MANUAL WHEELCHAIR/BASE	45	A			C			N
K0009	OTHER MANUAL WHEELCHAIR/BASE	46	A			C			N
K0010	STANDARD - WEIGHT FRAME MOTORIZED/POWER WHEELCHAIR	36	A			C			N
K0011	STANDARD - WEIGHT FRAME MOTORIZED/POWER WHEELCHAIR WITH PROGRAMMABLE CONTROL PARAMETERS FOR SPEED ADJUSTMENT, TREMOR DAMPENING, ACCELERATION CONTROL AND BRAKING	36	A			C			N
K0012	LIGHTWEIGHT PORTABLE MOTORIZED/POWER WHEELCHAIR	36	A			C			N
K0013	CUSTOM MOTORIZED/POWER WHEELCHAIR BASE	45	A			C			N
K0014	OTHER MOTORIZED/POWER WHEELCHAIR BASE	36	A			C			N
K0015	DETACHABLE, NON-ADJUSTABLE HEIGHT ARMREST, EACH	32	A			C			N
K0016	DETACHABLE, ADJUSTABLE HEIGHT ARMREST, COMPLETE ASSEMBLY, EACH	32	A		E0973	C			D
K0017	DETACHABLE, ADJUSTABLE HEIGHT ARMREST, BASE, EACH	32	A			C			N
K0018	DETACHABLE, ADJUSTABLE HEIGHT ARMREST, UPPER PORTION, EACH	32	A			C			N
K0019	ARM PAD, EACH	32	A			C			N
K0020	FIXED, ADJUSTABLE HEIGHT ARMREST, PAIR	32	A			C			N
K0021	ANTI-TIPPING DEVICE, EACH	32	A		E0971	C			N
K0022	REINFORCED BACK UPHOLSTERY	32	A		E0982	C			D
K0023	SOLID BACK INSERT, PLANAR BACK, SINGLE DENSITY FOAM, ATTACHED WITH STRAPS	32	A			C			N
K0024	SOLID BACK INSERT, PLANAR BACK, SINGLE DENSITY FOAM, WITH ADJUSTABLE HOOK-ON HARDWARE	32	A			C			N
K0025	HOOK-ON HEADREST EXTENSION	32	A		E0966	C			D
K0026	BACK UPHOLSTERY FOR ULTRALIGHTWEIGHT OR HIGH STRENGTH LIGHTWEIGHT WHEELCHAIR	32	A		E0982	C			D
K0027	BACK UPHOLSTERY FOR WHEELCHAIR TYPE OTHER THAN ULTRALIGHTWEIGHT OR HIGH STRENGTH LIGHTWEIGHT WHEELCHAIR	32	A		E0982	C			D
K0028	MANUAL, FULLY RECLINING BACK	32	A		E1226	C			D
K0029	REINFORCED SEAT UPHOLSTERY	32	A		E0981	C			D
K0030	SOLID SEAT INSERT, PLANAR SEAT, SINGLE DENSITY FOAM	32	A		E0992	C			D
K0031	SAFETY BELT/PELVIC STRAP, EACH	32	A		E0978	C			D
K0032	SEAT UPHOLSTERY FOR ULTRALIGHTWEIGHT OR HIGH STRENGTH LIGHTWEIGHT WHEELCHAIR	32	A		E0981	C			D
K0033	SEAT UPHOLSTERY FOR WHEELCHAIR TYPE OTHER THAN ULTRALIGHTWEIGHT OR HIGH STRENGTH LIGHTWEIGHT WHEELCHAIR	32	A		E0981	C			D
K0034	HEEL LOOP,EACH	32	A		E0951	C			N

HCPCS	Long Description	PTI	MPI	Statute	X-Refll	Coverage	ASC Pay Grp	ASC Pay Grp Eff Date	Action Code
K0035	HEEL LOOP WITH ANKLE STRAP, EACH	32	A		E0951	C			D
K0036	TOE LOOP, EACH	32	A		E0952	C			D
K0037	HIGH MOUNT FLIP-UP FOOTREST, EACH	32	A			C			N
K0038	LEG STRAP, EACH	32	A			C			N
K0039	LEG STRAP, H STYLE, EACH	32	A			C			N
K0040	ADJUSTABLE ANGLE FOOTPLATE, EACH	32	A			C			N
K0041	LARGE SIZE FOOTPLATE, EACH	32	A			C			N
K0042	STANDARD SIZE FOOTPLATE, EACH	32	A			C			N
K0043	FOOTREST, LOWER EXTENSION TUBE, EACH	32	A			C			N
K0044	FOOTREST, UPPER HANGER BRACKET, EACH	32	A			C			N
K0045	FOOTREST, COMPLETE ASSEMBLY	32	A			C			N
K0046	ELEVATING LEGREST, LOWER EXTENSION TUBE, EACH	32	A			C			N
K0047	ELEVATING LEGREST, UPPER HANGER BRACKET, EACH	32	A			C			N
K0048	ELEVATING LEGREST, COMPLETE ASSEMBLY	32	A		E0990	C			D
K0049	CALF PAD, EACH	32	A		E0995	C			D
K0050	RATCHET ASSEMBLY	32	A			C			N
K0051	CAM RELEASE ASSEMBLY, FOOTREST OR LEGREST, EACH	32	A			C			N
K0052	SWINGAWAY, DETACHABLE FOOTRESTS, EACH	32	A			C			N
K0053	ELEVATING FOOTRESTS, ARTICULATING (TELESCOPING), EACH	32	A			C			N
K0054	SEAT WIDTH OF 10", 11", 12", 15", 17", OR 20" FOR A HIGH STRENGTH, LIGHTWEIGHT OR ULTRALIGHTWEIGHT WHEELCHAIR	32	A			C			D
K0055	SEAT DEPTH OF 15", 17", OR 18" FOR A HIGH STRENGTH, LIGHTWEIGHT OR ULTRALIGHTWEIGHT WHEELCHAIR	32	A			C			D
K0056	SEAT HEIGHT LESS THAN 17" OR EQUAL TO OR GREATER THAN 21" FOR A HIGH STRENGTH, LIGHTWEIGHT, OR ULTRALIGHTWEIGHT WHEELCHAIR	32	A			C			N
K0057	SEAT WIDTH 19" OR 20" FOR HEAVY DUTY OR EXTRA HEAVY DUTY CHAIR	32	A			C			D
K0058	SEAT DEPTH 17" OR 18" FOR MOTORIZED/POWER WHEELCHAIR	32	A			C			D
K0059	PLASTIC COATED HANDRIM, EACH	32	A			C			N
K0060	STEEL HANDRIM, EACH	32	A			C			N

HCPCS	Long Description	PH	MPI	Statute	X-Ref	Coverage	ASC Pay Grp	ASC Pay Grp Eff Date	Action Code
K0061	ALUMINUM HANDRIM, EACH	32	A			C			N
K0062	HANDRIM WITH 8-10 VERTICAL OR OBLIQUE PROJECTIONS, EACH	32	A		E0967	C			D
K0063	HANDRIM WITH 12-16 VERTICAL OR OLBIQUE PROJECTIONS, EACH	32	A		E0967	C			D
K0064	ZERO PRESSURE TUBE (FLAT FREE INSERTS), ANY SIZE, EACH	32	A			C			N
K0065	SPOKE PROTECTORS, EACH	32	A			C			N
K0066	SOLID TIRE, ANY SIZE, EACH	32	A			C			N
K0067	PNEUMATIC TIRE, ANY SIZE, EACH	32	A			C			N
K0068	PNEUMATIC TIRE TUBE, EACH	32	A			C			N
K0069	REAR WHEEL ASSEMBLY, COMPLETE, WITH SOLID TIRE, SPOKES OR MOLDED, EACH	32	A			C			N
K0070	REAR WHEEL ASSEMBLY, COMPLETE, WITH PNEUMATIC TIRE, SPOKES OR MOLDED, EACH	32	A			C			N
K0071	FRONT CASTER ASSEMBLY, COMPLETE, WITH PNEUMATIC TIRE, EACH	32	A			C			N
K0072	FRONT CASTER ASSEMBLY, COMPLETE, WITH SEMI-PNEUMATIC TIRE, EACH	32	A			C			N
K0073	CASTER PIN LOCK,EACH	32	A			C			N
K0074	PNEUMATIC CASTER TIRE, ANY SIZE, EACH	32	A			C			N
K0075	SEMI-PNEUMATIC CASTER TIRE, ANY SIZE, EACH	32	A			C			N
K0076	SOLID CASTER TIRE, ANY SIZE, EACH	32	A			C			N
K0077	FRONT CASTER ASSEMBLY, COMPLETE, WITH SOLID TIRE, EACH	32	A			C			N
K0078	PNEUMATIC CASTER TIRE TUBE, EACH	32	A			C			N
K0079	WHEEL LOCK EXTENSION, PAIR	32	A		E0961	C			D
K0080	ANTI-ROLLBACK DEVICE, PAIR	32	A		E0974	C			D
K0081	WHEEL LOCK ASSEMBLY, COMPLETE, EACH	32	A			C			N
K0082	22 NF NON-SEALED LEAD ACID BATTERY, EACH	32	A		E2360	C			D
K0083	22 NF SEALED LEAD ACID BATTERY, EACH (E.G., GEL CELL, ABSORBED GLASS MAT)	32	A		E2361	C			D
K0084	GROUP 24 NON-SEALED LEAD ACID BATTERY, EACH	32	A		E2362	C			D
K0085	GROUP 24 SEALED LEAD ACID BATTERY, EACH (E.G., GEL CELL, ABSORBED GLASS MAT)	32	A		E2363	C			D
K0086	U-1 NON-SEALED LEAD ACID BATTERY, EACH	32	A		E2364	C			D
K0087	U-1 SEALED LEAD ACID BATTERY, EACH (E.G., GEL CELL, ABSORBED GLASS MAT)	32	A		E2365	C			D

HCPCS	Long Description	PTI	MPI	Statute	X-Ref1	Coverage	ASC Pay Grp	ASC Pay Grp Eff Date	Action Code
K0088	BATTERY CHARGER, SINGLE MODE, FOR USE WITH ONLY ONE BATTERY TYPE, SEALED OR NON-SEALED	32	A		E2366	C			D
K0089	BATTERY CHARGER, DUAL MODE, FOR USE WITH EITHER BATTERY TYPE, SEALED OR NON-SEALED	32	A		E2367	C			D
K0090	REAR WHEEL TIRE FOR POWER WHEELCHAIR, ANY SIZE, EACH	32	A			C			N
K0091	REAR WHEEL TIRE TUBE OTHER THAN ZERO PRESSURE FOR POWER WHEELCHAIR, ANY SIZE, EACH	32	A			C			N
K0092	REAR WHEEL ASSEMBLY FOR POWER WHEELCHAIR, COMPLETE, EACH	32	A			C			N
K0093	REAR WHEEL, ZERO PRESSURE TIRE TUBE (FLAT FREE INSERT) FOR POWER WHEELCHAIR, ANY SIZE, EACH	32	A			C			N
K0094	WHEEL TIRE FOR POWER BASE, ANY SIZE, EACH	32	A			C			N
K0095	WHEEL TIRE TUBE OTHER THAN ZERO PRESSURE FOR EACH BASE, ANY SIZE, EACH	32	A			C			N
K0096	WHEEL ASSEMBLY FOR POWER BASE, COMPLETE, EACH	32	A			C			N
K0097	WHEEL ZERO PRESSURE TIRE TUBE (FLAT FREE INSERT) FOR POWER BASE, ANY SIZE, EACH	32	A			C			N
K0098	DRIVE BELT FOR POWER WHEELCHAIR	32	A			C			N
K0099	FRONT CASTER FOR POWER WHEELCHAIR, EACH	32	A			C			N
K0100	WHEELCHAIR ADAPTER FOR AMPUTEE, PAIR (DEVICE USED TO COMPENSATE FOR TRANSFER OF WEIGHT DUE TO LOST LIMBS TO MAINTAIN PROPER BALANCE)	32	A		E0959	C			D
K0101	ONE-ARM DRIVE ATTACHMENT, EACH	36	A		E0958	C			N
K0102	CRUTCH AND CANE HOLDER, EACH	32	A			C			N
K0103	TRANSFER BOARD,<25"	32	A		E0972	C			D
K0104	CYLINDER TANK CARRIER, EACH	32	A			C			N
K0105	IV HANGER, EACH	32	A			C			N
K0106	ARM TROUGH, EACH	32	A			C			N
K0107	WHEELCHAIR TRAY	32	A		E0950	C			D
K0108	WHEELCHAIR COMPONENT OR ACCESSORY, NOT OTHERWISE SPECIFIED	46	A			C			N
K0112	TRUNK SUPPORT DEVICE, VEST TYPE, WITH INNER FRAME, PREFABRICATED	38	A			C			D
K0113	TRUNK SUPPORT DEVICE, VEST TYPE, WITHOUT INNER FRAME, PREFABRICATED	38	A			C			D
K0114	BACK SUPPORT SYSTEM FOR USE WITH A WHEELCHAIR, WITH INNER FRAME, PREFABRICATED	32	A			C			N
K0115	SEATING SYSTEM, BACK MODULE, POSTERIORLATERAL CONTROL, WITH OR WITHOUT LATERAL SUPPORTS, CUSTOM FABRICATED FOR ATTACHMENT TO WHEELCHAIR BASE	32	A			C			N
K0116	SEATING SYSTEM, COMBINED BACK AND SEAT MODULE, CUSTOM FABRICATED FOR ATTACHMENT TO WHEELCHAIR BASE	32	A			C			N

HCPCS	Long Description	PH	MPI	Statute	X-Ref1	Coverage	ASC Pay Grp	ASC Pay Grp Eff Date	Action Code
K0182	WATER, DISTILLED, USED WITH LARGE VOLUME NEBULIZER, 1000 ML	32	A		A7018	C			N
K0183	NASAL APPLICATION DEVICE USED WITH POSITIVE AIRWAY PRESSURE DEVICE	32	A		A7034	C			N
K0184	NASAL SINGLE PIECE INTERFACE, REPLACEMENT FOR NASAL APPLICATION DEVICE, PAIR OR SINGLE PIECE INTERFACE	32	A		A7032,3	C			N
K0185	HEADGEAR USED WITH POSITIVE AIRWAY PRESSURE DEVICE	32	A		A7035	C			N
K0186	CHIN STRAP USED WITH POSITIVE AIRWAY PRESSURE DEVICE	32	A		A7036	C			N
K0187	TUBING USED WITH POSITIVE AIRWAY PRESSURE DEVICE	32	A		A7037	C			N
K0188	FILTER, DISPOSABLE, USED WITH POSITIVE AIRWAY PRESSURE DEVICE	32	A		A7038	C			N
K0189	FILTER, NON DISPOSABLE, USED WITH POSITIVE AIRWAY PRESSURE DEVICE	32	A		A7039	C			N
K0195	ELEVATING LEG RESTS, PAIR (FOR USE WITH CAPPED RENTAL WHEELCHAIR BASE)	36	A			D			N
K0268	HUMIDIFIER, NON-HEATED, USED WITH POSITIVE AIRWAY PRESSURE DEVICE	32	A		E0561	C			D
K0269	AEROSOL COMPRESSOR, ADJUSTABLE PRESSURE, LIGHT DUTY FOR INTERMITTENT USE	36	A		E0572	C			N
K0270	ULTRASONIC GENERATOR WITH SMALL VOLUME ULTRASONIC NEBULIZER	36	A		E0574	C			N
K0280	EXTENSION DRAINAGE TUBING, ANY TYPE, ANY LENGTH, WITH CONNECTOR/ADAPTOR, FOR USE WITH URINARY LEG BAG OR UROSTOMY POUCH, EACH	37	A		A4331	C			N
K0281	LUBRICANT, INDIVIDUAL STERILE PACKET, FOR INSERTION OF URINARY CATHETER, EACH	37	A		A4332	C			N
K0283	SALINE SOLUTION, PER 10 ML, METERED DOSE DISPENSER, FOR USE WITH INHALATION DRUGS	34	A		A7019	C			N
K0407	URINARY CATHETER ANCHORING DEVICE, ADHESIVE SKIN ATTACHMENT	37	A		A4333	C			N
K0408	URINARY CATHETER ANCHORING DEVICE, LEG STRAP	37	A		A4334	C			N
K0409	STERILE WATER IRRIGATION SOLUTION, 1000 ML	37	A		A4319	C			N
K0410	MALE EXTERNAL CATHETER, WITH ADHESIVE COATING, EACH	37	A		A4324	C			N
K0411	MALE EXTERNAL CATHETER, WITH ADHESIVE STRIP, EACH	37	A		A4325	C			N
K0415	PRESCRIPTION ANTIEMETIC DRUG, ORAL, PER 1 MG, FOR USE IN CONJUNCTION WITH ORAL ANTI-CANCER DRUG, NOT OTHERWISE SPECIFIED	51	A			D			N
K0416	PRESCRIPTION ANTIEMETIC DRUG, RECTAL, PER 1 MG, FOR USE IN CONJUCTION WITH ORAL ANTI-CANCER DRUG, NOT OTHERWISE SPECIFIED	51	A			D			N
K0440	NASAL PROSTHESIS - PROVIDED BY A NON-PHYSICIAN	38	A		L8040	C			N
K0441	MIDFACIAL PROSTHESIS - PROVIDED BY A NON-PHYSICIAN	38	A		L8041	C			N
K0442	ORBITAL PROSTHESIS - PROVIDED BY A NON-PHYSICIAN	38	A		L8042	C			N
K0443	UPPER FACIAL PROSTHESIS - PROVIDED BY A NON-PHYSICIAN	38	A		L8043	C			N
K0444	HEMI-FACIAL PROSTHESIS - PROVIDED BY A NON-PHYSICIAN	38	A		L8044	C			N

HCPCS	Long Description	PII	MPI	Statute	X-Ref!	Coverage	ASC Pay Grp	ASC Pay Grp Eff Date	Action Code
K0445	AURICULAR PROSTHESIS - PROVIDED BY A NON-PHYSICIAN	38	A		L8045	C			N
K0446	PARTIAL FACIAL PROSTHESIS - PROVIDED BY A NON-PHYSICIAN	38	A		L8046	C			N
K0447	NASAL SEPTAL PROSTHESIS - PROVIDED BY A NON-PHYSICIAN	38	A		L8047	C			N
K0448	UNSPECIFIED MAXILLOFACIAL PROSTHESIS, BY REPORT - PROVIDED BY A NON-PHYSICIAN	46	A		L8048	C			N
K0449	REPAIR OR MODIFICATION OF MAXILLOFACIAL PROSTHESIS, LABOR COMPONENT, 15 MINUTE INCREMENTS - PROVIDED BY A NON-PHYSICIAN	46	A		L8049	C			N
K0450	ADHESIVE, LIQUID, FOR USE WITH FACIAL PROSTHESIS ONLY, PER OUNCE	38	A		A4364	C			N
K0451	ADHESIVE REMOVER, WIPES, FOR USE WITH FACIAL PROSTHESIS, PER BOX OF 50	38	A		A4365	C			N
K0452	WHEELCHAIR BEARINGS, ANY TYPE	32	A			C			N
K0455	INFUSION PUMP USED FOR UNINTERRUPTED PARENTERAL ADMINISTRATION OF MEDICATION, (E.G., EPOPROSTENOL OR TREPROSTINOL)	31	A			D			C
K0456	HOSPITAL BED, HEAVY DUTY, EXTRA WIDE, WITH ANY TYPE SIDE RAILS, WITH MATTRESS	36	A		E0298	C			N
K0457	EXTRA WIDE/HEAVY DUTY COMMODE CHAIR, EACH	32	A		E0168	C			N
K0458	HEAVY DUTY WALKER, WITHOUT WHEELS, EACH	32	A		E0148	C			N
K0459	HEAVY DUTY WHEELED WALKER, EACH	32	A		E0149	C			N
K0460	POWER ADD-ON, TO CONVERT MANUAL WHEELCHAIR TO MOTORIZED WHEELCHAIR, JOYSTICK CONTROL	36	A		E0983	C			D
K0461	POWER ADD-ON, TO CONVERT MANUAL WHEELCHAIR TO POWER OPERATED VEHICLE, TILLER CONTROL	32	A		E0984	C			D
K0462	TEMPORARY REPLACEMENT FOR PATIENT OWNED EQUIPMENT BEING REPAIRED, ANY TYPE	32	A			D			N
K0501	AEROSOL COMPRESSOR, BATTERY POWERED, FOR USE WITH SMALL VOLUME NEBULIZER	36	A		E0571	D			N
K0529	STERILE WATER OR STERILE SALINE, 1000 ML, USED WITH LARGE VOLUME NEBULIZER	34	A		A7020	C			N
K0531	HUMIDIFIER, HEATED, USED WITH POSITIVE AIRWAY PRESSURE DEVICE	32	A		E0562	D			D
K0532	RESPIRATORY ASSIST DEVICE, BI-LEVEL PRESSURE CAPABILITY, WITHOUT BACKUP RATE FEATURE, USED WITH NONINVASIVE INTERFACE, E.G., NASAL OR FACIAL MASK (INTERMITTENT ASSIST DEVICE WITH CONTINUOUS POSITIVE AIRWAY PRESSURE DEVICE)	36	A		E0470	D			D
K0533	RESPIRATORY ASSIST DEVICE, BI-LEVEL PRESSURE CAPABILITY, WITH BACKUP RATE FEATURE, USED WITH NONINVASIVE INTERFACE, E.G., NASAL OR FACIAL MASK (INTERMITTENT ASSIST DEVICE WITH CONTINUOUS POSITIVE AIRWAY PRESSURE DEVICE)	31	A		E0471	D			D
K0534	RESPIRATORY ASSIST DEVICE, BI-LEVEL PRESSURE CAPACITY, WITH BACK UP RATE FEATURE, USED WITH INVASIVE INTERFACE, E.G., TRACHEOSTOMY TUBE (INTERMITTENT ASSIST DEVICE WITH CONTINUOUS POSITIVE AIRWAY PRESSURE DEVICE)	31	A		E0472	D			D
K0535	GAUZE, IMPREGNATED, HYDROGEL, FOR DIRECT WOUND CONTACT PAD SIZE 16 SQUARE INCH OR LESS, WITHOUT ADHESIVE BORDER, EACH DRESSING	35	A		A6231	C			N
K0536	GAUZE, IMPREGNATED, HYDROGEL, FOR DIRECT WOUND CONTACT PAD SIZE MORE THAN 16 SQ IN, BUT LESS THAN OR EQUAL TO 48 SQ IN, WITHOUT ADHESIVE BORDER, EACH DRESSING	35	A		A6232	C			N

HCPCS	Long Description	PI	MPI	Statute	X-Ref†	Coverage	ASC Pay Grp	ASC Pay Grp Eff Date	Action Code
K0537	GAUZE, IMPREGNATED, HYDROGEL, FOR DIRECT WOUND CONTACT, PAD SIZE MORE THAN 48 SQ IN, WITHOUT ADHESIVE BORDER, EACH DRESSING	35	A		A6233	C			N
K0538	NEGATIVE PRESSURE WOUND THERAPY ELECTRICAL PUMP, STATIONARY OR PORTABLE	36	A		E2402	C			D
K0539	DRESSING SET FOR NEGATIVE PRESSURE WOUND THERAPY ELECTRICAL PUMP, STATIONARY OR PORTABLE, EACH	34	A		A6550	C			D
K0540	CANISTER SET FOR NEGATIVE PRESSURE WOUND THERAPY ELECTRICAL PUMP, STATIONARY OR PORTABLE, EACH	34	A		A6551	C			D
K0541	SPEECH GENERATING DEVICE, DIGITIZED SPEECH, USING PRE-RECORDED MESSAGES, LESS THAN OR EQUAL TO 8 MINUTES RECORDING TIME	32	A		E2500	D			D
K0542	SPEECH GENERATING DEVICE, DIGITIZED SPEECH, USING PRE-RECORDED MESSAGES, GREATER THAN 8 MINUTES RECORDING TIME	32	A			D			D
K0543	SPEECH GENERATING DEVICE, SYNTHESIZED SPEECH, REQUIRING MESSAGE FORMULATION BY SPELLING AND ACCESS BY PHYSICAL CONTACT WITH THE DEVICE	32	A		E2508	D			D
K0544	SPEECH GENERATING DEVICE, SYNTHESIZED SPEECH, PERMITTING MULTIPLE METHODS OF MESSAGE FORMULATION AND MULTIPLE METHODS OF DEVICE ACCESS	32	A		E2510	D			D
K0545	SPEECH GENERATING SOFTWARE PROGRAM, FOR PERSONAL COMPUTER OR PERSONAL DIGITAL ASSISTANT	32	A		E2511	D			D
K0546	ACCESSORY FOR SPEECH GENERATING DEVICE, MOUNTING SYSTEM	32	A		E2512	D			D
K0547	ACCESSORY FOR SPEECH GENERATING DEVICE, NOT OTHERWISE CLASSIFIED	46	A		E2599	D			D
K0548	INJECTION, INSULIN LISPRO, UP TO 50 UNITS	51	A		J1817	C			N
K0549	HOSPITAL BED, HEAVY DUTY, EXTRA WIDE, WITH WEIGHT CAPACITY GREATER THAN 350 POUNDS, BUT LESS THAN OR EQUAL TO 600 POUNDS, WITH ANY TYPE SIDE RAILS, WITH MATTRESS	36	A		E0303	D			D
K0550	HOSPITAL BED, EXTRA HEAVY DUTY, EXTRA WIDE, WITH WEIGHT CAPACITY GREATER THAN 600 POUNDS, WITH ANY TYPE SIDE RAILS, WITH MATTRESS	36	A		E0304	D			D
K0551	RESIDUAL LIMB SUPPORT SYSTEM, SOLID BASE WITH ADJUSTABLE DROP HOOKS, MOUNTS TO WHEELCHAIR FRAME, EACH	32	A		E1020	D			N
K0552	SUPPLIES FOR EXTERNAL DRUG INFUSION PUMP, SYRINGE TYPE CARTRIDGE, STERILE, EACH	34	A			D			A
K0556	ADDITION TO LOWER EXTREMITY, BELOW KNEE/ABOVE KNEE, CUSTOM FABRICATED FROM EXISTING MOLD OR PREFABRICATED, SOCKET INSERT, SILICONE GEL, ELASTOMERIC OR EQUAL, FOR USE WITH LOCKING MECHANISM	38	A		L5673	C			D
K0557	ADDITION TO LOWER EXTREMITY, BELOW KNEE/ABOVE KNEE, CUSTOM FABRICATED FROM EXISTING MOLD OR PREFABRICATED, SOCKET INSERT, SILICONE GEL, ELASTOMERIC OR EQUAL, NOT FOR USE WITH LOCKING MECHANISM	38	A		L5679	C			D
K0558	ADDITION TO LOWER EXTREMITY, BELOW KNEE/ABOVE KNEE, CUSTOM FABRICATED SOCKET INSERT FOR CONGENITAL OR ATYPICAL TRAUMATIC AMPUTEE, SILICONE GEL, ELASTOMERIC OR EQUAL, FOR USE WITH OR WITHOUT LOCKING MECHANISM, INITIAL ONLY (FOR OTHER THAN INITIAL, USE CODE K0556 OR K0557)	38	A		L5681	C			D
K0559	ADDITION TO LOWER EXTREMITY, BELOW KNEE/ABOVE KNEE, CUSTOM FABRICATED SOCKET INSERT FOR OTHER THAN CONGENITAL OR ATYPICAL TRAUMATIC AMPUTEE, SILICONE GEL, ELASTOMERIC OR EQUAL, FOR USE WITH OR WITHOUT LOCKING MECHANISM, INITIAL ONLY (FOR OTHER THAN INITIAL, USE CODE K0556 OR K0557)	38	A		L5683	C			D
K0560	METACARPAL PHALANGEAL JOINT REPLACEMENT, TWO PIECES, METAL (E.G., STAINLESS STEEL OR COBALT CHROME), CERAMIC-LIKE MATERIAL (E.G., PYROCARBON), FOR SURGICAL IMPLANTATION (ALL SIZES, INCLUDES ENTIRE SYSTEM)	38	A		L8631	D			D
K0561	OSTOMY SKIN BARRIER, NON-PECTIN BASED, PASTE, PER OUNCE	37	A		A4405	D			N
K0562	OSTOMY SKIN BARRIER, PECTIN-BASED, PASTE, PER OUNCE	37	A		A4406	D			N

HCPCS	Long Description	PII	MPI	Statute	X-Ref	Coverage	ASC Pay Grp	ASC Pay Grp Eff Date	Action Code
K0563	OSTOMY SKIN BARRIER WITH FLANGE (SOLID, FLEXIBLE OR ACCORDION), EXTENDED WEAR, WITH BUILT-IN CONVEXITY, 4X4 INCHES OR SMALLER, EACH	37	A		A4407	D			N
K0564	OSTOMY SKIN BARRIER, WITH FLANGE (SOLID, FLEXIBLE OR ACCORDION), EXTENDED WEAR, WITH BUILT-IN CONVEXITY, LARGER THAN 4X4 INCHES, EACH	37	A		A4408	D			N
K0565	OSTOMY SKIN BARRIER, WITH FLANGE (SOLID, FLEXIBLE OR ACCORDION), EXTENDED WEAR, WITHOUT BUILT-IN CONVEXITY, 4X4 INCHES OR SMALLER, EACH	37	A		A4409	D			N
K0566	OSTOMY SKIN BARRIER, WITH FLANGE (SOLID, FLEXIBLE OR ACCORDION), EXTENDED WEAR, WITHOUT BUILT-IN CONVEXITY, LARGER THAN 4X4 INCHES, EACH	37	A		A4410	D			N
K0567	OSTOMY POUCH, DRAINABLE, WITH KARAYA BASED BARRIER ATTACHED, WITHOUT BUILT-IN CONVEXITY, (1 PIECE), EACH	37	A			D			N
K0568	OSTOMY POUCH, DRAINABLE, WITH STANDARD WEAR BARRIER ATTACHED, WITHOUT BUILT-IN CONVEXITY, (1 PIECE), EACH	37	A			D			N
K0569	OSTOMY POUCH, DRAINABLE, HIGH OUTPUT, FOR USE ON BARRIER WITH FLANGE (2 PIECE SYSTEM), EACH	37	A		A4413	D			N
K0570	OSTOMY SKIN BARRIER, WITH FLANGE (SOLID, FLEXIBLE OR ACCORDION), WITHOUT BUILT-IN CONVEXITY, 4X4 INCHES OR SMALLER, EACH	37	A		A4414	D			N
K0571	OSTOMY SKIN BARRIER, WITH FLANGE (SOLID, FLEXIBLE OR ACCORDION), WITHOUT BUILT-IN CONVEXITY, LARGER THAN 4X4 INCHES, EACH	37	A		A4415	D			N
K0572	TAPE, NON-WATERPROOF, PER 18 SQUARE INCHES	37	A		A4450	D			N
K0573	TAPE, WATERPROOF, PER 18 SQUARE INCHES	37	A		A4452	D			N
K0574	ADDITION TO OSTOMY POUCH, FILTER, INTEGRAL OR ADDED SEPARATELY TO POUCH, EACH	37	A			D			N
K0575	ADDITION TO OSTOMY POUCH, RUSTLE-FREE MATERIAL, PER POUCH	37	A			D			N
K0576	ADDITION TO OSTOMY POUCH, FRICTION AND IRRITANT-REDUCING, ABSORBENT, INTERFACE LAYER (COMFORT PANEL), PER POUCH	37	A			D			N
K0577	ADDITION TO OSTOMY POUCH, ODOR BARRIER, INCORPORATED INTO POUCH LAMINATE, PER POUCH	37	A			D			N
K0578	ADDITION TO OSTOMY POUCH, FAUCET-TYPE TAP WITH VALVE FOR DRAINING URINARY POUCH, EACH	37	A			D			N
K0579	ADDITION TO OSTOMY POUCH, ABSORBENT MATERIAL (SHEET/PAD/CRYSTAL PACKET) TO THICKEN LIQUID STOMAL OUTPUT, FOR USE IN POUCH, EACH	37	A		A4422	D			N
K0580	ADDITION TO OSTOMY POUCH, FLANGE LOCKING	37	A			D			N
K0581	OSTOMY POUCH, CLOSED, WITH BARRIER ATTACHED, WITH FILTER (1 PIECE), EACH	37	A		A4416	C			D
K0582	OSTOMY POUCH, CLOSED, WITH BARRIER ATTACHED, WITH BUILT-IN CONVEXITY, WITH FILTER (1 PIECE), EACH	37	A		A4417	C			D
K0583	OSTOMY POUCH, CLOSED; WITHOUT BARRIER ATTACHED, WITH FILTER (1 PIECE), EACH	37	A		A4418	C			D
K0584	OSTOMY POUCH, CLOSED; FOR USE ON BARRIER WITH FLANGE, WITH FILTER (2 PIECE), EACH	37	A		A4419	C			D
K0585	OSTOMY POUCH, CLOSED; FOR USE ON BARRIER WITH LOCKING FLANGE (2 PIECE), EACH	37	A		A4420	C			D
K0586	OSTOMY POUCH, CLOSED; FOR USE ON BARRIER WITH LOCKING FLANGE, WITH FILTER (2 PIECE), EACH	37	A		A4423	C			D
K0587	OSTOMY POUCH, DRAINABLE, WITH BARRIER ATTACHED, WITH FILTER (1 PIECE), EACH	37	A		A4424	C			D
K0588	OSTOMY POUCH, DRAINABLE; FOR USE ON BARRIER WITH FLANGE, WITH FILTER (2 PIECE SYSTEM), EACH	37	A		A4425	C			D
K0589	OSTOMY POUCH, DRAINABLE; FOR USE ON BARRIER WITH LOCKING FLANGE (2 PIECE SYSTEM), EACH	37	A		A4426	C			D

HCPCS	Long Description	PI1	MPI	Statute	X-Ref	Coverage	ASC Pay Grp	ASC Pay Grp Eff Date	Action Code
K0590	OSTOMY POUCH, DRAINABLE; FOR USE ON BARRIER WITH LOCKING FLANGE, WITH FILTER (2 PIECE SYSTEM), EACH	37	A		A4427	C			D
K0591	OSTOMY POUCH, URINARY, WITH EXTENDED WEAR BARRIER ATTACHED, WITH FAUCET-TYPE TAP WITH VALVE (1 PIECE), EACH	37	A		A4428	C			D
K0592	OSTOMY POUCH, URINARY, WITH BARRIER ATTACHED, WITH BUILT-IN CONVEXITY, WITH FAUCET-TYPE TAP WITH VALVE (1 PIECE), EACH	37	A		A4429	C			D
K0593	OSTOMY POUCH, URINARY, WITH EXTENDED WEAR BARRIER ATTACHED, WITH BUILT-IN CONVEXITY, WITH FAUCET-TYPE TAP WITH VALVE (1 PIECE), EACH	37	A		A4430	C			D
K0594	OSTOMY POUCH, URINARY; WITH BARRIER ATTACHED, WITH FAUCET-TYPE TAP WITH VALVE (1 PIECE), EACH	37	A		A4431	C			D
K0595	OSTOMY POUCH, URINARY; FOR USE ON BARRIER WITH FLANGE, WITH FAUCET-TYPE TAP WITH VALVE (2 PIECE), EACH	37	A		A4432	C			D
K0596	OSTOMY POUCH, URINARY; FOR USE ON BARRIER WITH LOCKING FLANGE (2 PIECE), EACH OSTOMY POUCH, URINARY; FOR USE ON BARRIER WITH LOCKING FLANGE, WITH FAUCET-TYPE	37	A		A4433	C			D
K0597	OSTOMY POUCH, URINARY; FOR USE ON BARRIER WITH LOCKING FLANGE, WITH FAUCET-TYPE TAP WITH VALVE (2 PIECE), EACH FUNCTIONAL NEUROMUSCULAR STIMULATOR, TRANSCUTANEOUS STIMULATION OF MUSCLES OF								
K0600	FUNCTIONAL NEUROMUSCULAR STIMULATOR, TRANSCUTANEOUS STIMULATION OF MUSCLES OFAMBULATION WITH COMPUTER CONTROL, USED FOR WALKING BY SPINAL CORD INJURED, ENTIRE SYSTEM, AFTER COMPLETION OF TRAINING PROGRAM								
K0601	REPLACEMENT BATTERY FOR EXTERNAL INFUSION PUMP OWNED BY PATIENT, SILVER OXIDE, 1.5 VOLT, EACH	32	A			C			A
K0602	REPLACEMENT BATTERY FOR EXTERNAL INFUSION PUMP OWNED BY PATIENT, SILVER OXIDE, 3 VOLT, EACH	32	A			C			A
K0603	REPLACEMENT BATTERY FOR EXTERNAL INFUSION PUMP OWNED BY PATIENT, ALKALINE, 1.5 VOLT, EACH	32	A			C			A
K0604	REPLACEMENT BATTERY FOR EXTERNAL INFUSION PUMP OWNED BY PATIENT, LITHIUM, 3.6 VOLT, EACH	32	A			C			A
K0605	REPLACEMENT BATTERY FOR EXTERNAL INFUSION PUMP OWNED BY PATIENT, LITHIUM, 4.5 VOLT, EACH	32	A			C			A
K0606	AUTOMATIC EXTERNAL DEFIBRILLATOR, WITH INTEGRATED ELECTROCARDIOGRAM ANALYSIS, GARMENT TYPE	36	A			C			A
K0582	OSTOMY POUCH, CLOSED, WITH BARRIER ATTACHED, WITH BUILT-IN CONVEXITY, WITH FILTER (1 PIECE), EACH	37	A		A4417	C			D
K0583	OSTOMY POUCH, CLOSED; WITHOUT BARRIER ATTACHED, WITH FILTER (1 PIECE), EACH	37	A		A4418	C			D
K0584	OSTOMY POUCH, CLOSED; FOR USE ON BARRIER WITH FLANGE, WITH FILTER (2 PIECE), EACH	37	A		A4419	C			D
K0585	OSTOMY POUCH, CLOSED; FOR USE ON BARRIER WITH LOCKING FLANGE (2 PIECE), EACH	37	A		A4420	C			D
K0586	OSTOMY POUCH, CLOSED; FOR USE ON BARRIER WITH LOCKING FLANGE, WITH FILTER (2 PIECE), EACH	37	A		A4423	C			D
K0587	OSTOMY POUCH, DRAINABLE, WITH BARRIER ATTACHED, WITH FILTER (1 PIECE), EACH	37	A		A4424	C			D
K0588	OSTOMY POUCH, DRAINABLE; FOR USE ON BARRIER WITH FLANGE, WITH FILTER (2 PIECE SYSTEM), EACH	37	A		A4425	C			D
K0589	OSTOMY POUCH, DRAINABLE; FOR USE ON BARRIER WITH LOCKING FLANGE (2 PIECE SYSTEM), EACH	37	A		A4426	C			D
K0590	OSTOMY POUCH, DRAINABLE; FOR USE ON BARRIER WITH LOCKING FLANGE, WITH FILTER (2 PIECE SYSTEM), EACH	37	A		A4427	C			D
K0591	OSTOMY POUCH, URINARY, WITH EXTENDED WEAR BARRIER ATTACHED, WITH FAUCET-TYPE TAP WITH VALVE (1 PIECE), EACH	37	A		A4428	C			D
K0592	OSTOMY POUCH, URINARY, WITH BARRIER ATTACHED, WITH BUILT-IN CONVEXITY, WITH FAUCET-TYPE TAP WITH VALVE (1 PIECE), EACH	37	A		A4429	C			D

HCPCS	Long Description	PTI	MPI	Statute	X-Ref	Coverage	ASC Pay Grp	ASC Pay Grp Eff Date	Action Code
K0593	OSTOMY POUCH, URINARY, WITH EXTENDED WEAR BARRIER ATTACHED, WITH BUILT-IN CONVEXITY, WITH FAUCET-TYPE TAP WITH VALVE (1 PIECE), EACH	37	A		A4430	C			D
K0594	OSTOMY POUCH, URINARY; WITH BARRIER ATTACHED, WITH FAUCET-TYPE TAP WITH VALVE (1 PIECE), EACH	37	A		A4431	C			D
K0595	OSTOMY POUCH, URINARY; FOR USE ON BARRIER WITH FLANGE, WITH FAUCET-TYPE TAP WITH VALVE (2 PIECE), EACH	37	A		A4432	C			D
K0596	OSTOMY POUCH, URINARY; FOR USE ON BARRIER WITH LOCKING FLANGE (2 PIECE), EACH OSTOMY POUCH, URINARY; FOR USE ON BARRIER WITH LOCKING FLANGE, WITH FAUCET-TYPE	37	A		A4433	C			D
K0597	OSTOMY POUCH, URINARY; FOR USE ON BARRIER WITH LOCKING FLANGE WITH FAUCET-TYPE TAP WITH VALVE (2 PIECE), EACH	37	A		A4434	C			D
K0600	FUNCTIONAL NEUROMUSCULAR STIMULATOR, TRANSCUTANEOUS STIMULATION OF MUSCLES OF AMBULATION WITH COMPUTER CONTROL, USED FOR WALKING BY SPINAL CORD INJURED, ENTIRE SYSTEM, AFTER COMPLETION OF TRAINING PROGRAM	32	A			D			N
K0601	REPLACEMENT BATTERY FOR EXTERNAL INFUSION PUMP OWNED BY PATIENT, SILVER OXIDE, 1.5 VOLT, EACH	32	A			C			A
K0602	REPLACEMENT BATTERY FOR EXTERNAL INFUSION PUMP OWNED BY PATIENT, SILVER OXIDE, 3 VOLT, EACH	32	A			C			A
K0603	REPLACEMENT BATTERY FOR EXTERNAL INFUSION PUMP OWNED BY PATIENT, ALKALINE, 1.5 VOLT, EACH	32	A			C			A
K0604	REPLACEMENT BATTERY FOR EXTERNAL INFUSION PUMP OWNED BY PATIENT, LITHIUM, 3.6 VOLT, EACH	32	A			C			A
K0605	REPLACEMENT BATTERY FOR EXTERNAL INFUSION PUMP OWNED BY PATIENT, LITHIUM, 4.5 VOLT, EACH	32	A			C			A
K0606	AUTOMATIC EXTERNAL DEFIBRILLATOR, WITH INTEGRATED ELECTROCARDIOGRAM ANALYSIS, GARMENT TYPE	36	A			C			A
K0607	REPLACEMENT BATTERY FOR AUTOMATED EXTERNAL DEFIBRILLATOR, GARMENT TYPE ONLY, EACH	32	A			C			A
K0608	REPLACEMENT GARMENT FOR USE WITH AUTOMATED EXTERNAL DEFIBRILLATOR, EACH	32	A			C			A
K0609	REPLACEMENT ELECTRODES FOR USE WITH AUTOMATED EXTERNAL DEFIBRILLATOR, GARMENT TYPE ONLY, EACH	34	A			C			A
K0610	PERITONEAL DIALYSIS CLAMPS, EACH	52	A		E1634	D			D
K0611	DISPOSABLE CYCLER SET USED WITH CYCLER DIALYSIS MACHINE, EACH	52	A		A4671	D			D
K0612	DRAINAGE EXTENSION LINE, STERILE, FOR DIALYSIS, EACH	52	A		A4672	D			D
K0613	EXTENSION LINE WITH EASY LOCK CONNECTORS, USED WITH DIALYSIS	52	A		A4673	D			D
K0614	CHEMICALS/ANTISEPTICS SOLUTION USED TO CLEAN/STERILIZE DIALYSIS EQUIPMENT, PER 8 OZ	52	A		A4674	D			D
K0615	SPEECH GENERATING DEVICE, DIGITIZED SPEECH, USING PRE-RECORDED MESSAGES,	32	A		E2502	D			D
K0615	GREATER THAN 8 MINUTES BUT LESS THAN OR EQUAL TO 20 MINUTES RECORDING TIME								
K0616	SPEECH GENERATING DEVICE, DIGITIZED SPEECH, USING PRE-RECORDED MESSAGES,	32	A		E2504	D			D
K0616	GREATER THAN 20 MINUTES BUT LESS THAN OR EQUAL TO 40 MINUTES RECORDING TIME								
K0617	SPEECH GENERATING DEVICE, DIGITIZED SPEECH, USING PRE-RECORDED MESSAGES, GREATER THAN 40 MINUTES RECORDING TIME	32	A		E2506	D			D

HCPCS	Long Description	PH	MPI	Statute	X-Ref	Coverage	ASC Pay Grp	ASC Pay Grp Eff Date	Action Code
K0618	TLSO, SAGITTAL-CORONAL CONTROL, MODULAR SEGMENTED SPINAL SYSTEM, TWO RIGID PLASTIC SHELLS, POSTERIOR EXTENDS FROM THE SACROCOCCYGEAL JUNCTION AND TERMINATES JUST INFERIOR TO THE SCAPULAR SPINE, ANTERIOR EXTENDS FROM THE SYMPHYSIS PUBIS TO THE XIPHOID, SOFT LINER, RESTRICTS GROSS TRUNK MOTION IN THE SAGITTAL AND CORONAL PLANES, LATERAL STRENGTH IS PROVIDED BY OVERLAPPING PLASTIC AND STABILIZING CLOSURES, INCLUDES STRAPS AND CLOSURES, PREFABRICATED, INCLUDES FITTING AND ADJUSTMENT	38	A			C			A
K0619	TLSO, SAGITTAL-CORONAL CONTROL, MODULAR SEGMENTED SPINAL SYSTEM, THREE RIGID PLASTIC SHELLS, POSTERIOR EXTENDS FROM THE SACROCOCCYGEAL JUNCTION AND TERMINATES JUST INFERIOR TO THE SCAPULAR SPINE, ANTERIOR EXTENDS FROM THE SYMPHYSIS PUBIS TO THE XIPHOID, SOFT LINER, RESTRICTS GROSS TRUNK MOTION IN THE SAGITTAL AND CORONAL PLANES, LATERAL STRENGTH IS PROVIDED BY OVERLAPPING PLASTIC AND STABILIZING CLOSURES, INCLUDES STRAPS AND CLOSURES, PREFABRICATED, INCLUDES FITTING AND ADJUSTMENT	38	A			C			A
K0620	TUBULAR ELASTIC DRESSING, ANY WIDTH, PER LINEAR YARD	35	A			C			A
K0621	GAUZE, PACKING STRIPS, NON-IMPREGNATED, UP TO 2 INCHES IN WIDTH, PER LINEAR YARD	35	A			C			D
K0622	CONFORMING BANDAGE, NON-ELASTIC, KNITTED/WOVEN, NON-STERILE WIDTH LESS THAN THREE INCHES, PER ROLL	35	A			C			D
K0623	CONFORMING BANDAGE, NON-ELASTIC, KNITTED/WOVEN, STERILE WIDTH LESS THAN THREE INCHES, PER ROLL	35	A			C			D
K0624	LIGHT COMPRESSION BANDAGE, ELASTIC, KNITTED/WOVEN, WIDTH LESS THAN 3 INCHES, PER ROLL (AT LEAST 3 YARDS UNSTRETCHED)	35	A			C			D
K0625	SELF ADHERENT BANDAGE, ELASTIC, NON-KNITTED/NON-WOVEN, LOAD RESISTANCE GREATER THAN OR EQUAL TO 0.55 FOOT POUNDS AT 50% MAXIMUM STRETCH, WIDTH LESS THAN 3 INCHES, PER ROLL	35	A			C			D
K0626	SELF ADHERENT BANDAGE, ELASTIC, NON-KNITTED/NON-WOVEN, LOAD RESISTANCE GREATER THAN OR EQUAL TO 0.55 FOOT POUNDS AT 50% MAXIMUM STRETCH, WIDTH GREATER THAN OR EQUAL TO 5 INCHES, PER ROLL	35	A			C			D
L0100	CRANIAL ORTHOSIS (HELMET), WITH OR WITHOUT SOFT INTERFACE, MOLDED TO PATIENT MODEL	38	A			C			N
L0110	CRANIAL ORTHOSIS (HELMET), WITH OR WITHOUT SOFT-INTERFACE, NON-MOLDED	38	A			C			N
L0112	CRANIAL CERVICAL ORTHOSIS, CONGENITAL TORTICOLLIS TYPE, WITH OR WITHOUT SOFT INTERFACE MATERIAL, ADJUSTABLE RANGE OF MOTION JOINT, CUSTOM FABRICATED	38	A			C			A
L0120	CERVICAL, FLEXIBLE, NON-ADJUSTABLE (FOAM COLLAR)	38	A			C			N
L0130	CERVICAL, FLEXIBLE, THERMOPLASTIC COLLAR, MOLDED TO PATIENT	38	A			C			N
L0140	CERVICAL, SEMI-RIGID, ADJUSTABLE (PLASTIC COLLAR)	38	A			C			N
L0150	CERVICAL, SEMI-RIGID, ADJUSTABLE MOLDED CHIN CUP (PLASTIC COLLAR WITH MANDIBULAR/OCCIPITAL PIECE)	38	A			C			N
L0160	CERVICAL, SEMI-RIGID, WIRE FRAME OCCIPITAL/MANDIBULAR SUPPORT	38	A			C			N
L0170	CERVICAL, COLLAR, MOLDED TO PATIENT MODEL	38	A			C			N
L0172	CERVICAL, COLLAR, SEMI-RIGID THERMOPLASTIC FOAM, TWO PIECE	38	A			C			N
L0174	CERVICAL, COLLAR, SEMI-RIGID, THERMOPLASTIC FOAM, TWO PIECE WITH THORACIC EXTENSION	38	A			C			N

HCPCS	Long Description	PII	MP1	Statute	X-RefI	Coverage	ASC Pay Grp	ASC Pay Grp Eff Date	Action Code
L0180	CERVICAL, MULTIPLE POST COLLAR, OCCIPITAL/MANDIBULAR SUPPORTS, ADJUSTABLE	38	A			C			N
L0190	CERVICAL, MULTIPLE POST COLLAR, OCCIPITAL/MANDIBULAR SUPPORTS, ADJUSTABLE CERVICAL BARS (SOMI, GUILFORD, TAYLOR TYPES)	38	A			C			N
L0200	CERVICAL, MULTIPLE POST COLLAR, OCCIPITAL/MANDIBULAR SUPPORTS, ADJUSTABLE CERVICAL BARS, AND THORACIC EXTENSION	38	A			C			N
L0210	THORACIC, RIB BELT	38	A			C			N
L0220	THORACIC, RIB BELT, CUSTOM FABRICATED	38	A			C			N
L0300	THORACIC-LUMBAR-SACRAL-ORTHOSIS (TLSO), FLEXIBLE (DORSO-LUMBAR SURGICAL SUPPORT)	38	A			C			N
L0310	TLSO, FLEXIBLE, (DORSO-LUMBAR SURGICAL SUPPORT), CUSTOM FABRICATED	38	A			C			N
L0315	TLSO, FLEXIBLE DORSO-LUMBAR SURGICAL SUPPORT, ELASTIC TYPE, WITH RIGID POSTERIOR PANEL	38	A			C			N
L0317	TLSO, FLEXIBLE DORSO-LUMBAR SURGICAL SUPPORT, HYPEREXTENSION, ELASTIC TYPE, WITH RIGID POSTERIOR PANEL	38	A			C			N
L0320	TLSO, ANTERIOR-POSTERIOR CONTROL (TAYLOR TYPE), WITH APRON FRONT	38	A			C			N
L0321	TLSO, ANTERIOR-POSTERIOR CONTROL, WITH RIGID OR SEMI-RIGID POSTERIOR PANEL, PREFABRICATED (INCLUDES FITTING AND ADJUSTMENT)	38	A			C			N
L0330	TLSO, ANTERIOR-POSTERIOR-LATERAL CONTROL (KNIGHT-TAYLOR TYPE), WITH APRON FRONT	38	A			C			N
L0331	TLSO, ANTERIOR-POSTERIOR-LATERAL CONTROL, WITH RIGID OR SEMI-RIGID POSTERIOR PANEL, PREFABRICATED (INCLUDES FITTING AND ADJUSTMENT)	38	A			C			N
L0340	TLSO, ANTERIOR-POSTERIOR-LATERAL-ROTARY CONTROL (ARNOLD, MAGNUSON, STEINDLER TYPES), WITH APRON FRONT	38	A			C			N
L0350	TLSO, ANTERIOR-POSTERIOR-LATERAL-ROTARY CONTROL, FLEXION COMPRESSION JACKET, CUSTOM FITTED	38	A			C			N
L0360	TLSO, ANTERIOR-POSTERIOR-LATERAL-ROTARY CONTROL, FLEXION COMPRESSION JACKET MOLDED TO PATIENT MODEL	38	A			C			N
L0370	TLSO, ANTERIOR-POSTERIOR-LATERAL-ROTARY CONTROL, HYPEREXTENSION (JEWETT, LENNOX, BAKER, CASH TYPES)	38	A			C			N
L0380	TLSO, ANTERIOR-POSTERIOR-LATERAL-ROTARY CONTROL, WITH EXTENSIONS	38	A			C			N
L0390	TLSO, ANTERIOR-POSTERIOR-LATERAL CONTROL MOLDED TO PATIENT MODEL	38	A			C			N
L0391	TLSO, ANTERIOR-POSTERIOR-LATERAL-ROTARY CONTROL, WITH RIGID OR SEMI-RIGID POSTERIOR PANEL, PREFABRICATED (INCLUDES FITTING AND ADJUSTMENT)	38	A			C			N
L0400	TLSO, ANTERIOR-POSTERIOR-LATERAL CONTROL MOLDED TO PATIENT MODEL, WITH INTERFACE MATERIAL	38	A			C			N
L0410	TLSO, ANTERIOR-POSTERIOR-LATERAL CONTROL, TWO-PIECE CONSTRUCTION MOLDED TO PATIENT MODEL	38	A			C			N
L0420	TLSO, ANTERIOR-POSTERIOR-LATERAL CONTROL, TWO PIECE CONSTRUCTION MOLDED TO PATIENT MODEL, WITH INTERFACE MATERIAL	38	A			C			N
L0430	TLSO, ANTERIOR-POSTERIOR-LATERAL CONTROL, WITH INTERFACE MATERIAL CUSTOM FITTED	38	A			C			N
L0440	TLSO, ANTERIOR-POSTERIOR-LATERAL CONTROL, WITH OVERLAPPING FRONT SECTION, SPRING STEEL FRONT, CUSTOM FITTED	38	A			C			N

HCPCS	Long Description	PI	MPI	Statute	X-Ref	Coverage	ASC Pay Grp	ASC Pay Grp Eff Date	Action Code
L0450	TLSO, FLEXIBLE, PROVIDES TRUNK SUPPORT, UPPER THORACIC REGION, PRODUCES INTRACAVITARY PRESSURE TO REDUCE LOAD ON THE INTEVERTEBRAL DISKS WITH RIGID STAYS OR PANEL(S), INCLUDES SHOULDER STRAPS AND CLOSURES, PREFABRICATED, INCLUDES FITTING AND ADJUSTMENT	38	A			C			N
L0452	TLSO, FLEXIBLE, PROVIDES TRUNK SUPPORT, UPPER THORACIC REGION, PRODUCES INTRACAVITARY PRESSURE TO REDUCE LOAD ON THE INTERVERTEBRAL DISKS WITH RIGID STAYS OR PANEL(S), INCLUDES SHOULDER STRAPS AND CLOSURES, CUSTOM FABRICATED	38	A			C			N
L0454	TLSO FLEXIBLE, PROVIDES TRUNK SUPPORT, EXTENDS FROM SACROCOCCYGEAL JUNCTION TO ABOVE T-9 VERTEBRA, RESTRICTS GROSS TRUNK MOTION IN THE SAGITTAL PLANE, PRODUCES INTRACAVITARY PRESSURE TO REDUCE LOAD ON THE INTERVERTEBRAL DISKS WITH RIGID STAYS OR PANEL(S), INCLUDES SHOULDER STRAPS AND CLOSURES, PREFABRICATED, INCLUDES FITTING AND ADJUSTMENT	38	A			C			N
L0456	TLSO, FLEXIBLE, PROVIDES TRUNK SUPPORT, THORACIC REGION, RIGID POSTERIOR PANEL AND SOFT ANTERIOR APRON, EXTENDS FROM THE SACROCOCCYGEAL JUNCTION AND TERMINATES JUST INFERIOR TO THE SCAPULAR SPINE, RESTRICTS GROSS TRUNK MOTION IN THE SAGITTAL PLANE, PRODUCES INTRACAVITARY PRESSURE TO REDUCE LOAD ON THE INTERVERTEBRAL DISKS, INCLUDES STRAPS AND CLOSURES, PREFABRICATED, INCLUDES FITTING AND ADJUSTMENT	38	A			C			N
L0458	TLSO, TRIPLANAR CONTROL, MODULAR SEGMENTED SPINAL SYSTEM, TWO RIGID PLASTIC SHELLS, POSTERIOR EXTENDS FROM THE SACROCOCCYGEAL JUNCTION AND TERMINATES JUST INFERIOR TO THE SCAPULAR SPINE, ANTERIOR EXTENDS FROM THE SYMPHYSIS PUBIS TO THE XIPHOID, SOFT LINER, RESTRICTS GROSS TRUNK MOTION IN THE SAGITTAL, CORONAL, AND TRANVERSE PLANES, LATERAL STRENGTH IS PROVIDED BY OVERLAPPING PLASTIC AND STABILIZING CLOSURES, INCLUDES STRAPS AND CLOSURES, PREFABRICATED, INCLUDES FITTING AND ADJUSTMENT	38	A			C			N
L0460	TLSO, TRIPLANAR CONTROL, MODULAR SEGMENTED SPINAL SYSTEM, TWO RIGID PLASTIC SHELLS, POSTERIOR EXTENDS FROM THE SACROCOCCYGEAL JUNCTION AND TERMINATES JUST INFERIOR TO THE SCAPULAR SPINE, ANTERIOR EXTENDS FROM THE SYMPHYSIS PUBIS TO THE STERNAL NOTCH, SOFT LINER, RESTRICTS GROSS TRUNK MOTION IN THE SAGITTAL, CORONAL, AND TRANVERSE PLANES, LATERAL STRENGTH IS PROVIDED BY OVERLAPPING PLASTIC AND STABILIZING CLOSURES, INCLUDES STRAPS AND CLOSURES, PREFABRICATED, INCLUDES FITTING AND ADJUSTMENT	38	A			C			N
L0462	TLSO, TRIPLANAR CONTROL, MODULAR SEGMENTED SPINAL SYSTEM, THREE RIGID PLASTIC SHELLS, POSTERIOR EXTENDS FROM THE SACROCOCCYGEAL JUNCTION AND TERMINATES JUST INFERIOR TO THE SCAPULAR SPINE, ANTERIOR EXTENDS FROM THE SYMPHYSIS PUBIS TO THE STERNAL NOTCH, SOFT LINER, RESTRICTS GROSS TRUNK MOTION IN THE SAGITTAL, CORONAL, AND TRANSVERSE PLANES, LATERAL STRENGTH IS PROVIDED BY OVERLAPPING PLASTIC AND STABILIZING CLOSURES, INCLUDES STRAPS AND CLOSURES, PREFABRICATED, INCLUDES FITTING AND ADJUSTMENT	38	A			C			N
L0464	TLSO, TRIPLANAR CONTROL, MODULAR SEGMENTED SPINAL SYSTEM, FOUR RIGID PLASTIC SHELLS, POSTERIOR EXTENDS FROM SACROCOCCYGEAL JUNCTION AND TERMINATES JUST INFERIOR TO SCAPULAR SPINE, ANTERIOR EXTENDS FROM SYMPHYSIS PUBIS TO THE STERNAL NOTCH, SOFT LINER, RESTRICTS GROSS TRUNK MOTION IN SAGITTAL, CORONAL, AND TRANSVERSE PLANES, LATERAL STRENGTH IS PROVIDED BY OVERLAPPING PLASTIC AND STABILIZING CLOSURES, INCLUDES STRAPS AND CLOSURES, PREFABRICATED, INCLUDES FITTING AND ADJUSTMENT	38	A			C			N
L0466	TLSO, SAGITTAL CONTROL, RIGID POSTERIOR FRAME AND FLEXIBLE SOFT ANTERIOR APRON WITH STRAPS, CLOSURES AND PADDING, RESTRICTS GROSS TRUNK MOTION IN SAGITTAL PLANE, PRODUCES INTRACAVITARY PRESSURE TO REDUCE LOAD ON INTERVERTEBRAL DISKS, INCLUDES FITTING AND SHAPING THE FRAME, PREFABRICATED, INCLUDES FITTING AND ADJUSTMENT	38	A			C			N

HCPCS	Long Description	PTI	MPI	Statute	X-Ref1	Coverage	ASC Pay Grp	ASC Pay Grp Eff Date	Action Code
L0468	TLSO, SAGITTAL-CORONAL CONTROL, RIGID POSTERIOR FRAME AND FLEXIBLE SOFT ANTERIOR APRON WITH STRAPS, CLOSURES AND PADDING, EXTENDS FROM SACROCOCCYGEAL JUNCTION OVER SCAPULAE, LATERAL STRENGTH PROVIDED BY PELVIC, THORACIC, AND LATERAL FRAME PIECES, RESTRICTS GROSS TRUNK MOTION IN SAGITTAL, AND CORONAL PLANES, PRODUCES INTRACAVITARY PRESSURE TO REDUCE LOAD ON INTERVERTEBRAL DISKS, INCLUDES FITTING AND SHAPING THE FRAME, PREFABRICATED, INCLUDES FITTING AND ADJUSTMENT	38	A			C			N
L0470	TLSO, TRIPLANAR CONTROL, RIGID POSTERIOR FRAME AND FLEXIBLE SOFT ANTERIOR APRON WITH STRAPS, CLOSURES AND PADDING, EXTENDS FROM SACROCOCCYGEAL JUNCTION TO SCAPULA, LATERAL STRENGTH PROVIDED BY PELVIC, THORACIC, AND LATERAL FRAME PIECES, ROTATIONAL STRENGTH PROVIDED BY SUBCLAVICULAR EXTENSIONS, RESTRICTS GROSS TRUNK MOTION IN SAGITTAL, CORONAL, AND TRANVERSE PLANES, PRODUCES INTRACAVITARY PRESSURE TO REDUCE LOAD ON THE INTERVERTEBRAL DISKS, INCLUDES FITTING AND SHAPING THE FRAME, PREFABRICATED, INCLUDES FITTING AND ADJUSTMENT	38	A			C			N
L0472	TLSO, TRIPLANAR CONTROL, HYPEREXTENSION, RIGID ANTERIOR AND LATERAL FRAME EXTENDS FROM SYMPHYSIS PUBIS TO STERNAL NOTCH WITH TWO ANTERIOR COMPONENTS (ONE PUBIC AND ONE STERNAL), POSTERIOR AND LATERAL PADS WITH STRAPS AND CLOSURES, LIMITS SPINAL FLEXION, RESTRICTS GROSS TRUNK MOTION IN SAGITTAL, CORONAL, AND TRANSVERSE PLANES, INCLUDES FITTING AND SHAPING THE FRAME, PREFABRICATED, INCLUDES FITTING AND ADJUSTMENT	38	A			C			N
L0476	TLSO, SAGITTAL-CORONAL CONTROL, FLEXION COMPRESSION JACKET, TWO RIGID PLASTIC SHELLS WITH SOFT LINER, POSTERIOR EXTENDS FROM SACROCOCCYGEAL JUNCTION AND TERMINATES AT OR BEFORE THE T-9 VERTEBRA, ANTERIOR EXTENDS FROM SYMPHYSIS PUBIS TO XIPHOID, USUALLY LACED TOGETHER ON ONE SIDE, RESTRICTS GROSS TRUNK MOTION IN SAGITTAL AND CORONAL PLANES, ALLOWS FREE FLEXION AND COMPRESSION OF THE LS REGION, INCLUDES STRAPS AND CLOSURES, PREFABRICATED, INCLUDES FITTING AND ADJUSTMENT	38	A			C			N
L0478	TLSO, SAGITTAL-CORONAL CONTROL, FLEXION COMPRESSION JACKET, TWO RIGID PLASTIC SHELLS WITH SOFT LINER, POSTERIOR EXTENDS FROM SACROCOCCYGEAL JUNCTION AND TERMINATES AT OR BEFORE THE T-9 VERTEBRA, ANTERIOR EXTENDS FROM SYMPHYSIS PUBIS TO XIPHOID, USUALLY LACED TOGETHER ON ONE SIDE, RESTRICTS GROSS TRUNK MOTION IN SAGITTAL AND CORONAL PLANES, ALLOWS FREE FLEXION AND COMPRESSION OF LS REGION, INCLUDES STRAPS AND CLOSURES, CUSTOM FABRICATED	38	A			C			N
L0480	TLSO, TRIPLANAR CONTROL, ONE PIECE RIGID PLASTIC SHELL WITHOUT INTERFACE LINER, WITH MULTIPLE STRAPS AND CLOSURES, POSTERIOR EXTENDS FROM SACROCOCCYGEAL JUNCTION AND TERMINATES JUST INFERIOR TO SCAPULAR SPINE, ANTERIOR EXTENDS FROM SYMPHYSIS PUBIS TO STERNAL NOTCH, ANTERIOR OR POSTERIOR OPENING, RESTRICTS GROSS TRUNK MOTION IN SAGITTAL, CORONAL, AND TRANSVERSE PLANES, INCLUDES A CARVED PLASTER OR CAD-CAM MODEL, CUSTOM FABRICATED	38	A			C			T
L0482	TLSO, TRIPLANAR CONTROL, ONE PIECE RIGID PLASTIC SHELL WITH INTERFACE LINER, MULTIPLE STRAPS AND CLOSURES, POSTERIOR EXTENDS FROM SACROCOCCYGEAL JUNCTION AND TERMINATES JUST INFERIOR TO SCAPULAR SPINE, ANTERIOR EXTENDS FROM SYMPHYSIS PUBIS TO STERNAL NOTCH, ANTERIOR OR POSTERIOR OPENING, RESTRICTS GROSS TRUNK	38	A			C			N
L0484	TLSO, TRIPLANAR CONTROL, TWO PIECE RIGID PLASTIC SHELL WITHOUT INTERFACE LINER, WITH MULTIPLE STRAPS AND CLOSURES, POSTERIOR EXTENDS FROM SACROCOCCYGEAL JUNCTION AND TERMINATES JUST INFERIOR TO SCAPULAR SPINE, ANTERIOR EXTENDS FROM SYMPHYSIS PUBIS TO STERNAL NOTCH, LATERAL STRENGTH IS ENHANCED BY OVERLAPPING PLASTIC, RESTRICTS GROSS TRUNK MOTION IN THE SAGITTAL, CORONAL, AND TRANSVERSE PLANES, INCLUDES A CARVED PLASTER OR CAD-CAM MODEL, CUSTOM FABRICATED	38	A			C			N

HCPCS	Long Description	PTI	MPI	Statute	X-Ref1	Coverage	ASC Pay Grp	ASC Pay Grp Eff Date	Action Code
L0486	TLSO, TRIPLANAR CONTROL, TWO PIECE RIGID PLASTIC SHELL WITH INTERFACE LINER, MULTIPLE STRAPS AND CLOSURES, POSTERIOR EXTENDS FROM SACROCOCCYGEAL JUNCTION AND TERMINATES JUST INFERIOR TO SCAPULAR SPINE, ANTERIOR EXTENDS FROM SYMPHYSIS PUBIS TO STERNAL NOTCH, LATERAL STRENGTH IS ENHANCED BY OVERLAPPING PLASTIC, RESTRICTS GROSS TRUNK MOTION IN THE SAGITTAL, CORONAL, AND TRANSVERSE PLANES, INCLUDES A CARVED PLASTER OR CAD-CAM MODEL, CUSTOM FABRICATED	38	A			C			N
L0488	TLSO, TRIPLANAR CONTROL, ONE PIECE RIGID PLASTIC SHELL WITH INTERFACE LINER, MULTIPLE STRAPS AND CLOSURES, POSTERIOR EXTENDS FROM SACROCOCCYGEAL JUNCTION AND TERMINATES JUST INFERIOR TO SCAPULAR SPINE, ANTERIOR EXTENDS FROM SYMPHYSIS PUBIS TO STERNAL NOTCH, ANTERIOR OR POSTERIOR OPENING, RESTRICTS GROSS TRUNK MOTION IN SAGITTAL, CORONAL, AND TRANSVERSE PLANES, PREFABRICATED, INCLUDES FITTING AND ADJUSTMENT	38	A			C			N
L0490	TLSO, SAGITTAL-CORONAL CONTROL, ONE PIECE RIGID PLASTIC SHELL, WITH OVERLAPPING REINFORCED ANTERIOR, WITH MULTIPLE STRAPS AND CLOSURES, POSTERIOR EXTENDS FROM SACROCOCCYGEAL JUNCTION AND TERMINATES AT OR BEFORE THE T-9 VERTEBRA, ANTERIOR EXTENDS FROM SYMPHYSIS PUBIS TO XIPHOID, ANTERIOR OPENING, RESTRICTS GROSS TRUNK MOTION IN SAGITTAL AND CORONAL PLANES, PREFABRICATED, INCLUDES FITTING AND ADJUSTMENT	38	A			C			N
L0500	LUMBAR-SACRAL-ORTHOSIS (LSO), FLEXIBLE, (LUMBO-SACRAL SUPPORT)	38	A			C			N
L0510	LSO, FLEXIBLE (LUMBO-SACRAL SUPPORT), CUSTOM FABRICATED	38	A			C			N
L0515	LSO, ANTERIOR-POSTERIOR CONTROL, WITH RIGID OR SEMI-RIGID POSTERIOR PANEL, PREFABRICATED	38	A			C			N
L0520	LSO, ANTERIOR-POSTERIOR-LATERAL CONTROL (KNIGHT, WILCOX TYPES), WITH APRON FRONT	38	A			C			N
L0530	LSO, ANTERIOR-POSTERIOR CONTROL (MACAUSLAND TYPE), WITH APRON FRONT	38	A			C			N
L0540	LSO, LUMBAR FLEXION (WILLIAMS FLEXION TYPE)	38	A			C			N
L0550	LSO, ANTERIOR-POSTERIOR-LATERAL CONTROL, MOLDED TO PATIENT MODEL	38	A			C			N
L0560	LSO, ANTERIOR-POSTERIOR-LATERAL CONTROL, MOLDED TO PATIENT MODEL, WITH INTERFACE MATERIAL	38	A			C			N
L0561	LSO, ANTERIOR-POSTERIOR-LATERAL CONTROL, WITH RIGID OR SEMI-RIGID POSTERIOR PANEL, PREFABRICATED	38	A			C			N
L0565	LSO, ANTERIOR-POSTERIOR-LATERAL CONTROL, CUSTOM FITTED	38	A			C			N
L0600	SACROILIAC, FLEXIBLE (SACROILIAC SURGICAL SUPPORT),	38	A			C			N
L0610	SACROILIAC, FLEXIBLE (SACROILIAC SURGICAL SUPPORT), CUSTOM FABRICATED	38	A			C			N
L0620	SACROILIAC, SEMI-RIGID (GOLDTHWAITE, OSGOOD TYPES), WITH APRON FRONT	38	A			C			N
L0700	CERVICAL-THORACIC-LUMBAR-SACRAL-ORTHOSES (CTLSO), ANTERIOR-POSTERIOR-LATERAL CONTROL, MOLDED TO PATIENT MODEL, (MINERVA TYPE)	38	A			C			N
L0710	CTLSO, ANTERIOR-POSTERIOR-LATERAL-CONTROL, MOLDED TO PATIENT MODEL, WITH INTERFACE MATERIAL, (MINERVA TYPE)	38	A			C			N
L0810	HALO PROCEDURE, CERVICAL HALO INCORPORATED INTO JACKET VEST	38	A			C			N
L0820	HALO PROCEDURE, CERVICAL HALO INCORPORATED INTO PLASTER BODY JACKET	38	A			C			N

HCPCS	Long Description	PTI	MPI	Statute	X-Refl	Coverage	ASC Pay Grp	ASC Pay Grp Eff Date	Action Code
L0830	HALO PROCEDURE, CERVICAL HALO INCORPORATED INTO MILWAUKEE TYPE ORTHOSIS	38	A			C			N
L0860	ADDITION TO HALO PROCEDURES, MAGNETIC REASONANCE IMAGE COMPATIBLE SYSTEM	38	A			C			N
L0861	ADDITION TO HALO PROCEDURE, REPLACEMENT LINER/INTERFACE MATERIAL	38	A			C			A
L0900	TORSO SUPPORT, PTOSIS SUPPORT	38	A		L0500	C			N
L0910	TORSO SUPPORT, PTOSIS SUPPORT, CUSTOM FABRICATED	38	A		L0510	C			N
L0920	TORSO SUPPORT, PENDULOUS ABDOMEN SUPPORT	38	A		L0500	C			N
L0930	TORSO SUPPORT, PENDULOUS ABDOMEN SUPPORT, CUSTOM FABRICATED	38	A		L0510	C			N
L0940	TORSO SUPPORT, POSTSURGICAL SUPPORT	38	A		L0500	C			N
L0950	TORSO SUPPORT, POST SURGICAL SUPPORT, CUSTOM FABRICATED	38	A		L0510	C			N
L0960	TORSO SUPPORT, POST SURGICAL SUPPORT, PADS FOR POST SURGICAL SUPPORT	38	A			C			N
L0970	TLSO, CORSET FRONT	38	A			C			N
L0972	LSO, CORSET FRONT	38	A			C			N
L0974	TLSO, FULL CORSET	38	A			C			N
L0976	LSO, FULL CORSET	38	A			C			N
L0978	AXILLARY CRUTCH EXTENSION	38	A			C			N
L0980	PERONEAL STRAPS, PAIR	38	A			C			N
L0982	STOCKING SUPPORTER GRIPS, SET OF FOUR (4)	38	A			C			N
L0984	PROTECTIVE BODY SOCK, EACH	38	A			C			N
L0986	ADDITION TO SPINAL ORTHOSIS, RIGID OR SEMI-RIGID ABDOMINAL PANEL, PREFABRICATED	38	A			C			N
L0999	ADDITION TO SPINAL ORTHOSIS, NOT OTHERWISE SPECIFIED	46	A			C			N
L1000	CERVICAL-THORACIC-LUMBAR-SACRAL ORTHOSIS (CTLSO) (MILWAUKEE), INCLUSIVE OF FURNISHING INITIAL ORTHOSIS, INCLUDING MODEL	38	A			C			N
L1005	TENSION BASED SCOLIOSIS ORTHOSIS AND ACCESSORY PADS, INCLUDES FITTING AND ADJUSTMENT	38	A			C			N
L1010	ADDITION TO CERVICAL-THORACIC-LUMBAR-SACRAL ORTHOSIS (CTLSO) OR SCOLIOSIS ORTHOSIS, AXILLA SLING	38	A			C			N
L1020	ADDITION TO CTLSO OR SCOLIOSIS ORTHOSIS, KYPHOSIS PAD	38	A			C			N
L1025	ADDITION TO CTLSO OR SCOLIOSIS ORTHOSIS, KYPHOSIS PAD, FLOATING	38	A			C			N
L1030	ADDITION TO CTLSO OR SCOLIOSIS ORTHOSIS, LUMBAR BOLSTER PAD	38	A			C			N
L1040	ADDITION TO CTLSO OR SCOLIOSIS ORTHOSIS, LUMBAR OR LUMBAR RIB PAD	38	A			C			N
L1050	ADDITION TO CTLSO OR SCOLIOSIS ORTHOSIS, STERNAL PAD	38	A			C			N
L1060	ADDITION TO CTLSO OR SCOLIOSIS ORTHOSIS, THORACIC PAD	38	A			C			N
L1070	ADDITION TO CTLSO OR SCOLIOSIS ORTHOSIS, TRAPEZIUS SLING	38	A			C			N

HCPCS	Long Description	PH	MPI	Statute	X-Refl	Coverage	ASC Pay Grp	ASC Pay Grp Eff Date	Action Code
L1080	ADDITION TO CTLSO OR SCOLIOSIS ORTHOSIS, OUTRIGGER	38	A			C			N
L1085	ADDITION TO CTLSO OR SCOLIOSIS ORTHOSIS, OUTRIGGER, BILATERAL WITH VERTICAL EXTENSIONS	38	A			C			N
L1090	ADDITION TO CTLSO OR SCOLIOSIS ORTHOSIS, LUMBAR SLING	38	A			C			N
L1100	ADDITION TO CTLSO OR SCOLIOSIS ORTHOSIS, RING FLANGE, PLASTIC OR LEATHER	38	A			C			N
L1110	ADDITION TO CTLSO OR SCOLIOSIS ORTHOSIS, RING FLANGE, PLASTIC OR LEATHER, MOLDED TO PATIENT MODEL	38	A			C			N
L1120	ADDITION TO CTLSO, SCOLIOSIS ORTHOSIS, COVER FOR UPRIGHT, EACH	38	A			C			N
L1200	THORACIC-LUMBAR-SACRAL-ORTHOSIS (TLSO), INCLUSIVE OF FURNISHING INITIAL ORTHOSIS ONLY	38	A			C			N
L1210	ADDITION TO TLSO, (LOW PROFILE), LATERAL THORACIC EXTENSION	38	A			C			N
L1220	ADDITION TO TLSO, (LOW PROFILE), ANTERIOR THORACIC EXTENSION	38	A			C			N
L1230	ADDITION TO TLSO, (LOW PROFILE), MILWAUKEE TYPE SUPERSTRUCTURE	38	A			C			N
L1240	ADDITION TO TLSO, (LOW PROFILE), LUMBAR DEROTATION PAD	38	A			C			N
L1250	ADDITION TO TLSO, (LOW PROFILE), ANTERIOR ASIS PAD	38	A			C			N
L1260	ADDITION TO TLSO, (LOW PROFILE), ANTERIOR THORACIC DEROTATION PAD	38	A			C			N
L1270	ADDITION TO TLSO, (LOW PROFILE), ABDOMINAL PAD	38	A			C			N
L1280	ADDITION TO TLSO, (LOW PROFILE), RIB GUSSET (ELASTIC), EACH	38	A			C			N
L1290	ADDITION TO TLSO, (LOW PROFILE), LATERAL TROCHANTERIC PAD	38	A			C			N
L1300	OTHER SCOLIOSIS PROCEDURE, BODY JACKET MOLDED TO PATIENT MODEL	38	A			C			N
L1310	OTHER SCOLIOSIS PROCEDURE, POST-OPERATIVE BODY JACKET	38	A			C			N
L1499	SPINAL ORTHOSIS, NOT OTHERWISE SPECIFIED	46	A			C			N
L1500	THORACIC-HIP-KNEE-ANKLE ORTHOSIS (THKAO), MOBILITY FRAME (NEWINGTON, PARAPODIUM TYPES)	38	A			C			N
L1510	THKAO, STANDING FRAME, WITH OR WITHOUT TRAY AND ACCESSORIES	38	A			C			N
L1520	THKAO, SWIVEL WALKER	38	A			C			N
L1600	HIP ORTHOSIS, ABDUCTION CONTROL OF HIP JOINTS, FLEXIBLE, FREJKA TYPE WITH COVER, PREFABRICATED, INCLUDES FITTING AND ADJUSTMENT	38	A			C			N
L1610	HIP ORTHOSIS, ABDUCTION CONTROL OF HIP JOINTS, FLEXIBLE, (FREJKA COVER ONLY), PREFABRICATED, INCLUDES FITTING AND ADJUSTMENT	38	A			C			N
L1620	HIP ORTHOSIS, ABDUCTION CONTROL OF HIP JOINTS, FLEXIBLE, (PAVLIK HARNESS), PREFABRICATED, INCLUDES FITTING AND ADJUSTMENT	38	A			C			N
L1630	HIP ORTHOSIS, ABDUCTION CONTROL OF HIP JOINTS, SEMI-FLEXIBLE (VON ROSEN TYPE), CUSTOM-FABRICATED	38	A			C			N
L1640	HIP ORTHOSIS, ABDUCTION CONTROL OF HIP JOINTS, STATIC, PELVIC BAND OR SPREADER BAR, THIGH CUFFS, CUSTOM-FABRICATED	38	A			C			N

HCPCS	Long Description	PTI	MPI	Statute	X-Ref1	Coverage	ASC Pay Grp	ASC Pay Grp Eff Date	Action Code
L1650	HIP ORTHOSIS, ABDUCTION CONTROL OF HIP JOINTS, STATIC, ADJUSTABLE, (ILFLED TYPE), PREFABRICATED, INCLUDES FITTING AND ADJUSTMENT	38	A			C			N
L1652	HIP ORTHOSIS, BILATERAL THIGH CUFFS WITH ADJUSTABLE ABDUCTOR SPREADER BAR, ADULT SIZE, PREFABRICATED, INCLUDES FITTING AND ADJUSTMENT, ANY TYPE	38	A			C			N
L1660	HIP ORTHOSIS, ABDUCTION CONTROL OF HIP JOINTS, STATIC, PLASTIC, PREFABRICATED, INCLUDES FITTING AND ADJUSTMENT	38	A			C			N
L1680	HIP ORTHOSIS, ABDUCTION CONTROL OF HIP JOINTS, DYNAMIC, PELVIC CONTROL, ADJUSTABLE HIP MOTION CONTROL, THIGH CUFFS (RANCHO HIP ACTION TYPE), CUSTOM FABRICATED	38	A			C			N
L1685	HIP ORTHOSIS, ABDUCTION CONTROL OF HIP JOINT, POSTOPERATIVE HIP ABDUCTION TYPE, CUSTOM FABRICATED	38	A			C			N
L1686	HIP ORTHOSIS, ABDUCTION CONTROL OF HIP JOINT, POSTOPERATIVE HIP ABDUCTION TYPE, PREFABRICATED, INCLUDES FITTING AND ADJUSTMENT	38	A			C			N
L1690	COMBINATION, BILATERAL, LUMBO-SACRAL, HIP, FEMUR ORTHOSIS PROVIDING ADDUCTION AND INTERNAL ROTATION CONTROL, PREFABRICATED, INCLUDES FITTING AND ADJUSTMENT	38	A			C			N
L1700	LEGG PERTHES ORTHOSIS, (TORONTO TYPE), CUSTOM-FABRICATED	38	A			C			N
L1710	LEGG PERTHES ORTHOSIS, (NEWINGTON TYPE), CUSTOM FABRICATED	38	A			C			N
L1720	LEGG PERTHES ORTHOSIS, TRILATERAL, (TACHDIJAN TYPE), CUSTOM-FABRICATED	38	A			C			N
L1730	LEGG PERTHES ORTHOSIS, (SCOTTISH RITE TYPE), CUSTOM-FABRICATED	38	A			C			N
L1750	LEGG PERTHES ORTHOSIS, LEGG PERTHES SLING (SAM BROWN TYPE), PREFABRICATED, INCLUDES FITTING AND ADJUSTMENT	38	A			C			N
L1755	LEGG PERTHES ORTHOSIS, (PATTEN BOTTOM TYPE), CUSTOM-FABRICATED	38	A			C			N
L1800	KNEE ORTHOSIS, ELASTIC WITH STAYS, PREFABRICATED, INCLUDES FITTING AND ADJUSTMENT	38	A			C			N
L1810	KNEE ORTHOSIS, ELASTIC WITH JOINTS, PREFABRICATED, INCLUDES FITTING AND ADJUSTMENT	38	A			C			N
L1815	KNEE ORTHOSIS, ELASTIC OR OTHER ELASTIC TYPE MATERIAL WITH CONDYLAR PAD(S), PREFABRICATED, INCLUDES FITTING AND ADJUSTMENT	38	A			C			N
L1820	KNEE ORTHOSIS, ELASTIC WITH CONDYLAR PADS AND JOINTS, PREFABRICATED, INCLUDES FITTING AND ADJUSTMENT	38	A			C			N
L1825	KNEE ORTHOSIS, ELASTIC KNEE CAP, PREFABRICATED, INCLUDES FITTING AND ADJUSTMENT	38	A			C			N
L1830	KNEE ORTHOSIS, IMMOBILIZER, CANVAS LONGITUDINAL, PREFABRICATED, INCLUDES FITTING AND ADJUSTMENT	38	A			C			N
L1831	KNEE ORTHOSIS, LOCKING KNEE JOINT(S), POSITIONAL ORTHOSIS, PREFABRICATED, INCLUDES FITTING AND ADJUSTMENT	38	A			C			A
L1832	KNEE ORTHOSIS, ADJUSTABLE KNEE JOINTS, POSITIONAL ORTHOSIS, RIGID SUPPORT, PREFABRICATED, INCLUDES FITTING AND ADJUSTMENT	38	A			C			N
L1834	KNEE ORTHOSIS, WITHOUT KNEE JOINT, RIGID, CUSTOM-FABRICATED	38	A			C			N
L1836	KNEE ORTHOSIS, RIGID, WITHOUT JOINT(S), INCLUDES SOFT INTERFACE MATERIAL, PREFABRICATED, INCLUDES FITTING AND ADJUSTMENT	38	A			C			N
L1840	KNEE ORTHOSIS, DEROTATION, MEDIAL-LATERAL, ANTERIOR CRUCIATE LIGAMENT, CUSTOM FABRICATED	38	A			C			N
L1843	KNEE ORTHOSIS, SINGLE UPRIGHT, THIGH AND CALF, WITH ADJUSTABLE FLEXION AND EXTENSION JOINT, MEDIAL-LATERAL AND ROTATION CONTROL, WITH OR WITHOUT VARUS/VALGUS ADJUSTMENT, PREFABRICATED, INCLUDES FITTING AND ADJUSTMENT	38	A			C			C

HCPCS	Long Description	PII	MPI	Statute	X-Ref1	Coverage	ASC Pay Grp	ASC Pay Grp Eff Date	Action Code
L1844	KNEE ORTHOSIS, SINGLE UPRIGHT, THIGH AND CALF, WITH ADJUSTABLE FLEXION AND EXTENSION JOINT, MEDIAL-LATERAL AND ROTATION CONTROL, WITH OR WITHOUT VARUS/VALGUS ADJUSTMENT, CUSTOM FABRICATED	38	A			C			C
L1845	KNEE ORTHOSIS, DOUBLE UPRIGHT, THIGH AND CALF, WITH ADJUSTABLE FLEXION AND EXTENSION JOINT, MEDIAL-LATERAL AND ROTATION CONTROL, PREFABRICATED, INCLUDES FITTING AND ADJUSTMENT	38	A			C			N
L1846	KNEE ORTHOSIS, DOUBLE UPRIGHT, THIGH AND CALF, WITH ADJUSTABLE FLEXION AND EXTENSION JOINT, MEDIAL-LATERAL AND ROTATION CONTROL, CUSTOM FABRICATED	38	A			C			N
L1847	KNEE ORTHOSIS, DOUBLE UPRIGHT WITH ADJUSTABLE JOINT, WITH INFLATABLE AIR SUPPORT CHAMBER(S), PREFABRICATED, INCLUDES FITTING AND ADJUSTMENT	38	A			C			N
L1850	KNEE ORTHOSIS, SWEDISH TYPE, PREFABRICATED, INCLUDES FITTING AND ADJUSTMENT	38	A			C			N
L1855	KNEE ORTHOSIS, MOLDED PLASTIC, THIGH AND CALF SECTIONS, WITH DOUBLE UPRIGHT KNEE JOINTS, CUSTOM-FABRICATED	38	A			C			N
L1858	KNEE ORTHOSIS, MOLDED PLASTIC, POLYCENTRIC KNEE JOINTS, PNEUMATIC KNEE PADS (CTI), CUSTOM-FABRICATED	38	A			C			N
L1860	KNEE ORTHOSIS, MODIFICATION OF SUPRACONDYLAR PROSTHETIC SOCKET, CUSTOM-FABRICATED (SK)	38	A			C			N
L1870	KNEE ORTHOSIS, DOUBLE UPRIGHT, THIGH AND CALF LACERS WITH KNEE JOINTS, CUSTOM-FABRICATED	38	A			C			N
L1880	KNEE ORTHOSIS, DOUBLE UPRIGHT, NON-MOLDED THIGH AND CALF CUFFS/LACERS WITH KNEE JOINTS, CUSTOM-FABRICATED	38	A			C			N
L1885	KNEE ORTHOSIS, SINGLE OR DOUBLE UPRIGHT, THIGH AND CALF, WITH FUNCTIONAL ACTIVE RESISTANCE CONTROL, PREFABRICATED, INCLUDES FITTING AND ADJUSTMENT	38	A		E1810	C			D
L1900	ANKLE FOOT ORTHOSIS, SPRING WIRE, DORSIFLEXION ASSIST CALF BAND, CUSTOM-FABRICATED	38	A			C			N
L1901	ANKLE ORTHOSIS, ELASTIC, PREFABRICATED, INCLUDES FITTING AND ADJUSTMENT (E.G. NEOPRENE, LYCRA)	38	A			C			N
L1902	ANKLE FOOT ORTHOSIS, ANKLE GAUNTLET, PREFABRICATED, INCLUDES FITTING AND ADJUSTMENT	38	A			C			N
L1904	ANKLE FOOT ORTHOSIS, MOLDED ANKLE GAUNTLET, CUSTOM-FABRICATED	38	A			C			N
L1906	ANKLE FOOT ORTHOSIS, MULTILIGAMENTUS ANKLE SUPPORT, PREFABRICATED, INCLUDES FITTING AND ADJUSTMENT	38	A			C			N
L1907	AFO, SUPRAMALLEOLAR WITH STRAPS, WITH OR WITHOUT INTERFACE/PADS, CUSTOM FABRICATED	38	A			C			A
L1910	ANKLE FOOT ORTHOSIS, POSTERIOR, SINGLE BAR, CLASP ATTACHMENT TO SHOE COUNTER, PREFABRICATED, INCLUDES FITTING AND ADJUSTMENT	38	A			C			N
L1920	ANKLE FOOT ORTHOSIS, SINGLE UPRIGHT WITH STATIC OR ADJUSTABLE STOP (PHELPS OR PERLSTEIN TYPE), CUSTOM-FABRICATED	38	A			C			N
L1930	ANKLE FOOT ORTHOSIS, PLASTIC OR OTHER MATERIAL, PREFABRICATED, INCLUDES FITTING AND ADJUSTMENT	38	A			C			N
L1940	ANKLE FOOT ORTHOSIS, PLASTIC OR OTHER MATERIAL, CUSTOM-FABRICATED	38	A			C			N
L1945	ANKLE FOOT ORTHOSIS, PLASTIC, RIGID ANTERIOR TIBIAL SECTION (FLOOR REACTION), CUSTOM-FABRICATED	38	A			C			N
L1950	ANKLE FOOT ORTHOSIS, SPIRAL, (INSTITUTE OF REHABILITATIVE MEDICINE TYPE), PLASTIC, CUSTOM-FABRICATED	38	A			C			C
L1951	ANKLE FOOT ORTHOSIS, SPIRAL, (INSTITUTE OF REHABILITATIVE MEDICINE TYPE), PLASTIC OR OTHER MATERIAL, PREFABRICATED, INCLUDES FITTING AND ADJUSTMENT	38	A			C			A
L1960	ANKLE FOOT ORTHOSIS, POSTERIOR SOLID ANKLE, PLASTIC, CUSTOM-FABRICATED	38	A			C			N

HCPCS	Long Description	PFI	MPI	Statute	X-Ref1	Coverage	ASC Pay Grp	ASC Pay Grp Eff Date	Action Code
L1970	ANKLE FOOT ORTHOSIS, PLASTIC WITH ANKLE JOINT, CUSTOM-FABRICATED	38	A			C			N
L1971	ANKLE FOOT ORTHOSIS, PLASTIC OR OTHER MATERIAL WITH ANKLE JOINT, PREFABRICATED, INCLUDES FITTING AND ADJUSTMENT	38	A			C			A
L1980	ANKLE FOOT ORTHOSIS, SINGLE UPRIGHT FREE PLANTAR DORSIFLEXION, SOLID STIRRUP, CALF BAND/CUFF (SINGLE BAR BK ORTHOSIS), CUSTOM-FABRICATED	38	A			C			N
L1990	ANKLE FOOT ORTHOSIS, DOUBLE UPRIGHT FREE PLANTAR DORSIFLEXION, SOLID STIRRUP, CALF BAND/CUFF (DOUBLE BAR BK ORTHOSIS), CUSTOM-FABRICATED	38	A			C			N
L2000	KNEE ANKLE FOOT ORTHOSIS, SINGLE UPRIGHT, FREE KNEE, FREE ANKLE, SOLID STIRRUP, THIGH AND CALF BANDS/CUFFS (SINGLE BAR AK ORTHOSIS), CUSTOM-FABRICATED	38	A			C			N
L2010	KNEE ANKLE FOOT ORTHOSIS, SINGLE UPRIGHT, FREE ANKLE, SOLID STIRRUP, THIGH AND CALF BANDS/CUFFS (SINGLE BAR AK ORTHOSIS), WITHOUT KNEE JOINT, CUSTOM-FABRICATED	38	A			C			N
L2020	KNEE ANKLE FOOT ORTHOSIS, DOUBLE UPRIGHT, FREE ANKLE, SOLID STIRRUP, THIGH AND CALF BANDS/CUFFS (DOUBLE BAR AK ORTHOSIS), CUSTOM-FABRICATED	38	A			C			N
L2030	KNEE ANKLE FOOT ORTHOSIS, DOUBLE UPRIGHT, FREE ANKLE, SOLID STIRRUP, THIGH AND CALF BANDS/CUFFS, (DOUBLE BAR AK ORTHOSIS), WITHOUT KNEE JOINT, CUSTOM FABRICATED	38	A			C			N
L2035	KNEE ANKLE FOOT ORTHOSIS, FULL PLASTIC, STATIC (PEDIATRIC SIZE), PREFABRICATED, INCLUDES FITTING AND ADJUSTMENT	38	A			C			N
L2036	KNEE ANKLE FOOT ORTHOSIS, FULL PLASTIC, DOUBLE UPRIGHT, FREE KNEE, CUSTOM-FABRICATED	38	A			C			N
L2037	KNEE ANKLE FOOT ORTHOSIS, FULL PLASTIC, SINGLE UPRIGHT, FREE KNEE, CUSTOM-FABRICATED	38	A			C			N
L2038	KNEE ANKLE FOOT ORTHOSIS, FULL PLASTIC, WITH KNEE JOINT, MULTI-AXIS ANKLE, (LIVELY ORTHOSIS OR EQUAL), CUSTOM-FABRICATED	38	A			C			N
L2039	KNEE ANKLE FOOT ORTHOSIS, FULL PLASTIC, SINGLE UPRIGHT, POLY-AXIAL HINGE, MEDIAL LATERAL ROTATION CONTROL, CUSTOM-FABRICATED	38	A			C			N
L2040	HIP KNEE ANKLE FOOT ORTHOSIS, TORSION CONTROL, BILATERAL ROTATION STRAPS, PELVIC BAND/BELT, CUSTOM FABRICATED	38	A			C			N
L2050	HIP KNEE ANKLE FOOT ORTHOSIS, TORSION CONTROL, BILATERAL TORSION CABLES, HIP JOINT, PELVIC BAND/BELT, CUSTOM-FABRICATED	38	A			C			N
L2060	HIP KNEE ANKLE FOOT ORTHOSIS, TORSION CONTROL, BILATERAL TORSION CABLES, BALL BEARING HIP JOINT, PELVIC BAND/ BELT, CUSTOM-FABRICATED	38	A			C			N
L2070	HIP KNEE ANKLE FOOT ORTHOSIS, TORSION CONTROL, UNILATERAL ROTATION STRAPS, PELVIC BAND/BELT, CUSTOM FABRICATED	38	A			C			N
L2080	HIP KNEE ANKLE FOOT ORTHOSIS, TORSION CONTROL, UNILATERAL TORSION CABLE, HIP JOINT, PELVIC BAND/BELT, CUSTOM-FABRICATED	38	A			C			N
L2090	HIP KNEE ANKLE FOOT ORTHOSIS, TORSION CONTROL, UNILATERAL TORSION CABLE, BALL BEARING HIP JOINT, PELVIC BAND/ BELT, CUSTOM-FABRICATED	38	A			C			N
L2102	ANKLE FOOT ORTHOSIS, FRACTURE ORTHOSIS, TIBIAL FRACTURE CAST ORTHOSIS, PLASTER TYPE CASTING MATERIAL, CUSTOM-FABRICATED	00	9			I			D
L2104	ANKLE FOOT ORTHOSIS, FRACTURE ORTHOSIS, TIBIAL FRACTURE CAST ORTHOSIS, SYNTHETIC TYPE CASTING MATERIAL, CUSTOM-FABRICATED	00	9			I			D
L2106	ANKLE FOOT ORTHOSIS, FRACTURE ORTHOSIS, TIBIAL FRACTURE CAST ORTHOSIS, THERMOPLASTIC TYPE CASTING MATERIAL, CUSTOM-FABRICATED	38	A			C			N
L2108	ANKLE FOOT ORTHOSIS, FRACTURE ORTHOSIS, TIBIAL FRACTURE CAST ORTHOSIS, CUSTOM-FABRICATED	38	A			C			N
L2112	ANKLE FOOT ORTHOSIS, FRACTURE ORTHOSIS, TIBIAL FRACTURE ORTHOSIS, SOFT, PREFABRICATED, INCLUDES FITTING AND ADJUSTMENT	38	A			C			N
L2114	ANKLE FOOT ORTHOSIS, FRACTURE ORTHOSIS, TIBIAL FRACTURE ORTHOSIS, SEMI-RIGID, PREFABRICATED, INCLUDES FITTING AND ADJUSTMENT	38	A			C			N

HCPCS	Long Description	PI	MPI	Statute	X-Ref1	Coverage	ASC Pay Grp	ASC Pay Grp Eff Date	Action Code
L2116	ANKLE FOOT ORTHOSIS, FRACTURE ORTHOSIS, TIBIAL FRACTURE ORTHOSIS, RIGID, PREFABRICATED, INCLUDES FITTING AND ADJUSTMENT	38	A			C			N
L2122	KNEE ANKLE FOOT ORTHOSIS, FRACTURE ORTHOSIS, FEMORAL FRACTURE CAST ORTHOSIS, PLASTER TYPE CASTING MATERIAL, CUSTOM-FABRICATED	00	9			I			D
L2124	KNEE ANKLE FOOT ORTHOSIS, FRACTURE ORTHOSIS, FEMORAL FRACTURE CAST ORTHOSIS, SYNTHETIC TYPE CASTING MATERIAL, CUSTOM-FABRICATED	00	9			I			D
L2126	KNEE ANKLE FOOT ORTHOSIS, FRACTURE ORTHOSIS, FEMORAL FRACTURE CAST ORTHOSIS, THERMOPLASTIC TYPE CASTING MATERIAL, CUSTOM-FABRICATED	38	A			C			N
L2128	KNEE ANKLE FOOT ORTHOSIS, FRACTURE ORTHOSIS, FEMORAL FRACTURE CAST ORTHOSIS, CUSTOM-FABRICATED	38	A			C			N
L2132	KAFO, FRACTURE ORTHOSIS, FEMORAL FRACTURE CAST ORTHOSIS, SOFT, PREFABRICATED, INCLUDES FITTING AND ADJUSTMENT	38	A			C			N
L2134	KAFO, FRACTURE ORTHOSIS, FEMORAL FRACTURE CAST ORTHOSIS, SEMI-RIGID, PREFABRICATED, INCLUDES FITTING AND ADJUSTMENT	38	A			C			N
L2136	KAFO, FRACTURE ORTHOSIS, FEMORAL FRACTURE CAST ORTHOSIS, RIGID, PREFABRICATED, INCLUDES FITTING AND ADJUSTMENT	38	A			C			N
L2180	ADDITION TO LOWER EXTREMITY FRACTURE ORTHOSIS, PLASTIC SHOE INSERT WITH ANKLE JOINTS	38	A			C			N
L2182	ADDITION TO LOWER EXTREMITY FRACTURE ORTHOSIS, DROP LOCK KNEE JOINT	38	A			C			N
L2184	ADDITION TO LOWER EXTREMITY FRACTURE ORTHOSIS, LIMITED MOTION KNEE JOINT	38	A			C			N
L2186	ADDITION TO LOWER EXTREMITY FRACTURE ORTHOSIS, ADJUSTABLE MOTION KNEE JOINT, LERMAN TYPE	38	A			C			N
L2188	ADDITION TO LOWER EXTREMITY FRACTURE ORTHOSIS, QUADRILATERAL BRIM	38	A			C			N
L2190	ADDITION TO LOWER EXTREMITY FRACTURE ORTHOSIS, WAIST BELT	38	A			C			N
L2192	ADDITION TO LOWER EXTREMITY FRACTURE ORTHOSIS, HIP JOINT, PELVIC BAND, THIGH FLANGE, AND PELVIC BELT	38	A			C			N
L2200	ADDITION TO LOWER EXTREMITY, LIMITED ANKLE MOTION, EACH JOINT	38	A			C			N
L2210	ADDITION TO LOWER EXTREMITY, DORSIFLEXION ASSIST (PLANTAR FLEXION RESIST), EACH JOINT	38	A			C			N
L2220	ADDITION TO LOWER EXTREMITY, DORSIFLEXION AND PLANTAR FLEXION ASSIST/RESIST, EACH JOINT	38	A			C			N
L2230	ADDITION TO LOWER EXTREMITY, SPLIT FLAT CALIPER STIRRUPS AND PLATE ATTACHMENT	38	A			C			N
L2240	ADDITION TO LOWER EXTREMITY, ROUND CALIPER AND PLATE ATTACHMENT	38	A			C			N
L2250	ADDITION TO LOWER EXTREMITY, FOOT PLATE, MOLDED TO PATIENT MODEL, STIRRUP ATTACHMENT	38	A			C			N
L2260	ADDITION TO LOWER EXTREMITY, REINFORCED SOLID STIRRUP (SCOTT-CRAIG TYPE)	38	A			C			N
L2265	ADDITION TO LOWER EXTREMITY, LONG TONGUE STIRRUP	38	A			C			N
L2270	ADDITION TO LOWER EXTREMITY, VARUS/VALGUS CORRECTION (T) STRAP, PADDED/LINED OR MALLEOLUS PAD	38	A			C			N
L2275	ADDITION TO LOWER EXTREMITY, VARUS/VALGUS CORRECTION, PLASTIC MODIFICATION, PADDED/LINED	38	A			C			N
L2280	ADDITION TO LOWER EXTREMITY, MOLDED INNER BOOT	38	A			C			N
L2300	ADDITION TO LOWER EXTREMITY, ABDUCTION BAR (BILATERAL HIP INVOLVEMENT), JOINTED, ADJUSTABLE	38	A			C			N
L2310	ADDITION TO LOWER EXTREMITY, ABDUCTION BAR-STRAIGHT	38	A			C			N

HCPCS	Long Description	PIT	MPI	Statute	X-Ref	Coverage	ASC Pay Grp	ASC Pay Grp Eff Date	Action Code
L2320	ADDITION TO LOWER EXTREMITY, NON-MOLDED LACER	38	A			C			N
L2330	ADDITION TO LOWER EXTREMITY, LACER MOLDED TO PATIENT MODEL	38	A			C			N
L2335	ADDITION TO LOWER EXTREMITY, ANTERIOR SWING BAND	38	A			C			N
L2340	ADDITION TO LOWER EXTREMITY, PRE-TIBIAL SHELL, MOLDED TO PATIENT MODEL	38	A			C			N
L2350	ADDITION TO LOWER EXTREMITY, PROSTHETIC TYPE, (BK) SOCKET, MOLDED TO PATIENT MODEL, (USED FOR PTB AFO ORTHOSES)	38	A			C			N
L2360	ADDITION TO LOWER EXTREMITY, EXTENDED STEEL SHANK	38	A			C			N
L2370	ADDITION TO LOWER EXTREMITY, PATTEN BOTTOM ADDITION TO LOWER EXTREMITY, TORSION CONTROL, ANKLE JOINT AND HALF SOLID STIRRUP	38	A			C			N
L2380	ADDITION TO LOWER EXTREMITY, TORSION CONTROL, STRAIGHT KNEE JOINT, EACH JOINT	38	A			C			N
L2385	ADDITION TO LOWER EXTREMITY, STRAIGHT KNEE JOINT, HEAVY DUTY, EACH JOINT	38	A			C			N
L2390	ADDITION TO LOWER EXTREMITY, OFFSET KNEE JOINT, EACH JOINT	38	A			C			N
L2395	ADDITION TO LOWER EXTREMITY, OFFSET KNEE JOINT, HEAVY DUTY, EACH JOINT	38	A			C			N
L2397	ADDITION TO LOWER EXTREMITY ORTHOSIS, SUSPENSION SLEEVE	38	A			C			N
L2405	ADDITION TO KNEE JOINT, LOCK; DROP, STANCE OR SWING PHASE, EACH JOINT	38	A			C			C
L2415	ADDITION TO KNEE LOCK WITH INTEGRATED RELEASE MECHANISM (BAIL, CABLE, OR EQUAL), ANY MATERIAL, EACH JOINT	38	A			C			N
L2425	ADDITION TO KNEE JOINT, DISC OR DIAL LOCK FOR ADJUSTABLE KNEE FLEXION, EACH JOINT	38	A			C			N
L2430	ADDITION TO KNEE JOINT, RATCHET LOCK FOR ACTIVE AND PROGRESSIVE KNEE EXTENSION, EACH JOINT	38	A			C			N
L2435	ADDITION TO KNEE JOINT, POLYCENTRIC JOINT, EACH JOINT	38	A			C			N
L2492	ADDITION TO KNEE JOINT, LIFT LOOP FOR DROP LOCK RING	38	A			C			N
L2500	ADDITION TO LOWER EXTREMITY, THIGH/WEIGHT BEARING, GLUTEAL/ ISCHIAL WEIGHT BEARING, RING	38	A			C			N
L2510	ADDITION TO LOWER EXTREMITY, THIGH/WEIGHT BEARING, QUADRI- LATERAL BRIM, MOLDED TO PATIENT MODEL	38	A			C			N
L2520	ADDITION TO LOWER EXTREMITY, THIGH/WEIGHT BEARING, QUADRI- LATERAL BRIM, CUSTOM FITTED	38	A			C			N
L2525	ADDITION TO LOWER EXTREMITY, THIGH/WEIGHT BEARING, ISCHIAL CONTAINMENT/NARROW M-L BRIM MOLDED TO PATIENT MODEL	38	A			C			N
L2526	ADDITION TO LOWER EXTREMITY, THIGH/WEIGHT BEARING, ISCHIAL CONTAINMENT/NARROW M-L BRIM, CUSTOM FITTED	38	A			C			N
L2530	ADDITION TO LOWER EXTREMITY, THIGH-WEIGHT BEARING, LACER, NON- MOLDED	38	A			C			N
L2540	ADDITION TO LOWER EXTREMITY, THIGH/WEIGHT BEARING, LACER, MOLDED TO PATIENT MODEL	38	A			C			N
L2550	ADDITION TO LOWER EXTREMITY, THIGH/WEIGHT BEARING, HIGH ROLL CUFF	38	A			C			N

HCPCS	Long Description	PI	MPI	Statute	X-Ref1	Coverage	ASC Pay Grp	ASC Pay Grp Eff Date	Action Code
L2570	ADDITION TO LOWER EXTREMITY, PELVIC CONTROL, HIP JOINT, CLEVIS TYPE TWO POSITION JOINT, EACH	38	A			C			N
L2580	ADDITION TO LOWER EXTREMITY, PELVIC CONTROL, PELVIC SLING	38	A			C			N
L2600	ADDITION TO LOWER EXTREMITY, PELVIC CONTROL, HIP JOINT, CLEVIS TYPE, OR THRUST BEARING, FREE, EACH	38	A			C			N
L2610	ADDITION TO LOWER EXTREMITY, PELVIC CONTROL, HIP JOINT, CLEVIS OR THRUST BEARING, LOCK, EACH	38	A			C			N
L2620	ADDITION TO LOWER EXTREMITY, PELVIC CONTROL, HIP JOINT, HEAVY DUTY, EACH	38	A			C			N
L2622	ADDITION TO LOWER EXTREMITY, PELVIC CONTROL, HIP JOINT, ADJUSTABLE FLEXION, EACH	38	A			C			N
L2624	ADDITION TO LOWER EXTREMITY, PELVIC CONTROL, HIP JOINT, ADJUSTABLE FLEXION, EXTENSION, ABDUCTION CONTROL, EACH	38	A			C			N
L2627	ADDITION TO LOWER EXTREMITY, PELVIC CONTROL, PLASTIC, MOLDED TO PATIENT MODEL, RECIPROCATING HIP JOINT AND CABLES	38	A			C			N
L2628	ADDITION TO LOWER EXTREMITY, PELVIC CONTROL, METAL FRAME, RECIPROCATING HIP JOINT AND CABLES	38	A			C			N
L2630	ADDITION TO LOWER EXTREMITY, PELVIC CONTROL, BAND AND BELT, UNILATERAL	38	A			C			N
L2640	ADDITION TO LOWER EXTREMITY, PELVIC CONTROL, BAND AND BELT, BILATERAL	38	A			C			N
L2650	ADDITION TO LOWER EXTREMITY, PELVIC AND THORACIC CONTROL, GLUTEAL PAD, EACH	38	A			C			N
L2660	ADDITION TO LOWER EXTREMITY, THORACIC CONTROL, THORACIC BAND	38	A			C			N
L2670	ADDITION TO LOWER EXTREMITY, THORACIC CONTROL, PARASPINAL UPRIGHTS	38	A			C			N
L2680	ADDITION TO LOWER EXTREMITY, THORACIC CONTROL, LATERAL SUPPORT UPRIGHTS	38	A			C			N
L2750	ADDITION TO LOWER EXTREMITY ORTHOSIS, PLATING CHROME OR NICKEL, PER BAR	38	A			C			N
L2755	ADDITION TO LOWER EXTREMITY ORTHOSIS, HIGH STRENGTH, LIGHTWEIGHT MATERIAL, ALL HYBRID LAMINATION/PREPREG COMPOSITE, PER SEGMENT	38	A			C			N
L2760	ADDITION TO LOWER EXTREMITY ORTHOSIS, EXTENSION, PER EXTENSION, PER BAR (FOR LINEAL ADJUSTMENT FOR GROWTH)	38	A			C			N
L2768	ORTHOTIC SIDE BAR DISCONNECT DEVICE, PER BAR	38	A			C			N
L2770	ADDITION TO LOWER EXTREMITY ORTHOSIS, ANY MATERIAL - PER BAR OR JOINT	38	A			C			N
L2780	ADDITION TO LOWER EXTREMITY ORTHOSIS, NON-CORROSIVE FINISH, PER BAR	38	A			C			N
L2785	ADDITION TO LOWER EXTREMITY ORTHOSIS, DROP LOCK RETAINER, EACH	38	A			C			N
L2795	ADDITION TO LOWER EXTREMITY ORTHOSIS, KNEE CONTROL, FULL KNEECAP	38	A			C			N
L2800	ADDITION TO LOWER EXTREMITY ORTHOSIS, KNEE CONTROL, KNEE CAP, MEDIAL OR LATERAL PULL	38	A			C			N
L2810	ADDITION TO LOWER EXTREMITY ORTHOSIS, KNEE CONTROL, CONDYLAR PAD	38	A			C			N

HCPCS	Long Description	PII	MPI	Statute	X-Ref1	Coverage	ASC Pay Grp	ASC Pay Grp Eff Date	Action Code
L2820	ADDITION TO LOWER EXTREMITY ORTHOSIS, SOFT INTERFACE FOR MOLDED PLASTIC, BELOW KNEE SECTION	38	A			C			N
L2830	ADDITION TO LOWER EXTREMITY ORTHOSIS, SOFT INTERFACE FOR MOLDED PLASTIC, ABOVE KNEE SECTION	38	A			C			N
L2840	ADDITION TO LOWER EXTREMITY ORTHOSIS, TIBIAL LENGTH SOCK, FRACTURE OR EQUAL, EACH	38	A			C			N
L2850	ADDITION TO LOWER EXTREMITY ORTHOSIS, FEMORAL LENGTH SOCK, FRACTURE OR EQUAL, EACH	38	A			C			N
L2860	ADDITION TO LOWER EXTREMITY JOINT, KNEE OR ANKLE, CONCENTRIC ADJUSTABLE TORSION STYLE MECHANISM, EACH	00	9			C			N
L2999	LOWER EXTREMITY ORTHOSES, NOT OTHERWISE SPECIFIED	46	A			C			N
L3000	FOOT, INSERT, REMOVABLE, MOLDED TO PATIENT MODEL, UCB TYPE, BERKELEY SHELL, EACH	00	9			D			N
L3001	FOOT, INSERT, REMOVABLE, MOLDED TO PATIENT MODEL, SPENCO, EACH	00	9			D			N
L3002	FOOT, INSERT, REMOVABLE, MOLDED TO PATIENT MODEL, PLASTAZOTE OR EQUAL, EACH	00	9			D			N
L3003	FOOT, INSERT, REMOVABLE, MOLDED TO PATIENT MODEL, SILICONE GEL, EACH	00	9			D			N
L3010	FOOT, INSERT, REMOVABLE, MOLDED TO PATIENT MODEL, LONGITUDINAL ARCH SUPPORT, EACH	00	9			D			N
L3020	FOOT, INSERT, REMOVABLE, MOLDED TO PATIENT MODEL, LONGITUDINAL/ METATARSAL SUPPORT, EACH	00	9			D			N
L3030	FOOT, INSERT, REMOVABLE, FORMED TO PATIENT FOOT, EACH	00	9			D			N
L3031	FOOT, INSERT/PLATE, REMOVABLE, ADDITION TO LOWER EXTREMITY ORTHOSIS, HIGH STRENGTH, LIGHTWEIGHT MATERIAL, ALL HYBRID LAMINATION/PREPREG COMPOSITE, EACH	00	9			I			A
L3040	FOOT, ARCH SUPPORT, REMOVABLE, PREMOLDED, LONGITUDINAL, EACH	00	9			D			N
L3050	FOOT, ARCH SUPPORT, REMOVABLE, PREMOLDED, METATARSAL, EACH	00	9			D			N
L3060	FOOT, ARCH SUPPORT, REMOVABLE, PREMOLDED, LONGITUDINAL/ METATARSAL, EACH	00	9			D			N
L3070	FOOT, ARCH SUPPORT, NON-REMOVABLE ATTACHED TO SHOE, LONGITUDINAL, EACH	00	9			D			N
L3080	FOOT, ARCH SUPPORT, NON-REMOVABLE ATTACHED TO SHOE, METATARSAL, EACH	00	9			D			N
L3090	FOOT, ARCH SUPPORT, NON-REMOVABLE ATTACHED TO SHOE, LONGITUDINAL/METATARSAL,	00	9			D			N
L3100	HALLUS-VALGUS NIGHT DYNAMIC SPLINT	00	9			D			N
L3140	FOOT, ABDUCTION ROTATION BAR, INCLUDING SHOES	00	9			D			N
L3150	FOOT, ABDUCTION ROTATATION BAR, WITHOUT SHOES	00	9			D			N
L3160	FOOT, ADJUSTABLE SHOE-STYLED POSITIONING DEVICE	00	9			C			N

HCPCS	Long Description	PII	MPI	Statute	X-Ref	Coverage	ASC Pay Grp	ASC Pay Grp Eff Date	Action Code
L3170	FOOT, PLASTIC HEEL STABILIZER	00	9			D			N
L3201	ORTHOPEDIC SHOE, OXFORD WITH SUPINATOR OR PRONATOR, INFANT	00	9			D			N
L3202	ORTHOPEDIC SHOE, OXFORD WITH SUPINATOR OR PRONATOR, CHILD	00	9			D			N
L3203	ORTHOPEDIC SHOE, OXFORD WITH SUPINATOR OR PRONATOR, JUNIOR	00	9			D			N
L3204	ORTHOPEDIC SHOE, HIGHTOP WITH SUPINATOR OR PRONATOR, INFANT	00	9			D			N
L3206	ORTHOPEDIC SHOE, HIGHTOP WITH SUPINATOR OR PRONATOR, CHILD	00	9			D			N
L3207	ORTHOPEDIC SHOE, HIGHTOP WITH SUPINATOR OR PRONATOR, JUNIOR	00	9			D			N
L3208	SURGICAL BOOT, EACH, INFANT	00	9			D			N
L3209	SURGICAL BOOT, EACH, CHILD	00	9			D			N
L3211	SURGICAL BOOT, EACH, JUNIOR	00	9			D			N
L3212	BENESCH BOOT, PAIR, INFANT	00	9			D			N
L3213	BENESCH BOOT, PAIR, CHILD	00	9			D			N
L3214	BENESCH BOOT, PAIR, JUNIOR	00	9			D			N
L3215	ORTHOPEDIC FOOTWEAR, LADIES SHOES, OXFORD	00	9	1862A8		S			N
L3216	ORTHOPEDIC FOOTWEAR, LADIES SHOES, DEPTH INLAY	00	9	1862A8		S			N
L3217	ORTHOPEDIC FOOTWEAR, LADIES SHOES, HIGHTOP, DEPTH INLAY	00	9	1862A8		S			N
L3218	ORTHOPEDIC FOOTWEAR, LADIES SURGICAL BOOT, EACH	00	9		L3260	D			N
L3219	ORTHOPEDIC FOOTWEAR, MENS SHOES, OXFORD	00	9	1862A8		S			N
L3221	ORTHOPEDIC FOOTWEAR, MENS SHOES, DEPTH INLAY	00	9	1862A8		S			N
L3222	ORTHOPEDIC FOOTWEAR, MENS SHOES, HIGHTOP, DEPTH INLAY	00	9	1862A8		S			N
L3223	ORTHOPEDIC FOOTWEAR, MENS SURGICAL BOOT, EACH	00	9		L3260	D			N
L3224	ORTHOPEDIC FOOTWEAR, WOMANS SHOE, OXFORD, USED AS AN INTEGRAL PART OF A BRACE (ORTHOSIS)	38	A			D			N
L3225	ORTHOPEDIC FOOTWEAR, MANS SHOE, OXFORD, USED AS AN INTEGRAL PART OF A BRACE (ORTHOSIS)	38	A			D			N
L3230	ORTHOPEDIC FOOTWEAR, CUSTOM SHOES, DEPTH INLAY	00	9			D			N
L3250	ORTHOPEDIC FOOTWEAR, CUSTOM MOLDED SHOE, REMOVABLE INNER MOLD, PROSTHETIC SHOE, EACH	00	9			D			N

HCPCS	Long Description	PI	MPI	Statute	X-Refl	Coverage	ASC Pay Grp	ASC Pay Grp Eff Date	Action Code
L3251	FOOT, SHOE MOLDED TO PATIENT MODEL, SILICONE SHOE, EACH	00	9			D			N
L3252	FOOT, SHOE MOLDED TO PATIENT MODEL, PLASTAZOTE (OR SIMILAR), CUSTOM FABRICATED, EACH	00	9			D			N
L3253	FOOT, MOLDED SHOE PLASTAZOTE (OR SIMILAR) CUSTOM FITTED, EACH	00	9			D			N
L3254	NON-STANDARD SIZE OR WIDTH	00	9			D			N
L3255	NON-STANDARD SIZE OR LENGTH	00	9			D			N
L3257	ORTHOPEDIC FOOTWEAR, ADDITIONAL CHARGE FOR SPLIT SIZE	00	9			D			N
L3260	SURGICAL BOOT/SHOE, EACH	00	9			D			N
L3265	PLASTAZOTE SANDAL, EACH	00	9			C			N
L3300	LIFT, ELEVATION, HEEL, TAPERED TO METATARSALS, PER INCH	00	9			D			N
L3310	LIFT, ELEVATION, HEEL AND SOLE, NEOPRENE, PER INCH	00	9			D			N
L3320	LIFT, ELEVATION, HEEL AND SOLE, CORK, PER INCH	00	9			D			N
L3330	LIFT, ELEVATION, METAL EXTENSION (SKATE)	00	9			D			N
L3332	LIFT, ELEVATION, INSIDE SHOE, TAPERED, UP TO ONE-HALF INCH	00	9			D			N
L3334	LIFT, ELEVATION, HEEL, PER INCH	00	9			D			N
L3340	HEEL WEDGE, SACH	00	9			D			N
L3350	HEEL WEDGE	00	9			D			N
L3360	SOLE WEDGE, OUTSIDE SOLE	00	9			D			N
L3370	SOLE WEDGE, BETWEEN SOLE	00	9			D			N
L3380	CLUBFOOT WEDGE	00	9			D			N
L3390	OUTFLARE WEDGE	00	9			D			N
L3400	METATARSAL BAR WEDGE, ROCKER	00	9			D			N
L3410	METATARSAL BAR WEDGE, BETWEEN SOLE	00	9			D			N
L3420	FULL SOLE AND HEEL WEDGE, BETWEEN SOLE	00	9			D			N
L3430	HEEL, COUNTER, PLASTIC REINFORCED	00	9			D			N
L3440	HEEL, COUNTER, LEATHER REINFORCED	00	9			D			N
L3450	HEEL, SACH CUSHION TYPE	00	9			D			N
L3455	HEEL, NEW LEATHER, STANDARD	00	9			D			N

HCPCS	Long Description	PII	MPI	Statute	X-Ref	Coverage	ASC Pay Grp	ASC Pay Grp Eff Date	Action Code
L3460	HEEL, NEW RUBBER, STANDARD	00	9			D			N
L3465	HEEL, THOMAS WITH WEDGE	00	9			D			N
L3470	HEEL, THOMAS EXTENDED TO BALL	00	9			D			N
L3480	HEEL, PAD AND DEPRESSION FOR SPUR	00	9			D			N
L3485	HEEL, PAD, REMOVABLE FOR SPUR	00	9			D			N
L3500	ORTHOPEDIC SHOE ADDITION, INSOLE, LEATHER	00	9			D			N
L3510	ORTHOPEDIC SHOE ADDITION, INSOLE, RUBBER	00	9			D			N
L3520	ORTHOPEDIC SHOE ADDITION, INSOLE, FELT COVERED WITH LEATHER	00	9			D			N
L3530	ORTHOPEDIC SHOE ADDITION, SOLE, HALF	00	9			D			N
L3540	ORTHOPEDIC SHOE ADDITION, SOLE, FULL	00	9			D			N
L3550	ORTHOPEDIC SHOE ADDITION, TOE TAP STANDARD	00	9			D			N
L3560	ORTHOPEDIC SHOE ADDITION, TOE TAP, HORSESHOE	00	9			D			N
L3570	ORTHOPEDIC SHOE ADDITION, SPECIAL EXTENSION TO INSTEP (LEATHER WITH EYELETS)	00	9			D			N
L3580	ORTHOPEDIC SHOE ADDITION, CONVERT INSTEP TO VELCRO CLOSURE	00	9			D			N
L3590	ORTHOPEDIC SHOE ADDITION, CONVERT FIRM SHOE COUNTER TO SOFT COUNTER	00	9			D			N
L3595	ORTHOPEDIC SHOE ADDITION, MARCH BAR	00	9			D			N
L3600	TRANSFER OF AN ORTHOSIS FROM ONE SHOE TO ANOTHER, CALIPER PLATE, EXISTING	00	9			D			N
L3610	TRANSFER OF AN ORTHOSIS FROM ONE SHOE TO ANOTHER, CALIPER PLATE, NEW	00	9			D			N
L3620	TRANSFER OF AN ORTHOSIS FROM ONE SHOE TO ANOTHER, SOLID STIRRUP, EXISTING	00	9			D			N
L3630	TRANSFER OF AN ORTHOSIS FROM ONE SHOE TO ANOTHER, SOLID STIRRUP, NEW	00	9			D			N
L3640	TRANSFER OF AN ORTHOSIS FROM ONE SHOE TO ANOTHER, DENNIS BROWNE SPLINT (RIVETON), BOTH SHOES	00	9			D			N
L3649	ORTHOPEDIC SHOE, MODIFICATION, ADDITION OR TRANSFER, NOT OTHERWISE SPECIFIED	00	9			D			N
L3650	SHOULDER ORTHOSIS, FIGURE OF EIGHT DESIGN ABDUCTION RESTRAINER, PREFABRICATED, INCLUDES FITTING AND ADJUSTMENT	38	A			C			N

HCPCS	Long Description	PTI	MPI	Statute	X-Ref1	Coverage	ASC Pay Grp	ASC Pay Grp Eff Date	Action Code
L3651	SHOULDER ORTHOSIS, SINGLE SHOULDER, ELASTIC, PREFABRICATED, INCLUDES FITTING AND ADJUSTMENT (E.G. NEOPRENE, LYCRA)	38	A			C			N
L3652	SHOULDER ORTHOSIS, DOUBLE SHOULDER, ELASTIC, PREFABRICATED, INCLUDES FITTING AND ADJUSTMENT (E.G. NEOPRENE, LYCRA)	38	A			C			N
L3660	SHOULDER ORTHOSIS, FIGURE OF EIGHT DESIGN ABDUCTION RESTRAINER, CANVAS AND WEBBING, PREFABRICATED, INCLUDES FITTING AND ADJUSTMENT	38	A			C			N
L3670	SHOULDER ORTHOSIS, ACROMIO/CLAVICULAR (CANVAS AND WEBBING TYPE), PREFABRICATED, INCLUDES FITTING AND ADJUSTMENT	38	A			C			N
L3675	SHOULDER ORTHOSIS, VEST TYPE ABDUCTION RESTRAINER, CANVAS WEBBING TYPE OR EQUAL, PREFABRICATED, INCLUDES FITTING AND ADJUSTMENT	38	A			C			N
L3677	SHOULDER ORTHOSIS, HARD PLASTIC, SHOULDER STABILIZER, PRE-FABRICATED, INCLUDES FITTING AND ADJUSTMENT	00	9			D			N
L3700	ELBOW ORTHOSIS, ELASTIC WITH STAYS, PREFABRICATED, INCLUDES FITTING AND ADJUSTMENT	38	A			C			N
L3701	ELBOW ORTHOSIS, ELASTIC, PREFABRICATED, INCLUDES FITTING AND ADJUSTMENT (E.G. NEOPRENE, LYCRA)	38	A			C			N
L3710	ELBOW ORTHOSIS, ELASTIC WITH METAL JOINTS, PREFABRICATED, INCLUDES FITTING AND ADJUSTMENT	38	A			C			N
L3720	ELBOW ORTHOSIS, DOUBLE UPRIGHT WITH FOREARM/ARM CUFFS, FREE MOTION, CUSTOM-FABRICATED	38	A			C			N
L3730	ELBOW ORTHOSIS, DOUBLE UPRIGHT WITH FOREARM/ARM CUFFS, EXTENSION/ FLEXION ASSIST, CUSTOM-FABRICATED	38	A			C			N
L3740	ELBOW ORTHOSIS, DOUBLE UPRIGHT WITH FOREARM/ARM CUFFS, ADJUSTABLE POSITION LOCK WITH ACTIVE CONTROL, CUSTOM-FABRICATED	38	A			C			N
L3760	ELBOW ORTHOSIS, WITH ADJUSTABLE POSITION LOCKING JOINT(S), PREFABRICATED, INCLUDES FITTING AND ADJUSTMENTS, ANY TYPE	38	A			C			N
L3762	ELBOW ORTHOSIS, RIGID, WITHOUT JOINTS, INCLUDES SOFT INTERFACE MATERIAL, PREFABRICATED, INCLUDES FITTING AND ADJUSTMENT	38	A			C			N
L3800	WRIST HAND FINGER ORTHOSIS, SHORT OPPONENS, NO ATTACHMENTS, CUSTOM-FABRICATED	38	A			C			N
L3805	WRIST HAND FINGER ORTHOSIS, LONG OPPONENS, NO ATTACHMENT, CUSTOM-FABRICATED	38	A			C			N
L3807	WRIST HAND FINGER ORTHOSIS, WITHOUT JOINT(S), PREFABRICATED, INCLUDES FITTING AND ADJUSTMENTS, ANY TYPE	38	A			C			N
L3810	WHFO, ADDITION TO SHORT AND LONG OPPONENS, THUMB ABDUCTION (C) BAR	38	A			C			N
L3815	WHFO, ADDITION TO SHORT AND LONG OPPONENS, SECOND M.P. ABDUCTION ASSIST	38	A			C			N
L3820	WHFO, ADDITION TO SHORT AND LONG OPPONENS, I.P. EXTENSION ASSIST, WITH M.P. EXTENSION STOP	38	A			C			N
L3825	WHFO, ADDITION TO SHORT AND LONG OPPONENS, M.P. EXTENSION STOP	38	A			C			N
L3830	WHFO, ADDITION TO SHORT AND LONG OPPONENS, M.P. EXTENSION ASSIST	38	A			C			N
L3835	WHFO, ADDITION TO SHORT AND LONG OPPONENS, M.P. SPRING EXTENSION ASSIST	38	A			C			N
L3840	WHFO, ADDITION TO SHORT AND LONG OPPONENS, SPRING SWIVEL THUMB	38	A			C			N
L3845	WHFO, ADDITION TO SHORT AND LONG OPPONENS, THUMB I.P. EXTENSION ASSIST, WITH M.P. STOP	38	A			C			N

HCPCS	Long Description	PII	MPI	Statute	X-Ref1	Coverage	ASC Pay Grp	ASC Pay Grp Eff Date	Action Code
L3850	WHO, ADDITION TO SHORT AND LONG OPPONENS, ACTION WRIST, WITH DORSIFLEXION ASSIST	38	A			C			N
L3855	WHFO, ADDITION TO SHORT AND LONG OPPONENS, ADJUSTABLE M.P. FLEXION CONTROL	38	A			C			N
L3860	WHFO, ADDITION TO SHORT AND LONG OPPONENS, ADJUSTABLE M.P. FLEXION CONTROL AND I.P.	38	A			C			N
L3890	ADDITION TO UPPER EXTREMITY JOINT, WRIST OR ELBOW, CONCENTRIC ADJUSTABLE TORSION STYLE MECHANISM, EACH	00	9			C			N
L3900	WRIST HAND FINGER ORTHOSIS, DYNAMIC FLEXOR HINGE, RECIPROCAL WRIST EXTENSION/ FLEXION, FINGER FLEXION/EXTENSION, WRIST OR FINGER DRIVEN, CUSTOM-FABRICATED	38	A			C			N
L3901	WRIST HAND FINGER ORTHOSIS, DYNAMIC FLEXOR HINGE, RECIPROCAL WRIST EXTENSION/FLEXION, FINGER FLEXION/EXTENSION, CABLE DRIVEN, CUSTOM-FABRICATED	38	A			C			N
L3902	WRIST HAND FINGER ORTHOSIS, EXTERNAL POWERED, COMPRESSED GAS, CUSTOM-FABRICATED	00	9			I			F
L3904	WRIST HAND FINGER ORTHOSIS, EXTERNAL POWERED, ELECTRIC, CUSTOM-FABRICATED	38	A			C			N
L3906	WRIST HAND ORTHOSIS, WRIST GAUNTLET, CUSTOM-FABRICATED	38	A			C			N
L3907	WRIST HAND FINGER ORTHOSIS, WRIST GAUNTLET WITH THUMB SPICA, CUSTOM-FABRICATED	38	A			C			N
L3908	WRST HAND ORTHOSIS, WRIST EXTENSION CONTROL COCK-UP, NON MOLDED, PREFABRICATED, INCLUDES FITTING AND ADJUSTMENT	38	A			C			N
L3909	WRIST ORTHOSIS, ELASTIC, PREFABRICATED, INCLUDES FITTING AND ADJUSTMENT (E.G. NEOPRENE, LYCRA)	38	A			C			N
L3910	WRIST HAND FINGER ORTHOSIS, SWANSON DESIGN, PREFABRICATED, INCLUDES FITTING AND ADJUSTMENT	38	A			C			N
L3911	WRIST HAND FINGER ORTHOSIS, ELASTIC, PREFABRICATED, INCLUDES FITTING AND ADJUSTMENT (E.G. NEOPRENE, LYCRA)	38	A			C			N
L3912	HAND FINGER ORTHOSIS, FLEXION GLOVE WITH ELASTIC FINGER CONTROL, PREFABRICATED, INCLUDES FITTING AND ADJUSTMENT	38	A			C			N
L3914	WRIST HAND ORTHOSIS, WRIST EXTENSION COCK-UP, PREFABRICATED, INCLUDES FITTING/ADJUSTMENT	38	A			C			N
L3916	WRIST HAND FINGER ORTHOSIS, WRIST EXTENSION COCK-UP WITH OUTRIGGER, PREFABRICATED, INCLUDES FITTING AND ADJUSTMENT	38	A			C			N
L3917	HAND ORTHOSIS, METACARPAL FRACTURE ORTHOSIS, PREFABRICATED, INCLUDES FITTING AND ADJUSTMENT	38	A			C			A
L3918	HAND FINGER ORTHOSIS, KNUCKLE BENDER, PREFABRICATED, INCLUDES FITTING AND ADJUSTMENT	38	A			C			N
L3920	HAND FINGER ORTHOSIS, KNUCKLE BENDER WITH OUTRIGGER, PREFABRICATED, INCLUDES FITTING AND ADJUSTMENT	38	A			C			N
L3922	HAND FINGER ORTHOSIS, KNUCKLE BENDER, TWO SEGMENT TO FLEX JOINTS, PREFABRICATED, INCLUDES FITTING AND ADJUSTMENT	38	A			C			N
L3923	HAND FINGER ORTHOSIS, WITHOUT JOINT(S), PREFABRICATED, INCLUDES FITTING AND ADJUSTMENTS, ANY TYPE	38	A			C			N
L3924	WRIST HAND FINGER ORTHOSIS, OPPENHEIMER, PREFABRICATED, INCLUDES FITTING AND ADJUSTMENT	38	A			C			N
L3926	WRIST HAND FINGER ORTHOSIS, THOMAS SUSPENSION, PREFABRICATED, INCLUDES FITTING AND ADJUSTMENT	38	A			C			N
L3928	HAND FINGER ORTHOSIS, FINGER EXTENSION, WITH CLOCK SPRING, PREFABRICATED, INCLUDES FITTING AND ADJUSTMENT	38	A			C			N
L3930	WRIST HAND FINGER ORTHOSIS, FINGER EXTENSION, WITH WRIST SUPPORT, PREFABRICATED, INCLUDES FITTING AND ADJUSTMENT	38	A			C			N
L3932	FINGER ORTHOSIS, SAFETY PIN, SPRING WIRE, PREFABRICATED, INCLUDES FITTING AND ADJUSTMENT	38	A			C			N

HCPCS	Long Description	PII	MPI	Statute	X-Ref1	Coverage	ASC Pay Grp	ASC Pay Grp Eff Date	Action Code
L3934	FINGER ORTHOSIS, SAFETY PIN, MODIFIED, PREFABRICATED, INCLUDES FITTING AND ADJUSTMENT	38	A			C			N
L3936	WRIST HAND FINGER ORTHOSIS, PALMER, PREFABRICATED, INCLUDES FITTING AND ADJUSTMENT	38	A			C			N
L3938	WRIST HAND FINGER ORTHOSIS, DORSAL WRIST, PREFABRICATED, INCLUDES FITTING AND ADJUSTMENT	38	A			C			N
L3940	WRIST HAND FINGER ORTHOSIS, DORSAL WRIST, WITH OUTRIGGER ATTACHMENT, PREFABRICATED, INCLUDES FITTING AND ADJUSTMENT	38	A			C			N
L3942	HAND FINGER ORTHOSIS, REVERSE KNUCKLE BENDER, PREFABRICATED, INCLUDES FITTING AND ADJUSTMENT	38	A			C			N
L3944	HAND FINGER ORTHOSIS, REVERSE KNUCKLE BENDER, WITH OUTRIGGER, PREFABRICATED, INCLUDES FITTING AND ADJUSTMENT	38	A			C			N
L3946	HAND FINGER ORTHOSIS, COMPOSITE ELASTIC, PREFABRICATED, INCLUDES FITTING AND ADJUSTMENT	38	A			C			N
L3948	FINGER ORTHOSIS, FINGER KNUCKLE BENDER, PREFABRICATED, INCLUDES FITTING AND ADJUSTMENT	38	A			C			N
L3950	WRIST HAND FINGER ORTHOSIS, COMBINATION OPPENHEIMER, WITH KNUCKLE BENDER AND TWO ATTACHMENTS, PREFABRICATED, INCLUDES FITTING AND ADJUSTMENT	38	A			C			N
L3952	WRIST HAND FINGER ORTHOSIS, COMBINATION OPPENHEIMER, WITH REVERSE KNUCKLE AND TWO ATTACHMENTS, PREFABRICATED, INCLUDES FITTING AND ADJUSTMENT	38	A			C			N
L3954	HAND FINGER ORTHOSIS, SPREADING HAND, PREFABRICATED, INCLUDES FITTING AND ADJUSTMENT	38	A			C			N
L3956	ADDITION OF JOINT TO UPPER EXTREMITY ORTHOSIS, ANY MATERIAL; PER JOINT	38	A			C			N
L3960	SHOULDER ELBOW WRIST HAND ORTHOSIS, ABDUCTION POSITIONING, AIRPLANE DESIGN, PREFABRICATED, INCLUDES FITTING AND ADJUSTMENT	38	A			C			N
L3962	SHOULDER ELBOW WRIST HAND ORTHOSIS, ABDUCTION POSITIONING, ERBS PALSEY DESIGN, PREFABRICATED, INCLUDES FITTING AND ADJUSTMENT	38	A			C			N
L3963	SHOULDER ELBOW WRIST HAND ORTHOSIS, MOLDED SHOULDER, ARM, FOREARM AND WRIST, WITH ARTICULATING ELBOW JOINT, CUSTOM-FABRICATED	38	A			C			N
L3964	SHOULDER ELBOW ORTHOSIS, MOBILE ARM SUPPORT ATTACHED TO WHEELCHAIR, BALANCED, ADJUSTABLE, PREFABRICATED, INCLUDES FITTING AND ADJUSTMENT	32	A			C			N
L3965	SHOULDER ELBOW ORTHOSIS, MOBILE ARM SUPPORT ATTACHED TO WHEELCHAIR, BALANCED, ADJUSTABLE RANCHO TYPE, PREFABRICATED, INCLUDES FITTING AND ADJUSTMENT	32	A			C			N
L3966	SHOULDER ELBOW ORTHOSIS, MOBILE ARM SUPPORT ATTACHED TO WHEELCHAIR, BALANCED, RECLINING, PREFABRICATED, INCLUDES FITTING AND ADJUSTMENT	32	A			C			N
L3968	SHOULDER ELBOW ORTHOSIS, MOBILE ARM SUPPORT ATTACHED TO WHEELCHAIR, BALANCED, FRICTION ARM SUPPORT (FRICTION DAMPENING TO PROXIMAL AND DISTAL JOINTS), PREFABRICATED, INCLUDES FITTING AND ADJUSTMENT	32	A			C			N
L3969	SHOULDER ELBOW ORTHOSIS, MOBILE ARM SUPPORT, MONOSUSPENSION ARM AND HAND SUPPORT, OVERHEAD ELBOW FOREARM HAND SLING SUPPORT, YOKE TYPE SUSPENSION SUPPORT, PREFABRICATED, INCLUDES FITTING AND ADJUSTMENT	32	A			C			N
L3970	SEO, ADDITION TO MOBILE ARM SUPPORT, ELEVATING PROXIMAL ARM	32	A			C			N
L3972	SEO, ADDITION TO MOBILE ARM SUPPORT, OFFSET OR LATERAL ROCKER ARM WITH ELASTIC BALANCE CONTROL	32	A			C			N
L3974	SEO, ADDITION TO MOBILE ARM SUPPORT, SUPINATOR	32	A			C			N
L3980	UPPER EXTREMITY FRACTURE ORTHOSIS, HUMERAL, PREFABRICATED, INCLUDES FITTING AND ADJUSTMENT	38	A			C			N

HCPCS	Long Description	PH	MPI	Statute	X-Ref	Coverage	ASC Pay Grp	ASC Pay Grp Eff Date	Action Code
L3982	UPPER EXTREMITY FRACTURE ORTHOSIS, RADIUS/ULNAR, PREFABRICATED, INCLUDES FITTING AND ADJUSTMENT	38	A			C			N
L3984	UPPER EXTREMITY FRACTURE ORTHOSIS, WRIST, PREFABRICATED, INCLUDES FITTING AND ADJUSTMENT	38	A			C			N
L3985	UPPER EXTREMITY FRACTURE ORTHOSIS, FOREARM, HAND WITH WRIST HINGE, CUSTOM-FABRICATED	38	A			C			N
L3986	UPPER EXTREMITY FRACTURE ORTHOSIS, COMBINATION OF HUMERAL, RADIUS/ULNAR, WRIST, (EXAMPLE--COLLES FRACTURE), CUSTOM FABRICATED	38	A			C			N
L3995	ADDITION TO UPPER EXTREMITY ORTHOSIS, SOCK, FRACTURE OR EQUAL, EACH	38	A			C			N
L3999	UPPER LIMB ORTHOSIS, NOT OTHERWISE SPECIFIED	46	A			C			N
L4000	REPLACE GIRDLE FOR SPINAL ORTHOSIS (CTLSO OR SO)	38	A			C			N
L4010	REPLACE TRILATERAL SOCKET BRIM	38	A			C			N
L4020	REPLACE QUADRILATERAL SOCKET BRIM, MOLDED TO PATIENT MODEL	38	A			C			N
L4030	REPLACE QUADRILATERAL SOCKET BRIM, CUSTOM FITTED	38	A			C			N
L4040	REPLACE MOLDED THIGH LACER	38	A			C			N
L4045	REPLACE NON-MOLDED THIGH LACER	38	A			C			N
L4050	REPLACE MOLDED CALF LACER	38	A			C			N
L4055	REPLACE NON-MOLDED CALF LACER	38	A			C			N
L4060	REPLACE HIGH ROLL CUFF	38	A			C			N
L4070	REPLACE PROXIMAL AND DISTAL UPRIGHT FOR KAFO	38	A			C			N
L4080	REPLACE METAL BANDS KAFO, PROXIMAL THIGH	38	A			C			N
L4090	REPLACE METAL BANDS KAFO-AFO, CALF OR DISTAL THIGH	38	A			C			N
L4100	REPLACE LEATHER CUFF KAFO, PROXIMAL THIGH	38	A			C			N
L4110	REPLACE LEATHER CUFF KAFO-AFO, CALF OR DISTAL THIGH	38	A			C			N
L4130	REPLACE PRETIBIAL SHELL	38	A			C			N
L4205	REPAIR OF ORTHOTIC DEVICE, LABOR COMPONENT, PER 15 MINUTES	46	A			D			N
L4210	REPAIR OF ORTHOTIC DEVICE, REPAIR OR REPLACE MINOR PARTS	46	A			D			N
L4350	ANKLE CONTROL ORTHOSIS, STIRRUP STYLE, RIGID, INCLUDES ANY TYPE INTERFACE (E.G., PNEUMATIC, GEL), PREFABRICATED, INCLUDES FITTING AND ADJUSTMENT	38	A			C			C
L4360	WALKING BOOT, PNEUMATIC, WITH OR WITHOUT JOINTS, WITH OR WITHOUT INTERFACE MATERIAL, PREFABRICATED, INCLUDES FITTING AND ADJUSTMENT	38	A			C			C
L4370	PNEUMATIC FULL LEG SPLINT, PREFABRICATED, INCLUDES FITTING AND ADJUSTMENT	38	A			C			N

HCPCS	Long Description	PTI	MPI	Statute	X-Ref1	Coverage	ASC Pay Grp	ASC Pay Grp Eff Date	Action Code
L4380	PNEUMATIC KNEE SPLINT, PREFABRICATED, INCLUDES FITTING AND ADJUSTMENT	38	A			C			N
L4386	WALKING BOOT, NON-PNEUMATIC, WITH OR WITHOUT JOINTS, WITH OR WITHOUT INTERFACE MATERIAL, PREFABRICATED, INCLUDES FITTING AND ADJUSTMENT	38	A			C			C
L4392	REPLACEMENT, SOFT INTERFACE MATERIAL, STATIC AFO	38	A			C			N
L4394	REPLACE SOFT INTERFACE MATERIAL, FOOT DROP SPLINT	38	A			C			N
L4396	STATIC ANKLE FOOT ORTHOSIS, INCLUDING SOFT INTERFACE MATERIAL, ADJUSTABLE FOR FIT, FOR POSITIONING, PRESSURE REDUCTION, MAY BE USED FOR MINIMAL AMBULATION, PREFABRICATED, INCLUDES FITTING AND ADJUSTMENT	38	A			C			N
L4398	FOOT DROP SPLINT, RECUMBENT POSITIONING DEVICE, PREFABRICATED, INCLUDES FITTING AND ADJUSTMENT	38	A			C			N
L5000	PARTIAL FOOT, SHOE INSERT WITH LONGITUDINAL ARCH, TOE FILLER	38	A			D			N
L5010	PARTIAL FOOT, MOLDED SOCKET, ANKLE HEIGHT, WITH TOE FILLER	38	A			D			N
L5020	PARTIAL FOOT, MOLDED SOCKET, TIBIAL TUBERCLE HEIGHT, WITH TOE FILLER	38	A			D			N
L5050	ANKLE, SYMES, MOLDED SOCKET, SACH FOOT	38	A			C			N
L5060	ANKLE, SYMES, METAL FRAME, MOLDED LEATHER SOCKET, ARTICULATED ANKLE/FOOT	38	A			C			N
L5100	BELOW KNEE, MOLDED SOCKET, SHIN, SACH FOOT	38	A			C			N
L5105	BELOW KNEE, PLASTIC SOCKET, JOINTS AND THIGH LACER, SACH FOOT	38	A			C			N
L5150	KNEE DISARTICULATION (OR THROUGH KNEE), MOLDED SOCKET, EXTERNAL KNEE JOINTS, SHIN, SACH FOOT	38	A			C			N
L5160	KNEE DISARTICULATION (OR THROUGH KNEE), MOLDED SOCKET, BENT KNEE CONFIGURATION, EXTERNAL KNEE JOINTS, SHIN, SACH FOOT	38	A			C			N
L5200	ABOVE KNEE, MOLDED SOCKET, SINGLE AXIS CONSTANT FRICTION KNEE, SHIN, SACH FOOT	38	A			C			N
L5210	ABOVE KNEE, SHORT PROSTHESIS, NO KNEE JOINT (STUBBIES), WITH FOOT BLOCKS, NO ANKLE JOINTS, EACH	38	A			C			N
L5220	ABOVE KNEE, SHORT PROSTHESIS, NO KNEE JOINT (STUBBIES), WITH ARTICULATED ANKLE/FOOT, DYNAMICALLY ALIGNED, EACH	38	A			C			N
L5230	ABOVE KNEE, FOR PROXIMAL FEMORAL FOCAL DEFICIENCY, CONSTANT FRICTION KNEE, SHIN, SACH FOOT	38	A			C			N
L5250	HIP DISARTICULATION, CANADIAN TYPE; MOLDED SOCKET, HIP JOINT, SINGLE AXIS CONSTANT FRICTION KNEE, SHIN, SACH FOOT	38	A			C			N
L5270	HIP DISARTICULATION, TILT TABLE TYPE; MOLDED SOCKET, LOCKING HIP JOINT, SINGLE AXIS CONSTANT FRICTION KNEE, SHIN, SACH FOOT	38	A			C			N
L5280	HEMIPELVECTOMY, CANADIAN TYPE; MOLDED SOCKET, HIP JOINT, SINGLE AXIS CONSTANT FRICTION KNEE, SHIN, SACH FOOT	38	A			C			N
L5300	BELOW KNEE, MOLDED SOCKET, SACH FOOT, ENDOSKELETAL SYSTEM, INCLUDING SOFT COVER AND FINISHING	38	A		L5301	C			N
L5301	BELOW KNEE, MOLDED SOCKET, SHIN, SACH FOOT, ENDOSKELETAL SYSTEM	38	A			C			N
L5310	KNEE DISARTICULATION (OR THROUGH KNEE), MOLDED SOCKET, SACH FOOT ENDOSKELETAL SYSTEM, INCLUDING SOFT COVER AND FINISHING	38	A		L5311	C			N
L5311	KNEE DISARTICULATION (OR THROUGH KNEE), MOLDED SOCKET, EXTERNAL KNEE JOINTS, SHIN, SACH FOOT, ENDOSKELETAL SYSTEM	38	A			C			N

HCPCS	Long Description	PTI	MPI	Statute	X-Reft	Coverage	ASC Pay Grp	ASC Pay Grp Eff Date	Action Code
L5320	ABOVE KNEE, MOLDED SOCKET, OPEN END, SACH FOOT, ENDOSKELETAL SYSTEM, SINGLE AXIS KNEE, INCLUDING SOFT COVER AND FINISHING	38	A		L5321	C			N
L5321	ABOVE KNEE, MOLDED SOCKET, OPEN END, SACH FOOT, ENDOSKELETAL SYSTEM, SINGLE AXIS KNEE	38	A			C			N
L5330	HIP DISARTICULATION, CANADIAN TYPE; MOLDED SOCKET, ENDOSKELETAL SYSTEM, HIP JOINT, SINGLE AXIS KNEE, SACH FOOT, INCLUDING SOFT COVER AND FINISHING	38	A		L5331	C			N
L5331	HIP DISARTICULATION, CANADIAN TYPE, MOLDED SOCKET, ENDOSKELETAL SYSTEM, HIP JOINT, SINGLE AXIS KNEE, SACH FOOT	38	A			C			N
L5340	HEMIPELVECTOMY, CANADIAN TYPE; MOLDED SOCKET, ENDOSKELETAL SYSTEM, HIP JOINT, SINGLE AXIS KNEE, SACH FOOT, INCLUDING SOFT COVER AND FINISHING	38	A		L5341	C			N
L5341	HEMIPELVECTOMY, CANADIAN TYPE, MOLDED SOCKET, ENDOSKELETAL SYSTEM, HIP JOINT, SINGLE AXIS KNEE, SACH FOOT	38	A			C			N
L5400	IMMEDIATE POST SURGICAL OR EARLY FITTING, APPLICATION OF INITIAL RIGID DRESSING, INCLUDING FITTING, ALIGNMENT, SUSPENSION, AND ONE CAST CHANGE, BELOW KNEE	38	A			C			N
L5410	IMMEDIATE POST SURGICAL OR EARLY FITTING, APPLICATION OF INITIAL RIGID DRESSING, INCLUDING FITTING, ALIGNMENT AND SUSPENSION, BELOW KNEE, EACH ADDITIONAL CAST CHANGE AND REALIGNMENT	38	A			C			N
L5420	IMMEDIATE POST SURGICAL OR EARLY FITTING, APPLICATION OF INITIAL RIGID DRESSING, INCLUDING FITTING, ALIGNMENT AND SUSPENSION AND ONE CAST CHANGE AK OR KNEE DISARTICULATION	38	A			C			N
L5430	IMMEDIATE POST SURGICAL OR EARLY FITTING, APPLICATION OF INITIAL RIGID DRESSING, INCL. FITTING, ALIGNMENT AND SUPENSION, AK OR KNEE DISARTICULATION, EACH ADDITIONAL CAST CHANGE AND REALIGNMENT	38	A			C			N
L5450	IMMEDIATE POST SURGICAL OR EARLY FITTING, APPLICATION OF NON-WEIGHT BEARING RIGID DRESSING, BELOW KNEE	38	A			C			N
L5460	IMMEDIATE POST SURGICAL OR EARLY FITTING, APPLICATION OF NON-WEIGHT BEARING RIGID DRESSING, ABOVE KNEE	38	A			C			N
L5500	INITIAL, BELOW KNEE PTB TYPE SOCKET, NON-ALIGNABLE SYSTEM, PYLON, NO COVER, SACH FOOT, PLASTER SOCKET, DIRECT FORMED	38	A			C			N
L5505	INITIAL, ABOVE KNEE - KNEE DISARTICULATION, ISCHIAL LEVEL SOCKET, NON-ALIGNABLE SYSTEM, PYLON, NO COVER, SACH FOOT, PLASTER SOCKET, DIRECT FORMED	38	A			C			N
L5510	PREPARATORY, BELOW KNEE PTB TYPE SOCKET, NON-ALIGNABLE SYSTEM, PYLON, NO COVER, SACH FOOT, PLASTER SOCKET, MOLDED TO MODEL	38	A			C			N
L5520	PREPARATORY, BELOW KNEE PTB TYPE SOCKET, NON-ALIGNABLE SYSTEM, PYLON, NO COVER, SACH FOOT, THERMOPLASTIC OR EQUAL, DIRECT FORMED	38	A			C			N
L5530	PREPARATORY, BELOW KNEE PTB TYPE SOCKET, NON-ALIGNABLE SYSTEM, PYLON, NO COVER, SACH FOOT, THERMOPLASTIC OR EQUAL, MOLDED TO MODEL	38	A			C			N
L5535	PREPARATORY, BELOW KNEE PTB TYPE SOCKET, NON-ALIGNABLE SYSTEM, NO COVER, SACH FOOT, PREFABRICATED, ADJUSTABLE OPEN END SOCKET	38	A			C			N
L5540	PREPARATORY, BELOW KNEE PTB TYPE SOCKET, NON-ALIGNABLE SYSTEM, PYLON, NO COVER, SACH FOOT, LAMINATED SOCKET, MOLDED TO MODEL	38	A			C			N
L5560	PREPARATORY, ABOVE KNEE- KNEE DISARTICULATION, ISCHIAL LEVEL SOCKET, NON-ALIGNABLE SYSTEM, PYLON, NO COVER, SACH FOOT, PLASTER SOCKET, MOLDED TO MODEL	38	A			C			N
L5570	PREPARATORY, ABOVE KNEE - KNEE DISARTICULATION, ISCHIAL LEVEL SOCKET, NON-ALIGNABLE SYSTEM, PYLON, NO COVER, SACH FOOT, THERMOPLASTIC OR EQUAL, DIRECT FORMED	38	A			C			N
L5580	PREPARATORY, ABOVE KNEE - KNEE DISARTICULATION ISCHIAL LEVEL SOCKET, NON-ALIGNABLE SYSTEM, PYLON, NO COVER, SACH FOOT, THERMOPLASTIC OR EQUAL, MOLDED TO MODEL	38	A			C			N
L5585	PREPARATORY, ABOVE KNEE - KNEE DISARTICULATION, ISCHIAL LEVEL SOCKET, NON-ALIGNABLE SYSTEM, PYLON, NO COVER, SACH FOOT, PREFABRICATED ADJUSTABLE OPEN END SOCKET	38	A			C			N

HCPCS	Long Description	PII	MPI	Statute	X-Ref	Coverage	ASC Pay Grp	ASC Pay Grp Eff Date	Action Code
L5590	PREPARATORY, ABOVE KNEE - KNEE DISARTICULATION ISCHIAL LEVEL SOCKET, NON-ALIGNABLE SYSTEM, PYLON NO COVER, SACH FOOT, LAMINATED SOCKET, MOLDED TO MODEL	38	A			C			N
L5595	PREPARATORY, HIP DISARTICULATION-HEMIPELVECTOMY, PYLON, NO COVER, SACH FOOT, THERMOPLASTIC OR EQUAL, MOLDED TO PATIENT MODEL	38	A			C			N
L5600	PREPARATORY, HIP DISARTICULATION-HEMIPELVECTOMY, PYLON, NO COVER, SACH FOOT, LAMINATED SOCKET, MOLDED TO PATIENT MODEL	38	A			C			N
L5610	ADDITION TO LOWER EXTREMITY, ENDOSKELETAL SYSTEM, ABOVE KNEE, HYDRACADENCE SYSTEM	38	A			C			N
L5611	ADDITION TO LOWER EXTREMITY, ENDOSKELETAL SYSTEM, ABOVE KNEE - KNEE DISARTICULATION, 4 BAR LINKAGE, WITH FRICTION SWING PHASE CONTROL	38	A			C			N
L5613	ADDITION TO LOWER EXTREMITY, ENDOSKELETAL SYSTEM, ABOVE KNEE-KNEE DISARTICULATION, 4 BAR LINKAGE, WITH HYDRAULIC SWING PHASE CONTROL	38	A			C			N
L5614	ADDITION TO LOWER EXTREMITY, EXOSKELETAL SYSTEM, ABOVE KNEE-KNEE DISARTICULATION, 4 BAR LINKAGE, WITH PNEUMATIC SWING PHASE CONTROL	38	A			C			N
L5616	ADDITION TO LOWER EXTREMITY, ENDOSKELETAL SYSTEM, ABOVE KNEE, UNIVERSAL MULTIPLEX SYSTEM, FRICTION SWING PHASE CONTROL	38	A			C			N
L5617	ADDITION TO LOWER EXTREMITY, QUICK CHANGE SELF-ALIGNING UNIT, ABOVE KNEE OR BELOW KNEE, EACH	38	A			C			N
L5618	ADDITION TO LOWER EXTREMITY, TEST SOCKET, SYMES	38	A			C			N
L5620	ADDITION TO LOWER EXTREMITY, TEST SOCKET, BELOW KNEE	38	A			C			N
L5622	ADDITION TO LOWER EXTREMITY, TEST SOCKET, KNEE DISARTICULATION	38	A			C			N
L5624	ADDITION TO LOWER EXTREMITY, TEST SOCKET, ABOVE KNEE	38	A			C			N
L5626	ADDITION TO LOWER EXTREMITY, TEST SOCKET, HIP DISARTICULATION	38	A			C			N
L5628	ADDITION TO LOWER EXTREMITY, TEST SOCKET, HEMIPELVECTOMY	38	A			C			N
L5629	ADDITION TO LOWER EXTREMITY, BELOW KNEE, ACRYLIC SOCKET	38	A			C			N
L5630	ADDITION TO LOWER EXTREMITY, SYMES TYPE, EXPANDABLE WALL SOCKET	38	A			C			N
L5631	ADDITION TO LOWER EXTREMITY, ABOVE KNEE OR KNEE DISARTICULATION, ACRYLIC SOCKET	38	A			C			N
L5632	ADDITION TO LOWER EXTREMITY, SYMES TYPE, PTB BRIM DESIGN SOCKET	38	A			C			N
L5634	ADDITION TO LOWER EXTREMITY, SYMES TYPE, POSTERIOR OPENING (CANADIAN) SOCKET	38	A			C			N
L5636	ADDITION TO LOWER EXTREMITY, SYMES TYPE, MEDIAL OPENING SOCKET	38	A			C			N
L5637	ADDITION TO LOWER EXTREMITY, BELOW KNEE, TOTAL CONTACT	38	A			C			N
L5638	ADDITION TO LOWER EXTREMITY, BELOW KNEE, LEATHER SOCKET	38	A			C			N
L5639	ADDITION TO LOWER EXTREMITY, BELOW KNEE, WOOD SOCKET	38	A			C			N
L5640	ADDITION TO LOWER EXTREMITY, KNEE DISARTICULATION, LEATHER SOCKET	38	A			C			N
L5642	ADDITION TO LOWER EXTREMITY, ABOVE KNEE, LEATHER SOCKET	38	A			C			N

HCPCS	Long Description	PII	MPI	Statute	X-Refl	Coverage	ASC Pay Grp	ASC Pay Grp Eff Date	Action Code
L5643	ADDITION TO LOWER EXTREMITY, HIP DISARTICULATION, FLEXIBLE INNER SOCKET, EXTERNAL FRAME	38	A			C			N
L5644	ADDITION TO LOWER EXTREMITY, ABOVE KNEE, WOOD SOCKET	38	A			C			N
L5645	ADDITION TO LOWER EXTREMITY, BELOW KNEE, FLEXIBLE INNER SOCKET, EXTERNAL FRAME	38	A			C			N
L5646	ADDITION TO LOWER EXTREMITY, BELOW KNEE, AIR, FLUID, GEL OR EQUAL, CUSHION SOCKET	38	A			C			C
L5647	ADDITION TO LOWER EXTREMITY, BELOW KNEE SUCTION SOCKET	38	A			C			N
L5648	ADDITION TO LOWER EXTREMITY, ABOVE KNEE, AIR, FLUID, GEL OR EQUAL, CUSHION SOCKET	38	A			C			C
L5649	ADDITION TO LOWER EXTREMITY, ISCHIAL CONTAINMENT/NARROW M-L SOCKET	38	A			C			N
L5650	ADDITIONS TO LOWER EXTREMITY, TOTAL CONTACT, ABOVE KNEE OR KNEE DISARTICULATION SOCKET	38	A			C			N
L5651	ADDITION TO LOWER EXTREMITY, ABOVE KNEE, FLEXIBLE INNER SOCKET, EXTERNAL FRAME	38	A			C			N
L5652	ADDITION TO LOWER EXTREMITY, SUCTION SUSPENSION, ABOVE KNEE OR KNEE DISARTICULATION SOCKET	38	A			C			N
L5653	ADDITION TO LOWER EXTREMITY, KNEE DISARTICULATION, EXPANDABLE WALL SOCKET	38	A			C			N
L5654	ADDITION TO LOWER EXTREMITY, SOCKET INSERT, SYMES, (KEMBLO, PELITE, ALIPLAST, PLASTAZOTE OR EQUAL)	38	A			C			N
L5655	ADDITION TO LOWER EXTREMITY, SOCKET INSERT, BELOW KNEE (KEMBLO, PELITE, ALIPLAST, PLASTAZOTE OR EQUAL)	38	A			C			N
L5656	ADDITION TO LOWER EXTREMITY, SOCKET INSERT, KNEE DISARTICULATION (KEMBLO, PELITE, ALIPLAST, PLASTAZOTE OR EQUAL)	38	A			C			N
L5658	ADDITION TO LOWER EXTREMITY, SOCKET INSERT, ABOVE KNEE (KEMBLO, PELITE, ALIPLAST, PLASTAZOTE OR EQUAL)	38	A			C			N
L5660	ADDITION TO LOWER EXTREMITY, SOCKET INSERT, SYMES, SILICONE GEL OR EQUAL	00	9			G			N
L5661	ADDITION TO LOWER EXTREMITY, SOCKET INSERT, MULTI-DUROMETER SYMES	38	A			C			N
L5662	ADDITION TO LOWER EXTREMITY, SOCKET INSERT, BELOW KNEE, SILICONE GEL OR EQUAL	00	9			G			N
L5663	ADDITION TO LOWER EXTREMITY, SOCKET INSERT, KNEE DISARTICULATION, SILICONE GEL OR EQUAL	00	9			G			N
L5664	ADDITION TO LOWER EXTREMITY, SOCKET INSERT, ABOVE KNEE, SILICONE GEL OR EQUAL	00	9			G			N
L5665	ADDITION TO LOWER EXTREMITY, SOCKET INSERT, MULTI-DUROMETER, BELOW KNEE	38	A			C			N
L5666	ADDITION TO LOWER EXTREMITY, BELOW KNEE, CUFF SUSPENSION	38	A			C			N
L5667	ADDITION TO LOWER EXTREMITY, BELOW KNEE/ABOVE KNEE, SOCKET INSERT, SUCTION SUSPENSION WITH LOCKING MECHANISM	38	A			C			N
L5668	ADDITION TO LOWER EXTREMITY, BELOW KNEE, MOLDED DISTAL CUSHION	38	A			C			N
L5669	ADDITION TO LOWER EXTREMITY, BELOW KNEE/ABOVE KNEE, SOCKET INSERT, SUCTION SUSPENSION WITHOUT LOCKING MECHANISM	38	A		L5660,2-4	C			N
L5670	ADDITION TO LOWER EXTREMITY, BELOW KNEE, MOLDED SUPRACONDYLAR SUSPENSION (PTS OR SIMILAR)	38	A			C			N
L5671	ADDITION TO LOWER EXTREMITY, BELOW KNEE / ABOVE KNEE SUSPENSION LOCKING MECHANISM (SHUTTLE, LANYARD OR EQUAL), EXCLUDES SOCKET INSERT	38	A			C			N

HCPCS	Long Description	PI	MPI	Statute	X-Ref	Coverage	ASC Pay Grp	ASC Pay Grp Eff Date	Action Code
L5672	ADDITION TO LOWER EXTREMITY, BELOW KNEE, REMOVABLE MEDIAL BRIM SUSPENSION	38	A			C			N
L5673	ADDITION TO LOWER EXTREMITY, BELOW KNEE/ABOVE KNEE, CUSTOM FABRICATED FROM EXISTING MOLD OR PREFABRICATED, SOCKET INSERT, SILICONE GEL, ELASTOMERIC OR EQUAL, FOR USE WITH LOCKING MECHANISM	38	A			C			A
L5674	ADDITION TO LOWER EXTREMITY, BELOW KNEE, SUSPENSION SLEEVE, ANY MATERIAL, EACH	38	A			C			N
L5675	ADDITION TO LOWER EXTREMITY, BELOW KNEE, SUSPENSION SLEEVE, HEAVY DUTY, ANY MATERIAL, EACH	38	A			C			N
L5676	ADDITIONS TO LOWER EXTREMITY, BELOW KNEE, KNEE JOINTS, SINGLE AXIS, PAIR	38	A			C			N
L5677	ADDITIONS TO LOWER EXTREMITY, BELOW KNEE, KNEE JOINTS, POLYCENTRIC, PAIR	38	A			C			N
L5678	ADDITIONS TO LOWER EXTREMITY, BELOW KNEE, JOINT COVERS, PAIR	38	A			C			N
L5679	ADDITION TO LOWER EXTREMITY, BELOW KNEE/ABOVE KNEE, CUSTOM FABRICATED FROM EXISTING MOLD OR PREFABRICATED, SOCKET INSERT, SILICONE GEL, ELASTOMERIC OR EQUAL, NOT FOR USE WITH LOCKING MECHANISM	38	A			C			A
L5680	ADDITION TO LOWER EXTREMITY, BELOW KNEE, THIGH LACER, NONMOLDED	38	A			C			N
L5681	ADDITION TO LOWER EXTREMITY, BELOW KNEE/ABOVE KNEE, CUSTOM FABRICATED SOCKET INSERT FOR CONGENITAL OR ATYPICAL TRAUMATIC AMPUTEE, SILICONE GEL, ELASTOMERIC OR EQUAL, FOR USE WITH OR WITHOUT LOCKING MECHANISM, INITIAL ONLY (FOR OTHER THAN INITIAL, USE CODE L5673 OR L5679)	38	A			C			A
L5682	ADDITION TO LOWER EXTREMITY, BELOW KNEE, THIGH LACER, GLUTEAL/ISCHIAL, MOLDED	38	A			C			N
L5683	ADDITION TO LOWER EXTREMITY, BELOW KNEE/ABOVE KNEE, CUSTOM FABRICATED SOCKET INSERT FOR OTHER THAN CONGENITAL OR ATYPICAL TRAUMATIC AMPUTEE, SILICONE GEL, ELASTOMERIC OR EQUAL, FOR USE WITH OR WITHOUT LOCKING MECHANISM, INITIAL ONLY (FOR OTHER THAN INITIAL, USE CODE L5673 OR L5679)	38	A			C			A
L5684	ADDITION TO LOWER EXTREMITY, BELOW KNEE, FORK STRAP	38	A			C			N
L5686	ADDITION TO LOWER EXTREMITY, BELOW KNEE, BACK CHECK (EXTENSION CONTROL)	38	A			C			N
L5688	ADDITION TO LOWER EXTREMITY, BELOW KNEE, WAIST BELT, WEBBING	38	A			C			N
L5690	ADDITION TO LOWER EXTREMITY, BELOW KNEE, WAIST BELT, PADDED AND LINED	38	A			C			N
L5692	ADDITION TO LOWER EXTREMITY, ABOVE KNEE, PELVIC CONTROL BELT, LIGHT	38	A			C			N
L5694	ADDITION TO LOWER EXTREMITY, ABOVE KNEE, PELVIC CONTROL BELT, PADDED AND LINED	38	A			C			N
L5695	ADDITION TO LOWER EXTREMITY, ABOVE KNEE, PELVIC CONTROL, SLEEVE SUSPENSION, NEOPRENE OR EQUAL, EACH	38	A			C			N
L5696	ADDITION TO LOWER EXTREMITY, ABOVE KNEE OR KNEE DISARTICULATION, PELVIC JOINT	38	A			C			N
L5697	ADDITION TO LOWER EXTREMITY, ABOVE KNEE OR KNEE DISARTICULATION, PELVIC BAND	38	A			C			N
L5698	ADDITION TO LOWER EXTREMITY, ABOVE KNEE OR KNEE DISARTICULATION, SILESIAN BANDAGE	38	A			C			N
L5699	ALL LOWER EXTREMITY PROSTHESES, SHOULDER HARNESS	38	A			C			N
L5700	REPLACEMENT, SOCKET, BELOW KNEE, MOLDED TO PATIENT MODEL	38	A			C			N

HCPCS	Long Description	PII	MPI	Statute	X-Refl	Coverage	ASC Pay Grp	ASC Pay Grp Eff Date	Action Code
L5701	REPLACEMENT, SOCKET, ABOVE KNEE/KNEE DISARTICULATION, INCLUDING ATTACHMENT PLATE, MOLDED TO PATIENT MODEL	38	A			C			N
L5702	REPLACEMENT, SOCKET, HIP DISARTICULATION, INCLUDING HIP JOINT, MOLDED TO PATIENT MODEL	38	A			C			N
L5704	CUSTOM SHAPED PROTECTIVE COVER, BELOW KNEE	38	A			C			N
L5705	CUSTOM SHAPED PROTECTIVE COVER, ABOVE KNEE	38	A			C			N
L5706	CUSTOM SHAPED PROTECTIVE COVER, KNEE DISARTICULATION	38	A			C			N
L5707	CUSTOM SHAPED PROTECTIVE COVER, HIP DISARTICULATION	38	A			C			N
L5710	ADDITION, EXOSKELETAL KNEE-SHIN SYSTEM, SINGLE AXIS, MANUAL LOCK	38	A			C			N
L5711	ADDITIONS EXOSKELETAL KNEE-SHIN SYSTEM, SINGLE AXIS, MANUAL LOCK, ULTRA-LIGHT MATERIAL	38	A			C			N
L5712	ADDITION, EXOSKELETAL KNEE-SHIN SYSTEM, SINGLE AXIS, FRICTION SWING AND STANCE PHASE CONTROL (SAFETY KNEE)	38	A			C			N
L5714	ADDITION, EXOSKELETAL KNEE-SHIN SYSTEM, SINGLE AXIS, VARIABLE FRICTION SWING PHASE CONTROL	38	A			C			N
L5716	ADDITION, EXOSKELETAL KNEE-SHIN SYSTEM, POLYCENTRIC, MECHANICAL STANCE PHASE LOCK	38	A			C			N
L5718	ADDITION, EXOSKELETAL KNEE-SHIN SYSTEM, POLYCENTRIC, FRICTION SWING AND STANCE PHASE CONTROL	38	A			C			N
L5722	ADDITION, EXOSKELETAL KNEE-SHIN SYSTEM, SINGLE AXIS, PNEUMATIC SWING, FRICTION STANCE PHASE CONTROL	38	A			C			N
L5724	ADDITION, EXOSKELETAL KNEE-SHIN SYSTEM, SINGLE AXIS, FLUID SWING PHASE CONTROL	38	A			C			N
L5726	ADDITION, EXOSKELETAL KNEE-SHIN SYSTEM, SINGLE AXIS, EXTERNAL JOINTS FLUID SWING PHASE CONTROL	38	A			C			N
L5728	ADDITION, EXOSKELETAL KNEE-SHIN SYSTEM, SINGLE AXIS, FLUID SWING AND STANCE PHASE CONTROL	38	A			C			N
L5780	ADDITION, EXOSKELETAL KNEE-SHIN SYSTEM, SINGLE AXIS, PNEUMATIC/HYDRA PNEUMATIC SWING PHASE CONTROL	38	A			C			N
L5781	ADDITION TO LOWER LIMB PROSTHESIS, VACUUM PUMP, RESIDUAL LIMB VOLUME MANAGEMENT AND MOISTURE EVACUATION SYSTEM	38	A			C			N
L5782	ADDITION TO LOWER LIMB PROSTHESIS, VACUUM PUMP, RESIDUAL LIMB VOLUME MANAGEMENT AND MOISTURE EVACUATION SYSTEM, HEAVY DUTY	38	A			C			N
L5785	ADDITION, EXOSKELETAL SYSTEM, BELOW KNEE, ULTRA-LIGHT MATERIAL (TITANIUM, CARBON FIBER OR EQUAL)	38	A			C			N
L5790	ADDITION, EXOSKELETAL SYSTEM, ABOVE KNEE, ULTRA-LIGHT MATERIAL (TITANIUM, CARBON FIBER OR EQUAL)	38	A			C			N
L5795	ADDITION, EXOSKELETAL SYSTEM, HIP DISARTICULATION, ULTRA-LIGHT MATERIAL (TITANIUM, CARBON FIBER OR EQUAL)	38	A			C			N
L5810	ADDITION, ENDOSKELETAL KNEE-SHIN SYSTEM, SINGLE AXIS, MANUAL LOCK	38	A			C			N
L5811	ADDITION, ENDOSKELETAL KNEE-SHIN SYSTEM, SINGLE AXIS, MANUAL LOCK, ULTRA-LIGHT MATERIAL	38	A			C			N

HCPCS	Long Description	PII	MPI	Statute	X-Ref	Coverage	ASC Pay Grp	ASC Pay Grp Eff Date	Action Code
L5812	ADDITION, ENDOSKELETAL KNEE-SHIN SYSTEM, SINGLE AXIS, FRICTION SWING AND STANCE PHASE CONTROL (SAFETY KNEE)	38	A			C			N
L5814	ADDITION, ENDOSKELETAL KNEE-SHIN SYSTEM, POLYCENTRIC, HYDRAULIC SWING PHASE CONTROL, MECHANICAL STANCE PHASE LOCK	38	A			C			N
L5816	ADDITION, ENDOSKELETAL KNEE-SHIN SYSTEM, POLYCENTRIC, MECHANICAL STANCE PHASE LOCK	38	A			C			N
L5818	ADDITION, ENDOSKELETAL KNEE-SHIN SYSTEM, POLYCENTRIC, FRICTION SWING, AND STANCE PHASE CONTROL	38	A			C			N
L5822	ADDITION, ENDOSKELETAL KNEE-SHIN SYSTEM, SINGLE AXIS, PNEUMATIC SWING, FRICTION STANCE PHASE CONTROL	38	A			C			N
L5824	ADDITION, ENDOSKELETAL KNEE-SHIN SYSTEM, SINGLE AXIS, FLUID SWING PHASE CONTROL	38	A			C			N
L5826	ADDITION, ENDOSKELETAL KNEE-SHIN SYSTEM, SINGLE AXIS, HYDRAULIC SWING PHASE CONTROL, WITH MINIATURE HIGH ACTIVITY FRAME	38	A			C			N
L5828	ADDITION, ENDOSKELETAL KNEE-SHIN SYSTEM, SINGLE AXIS, FLUID SWING AND STANCE PHASE CONTROL	38	A			C			N
L5830	ADDITION, ENDOSKELETAL KNEE-SHIN SYSTEM, SINGLE AXIS, PNEUMATIC/ SWING PHASE CONTROL	38	A			C			N
L5840	ADDITION, ENDOSKELETAL KNEE/SHIN SYSTEM, 4-BAR LINKAGE OR MULTIAXIAL, PNEUMATIC SWING PHASE CONTROL	38	A			C			N
L5845	ADDITION, ENDOSKELETAL, KNEE-SHIN SYSTEM, STANCE FLEXION FEATURE, ADJUSTABLE	38	A			C			N
L5846	ADDITION, ENDOSKELETAL, KNEE-SHIN SYSTEM, MICROPROCESSOR CONTROL FEATURE, SWING PHASE ONLY	38	A			C			N
L5847	ADDITION, ENDOSKELETAL KNEE-SHIN SYSTEM, MICROPROCESSOR CONTROL FEATURE, STANCE PHASE	38	A			C			N
L5848	ADDITION TO ENDOSKELETAL, KNEE-SHIN SYSTEM, HYDRAULIC STANCE EXTENSION, DAMPENING FEATURE, WITH OR WITHOUT ADJUSTABILITY	38	A			C			C
L5850	ADDITION, ENDOSKELETAL SYSTEM, ABOVE KNEE OR HIP DISARTICULATION, KNEE EXTENSION ASSIST	38	A			C			N
L5855	ADDITION, ENDOSKELETAL SYSTEM, HIP DISARTICULATION, MECHANICAL HIP EXTENSION ASSIST	38	A			C			N
L5910	ADDITION, ENDOSKELETAL SYSTEM, BELOW KNEE, ALIGNABLE SYSTEM	38	A			C			N
L5920	ADDITION, ENDOSKELETAL SYSTEM, ABOVE KNEE OR HIP DISARTICULATION, ALIGNABLE SYSTEM	38	A			C			N
L5925	ADDITION, ENDOSKELETAL SYSTEM, ABOVE KNEE, KNEE DISARTICULATION OR HIP DISARTICULATION, MANUAL LOCK	38	A			C			N
L5930	ADDITION, ENDOSKELETAL SYSTEM, HIGH ACTIVITY KNEE CONTROL FRAME	38	A			C			N
L5940	ADDITION, ENDOSKELETAL SYSTEM, BELOW KNEE, ULTRA-LIGHT MATERIAL (TITANIUM, CARBON FIBER OR EQUAL)	38	A			C			N
L5950	ADDITION, ENDOSKELETAL SYSTEM, ABOVE KNEE, ULTRA-LIGHT MATERIAL (TITANIUM, CARBON FIBER OR EQUAL)	38	A			C			N
L5960	ADDITION, ENDOSKELETAL SYSTEM, HIP DISARTICULATION, ULTRA-LIGHT MATERIAL (TITANIUM, CARBON FIBER OR EQUAL)	38	A			C			N
L5962	ADDITION, ENDOSKELETAL SYSTEM, BELOW KNEE, FLEXIBLE PROTECTIVE OUTER SURFACE COVERING SYSTEM	38	A			C			N
L5964	ADDITION, ENDOSKELETAL SYSTEM, ABOVE KNEE, FLEXIBLE PROTECTIVE OUTER SURFACE COVERING SYSTEM	38	A			C			N

HCPCS	Long Description	PTI	MPI	Statute	X-Ref1	Coverage	ASC Pay Grp	ASC Pay Grp Eff Date	Action Code
L5966	ADDITION, ENDOSKELETAL SYSTEM, HIP DISARTICULATION, FLEXIBLE PROTECTIVE OUTER SURFACE COVERING SYSTEM	38	A			C			N
L5968	ADDITION TO LOWER LIMB PROSTHESIS, MULTIAXIAL ANKLE WITH SWING PHASE ACTIVE DORSIFLEXION FEATURE	38	A			C			N
L5970	ALL LOWER EXTREMITY PROSTHESES, FOOT, EXTERNAL KEEL, SACH FOOT	38	A			C			N
L5972	ALL LOWER EXTREMITY PROSTHESES, FLEXIBLE KEEL FOOT (SAFE, STEN, BOCK DYNAMIC OR EQUAL)	38	A			C			N
L5974	ALL LOWER EXTREMITY PROSTHESES, FOOT, SINGLE AXIS ANKLE/FOOT	38	A			C			N
L5975	ALL LOWER EXTREMITY PROSTHESIS, COMBINATION SINGLE AXIS ANKLE AND FLEXIBLE KEEL FOOT	38	A			C			N
L5976	ALL LOWER EXTREMITY PROSTHESES, ENERGY STORING FOOT (SEATTLE CARBON COPY II OR EQUAL)	38	A			C			N
L5978	ALL LOWER EXTREMITY PROSTHESES, FOOT, MULTIAXIAL ANKLE/FOOT	38	A			C			N
L5979	ALL LOWER EXTREMITY PROSTHESIS, MULTI-AXIAL ANKLE, DYNAMIC RESPONSE FOOT, ONE PIECE SYSTEM	38	A			C			N
L5980	ALL LOWER EXTREMITY PROSTHESES, FLEX FOOT SYSTEM	38	A			C			N
L5981	ALL LOWER EXTREMITY PROSTHESES, FLEX-WALK SYSTEM OR EQUAL	38	A			C			N
L5982	ALL EXOSKELETAL LOWER EXTREMITY PROSTHESES, AXIAL ROTATION UNIT	38	A			C			N
L5984	ALL ENDOSKELETAL LOWER EXTREMITY PROSTHESIS, AXIAL ROTATION UNIT, WITH OR WITHOUT ADJUSTABILITY	38	A			C			C
L5985	ALL ENDOSKELETAL LOWER EXTREMITY PROTHESES, DYNAMIC PROSTHETIC PYLON	38	A			C			N
L5986	ALL LOWER EXTREMITY PROSTHESES, MULTI-AXIAL ROTATION UNIT (MCP OR EQUAL)	38	A			C			N
L5987	ALL LOWER EXTREMITY PROSTHESIS, SHANK FOOT SYSTEM WITH VERTICAL LOADING PYLON	38	A			C			N
L5988	ADDITION TO LOWER LIMB PROSTHESIS, VERTICAL SHOCK REDUCING PYLON FEATURE	38	A			C			N
L5989	ADDITION TO LOWER EXTREMITY PROSTHESIS, ENDOSKELETAL SYSTEM, PYLON WITH INTEGRATED ELECTRONIC FORCE SENSORS	38	A			C			N
L5990	ADDITION TO LOWER EXTREMITY PROSTHESIS, USER ADJUSTABLE HEEL HEIGHT	38	A			C			N
L5995	ADDITION TO LOWER EXTREMITY PROSTHESIS, HEAVY DUTY FEATURE (FOR PATIENT WEIGHT > 300 LBS)	38	A			C			N
L5999	LOWER EXTREMITY PROSTHESIS, NOT OTHERWISE SPECIFIED	46	A			C			N
L6000	PARTIAL HAND, ROBIN-AIDS, THUMB REMAINING (OR EQUAL)	38	A			C			N
L6010	PARTIAL HAND, ROBIN-AIDS, LITTLE AND/OR RING FINGER REMAINING (OR EQUAL)	38	A			C			N
L6020	PARTIAL HAND, ROBIN-AIDS, NO FINGER REMAINING (OR EQUAL)	38	A			C			N
L6025	TRANSCARPAL/METACARPAL OR PARTIAL HAND DISARTICULATION PROSTHESIS, EXTERNAL POWER, SELF-SUSPENDED, INNER SOCKET WITH REMOVABLE FOREARM SECTION, ELECTRODES AND CABLES, TWO BATTERIES, CHARGER, MYOELECTRIC CONTROL OF TERMINAL DEVICE	38	A			C			N

HCPCS	Long Description	PII	MPI	Statute	X-Refl	Coverage	ASC Pay Grp	ASC Pay Grp Eff Date	Action Code
L6050	WRIST DISARTICULATION, MOLDED SOCKET, FLEXIBLE ELBOW HINGES, TRICEPS PAD	38	A			C			N
L6055	WRIST DISARTICULATION, MOLDED SOCKET WITH EXPANDABLE INTERFACE, FLEXIBLE ELBOW HINGES, TRICEPS PAD	38	A			C			N
L6100	BELOW ELBOW, MOLDED SOCKET, FLEXIBLE ELBOW HINGE, TRICEPS PAD	38	A			C			N
L6110	BELOW ELBOW, MOLDED SOCKET, (MUENSTER OR NORTHWESTERN SUSPENSION TYPES)	38	A			C			N
L6120	BELOW ELBOW, MOLDED DOUBLE WALL SPLIT SOCKET, STEP-UP HINGES, HALF CUFF	38	A			C			N
L6130	BELOW ELBOW, MOLDED DOUBLE WALL SPLIT SOCKET, STUMP ACTIVATED LOCKING HINGE, HALF CUFF	38	A			C			N
L6200	ELBOW DISARTICULATION, MOLDED SOCKET, OUTSIDE LOCKING HINGE, FOREARM	38	A			C			N
L6205	ELBOW DISARTICULATION, MOLDED SOCKET WITH EXPANDABLE INTERFACE, OUTSIDE LOCKING HINGES, FOREARM	38	A			C			N
L6250	ABOVE ELBOW, MOLDED DOUBLE WALL SOCKET, INTERNAL LOCKING ELBOW, FOREARM	38	A			C			N
L6300	SHOULDER DISARTICULATION, MOLDED SOCKET, SHOULDER BULKHEAD, HUMERAL SECTION, INTERNAL LOCKING ELBOW, FOREARM	38	A			C			N
L6310	SHOULDER DISARTICULATION, PASSIVE RESTORATION (COMPLETE PROSTHESIS)	38	A			C			N
L6320	SHOULDER DISARTICULATION, PASSIVE RESTORATION (SHOULDER CAP ONLY)	38	A			C			N
L6350	INTERSCAPULAR THORACIC, MOLDED SOCKET, SHOULDER BULKHEAD, HUMERAL SECTION, INTERNAL LOCKING ELBOW, FOREARM	38	A			C			N
L6360	INTERSCAPULAR THORACIC, PASSIVE RESTORATION (COMPLETE PROSTHESIS)	38	A			C			N
L6370	INTERSCAPULAR THORACIC, PASSIVE RESTORATION (SHOULDER CAP ONLY)	38	A			C			N
L6380	IMMEDIATE POST SURGICAL OR EARLY FITTING, APPLICATION OF INITIAL RIGID DRESSING, INCLUDING FITTING ALIGNMENT AND SUSPENSION OF COMPONENTS, AND ONE CAST CHANGE, WRIST DISARTICULATION OR BELOW ELBOW	38	A			C			N
L6382	IMMEDIATE POST SURGICAL OR EARLY FITTING, APPLICATION OF INITIAL RIGID DRESSING INCLUDING FITTING ALIGNMENT AND SUSPENSION OF COMPONENTS, AND ONE CAST CHANGE, ELBOW DISARTICULATION OR ABOVE ELBOW	38	A			C			N
L6384	IMMEDIATE POST SURGICAL OR EARLY FITTING, APPLICATION OF INITIAL RIGID DRESSING INCLUDING FITTING ALIGNMENT AND SUSPENSION OF COMPONENTS, AND ONE CAST CHANGE, SHOULDER DISARTICULATION OR INTERSCAPULAR THORACIC	38	A			C			N
L6386	IMMEDIATE POST SURGICAL OR EARLY FITTING, EACH ADDITIONAL CAST CHANGE AND REALIGNMENT	38	A			C			N
L6388	IMMEDIATE POST SURGICAL OR EARLY FITTING, APPLICATION OF RIGID DRESSING ONLY	38	A			C			N
L6400	BELOW ELBOW, MOLDED SOCKET, ENDOSKELETAL SYSTEM, INCLUDING SOFT PROSTHETIC TISSUE SHAPING	38	A			C			N
L6450	ELBOW DISARTICULATION, MOLDED SOCKET, ENDOSKELETAL SYSTEM, INCLUDING SOFT PROSTHETIC TISSUE SHAPING	38	A			C			N
L6500	ABOVE ELBOW, MOLDED SOCKET, ENDOSKELETAL SYSTEM, INCLUDING SOFT PROSTHETIC TISSUE SHAPING	38	A			C			N

HCPCS	Long Description	PTI	MPI	Statute	X-Ref1	Coverage	ASC Pay Grp	ASC Pay Grp Eff Date	Action Code
L6550	SHOULDER DISARTICULATION, MOLDED SOCKET, ENDOSKELETAL SYSTEM, INCLUDING SOFT PROSTHETIC TISSUE SHAPING	38	A			C			N
L6570	INTERSCAPULAR THORACIC, MOLDED SOCKET, ENDOSKELETAL SYSTEM, INCLUDING SOFT PROSTHETIC TISSUE SHAPING	38	A			C			N
L6580	PREPARATORY, WRIST DISARTICULATION OR BELOW ELBOW, SINGLE WALL PLASTIC SOCKET, FRICTION WRIST, FLEXIBLE ELBOW HINGES, FIGURE OF EIGHT HARNESS, HUMERAL CUFF, BOWDEN CABLE CONTROL, USMC OR EQUAL PYLON, NO COVER, MOLDED TO PATIENT MODEL	38	A			C			N
L6582	PREPARATORY, WRIST DISARTICULATION OR BELOW ELBOW, SINGLE WALL SOCKET, FRICTION WRIST, FLEXIBLE ELBOW HINGES, FIGURE OF EIGHT HARNESS, HUMERAL CUFF, BOWDEN CABLE CONTROL, USMC OR EQUAL PYLON, NO COVER, DIRECT FORMED	38	A			C			N
L6584	PREPARATORY, ELBOW DISARTICULATION OR ABOVE ELBOW, SINGLE WALL PLASTIC SOCKET, FRICTION WRIST, LOCKING ELBOW, FIGURE OF EIGHT HARNESS, FAIR LEAD CABLE CONTROL, USMC OR EQUAL PYLON, NO COVER, MOLDED TO PATIENT MODEL	38	A			C			N
L6586	PREPARATORY, ELBOW DISARTICULATION OR ABOVE ELBOW, SINGLE WALL SOCKET, FRICTION WRIST, LOCKING ELBOW, FIGURE OF EIGHT HARNESS, FAIR LEAD CABLE CONTROL, USMC OR EQUAL PYLON, NO COVER, DIRECT FORMED	38	A			C			N
L6588	PREPARATORY, SHOULDER DISARTICULATION OR INTERSCAPULAR THORACIC, SINGLE WALL PLASTIC SOCKET, SHOULDER JOINT, LOCKING ELBOW, FRICTION WRIST, CHEST STRAP, FAIR LEAD CABLE CONTROL, USMC OR EQUAL PYLON, NO COVER, MOLDED TO PATIENT MODEL	38	A			C			N
L6590	PREPARATORY, SHOULDER DISARTICULATION OR INTERSCAPULAR THORACIC, SINGLE WALL SOCKET, SHOULDER JOINT, LOCKING ELBOW, FRICTION WRIST, CHEST STRAP, FAIR LEAD CABLE CONTROL, USMC OR EQUAL PYLON, NO COVER, DIRECT FORMED	38	A			C			N
L6600	UPPER EXTREMITY ADDITIONS, POLYCENTRIC HINGE, PAIR	38	A			C			N
L6605	UPPER EXTREMITY ADDITIONS, SINGLE PIVOT HINGE, PAIR	38	A			C			N
L6610	UPPER EXTREMITY ADDITIONS, FLEXIBLE METAL HINGE, PAIR	38	A			C			N
L6615	UPPER EXTREMITY ADDITION, DISCONNECT LOCKING WRIST UNIT	38	A			C			N
L6616	UPPER EXTREMITY ADDITION, ADDITIONAL DISCONNECT INSERT FOR LOCKING WRIST UNIT, EACH	38	A			C			N
L6620	UPPER EXTREMITY ADDITION, FLEXION/EXTENSION WRIST UNIT, WITH OR WITHOUT FRICTION	38	A			C			C
L6623	UPPER EXTREMITY ADDITION, SPRING ASSISTED ROTATIONAL WRIST UNIT WITH LATCH RELEASE	38	A			C			N
L6625	UPPER EXTREMITY ADDITION, ROTATION WRIST UNIT WITH CABLE LOCK	38	A			C			N
L6628	UPPER EXTREMITY ADDITION, QUICK DISCONNECT HOOK ADAPTER, OTTO BOCK OR EQUAL	38	A			C			N
L6629	UPPER EXTREMITY ADDITION, QUICK DISCONNECT LAMINATION COLLAR WITH COUPLING PIECE, OTTO BOCK OR EQUAL	38	A			C			N
L6630	UPPER EXTREMITY ADDITION, STAINLESS STEEL, ANY WRIST	38	A			C			N
L6632	UPPER EXTREMITY ADDITION, LATEX SUSPENSION SLEEVE, EACH	38	A			C			N
L6635	UPPER EXTREMITY ADDITION, LIFT ASSIST FOR ELBOW	38	A			C			N
L6637	UPPER EXTREMITY ADDITION, NUDGE CONTROL ELBOW LOCK	38	A			C			N
L6638	UPPER EXTREMITY ADDITION TO PROSTHESIS, ELECTRIC LOCKING FEATURE, ONLY FOR USE WITH MANUALLY POWERED ELBOW	38	A			C			N

HCPCS	Long Description	PII	MPI	Statute	X-Ref	Coverage	ASC Pay Grp	ASC Pay Grp Eff Date	Action Code
L6640	UPPER EXTREMITY ADDITIONS, SHOULDER ABDUCTION JOINT, PAIR	38	A			C			N
L6641	UPPER EXTREMITY ADDITION, EXCURSION AMPLIFIER, PULLEY TYPE	38	A			C			N
L6642	UPPER EXTREMITY ADDITION, EXCURSION AMPLIFIER, LEVER TYPE	38	A			C			N
L6645	UPPER EXTREMITY ADDITION, SHOULDER FLEXION-ABDUCTION JOINT, EACH	38	A			C			N
L6646	UPPER EXTREMITY ADDITION, SHOULDER JOINT, MULTIPOSITIONAL LOCKING, FLEXION, ADJUSTABLE ABDUCTION FRICTION CONTROL, FOR USE WITH BODY POWERED OR EXTERNAL POWERED SYSTEM	38	A			C			N
L6647	UPPER EXTREMITY ADDITION, SHOULDER LOCK MECHANISM, BODY POWERED ACTUATOR	38	A			C			N
L6648	UPPER EXTREMITY ADDITION, SHOULDER LOCK MECHANISM, EXTERNAL POWERED ACTUATOR	38	A			C			N
L6650	UPPER EXTREMITY ADDITION, SHOULDER UNIVERSAL JOINT, EACH	38	A			C			N
L6655	UPPER EXTREMITY ADDITION, STANDARD CONTROL CABLE, EXTRA	38	A			C			N
L6660	UPPER EXTREMITY ADDITION, HEAVY DUTY CONTROL CABLE	38	A			C			N
L6665	UPPER EXTREMITY ADDITION, TEFLON, OR EQUAL, CABLE LINING	38	A			C			N
L6670	UPPER EXTREMITY ADDITION, HOOK TO HAND, CABLE ADAPTER	38	A			C			N
L6672	UPPER EXTREMITY ADDITION, HARNESS, CHEST OR SHOULDER, SADDLE TYPE	38	A			C			N
L6675	UPPER EXTREMITY ADDITION, HARNESS, (E.G. FIGURE OF EIGHT TYPE), SINGLE CABLE DESIGN	38	A			C			C
L6676	UPPER EXTREMITY ADDITION, HARNESS, (E.G. FIGURE OF EIGHT TYPE), DUAL CABLE DESIGN	38	A			C			C
L6680	UPPER EXTREMITY ADDITION, TEST SOCKET, WRIST DISARTICULATION OR BELOW ELBOW	38	A			C			N
L6682	UPPER EXTREMITY ADDITION, TEST SOCKET, ELBOW DISARTICULATION OR ABOVE ELBOW	38	A			C			N
L6684	UPPER EXTREMITY ADDITION, TEST SOCKET, SHOULDER DISARTICULATION OR INTERSCAPULAR THORACIC	38	A			C			N
L6686	UPPER EXTREMITY ADDITION, SUCTION SOCKET	38	A			C			N
L6687	UPPER EXTREMITY ADDITION, FRAME TYPE SOCKET, BELOW ELBOW OR WRIST DISARTICULATION	38	A			C			N
L6688	UPPER EXTREMITY ADDITION, FRAME TYPE SOCKET, ABOVE ELBOW OR ELBOW DISARTICULATION	38	A			C			N
L6689	UPPER EXTREMITY ADDITION, FRAME TYPE SOCKET, SHOULDER DISARTICULATION	38	A			C			N
L6690	UPPER EXTREMITY ADDITION, FRAME TYPE SOCKET, INTERSCAPULAR-THORACIC	38	A			C			N
L6691	UPPER EXTREMITY ADDITION, REMOVABLE INSERT, EACH	38	A			C			N
L6692	UPPER EXTREMITY ADDITION, SILICONE GEL INSERT OR EQUAL, EACH	38	A			C			N

HCPCS	Long Description	PI1	MPI	Statute	X-Refl	Coverage	ASC Pay Grp	ASC Pay Grp Eff Date	Action Code
L6693	UPPER EXTREMITY ADDITION, LOCKING ELBOW, FOREARM COUNTERBALANCE	38	A			C			N
L6700	TERMINAL DEVICE, HOOK, DORRANCE, OR EQUAL, MODEL #3	38	A			D			N
L6705	TERMINAL DEVICE, HOOK, DORRANCE, OR EQUAL, MODEL #5	38	A			D			N
L6710	TERMINAL DEVICE, HOOK, DORRANCE, OR EQUAL, MODEL #5X	38	A			D			N
L6715	TERMINAL DEVICE, HOOK, DORRANCE, OR EQUAL, MODEL #5XA	38	A			D			N
L6720	TERMINAL DEVICE, HOOK, DORRANCE, OR EQUAL, MODEL #6	38	A			D			N
L6725	TERMINAL DEVICE, HOOK, DORRANCE, OR EQUAL, MODEL #7	38	A			D			N
L6730	TERMINAL DEVICE, HOOK, DORRANCE, OR EQUAL, MODEL #7LO	38	A			D			N
L6735	TERMINAL DEVICE, HOOK, DORRANCE, OR EQUAL, MODEL #8	38	A			D			N
L6740	TERMINAL DEVICE, HOOK, DORRANCE, OR EQUAL, MODEL #8X	38	A			D			N
L6745	TERMINAL DEVICE, HOOK, DORRANCE, OR EQUAL, MODEL #88X	38	A			D			N
L6750	TERMINAL DEVICE, HOOK, DORRANCE, OR EQUAL, MODEL #10P	38	A			D			N
L6755	TERMINAL DEVICE, HOOK, DORRANCE, OR EQUAL, MODEL #10X	38	A			D			N
L6765	TERMINAL DEVICE, HOOK, DORRANCE, OR EQUAL, MODEL #12P	38	A			D			N
L6770	TERMINAL DEVICE, HOOK, DORRANCE, OR EQUAL, MODEL #99X	38	A			D			N
L6775	TERMINAL DEVICE, HOOK, DORRANCE, OR EQUAL, MODEL #555	38	A			D			N
L6780	TERMINAL DEVICE, HOOK, DORRANCE, OR EQUAL, MODEL #SS555	38	A			D			N
L6790	TERMINAL DEVICE, HOOK-ACCU HOOK, OR EQUAL	38	A			D			N
L6795	TERMINAL DEVICE, HOOK-2 LOAD, OR EQUAL	38	A			D			N
L6800	TERMINAL DEVICE, HOOK-APRL VC, OR EQUAL	38	A			D			N
L6805	TERMINAL DEVICE, MODIFIER WRIST FLEXION UNIT	38	A			D			N
L6806	TERMINAL DEVICE, HOOK, TRS GRIP, GRIP III, VC, OR EQUAL	38	A			D			N
L6807	TERMINAL DEVICE, HOOK, GRIP I, GRIP II, VC, OR EQUAL	38	A			D			N
L6808	TERMINAL DEVICE, HOOK, TRS ADEPT, INFANT OR CHILD, VC, OR EQUAL	38	A			D			N
L6809	TERMINAL DEVICE, HOOK, TRS SUPER SPORT, PASSIVE	38	A			D			N
L6810	TERMINAL DEVICE, PINCHER TOOL, OTTO BOCK OR EQUAL	38	A			D			N

HCPCS	Long Description	PII	MPI	Statute	X-Ref1	Coverage	ASC Pay Grp	ASC Pay Grp Eff Date	Action Code
L6825	TERMINAL DEVICE, HAND, DORRANCE, VO	38	A			D			N
L6830	TERMINAL DEVICE, HAND, APRL, VC	38	A			D			N
L6835	TERMINAL DEVICE, HAND, SIERRA, VO	38	A			D			N
L6840	TERMINAL DEVICE, HAND, BECKER IMPERIAL	38	A			D			N
L6845	TERMINAL DEVICE, HAND, BECKER LOCK GRIP	38	A			D			N
L6850	TERMINAL DEVICE, HAND, BECKER PLYLITE	38	A			D			N
L6855	TERMINAL DEVICE, HAND, ROBIN-AIDS, VO	38	A			D			N
L6860	TERMINAL DEVICE, HAND, ROBIN-AIDS, VO SOFT	38	A			D			N
L6865	TERMINAL DEVICE, HAND, PASSIVE HAND	38	A			D			N
L6867	TERMINAL DEVICE, HAND, DETROIT INFANT HAND (MECHANICAL)	38	A			D			N
L6868	TERMINAL DEVICE, HAND, PASSIVE INFANT HAND, (STEEPER, HOSMER OR EQUAL)	38	A			D			N
L6870	TERMINAL DEVICE, HAND, CHILD MITT	38	A			D			N
L6872	TERMINAL DEVICE, HAND, NYU CHILD HAND	38	A			D			N
L6873	TERMINAL DEVICE, HAND, MECHANICAL INFANT HAND, STEEPER OR EQUAL	38	A			D			N
L6875	TERMINAL DEVICE, HAND, BOCK, VC	38	A			D			N
L6880	TERMINAL DEVICE, HAND, BOCK, VO	38	A			D			N
L6881	AUTOMATIC GRASP FEATURE, ADDITION TO UPPER LIMB PROSTHETIC TERMINAL DEVICE	38	A			C			N
L6882	MICROPROCESSOR CONTROL FEATURE, ADDITION TO UPPER LIMB PROSTHETIC TERMINAL DEVICE	38	A			D			N
L6890	TERMINAL DEVICE, GLOVE FOR ABOVE HANDS, PRODUCTION GLOVE	38	A			C			N
L6895	TERMINAL DEVICE, GLOVE FOR ABOVE HANDS, CUSTOM GLOVE	38	A			C			N
L6900	HAND RESTORATION (CASTS, SHADING AND MEASUREMENTS INCLUDED), PARTIAL HAND, WITH GLOVE, THUMB OR ONE FINGER REMAINING	38	A			C			N
L6905	HAND RESTORATION (CASTS, SHADING AND MEASUREMENTS INCLUDED), PARTIAL HAND, WITH GLOVE, MULTIPLE FINGERS REMAINING	38	A			C			N
L6910	HAND RESTORATION (CASTS, SHADING AND MEASUREMENTS INCLUDED), PARTIAL HAND, WITH GLOVE, NO FINGERS REMAINING	38	A			C			N
L6915	HAND RESTORATION (SHADING, AND MEASUREMENTS INCLUDED), REPLACEMENT GLOVE FOR ABOVE	38	A			C			N
L6920	WRIST DISARTICULATION, EXTERNAL POWER, SELF-SUSPENDED INNER SOCKET, REMOVABLE FOREARM SHELL, OTTO BOCK OR EQUAL, SWITCH, CABLES, TWO BATTERIES AND ONE CHARGER, SWITCH CONTROL OF TERMINAL DEVICE	38	A			C			N
L6925	WRIST DISARTICULATION, EXTERNAL POWER, SELF-SUSPENDED INNER SOCKET, REMOVABLE FOREARM SHELL, OTTO BOCK OR EQUAL ELECTRODES, CABLES, TWO BATTERIES AND ONE CHARGER, MYOELECTRONIC CONTROL OF TERMINAL DEVICE	38	A			C			N
L6930	BELOW ELBOW, EXTERNAL POWER, SELF-SUSPENDED INNER SOCKET, REMOVABLE FOREARM SHELL, OTTO BOCK OR EQUAL SWITCH, CABLES, TWO BATTERIES AND ONE CHARGER, SWITCH CONTROL OF TERMINAL DEVICE	38	A			C			N

HCPCS	Long Description	PTI	MPI	Statute	X-Ref	Coverage	ASC Pay Grp	ASC Pay Grp Eff Date	Action Code
L6935	BELOW ELBOW, EXTERNAL POWER, SELF-SUSPENDED INNER SOCKET, REMOVABLE FOREARM SHELL, OTTO BOCK OR EQUAL ELECTRODES, CABLES, TWO BATTERIES AND ONE CHARGER, MYOELECTRONIC CONTROL OF TERMINAL DEVICE	38	A			C			N
L6940	ELBOW DISARTICULATION, EXTERNAL POWER, MOLDED INNER SOCKET, REMOVABLE HUMERAL SHELL, OUTSIDE LOCKING HINGES, FOREARM, OTTO BOCK OR EQUAL SWITCH, CABLES, TWO BATTERIES AND ONE CHARGER, SWITCH CONTROL OF TERMINAL DEVICE	38	A			C			N
L6945	ELBOW DISARTICULATION, EXTERNAL POWER, MOLDED INNER SOCKET, REMOVABLE HUMERAL SHELL, OUTSIDE LOCKING HINGES, FOREARM, OTTO BOCK OR EQUAL ELECTRODES, CABLES, TWO BATTERIES AND ONE CHARGER, MYOELECTRONIC CONTROL OF TERMINAL DEVICE	38	A			C			N
L6950	ABOVE ELBOW, EXTERNAL POWER, MOLDED INNER SOCKET, REMOVABLE HUMERAL SHELL, INTERNAL LOCKING ELBOW, FOREARM, OTTO BOCK OR EQUAL SWITCH, CABLES, TWO BATTERIES AND ONE CHARGER, SWITCH CONTROL OF TERMINAL DEVICE	38	A			C			N
L6955	ABOVE ELBOW, EXTERNAL POWER, MOLDED INNER SOCKET, REMOVABLE HUMERAL SHELL, INTERNAL LOCKING ELBOW, FOREARM, OTTO BOCK OR EQUAL ELECTRODES, CABLES, TWO BATTERIES AND ONE CHARGER, MYOELECTRONIC CONTROL OF TERMINAL DEVICE	38	A			C			N
L6960	SHOULDER DISARTICULATION, EXTERNAL POWER, MOLDED INNER SOCKET, REMOVABLE SHOULDER SHELL, SHOULDER BULKHEAD, HUMERAL SECTION, MECHANICAL ELBOW, FOREARM, OTTO BOCK OR EQUAL SWITCH, CABLES, TWO BATTERIES AND ONE CHARGER, SWITCH CONTROL OF TERMINAL DEVICE	38	A			C			N
L6965	SHOULDER DISARTICULATION, EXTERNAL POWER, MOLDED INNER SOCKET, REMOVABLE SHOULDER SHELL, SHOULDER BULKHEAD, HUMERAL SECTION, MECHANICAL ELBOW, FOREARM, OTTO BOCK OR EQUAL ELECTRODES, CABLES, TWO BATTERIES AND ONE CHARGER, MYOELECTRONIC CONTROL OF TERMINAL DEVICE	38	A			C			N
L6970	INTERSCAPULAR-THORACIC, EXTERNAL POWER, MOLDED INNER SOCKET, REMOVABLE SHOULDER SHELL, SHOULDER BULKHEAD, HUMERAL SECTION, MECHANICAL ELBOW, FOREARM, OTTO BOCK OR EQUAL SWITCH, CABLES, TWO BATTERIES AND ONE CHARGER, SWITCH CONTROL OF TERMINAL DEVICE	38	A			C			N
L6975	INTERSCAPULAR-THORACIC, EXTERNAL POWER, MOLDED INNER SOCKET, REMOVABLE SHOULDER SHELL, SHOULDER BULKHEAD, HUMERAL SECTION, MECHANICAL ELBOW, FOREARM, OTTO BOCK OR EQUAL ELECTRODES, CABLES, TWO BATTERIES AND ONE CHARGER, MYOELECTRONIC CONTROL OF TERMINAL DEVICE	38	A			C			N
L7010	ELECTRONIC HAND, OTTO BOCK, STEEPER OR EQUAL, SWITCH CONTROLLED	38	A			C			N
L7015	ELECTRONIC HAND, SYSTEM TEKNIK, VARIETY VILLAGE OR EQUAL, SWITCH CONTROLLED	38	A			C			N
L7020	ELECTRONIC GREIFER, OTTO BOCK OR EQUAL, SWITCH CONTROLLED	38	A			C			N
L7025	ELECTRONIC HAND, OTTO BOCK OR EQUAL, MYOELECTRONICALLY CONTROLLED	38	A			C			N
L7030	ELECTRONIC HAND, SYSTEM TEKNIK, VARIETY VILLAGE OR EQUAL, MYOELECTRONICALLY CONTROLLED	38	A			C			N
L7035	ELECTRONIC GREIFER, OTTO BOCK OR EQUAL, MYOELECTRONICALLY CONTROLLED	38	A			C			N
L7040	PREHENSILE ACTUATOR, HOSMER OR EQUAL, SWITCH CONTROLLED	38	A			C			N
L7045	ELECTRONIC HOOK, CHILD, MICHIGAN OR EQUAL, SWITCH CONTROLLED	38	A			C			N
L7170	ELECTRONIC ELBOW, HOSMER OR EQUAL, SWITCH CONTROLLED	38	A			C			N
L7180	ELECTRONIC ELBOW, BOSTON, UTAH OR EQUAL, MYOELECTRONICALLY CONTROLLED	38	A			C			N

HCPCS	Long Description	PII	MPI	Statute	X-Ref	Coverage	ASC Pay Grp	ASC Pay Grp Eff Date	Action Code
L7185	ELECTRONIC ELBOW, ADOLESCENT, VARIETY VILLAGE OR EQUAL, SWITCH CONTROLLED	38	A			C			N
L7186	ELECTRONIC ELBOW, CHILD, VARIETY VILLAGE OR EQUAL, SWITCH CONTROLLED	38	A			C			N
L7190	ELECTRONIC ELBOW, ADOLESCENT, VARIETY VILLAGE OR EQUAL, MYOELECTRONICALLY CONTROLLED	38	A			C			N
L7191	ELECTRONIC ELBOW, CHILD, VARIETY VILLAGE OR EQUAL, MYOELECTRONICALLY CONTROLLED	38	A			C			N
L7260	ELECTRONIC WRIST ROTATOR, OTTO BOCK OR EQUAL	38	A			C			N
L7261	ELECTRONIC WRIST ROTATOR, FOR UTAH ARM	38	A			C			N
L7266	SERVO CONTROL, STEEPER OR EQUAL	38	A			C			N
L7272	ANALOGUE CONTROL, UNB OR EQUAL	38	A			C			N
L7274	PROPORTIONAL CONTROL, 6-12 VOLT, LIBERTY, UTAH OR EQUAL	38	A			C			N
L7360	SIX VOLT BATTERY, OTTO BOCK OR EQUAL, EACH	38	A			C			N
L7362	BATTERY CHARGER, SIX VOLT, OTTO BOCK OR EQUAL	38	A			C			N
L7364	TWELVE VOLT BATTERY, UTAH OR EQUAL, EACH	38	A			C			N
L7366	BATTERY CHARGER, TWELVE VOLT, UTAH OR EQUAL	38	A			C			N
L7367	LITHIUM ION BATTERY, REPLACEMENT	38	A			C			N
L7368	LITHIUM ION BATTERY CHARGER	38	A			C			N
L7499	UPPER EXTREMITY PROSTHESIS, NOT OTHERWISE SPECIFIED	46	A			C			N
L7500	REPAIR OF PROSTHETIC DEVICE, HOURLY RATE (EXCLUDES V5335 REPAIR OF ORAL OR LARYNGEAL PROSTHESIS OR ARTIFICIAL LARYNX)	46	A			D			N
L7510	REPAIR OF PROSTHETIC DEVICE, REPAIR OR REPLACE MINOR PARTS	46	A			D			N
L7520	REPAIR PROSTHETIC DEVICE, LABOR COMPONENT, PER 15 MINUTES	46	A			C			N
L7900	MALE VACUUM ERECTION SYSTEM	38	A			C			N
L8000	BREAST PROSTHESIS, MASTECTOMY BRA	38	A			D			N
L8001	BREAST PROSTHESIS, MASTECTOMY BRA, WITH INTEGRATED BREAST PROSTHESIS FORM, UNILATERAL	38	A			D			N
L8002	BREAST PROSTHESIS, MASTECTOMY BRA, WITH INTEGRATED BREAST PROSTHESIS FORM, BILATERAL	38	A			D			N
L8010	BREAST PROSTHESIS, MASTECTOMY SLEEVE	38	A			D			N
L8015	EXTERNAL BREAST PROSTHESIS GARMENT, WITH MASTECTOMY FORM, POST MASTECTOMY	38	A			D			N
L8020	BREAST PROSTHESIS, MASTECTOMY FORM	38	A			D			N

HCPCS	Long Description	PH	MPI	Statute	X-Ref	Coverage	ASC Pay Grp	ASC Pay Grp Eff Date	Action Code
L8030	BREAST PROSTHESIS, SILICONE OR EQUAL	38	A			D			N
L8035	CUSTOM BREAST PROSTHESIS, POST MASTECTOMY, MOLDED TO PATIENT MODEL	38	A			D			N
L8039	BREAST PROSTHESIS, NOT OTHERWISE SPECIFIED	46	A			C			N
L8040	NASAL PROSTHESIS, PROVIDED BY A NON-PHYSICIAN	38	A			C			N
L8041	MIDFACIAL PROSTHESIS, PROVIDED BY A NON-PHYSICIAN	38	A			C			N
L8042	ORBITAL PROSTHESIS, PROVIDED BY A NON-PHYSICIAN	38	A			C			N
L8043	UPPER FACIAL PROSTHESIS, PROVIDED BY A NON-PHYSICIAN	38	A			C			N
L8044	HEMI-FACIAL PROSTHESIS, PROVIDED BY A NON-PHYSICIAN	38	A			C			N
L8045	AURICULAR PROSTHESIS, PROVIDED BY A NON-PHYSICIAN	38	A			C			N
L8046	PARTIAL FACIAL PROSTHESIS, PROVIDED BY A NON-PHYSICIAN	38	A			C			N
L8047	NASAL SEPTAL PROSTHESIS, PROVIDED BY A NON-PHYSICIAN	38	A			C			N
L8048	UNSPECIFIED MAXILLOFACIAL PROSTHESIS, BY REPORT, PROVIDED BY A NON-PHYSICIAN	46	A			C			N
L8049	REPAIR OR MODIFICATION OF MAXILLOFACIAL PROSTHESIS, LABOR COMPONENT, 15 MINUTE INCREMENTS, PROVIDED BY A NON-PHYSICIAN	46	A			C			N
L8100	GRADIENT COMPRESSION STOCKING, BELOW KNEE, 18-30 MMHG, EACH	00	9			M			N
L8110	GRADIENT COMPRESSION STOCKING, BELOW KNEE, 30-40 MMHG, EACH	35	A			D			F
L8120	GRADIENT COMPRESSION STOCKING, BELOW KNEE, 40-50 MMHG, EACH	35	A			D			F
L8130	GRADIENT COMPRESSION STOCKING, THIGH LENGTH, 18-30 MMHG, EACH	00	9			M			N
L8140	GRADIENT COMPRESSION STOCKING, THIGH LENGTH, 30-40 MMHG, EACH	00	9			M			N
L8150	GRADIENT COMPRESSION STOCKING, THIGH LENGTH, 40-50 MMHG, EACH	00	9			M			N
L8160	GRADIENT COMPRESSION STOCKING, FULL LENGTH/CHAP STYLE, 18-30 MMHG, EACH	00	9			M			N
L8170	GRADIENT COMPRESSION STOCKING, FULL LENGTH/CHAP STYLE, 30-40 MMHG, EACH	00	9			M			N
L8180	GRADIENT COMPRESSION STOCKING, FULL LENGTH/CHAP STYLE, 40-50 MMHG, EACH	00	9			M			N
L8190	GRADIENT COMPRESSION STOCKING, WAIST LENGTH, 18-30 MMHG, EACH	00	9			M			N
L8195	GRADIENT COMPRESSION STOCKING, WAIST LENGTH, 30-40 MMHG, EACH	00	9			M			N
L8200	GRADIENT COMPRESSION STOCKING, WAIST LENGTH, 40-50 MMHG, EACH	00	9			M			N
L8210	GRADIENT COMPRESSION STOCKING, CUSTOM MADE	00	9			M			N
L8220	GRADIENT COMPRESSION STOCKING, LYMPHEDEMA	00	9			M			N

HCPCS	Long Description	PII	MPI	Statute	X-Ref	Coverage	ASC Pay Grp	ASC Pay Grp Eff Date	Action Code
L8230	GRADIENT COMPRESSION STOCKING, GARTER BELT	00	9			M			N
L8239	GRADIENT COMPRESSION STOCKING, NOT OTHERWISE SPECIFIED	46	A			C			N
L8300	TRUSS, SINGLE WITH STANDARD PAD	38	A			D			N
L8310	TRUSS, DOUBLE WITH STANDARD PADS	38	A			D			N
L8320	TRUSS, ADDITION TO STANDARD PAD, WATER PAD	38	A			D			N
L8330	TRUSS, ADDITION TO STANDARD PAD, SCROTAL PAD	38	A			D			N
L8400	PROSTHETIC SHEATH, BELOW KNEE, EACH	38	A			D			N
L8410	PROSTHETIC SHEATH, ABOVE KNEE, EACH	38	A			D			N
L8415	PROSTHETIC SHEATH, UPPER LIMB, EACH	38	A			D			N
L8417	PROSTHETIC SHEATH/SOCK, INCLUDING A GEL CUSHION LAYER, BELOW KNEE OR ABOVE	38	A			C			N
L8417	KNEE, EACH								
L8420	PROSTHETIC SOCK, MULTIPLE PLY, BELOW KNEE, EACH	38	A			D			N
L8430	PROSTHETIC SOCK, MULTIPLE PLY, ABOVE KNEE, EACH	38	A			D			N
L8435	PROSTHETIC SOCK, MULTIPLE PLY, UPPER LIMB, EACH	38	A			D			N
L8440	PROSTHETIC SHRINKER, BELOW KNEE, EACH	38	A			D			N
L8460	PROSTHETIC SHRINKER, ABOVE KNEE, EACH	38	A			D			N
L8465	PROSTHETIC SHRINKER, UPPER LIMB, EACH	38	A			D			N
L8470	PROSTHETIC SOCK, SINGLE PLY, FITTING, BELOW KNEE, EACH	38	A			D			N
L8480	PROSTHETIC SOCK, SINGLE PLY, FITTING, ABOVE KNEE, EACH	38	A			D			N
L8485	PROSTHETIC SOCK, SINGLE PLY, FITTING, UPPER LIMB, EACH	38	A			D			N
L8490	ADDITION TO PROSTHETIC SHEATH/SOCK, AIR SEAL SUCTION RETENTION SYSTEM	38	A			C			N
L8499	UNLISTED PROCEDURE FOR MISCELLANEOUS PROSTHETIC SERVICES	46	A			C			N
L8500	ARTIFICIAL LARYNX, ANY TYPE	38	A			D			N
L8501	TRACHEOSTOMY SPEAKING VALVE	38	A			D			N
L8505	ARTIFICIAL LARYNX REPLACEMENT BATTERY / ACCESSORY, ANY TYPE	46	A			C			N
L8507	TRACHEO-ESOPHAGEAL VOICE PROSTHESIS, PATIENT INSERTED, ANY TYPE, EACH	38	A			C			N
L8509	TRACHEO-ESOPHAGEAL VOICE PROSTHESIS, INSERTED BY A LICENSED HEALTH CARE PROVIDER, ANY TYPE	38	A			C			N
L8510	VOICE AMPLIFIER	38	A			D			N

HCPCS	Long Description	PI	MPI	Statute	X-Ref	Coverage	ASC Pay Grp	ASC Pay Grp Eff Date	Action Code
L8511	INSERT FOR INDWELLING TRACHEOESOPHAGEAL PROSTHESIS, WITH OR WITHOUT VALVE, REPLACEMENT ONLY, EACH	38	A			C			A
L8512	GELATIN CAPSULES OR EQUIVALENT, FOR USE WITH TRACHEOESOPHAGEAL VOICE PROSTHESIS, REPLACEMENT ONLY, PER 10	38	A			C			A
L8513	CLEANING DEVICE USED WITH TRACHEOESOPHAGEAL VOICE PROSTHESIS, PIPET, BRUSH, OR EQUAL, REPLACEMENT ONLY, EACH	38	A			C			A
L8514	TRACHEOESOPHAGEAL PUNCTURE DILATOR, REPLACEMENT ONLY, EACH	38	A			C			A
L8600	IMPLANTABLE BREAST PROSTHESIS, SILICONE OR EQUAL	38	A			D			N
L8603	INJECTABLE BULKING AGENT, COLLAGEN IMPLANT, URINARY TRACT, 2.5 ML SYRINGE, INCLUDES SHIPPING AND NECESSARY SUPPLIES	38	A			D			N
L8606	INJECTABLE BULKING AGENT, SYNTHETIC IMPLANT, URINARY TRACT, 1 ML SYRINGE, INCLUDES SHIPPING AND NECESSARY SUPPLIES	38	A			D			N
L8610	OCULAR IMPLANT	38	A			D			N
L8612	AQUEOUS SHUNT	38	A		Q0074	D			N
L8613	OSSICULA IMPLANT	38	A			D			N
L8614	COCHLEAR DEVICE/SYSTEM	38	A			D			N
L8619	COCHLEAR IMPLANT EXTERNAL SPEECH PROCESSOR, REPLACEMENT	38	A			D			N
L8630	METACARPOPHALANGEAL JOINT IMPLANT	38	A			D			N
L8631	METACARPAL PHALANGEAL JOINT REPLACEMENT, TWO OR MORE PIECES, METAL (E.G., STAINLESS STEEL OR COBALT CHROME), CERAMIC-LIKE MATERIAL (E.G., PYROCARBON), FOR SURGICAL IMPLANTATION (ALL SIZES, INCLUDES ENTIRE SYSTEM)	38	A			D			A
L8641	METATARSAL JOINT IMPLANT	38	A			D			N
L8642	HALLUX IMPLANT	38	A		Q0073	D			N
L8658	INTERPHALANGEAL JOINT SPACER, SILICONE OR EQUAL, EACH	38	A			D			C
L8659	INTERPHALANGEAL FINGER JOINT REPLACEMENT, 2 OR MORE PIECES, METAL (E.G., STAINLESS STEEL OR COBALT CHROME), CERAMIC-LIKE MATERIAL (E.G., PYROCARBON) FOR SURGICAL IMPLANTATION, ANY SIZE	38	A			D			A
L8670	VASCULAR GRAFT MATERIAL, SYNTHETIC, IMPLANT	38	A			D			N
L8699	PROSTHETIC IMPLANT, NOT OTHERWISE SPECIFIED	46	A			C			N
L9900	ORTHOTIC AND PROSTHETIC SUPPLY, ACCESSORY, AND/OR SERVICE COMPONENT OF ANOTHER HCPCS "L" CODE	46	A			C			N
M0064	BRIEF OFFICE VISIT FOR THE SOLE PURPOSE OF MONITORING OR CHANGING DRUG PRESCRIPTIONS USED IN THE TREATMENT OF MENTAL PSYCHONEUROTIC AND PERSONALITY DISORDERS	11	A			D			N
M0075	CELLULAR THERAPY	00	9			M			N
M0076	PROLOTHERAPY	00	9			M			N
M0100	INTRAGASTRIC HYPOTHERMIA USING GASTRIC FREEZING	00	9			M			C
M0300	IV CHELATION THERAPY (CHEMICAL ENDARTERECTOMY)	00	9			M			N
M0301	FABRIC WRAPPING OF ABDOMINAL ANEURYSM	00	9			M			C

HCPCS	Long Description	PH	MPI	Statute	X-Ref	Coverage	ASC Pay Grp	ASC Pay Grp Eff Date	Action Code
M0302	ASSESSMENT OF CARDIAC OUTPUT BY ELECTRICAL BIOIMPEDANCE	57	A		CPT	D			N
P2028	CEPHALIN FLOCULATION, BLOOD	57	A			D			N
P2029	CONGO RED, BLOOD	57	A			D			N
P2031	HAIR ANALYSIS (EXCLUDING ARSENIC)	00	9			M			N
P2033	THYMOL TURBIDITY, BLOOD	57	A			D			N
P2038	MUCOPROTEIN, BLOOD (SEROMUCOID) (MEDICAL NECESSITY PROCEDURE)	21	A			D			N
P3000	SCREENING PAPANICOLAOU SMEAR, CERVICAL OR VAGINAL, UP TO THREE SMEARS, BY TECHNICIAN UNDER PHYSICIAN SUPERVISION	21	A			D			N
P3001	SCREENING PAPANICOLAOU SMEAR, CERVICAL OR VAGINAL, UP TO THREE SMEARS, REQUIRING INTERPRETATION BY PHYSICIAN	11	C			D			N
P7001	CULTURE, BACTERIAL, URINE; QUANTITATIVE, SENSITIVITY STUDY	00	9		CPT	I			N
P9010	BLOOD (WHOLE), FOR TRANSFUSION, PER UNIT	52	A			D			N
P9011	BLOOD (SPLIT UNIT), SPECIFY AMOUNT	52	A			D			N
P9012	CRYOPRECIPITATE, EACH UNIT	52	A			D			N
P9013	FIBRINOGEN UNIT	52	A			D			N
P9016	RED BLOOD CELLS, LEUKOCYTES REDUCED, EACH UNIT	52	A			D			N
P9017	FRESH FROZEN PLASMA (SINGLE DONOR), FROZEN WITHIN 8 HOURS OF COLLECTION, EACH UNIT	52	A			D			C
P9018	PLASMA PROTEIN FRACTION, EACH UNIT	52	A			D			N
P9019	PLATELETS, EACH UNIT	52	A			D			N
P9020	PLATELET RICH PLASMA, EACH UNIT	52	A			D			N
P9021	RED BLOOD CELLS, EACH UNIT	52	A			D			N
P9022	RED BLOOD CELLS, WASHED, EACH UNIT	52	A			D			N
P9023	PLASMA, POOLED MULTIPLE DONOR, SOLVENT/DETERGENT TREATED, FROZEN, EACH UNIT	52	A			D			N
P9031	PLATELETS, LEUKOCYTES REDUCED, EACH UNIT	52	A			D			N
P9032	PLATELETS, IRRADIATED, EACH UNIT	52	A			D			N
P9033	PLATELETS, LEUKOCYTES REDUCED, IRRADIATED, EACH UNIT	52	A			D			N
P9034	PLATELETS, PHERESIS, EACH UNIT	52	A			D			N
P9035	PLATELETS, PHERESIS, LEUKOCYTES REDUCED, EACH UNIT	52	A			D			N
P9036	PLATELETS, PHERESIS, IRRADIATED, EACH UNIT	52	A			D			N
P9037	PLATELETS, PHERESIS, LEUKOCYTES REDUCED, IRRADIATED, EACH UNIT	52	A			D			N

HCPCS	Long Description	PTI	MPI	Statute	X-Ref1	Coverage	ASC Pay Grp	ASC Pay Grp Eff Date	Action Code
P9038	RED BLOOD CELLS, IRRADIATED, EACH UNIT	52	A			D			N
P9039	RED BLOOD CELLS, DEGLYCEROLIZED, EACH UNIT	52	A			D			N
P9040	RED BLOOD CELLS, LEUKOCYTES REDUCED, IRRADIATED, EACH UNIT	52	A			D			N
P9041	INFUSION, ALBUMIN (HUMAN), 5%, 50 ML	52	A			C			N
P9042	INFUSION, ALBUMIN (HUMAN), 25%, 10 ML	52	A		P9046	C			N
P9043	INFUSION, PLASMA PROTEIN FRACTION (HUMAN), 5%, 50 ML	52	A			D			N
P9044	PLASMA, CRYOPRECIPITATE REDUCED, EACH UNIT	52	A			D			N
P9045	INFUSION, ALBUMIN (HUMAN), 5%, 250 ML	52	A			C			N
P9046	INFUSION, ALBUMIN (HUMAN), 25%, 20 ML	52	A			C			N
P9047	INFUSION, ALBUMIN (HUMAN), 25%, 50 ML	52	A			C			N
P9048	INFUSION, PLASMA PROTEIN FRACTION (HUMAN), 5%, 250ML	52	A			C			N
P9050	GRANULOCYTES, PHERESIS, EACH UNIT	52	A			C			N
P9051	WHOLE BLOOD OR RED BLOOD CELLS, LEUKOCYTES REDUCED, CMV-NEGATIVE, EACH UNIT	52	A	1833T		D			A
P9052	PLATELETS, HLA-MATCHED LEUKOCYTES REDUCED, APHERESIS/PHERESIS, EACH UNIT	52	A	1833T		D			A
P9053	PLATELETS, PHERESIS, LEUKOCYTES REDUCED, CMV-NEGATIVE, IRRADIATED, EACH UNIT	52	A	1833T		D			A
P9054	WHOLE BLOOD OR RED BLOOD CELLS, LEUKOCYTES REDUCED, FROZEN, DEGLYCEROL, WASHED, EACH UNIT	52	A	1833T		D			A
P9055	PLATELETS, LEUKOCYTES REDUCED, CMV-NEGATIVE, APHERESIS/PHERESIS, EACH UNIT	52	A	1833T		D			A
P9056	WHOLE BLOOD, LEUKOCYTES REDUCED, IRRADIATED, EACH UNIT	52	A	1833T		D			A
P9057	RED BLOOD CELLS, FROZEN/DEGLYCEROLIZED/WASHED, LEUKOCYTES REDUCED, IRRADIATED, EACH UNIT	52	A	1833T		D			A
P9058	RED BLOOD CELLS, LEUKOCYTES REDUCED, CMV-NEGATIVE, IRRADIATED, EACH UNIT	52	A	1833T		D			A
P9059	FRESH FROZEN PLASMA BETWEEN 8-24 HOURS OF COLLECTION, EACH UNIT	52	A	1833T		D			A
P9060	FRESH FROZEN PLASMA, DONOR RETESTED, EACH UNIT	52	A	1833T		D			A
P9603	TRAVEL ALLOWANCE ONE WAY IN CONNECTION WITH MEDICALLY NECESSARY LABORATORY SPECIMEN COLLECTION DRAWN FROM HOME BOUND OR NURSING HOME BOUND PATIENT; PRORATED MILES ACTUALLY TRAVELLED.	22	A			D			N
P9604	TRAVEL ALLOWANCE ONE WAY IN CONNECTION WITH MEDICALLY NECESSARY LABORATORY SPECIMEN COLLECTION DRAWN FROM HOME BOUND OR NURSING HOME BOUND PATIENT; PRORATED TRIP CHARGE.	22	A			D			N
P9612	CATHETERIZATION FOR COLLECTION OF SPECIMEN, SINGLE PATIENT, ALL PLACES OF SERVICE	57	A			D			N
P9615	CATHETERIZATION FOR COLLECTION OF SPECIMEN (S) (MULTIPLE PATIENTS)	57	A			D			N

HCPCS	Long Description	PTI	MPI	Statute	X-Ref1	Coverage	ASC Pay Grp	ASC Pay Grp Eff Date	Action Code
Q0034	ADMINISTRATION OF INFLUENZA VACCINE TO MEDICARE BENEFICIARIES BY PARTICIPATING	54	A			C			N
Q0035	DEMONSTRATION SITES CARDIOKYMOGRAPHY	11	A			D			N
Q0081	INFUSION THERAPY, USING OTHER THAN CHEMOTHERAPEUTIC DRUGS, PER VISIT	00	9			D			N
Q0082	ACTIVITY THERAPY FURNISHED IN CONNECTION WITH PARTIAL HOSPITALIZATION (EG MUSIC, DANCE, ART OR PLAY THERAPIES THAT ARE NOT PRIMARILY RECREATIONAL), PER VISIT	00	9		G0176	C			N
Q0083	CHEMOTHERAPY ADMINISTRATION BY OTHER THAN INFUSION TECHNIQUE ONLY (EG SUBCUTANEOUS, INTRAMUSCULAR, PUSH), PER VISIT	00	9			C			N
Q0084	CHEMOTHERAPY ADMINISTRATION BY INFUSION TECHNIQUE ONLY, PER VISIT	00	9			D			N
Q0085	CHEMOTHERAPY ADMINISTRATION BY BOTH INFUSION TECHNIQUE AND OTHER TECHIQUE(S) (EG SUBCUTANEOUS, INTRAMUSCULAR, PUSH), PER VISIT	00	9			C			N
Q0086	PHYSICAL THERAPY EVALUATION/TREATMENT, PER VISIT	00	9			D			D
Q0091	SCREENING PAPANICOLAOU SMEAR; OBTAINING, PREPARING AND CONVEYANCE OF CERVICAL OR VAGINAL SMEAR TO LABORATORY	11	A			D			N
Q0092	SET-UP PORTABLE X-RAY EQUIPMENT	11	A			D			N
Q0111	WET MOUNTS, INCLUDING PREPARATIONS OF VAGINAL, CERVICAL OR SKIN SPECIMENS	21	A			C			N
Q0112	ALL POTASSIUM HYDROXIDE (KOH) PREPARATIONS	21	A			C			N
Q0113	PINWORM EXAMINATIONS	21	A			C			N
Q0114	FERN TEST	21	A			C			N
Q0115	POST-COITAL DIRECT, QUALITATIVE EXAMINATIONS OF VAGINAL OR CERVICAL MUCOUS	21	A			C			N
Q0136	INJECTION, EPOETIN ALPHA, (FOR NON ESRD USE), PER 1000 UNITS	51	A			D			N
Q0137	INJECTION, DARBEPOETIN ALFA, 1 MCG (NON-ESRD USE)	57	A			D			A
Q0144	AZITHROMYCIN DIHYDRATE, ORAL, CAPSULES/POWDER, 1 GRAM	00	9			M			N
Q0156	INFUSION, ALBUMIN (HUMAN), 5%, 500 ML	51	A			C			N
Q0157	INFUSION, ALBUMIN (HUMAN), 25%, 50 ML	51	A			C			N
Q0160	FACTOR IX (ANTIHEMOPHILIC FACTOR, PURIFIED, NON-RECOMBINANT) PER I.U.	51	A		J7193	D			N
Q0161	FACTOR IX (ANTIHEMOPHILIC FACTOR, RECOMBINANT) PER I.U.	51	A		J7195	D			N
Q0163	DIPHENHYDRAMINE HYDROCHLORIDE, 50 MG, ORAL, FDA APPROVED PRESCRIPTION ANTI-EMETIC, FOR USE AS A COMPLETE THERAPEUTIC SUBSTITUTE FOR AN IV ANTI-EMETIC AT TIME OF CHEMOTHERAPY TREATMENT NOT TO EXCEED A 48 HOUR DOSAGE REGIMEN	51	A	4557		D			N
Q0164	PROCHLORPERAZINE MALEATE, 5 MG, ORAL, FDA APPROVED PRESCRIPTION ANTI-EMETIC, FOR USE AS A COMPLETE THERAPEUTIC SUBSTITUTE FOR AN IV ANTI-EMETIC AT THE TIME OF CHEMOTHERAPY TREATMENT, NOT TO EXCEED A 48 HOUR DOSAGE REGIMEN	51	A	4557		D			N
Q0165	PROCHLORPERAZINE MALEATE, 10 MG, ORAL, FDA APPROVED PRESCRIPTION ANTI-EMETIC, FOR USE AS A COMPLETE THERAPEUTIC SUBSTITUTE FOR AN IV ANTI-EMETIC AT THE TIME OF CHEMOTHERAPY TREATMENT, NOT TO EXCEED A 48 HOUR DOSAGE REGIMEN	51	A	4557		D			N
Q0166	GRANISETRON HYDROCHLORIDE, 1 MG, ORAL, FDA APPROVED PRESCRIPTION ANTI-EMETIC, FOR USE AS A COMPLETE THERAPEUTIC SUBSTITUTE FOR AN IV ANTI-EMETIC AT THE TIME OF CHEMOTHERAPY TREATMENT, NOT TO EXCEED A 24 HOUR DOSAGE REGIMEN	51	A	4557		D			N

HCPCS	Long Description	PI	MPI	Statute	X-Ref1	Coverage	ASC Pay Grp	ASC Pay Grp Eff Date	Action Code
Q0167	DRONABINOL, 2.5 MG, ORAL, FDA APPROVED PRESCRIPTION ANTI-EMETIC, FOR USE AS A COMPLETE THERAPEUTIC SUBSTITUTE FOR AN IV ANTI-EMETIC AT THE TIME OF CHEMOTHERAPY TREATMENT, NOT TO EXCEED A 48 HOUR DOSAGE REGIMEN	51	A	4557		D			N
Q0168	DRONABINOL, 5 MG, ORAL, FDA APPROVED PRESCRIPTION ANTI-EMETIC, FOR USE AS A ANTI-EMETIC, FOR USE AS A COMPLETE THERAPEUTIC SUBSTITUTE FOR AN IV ANTI-EMETIC AT THE TIME OF CHEMOTHERAPY TREATMENT, NOT TO EXCEED A 48 HOUR DOSAGE REGIMEN	51	A	4557		D			N
Q0169	PROMETHAZINE HYDROCHLORIDE, 12.5 MG, ORAL, FDA APPROVED PRESCRIPTION ANTI-EMETIC, FOR USE AS A COMPLETE THERAPEUTIC SUBSTITUTE FOR AN IV ANTI-EMETIC AT THE TIME OF CHEMOTHERAPY TREATMENT, NOT TO EXCEED A 48 HOUR DOSAGE REGIMEN	51	A	4557		D			N
Q0170	PROMETHAZINE HYDROCHLORIDE, 25 MG, ORAL, FDA APPROVED PRESCRIPTION ANTI-EMETIC, FOR USE AS A COMPLETE THERAPEUTIC SUBSTITUTE FOR AN IV ANTI-EMETIC AT THE TIME OF CHEMOTHERAPY TREATMENT, NOT TO EXCEED A 48 HOUR DOSAGE REGIMEN	51	A	4557		D			N
Q0171	CHLORPROMAZINE HYDROCHLORIDE, 10 MG, ORAL, FDA APPROVED PRESCRIPTION ANTI-EMETIC, FOR USE AS A COMPLETE THERAPEUTIC SUBSTITUTE FOR AN IV ANTI-EMETIC AT THE TIME OF CHEMOTHERAPY TREATMENT, NOT TO EXCEED A 48 HOUR DOSAGE REGIMEN	51	A	4557		D			N
Q0172	CHLORPROMAZINE HYDROCHLORIDE, 25 MG, ORAL, FDA APPROVED PRESCRIPTION ANTI-EMETIC, FOR USE AS A COMPLETE THERAPEUTIC SUBSTITUTE FOR AN IV ANTI-EMETIC AT THE TIME OF CHEMOTHERAPY TREATMENT, NOT TO EXCEED A 48 HOUR DOSAGE REGIMEN	51	A	4557		D			N
Q0173	TRIMETHOBENZAMIDE HYDROCHLORIDE, 250 MG, ORAL, FDA APPROVED PRESCRIPTION ANTI-EMETIC, FOR USE AS A COMPLETE THERAPEUTIC SUBSTITUTE FOR AN IV ANTI-EMETIC AT THE TIME OF CHEMOTHERAPY TREATMENT, NOT TO EXCEED A 48 HOUR DOSAGE REGIMEN	51	A	4557		D			N
Q0174	THIETHYLPERAZINE MALEATE, 10 MG, ORAL, FDA APPROVED PRESCRIPTION ANTI-EMETIC, COMPLETE THERAPEUTIC SUBSTITUTE FOR AN IV ANTI-EMETIC AT THE TIME OF CHEMOTHERAPY TREATMENT, NOT TO EXCEED A 48 HOUR DOSAGE REGIMEN	51	A	4557		D			N
Q0175	PERPHENAZINE, 4 MG, ORAL, FDA APPROVED PRESCRIPTION ANTI-EMETIC, FOR USE AS A COMPLETE THERAPEUTIC SUBSTITUTE FOR AN IV ANTI-EMETIC AT THE TIME OF CHEMOTHERAPY TREATMENT, NOT TO EXCEED A 48 HOUR DOSAGE REGIMEN	51	A	4557		D			N
Q0176	PERPHENAZINE, 8MG, ORAL, FDA APPROVED PRESCRIPTION ANTI-EMETIC, FOR USE AS A COMPLETE THERAPEUTIC SUBSTITUTE FOR AN IV ANTI-EMETIC AT THE TIME OF CHEMOTHERAPY TREATMENT, NOT TO EXCEED A 48 HOUR DOSAGE REGIMEN	51	A	4557		D			N
Q0177	HYDROXYZINE PAMOATE, 25 MG, ORAL, FDA APPROVED PRESCRIPTION ANTI-EMETIC, FOR USE AS A COMPLETE THERAPEUTIC SUBSTITUTE FOR AN IV ANTI-EMETIC AT THE TIME OF CHEMOTHERAPY TREATMENT, NOT TO EXCEED A 48 HOUR DOSAGE REGIMEN	51	A	4557		D			N
Q0178	HYDROXYZINE PAMOATE, 50 MG, ORAL, FDA APPROVED PRESCRIPTION ANTI-EMETIC, FOR USE AS A COMPLETE THERAPEUTIC SUBSTITUTE FOR AN IV ANTI-EMETIC AT THE TIME OF CHEMOTHERAPY TREATMENT, NOT TO EXCEED A 48 HOUR DOSAGE REGIMEN	51	A	4557		D			N
Q0179	ONDANSETRON HYDROCHLORIDE 8 MG, ORAL, FDA APPROVED PRESCRIPTION ANTI-EMETIC, USE AS A COMPLETE THERAPEUTIC SUBSTITUTE FOR AN IV ANTI-EMETIC AT THE TIME OF CHEMOTHERAPY TREATMENT, NOT TO EXCEED A 48 HOUR DOSAGE REGIMEN	51	A	4557		D			N
Q0180	DOLASETRON MESYLATE, 100 MG, ORAL, FDA APPROVED PRESCRIPTION ANTI-EMETIC, FOR USE AS A COMPLETE THERAPEUTIC SUBSTITUTE FOR AN IV ANTI-EMETIC AT THE TIME OF CHEMOTHERAPY TREATMENT, NOT TO EXCEED A 24 HOUR DOSAGE REGIMEN	51	A	4557		D			N
Q0181	UNSPECIFIED ORAL DOSAGE FORM, FDA APPROVED PRESCRIPTION ANTI-EMETIC, FOR USE AS A COMPLETE THERAPEUTIC SUBSTITUTE FOR A IV ANTI-EMETIC AT THE TIME OF CHEMOTHERAPY TREATMENT, NOT TO EXCEED A 48 HOUR DOSAGE REGIMEN	51	A	4557		D			N
Q0182	DERMAL AND EPIDERMAL, TISSUE OF NON-HUMAN ORIGIN, WITH OR WITHOUT OTHER BIOENGINEERED OR PROCESSED ELEMENTS, WITHOUT METABOLICALLY ACTIVE ELEMENTS, PER SQUARE CENTIMETER	51	A			C			A
Q0183	DERMAL TISSUE, OF HUMAN ORIGIN, WITH AND WITHOUT OTHER BIOENGINEERED OR PROCESSED ELEMENTS, BUT WITHOUT METABOLICALLY ACTIVE ELEMENTS, PER SQUARE CENTIMETER	51	A			C			N

HCPCS	Long Description	PH	MPI	Statute	X-Ref	Coverage	ASC Pay Grp	ASC Pay Grp Eff Date	Action Code
Q0184	DERMAL TISSUE, OF HUMAN ORIGIN, WITH OR WITHOUT OTHER BIOENGINEERED OR PROCESSED ELEMENTS, WITH METABOLICALLY ACTIVE ELEMENTS, PER SQUARE CENTIMETER	51	A		J7342	C			N
Q0185	DERMAL AND EPIDERMAL, TISSUE OF HUMAN ORIGIN, WITH OR WITHOUT BIOENGINEERED OR PROCESSED ELEMENTS, WITH METABOLICALLY ACTIVE ELEMENTS, PER SQUARE CENTIMETER	46	A		J7340	C			N
Q0186	PARAMEDIC INTERCEPT, RURAL AREA, TRANSPORT FURNISHED BY A VOLUNTEER AMBULANCE COMPANY WHICH IS PROHIBITED BY STATE LAW FROM BILLING THIRD PARTY PAYERS	52	A		A0432	D			N
Q0187	FACTOR VIIA (COAGULATION FACTOR, RECOMBINANT) PER 1.2 MG	51	A			D			N
Q0188	SUPPLY OF INJECTABLE CONTRAST MATERIAL FOR USE IN ECHOCARDIOGRAPHY, PER STUDY	57	A		A9700	D			N
Q1001	NEW TECHNOLOGY INTRAOCULAR LENS CATEGORY 1 AS DEFINED IN FEDERAL REGISTER NOTICE, VOL 65, DATED MAY 3, 2000	57	A			D			T
Q1002	NEW TECHNOLOGY INTRAOCULAR LENS CATEGORY 2 AS DEFINED IN FEDERAL REGISTER NOTICE, VOL 65, DATED MAY 3, 2000	57	A			D			T
Q1003	NEW TECHNOLOGY INTRAOCULAR LENS CATEGORY 3 AS DEFINED IN FEDERAL REGISTER NOTICE	57	A			D			T
Q1004	NEW TECHNOLOGY INTRAOCULAR LENS CATEGORY 4 AS DEFINED IN FEDERAL REGISTER NOTICE	57	A			D			T
Q1005	NEW TECHNOLOGY INTRAOCULAR LENS CATEGORY 5 AS DEFINED IN FEDERAL REGISTER NOTICE	57	A			D			T
Q2001	ORAL, CABERGOLINE, 0.5 MG	00	9			M			N
Q2002	INJECTION, ELLIOTTS B SOLUTION, PER ML	51	A	1861S2B		D			N
Q2003	INJECTION, APROTININ, 10,000 KIU	51	A	1861S2B		D			N
Q2004	IRRIGATION SOLUTION FOR TREATMENT OF BLADDER CALCULI, FOR EXAMPLE RENACIDIN, PER 500 ML	51	A	1861S2B		D			N
Q2005	INJECTION, CORTICORELIN OVINE TRIFLUTATE, PER DOSE	51	A	1861S2B		D			N
Q2006	INJECTION, DIGOXIN IMMUNE FAB (OVINE), PER VIAL	51	A	1861S2B		D			N
Q2007	INJECTION, ETHANOLAMINE OLEATE, 100 MG	51	A	1861S2B		D			N
Q2008	INJECTION, FOMEPIZOLE, 15 MG	51	A	1861S2B		D			N
Q2009	INJECTION, FOSPHENYTOIN, 50 MG	51	A	1861S2B		D			N
Q2010	INJECTION, GLATIRAMER ACETATE, PER DOSE	51	A	1861S2B		D			D
Q2011	INJECTION, HEMIN, PER 1 MG	51	A	1861S2B		D			N
Q2012	INJECTION, PEGADEMASE BOVINE, 25 IU	51	A	1861S2B		D			N
Q2013	INJECTION, PENTASTARCH, 10% SOLUTION, PER 100 ML	51	A	1861S2B		D			N
Q2014	INJECTION, SERMORELIN ACETATE, 0.5 MG	51	A	1861S2B		D			N
Q2015	INJECTION, SOMATREM, 5 MG	51	A	1861S2B		D			N
Q2016	INJECTION, SOMATROPIN, 1 MG	51	A	1861S2B		D			N
Q2017	INJECTION, TENIPOSIDE, 50 MG	51	A	1861S2B		D			N
Q2018	INJECTION, UROFOLLITROPIN, 75 IU	51	A	1861S2B		D			N
Q2019	INJECTION, BASILIXIMAB, 20 MG	51	A			D			N
Q2020	INJECTION, HISTRELIN ACETATE, 10 MCG	51	A	1861S2B		D			N

HCPCS	Long Description	PH	MPI	Statute	X-Ref	Coverage	ASC Pay Grp	ASC Pay Grp Eff Date	Action Code
Q2021	INJECTION, LEPIRUDIN, 50 MG	51	A	1861S2B		D			N
Q2022	VON WILLEBRAND FACTOR COMPLEX, HUMAN, PER IU	51	A			D			N
Q3000	SUPPLY OF RADIOPHARMACEUTICAL DIAGNOSTIC IMAGING AGENT, RUBIDIUM RB-82, PER DOSE	99	9			D			N
Q3001	RADIOELEMENTS FOR BRACHYTHERAPY, ANY TYPE, EACH	57	A			D			N
Q3002	SUPPLY OF RADIOPHARMACEUTICAL DIAGNOSTIC IMAGING AGENT, GALLIUM GA 67, PER MCI	57	A			D			N
Q3003	SUPPLY OF RADIOPHARMACEUTICAL DIAGNOSTIC IMAGING AGENT, TECHNETIUM TC99M BICISATE, PER UNIT DOSE	57	A			D			N
Q3004	SUPPLY OF RADIOPHARMACEUTICAL DIAGNOSTIC IMAGING AGENT, XENON XE 133, PER 10 MCI	57	A			D			N
Q3005	SUPPLY OF RADIOPHARMACEUTICAL DIAGNOSTIC IMAGING AGENT, TECHNETIUM TC-99M MERTIATIDE, PER MCI	57	A			D			N
Q3006	SUPPLY OF RADIOPHARMACEUTICAL DIAGNOSTIC IMAGING AGENT, TECHNETIUM TC 99M GLUCEPATATE, PER 5 MCI	57	A			D			N
Q3007	SUPPLY OF RADIOPHARMACEUTICAL DIAGNOSTIC IMAGING AGENT, SODIUM PHOSPHATE P32, PER MCI	57	A			D			N
Q3008	SUPPLY OF RADIOPHARMACEUTICAL DIAGNOSTIC IMAGING AGENT, INDIUM 111-IN PENTETREOTIDE, PER 3 MCI	57	A			D			N
Q3009	SUPPLY OF RADIOPHARMACEUTICAL DIAGNOSTIC IMAGING AGENT, TECHNETIUM TC99M OXIDRONATE, PER MCI	57	A			D			N
Q3010	SUPPLY OF RADIOPHARMACEUTICAL DIAGNOSTIC IMAGING AGENT, TECHNETIUM TC99M - LABELED RED BLOOD CELLS, PER MCI	57	A			D			N
Q3011	SUPPLY OF RADIOPHARMACEUTICAL DIAGNOSTIC IMAGING AGENT, CHROMIC PHOSPHATE P32 SUSPENSION, PER MCI	57	A			D			N
Q3012	SUPPLY OF ORAL RADIOPHARMACEUTICAL DIAGNOSTIC IMAGING AGENT, CYANOCOBALAMIN COBALT CO57, PER 0.5 MCI	57	A			D			N
Q3013	INJECTION, VERTEPORFIN, 15 MG	51	A		J3395	D			N
Q3014	TELEHEALTH ORIGINATING SITE FACILITY FEE	53	A			C			N
Q3017	AMBULANCE SERVICE, ADVANCED LIFE SUPPORT (ALS) ASSESSMENT, NO OTHER ALS SERVICES PROVIDED	52	A			C			N
Q3019	ALS VEHICLE USED, EMERGENCY TRANSPORT, NO ALS LEVEL SERVICES FURNISHED	52	A			C			N
Q3020	ALS VEHICLE USED, NON-EMERGENCY TRANSPORT, NO ALS LEVEL SERVICE FURNISHED	52	A			C			N
Q3025	INJECTION, INTERFERON BETA-1A, 11 MCG FOR INTRAMUSCULAR USE	51	A			D			N
Q3026	INJECTION, INTERFERON BETA-1A, 11 MCG FOR SUBCUTANEOUS USE	00	9			I			N
Q3030	SODIUM HYALURONATE PER 20 TO 25 MG DOSE, FOR INTRA-ARTICULAR INJECTION	51	A		J7317	C			N
Q3031	COLLAGEN SKIN TEST	11	A			D			A
Q4001	CASTING SUPPLIES, BODY CAST ADULT, WITH OR WITHOUT HEAD, PLASTER	52	A			C			N
Q4002	CAST SUPPLIES, BODY CAST ADULT, WITH OR WITHOUT HEAD, FIBERGLASS	52	A			C			N

HCPCS	Long Description	PTI	MPI	Statute	X-Ref1	Coverage	ASC Pay Grp	ASC Pay Grp Eff Date	Action Code
Q4003	CAST SUPPLIES, SHOULDER CAST, ADULT (11 YEARS +), PLASTER	52	A			C			N
Q4004	CAST SUPPLIES, SHOULDER CAST, ADULT (11 YEARS +), FIBERGLASS	52	A			C			N
Q4005	CAST SUPPLIES, LONG ARM CAST, ADULT (11 YEARS +), PLASTER	52	A			C			N
Q4006	CAST SUPPLIES, LONG ARM CAST, ADULT (11 YEARS +), FIBERGLASS	52	A			C			N
Q4007	CAST SUPPLIES, LONG ARM CAST, PEDIATRIC (0-10 YEARS), PLASTER	52	A			C			N
Q4008	CAST SUPPLIES, LONG ARM CAST, PEDIATRIC (0-10 YEARS), FIBERGLASS	52	A			C			N
Q4009	CAST SUPPLIES, SHORT ARM CAST, ADULT (11 YEARS +), PLASTER	52	A			C			N
Q4010	CAST SUPPLIES, SHORT ARM CAST, ADULT (11 YEARS +), FIBERGLASS	52	A			C			N
Q4011	CAST SUPPLIES, SHORT ARM CAST, PEDIATRIC (0-10 YEARS), PLASTER	52	A			C			N
Q4012	CAST SUPPLIES, SHORT ARM CAST, PEDIATRIC (0-10 YEARS), FIBERGLASS	52	A			C			N
Q4013	CAST SUPPLIES, GAUNTLET CAST (INCLUDES LOWER FOREARM AND HAND), ADULT (11 YEARS +), PLASTER	52	A			C			N
Q4014	CAST SUPPLIES, GAUNTLET CAST (INCLUDES LOWER FOREARM AND HAND), ADULT (11 YEARS +), FIBERGLASS	52	A			C			N
Q4015	CAST SUPPLIES, GAUNTLET CAST (INCLUDES LOWER FOREARM AND HAND), PEDIATRIC (0-10 YEARS), PLASTER	52	A			C			N
Q4016	CAST SUPPLIES, GAUNTLET CAST (INCLUDES LOWER FOREARM AND HAND), PEDIATRIC (0-10 YEARS), FIBERGLASS	52	A			C			N
Q4017	CAST SUPPLIES, LONG ARM SPLINT, ADULT (11 YEARS +), PLASTER	52	A			C			N
Q4018	CAST SUPPLIES, LONG ARM SPLINT, ADULT (11 YEARS +), FIBERGLASS	52	A			C			N
Q4019	CAST SUPPLIES, LONG ARM SPLINT, PEDIATRIC (0-10 YEARS), PLASTER	52	A			C			N
Q4020	CAST SUPPLIES, LONG ARM SPLINT, PEDIATRIC (0-10 YEARS), FIBERGLASS	52	A			C			N
Q4021	CAST SUPPLIES, SHORT ARM SPLINT, ADULT (11 YEARS +), PLASTER	52	A			C			N
Q4022	CAST SUPPLIES, SHORT ARM SPLINT, ADULT (11 YEARS +), FIBERGLASS	52	A			C			N
Q4023	CAST SUPPLIES, SHORT ARM SPLINT, PEDIATRIC (0-10 YEARS), PLASTER	52	A			C			N
Q4024	CAST SUPPLIES, SHORT ARM SPLINT, PEDIATRIC (0-10 YEARS), FIBERGLASS	52	A			C			N
Q4025	CAST SUPPLIES, HIP SPICA (ONE OR BOTH LEGS), ADULT (11 YEARS +), PLASTER	52	A			C			N
Q4026	CAST SUPPLIES, HIP SPICA (ONE OR BOTH LEGS), ADULT (11 YEARS +), FIBERGLASS	52	A			C			N
Q4027	CAST SUPPLIES, HIP SPICA (ONE OR BOTH LEGS), PEDIATRIC (0-10 YEARS), PLASTER	52	A			C			N

HCPCS	Long Description	PII	MPI	Statute	X-Refl	Coverage	ASC Pay Grp	ASC Pay Grp Eff Date	Action Code
Q4028	CAST SUPPLIES, HIP SPICA (ONE OR BOTH LEGS), PEDIATRIC (0-10 YEARS), FIBERGLASS	52	A			C			N
Q4029	CAST SUPPLIES, LONG LEG CAST, ADULT (11 YEARS +), PLASTER	52	A			C			N
Q4030	CAST SUPPLIES, LONG LEG CAST, ADULT (11 YEARS +), FIBERGLASS	52	A			C			N
Q4031	CAST SUPPLIES, LONG LEG CAST, PEDIATRIC (0-10 YEARS), PLASTER	52	A			C			N
Q4032	CAST SUPPLIES, LONG LEG CAST, PEDIATRIC (0-10 YEARS), FIBERGLASS	52	A			C			N
Q4033	CAST SUPPLIES, LONG LEG CYLINDER CAST, ADULT (11 YEARS +), PLASTER	52	A			C			N
Q4034	CAST SUPPLIES, LONG LEG CYLINDER CAST, ADULT (11 YEARS +), FIBERGLASS	52	A			C			N
Q4035	CAST SUPPLIES, LONG LEG CYLINDER CAST, PEDIATRIC (0-10 YEARS), PLASTER	52	A			C			N
Q4036	CAST SUPPLIES, LONG LEG CYLINDER CAST, PEDIATRIC (0-10 YEARS), FIBERGLASS	52	A			C			N
Q4037	CAST SUPPLIES, SHORT LEG CAST, ADULT (11 YEARS +), PLASTER	52	A			C			N
Q4038	CAST SUPPLIES, SHORT LEG CAST, ADULT (11 YEARS +), FIBERGLASS	52	A			C			N
Q4039	CAST SUPPLIES, SHORT LEG CAST, PEDIATRIC (0-10 YEARS), PLASTER	52	A			C			N
Q4040	CAST SUPPLIES, SHORT LEG CAST, PEDIATRIC (0-10 YEARS), FIBERGLASS	52	A			C			N
Q4041	CAST SUPPLIES, LONG LEG SPLINT, ADULT (11 YEARS +), PLASTER	52	A			C			N
Q4042	CAST SUPPLIES, LONG LEG SPLINT, ADULT (11 YEARS +), FIBERGLASS	52	A			C			N
Q4043	CAST SUPPLIES, LONG LEG SPLINT, PEDIATRIC (0-10 YEARS), PLASTER	52	A			C			N
Q4044	CAST SUPPLIES, LONG LEG SPLINT, PEDIATRIC (0-10 YEARS), FIBERGLASS	52	A			C			N
Q4045	CAST SUPPLIES, SHORT LEG SPLINT, ADULT (11 YEARS +), PLASTER	52	A			C			N
Q4046	CAST SUPPLIES, SHORT LEG SPLINT, ADULT (11 YEARS +), FIBERGLASS	52	A			C			N
Q4047	CAST SUPPLIES, SHORT LEG SPLINT, PEDIATRIC (0-10 YEARS), PLASTER	52	A			C			N
Q4048	CAST SUPPLIES, SHORT LEG SPLINT, PEDIATRIC (0-10 YEARS), FIBERGLASS	52	A			C			N
Q4049	FINGER SPLINT, STATIC	52	A			C			N
Q4050	CAST SUPPLIES, FOR UNLISTED TYPES AND MATERIALS OF CASTS	57	A			C			N
Q4051	SPLINT SUPPLIES, MISCELLANEOUS (INCLUDES THERMOPLASTICS, STRAPPING, FASTENERS, PADDING AND OTHER SUPPLIES)	57	A			C			N
Q4052	INJECTION, OCTREOTIDE, DEPOT FORM FOR INTRAMUSCULAR INJECTION, 1 MG	51	A		J2353	C			D
Q4053	INJECTION, PEGFILGRASTIM, 1 MG	51	A		J2505	D			D
Q4054	INJECTION, DARBEPOETIN ALFA, 1 MCG (FOR ESRD ON DIALYSIS)	57	A			D			A
Q4055	INJECTION, EPOETIN ALFA, 1000 UNITS (FOR ESRD ON DIALYSIS)	57	A			D			A
Q4075	INJECTION, ACYCLOVIR, 5 MG	51	A			C			A
Q4076	INJECTION, DOPAMINE HCL, 40 MG	51	A			C			A
Q4077	INJECTION, TREPROSTINIL, 1 MG	51	A			C			A
Q4078	SUPPLY OF RADIOPHARMACEUTICAL DIAGNOSTIC IMAGING AGENT, AMMONIA N-13, PER DOSE	53	A		A9526	D			D

HCPCS	Long Description	PTI	MPI	Statute	X-Reff	Coverage	ASC Pay Grp	ASC Pay Grp Eff Date	Action Code
Q9920	INJECTION OF EPO, PER 1000 UNITS, AT PATIENT HCT OF 20 OR LESS	57	A			D			D
Q9921	INJECTION OF EPO, PER 1000 UNITS, AT PATIENT HCT OF 21	57	A			D			D
Q9922	INJECTION OF EPO, PER 1000 UNITS, AT PATIENT HCT OF 22	57	A			D			D
Q9923	INJECTION OF EPO, PER 1000 UNITS, AT PATIENT HCT OF 23	57	A			D			D
Q9924	INJECTION OF EPO, PER 1000 UNITS, AT PATIENT HCT OF 24	57	A			D			D
Q9925	INJECTION OF EPO, PER 1000 UNITS, AT PATIENT HCT OF 25	57	A			D			D
Q9926	INJECTION OF EPO, PER 1000 UNITS, AT PATIENT HCT OF 26	57	A			D			D
Q9927	INJECTION OF EPO, PER 1000 UNITS, AT PATIENT HCT OF 27	57	A			D			D
Q9928	INJECTION OF EPO, PER 1000 UNITS, AT PATIENT HCT OF 28	57	A			D			D
Q9929	INJECTION OF EPO, PER 1000 UNITS, AT PATIENT HCT OF 29	57	A			D			D
Q9930	INJECTION OF EPO, PER 1000 UNITS, AT PATIENT HCT OF 30	57	A			D			D
Q9931	INJECTION OF EPO, PER 1000 UNITS, AT PATIENT HCT OF 31	57	A			D			D
Q9932	INJECTION OF EPO, PER 1000 UNITS, AT PATIENT HCT OF 32	57	A			D			D
Q9933	INJECTION OF EPO, PER 1000 UNITS, AT PATIENT HCT OF 33	57	A			D			D
Q9934	INJECTION OF EPO, PER 1000 UNITS, AT PATIENT HCT OF 34	57	A			D			D
Q9935	INJECTION OF EPO, PER 1000 UNITS, AT PATIENT HCT OF 35	57	A			D			D
Q9936	INJECTION OF EPO, PER 1000 UNITS, AT PATIENT HCT OF 36	57	A			D			D
Q9937	INJECTION OF EPO, PER 1000 UNITS, AT PATIENT HCT OF 37	57	A			D			D
Q9938	INJECTION OF EPO, PER 1000 UNITS, AT PATIENT HCT OF 38	57	A			D			D
Q9939	INJECTION OF EPO, PER 1000 UNITS, AT PATIENT HCT OF 39	57	A			D			D
Q9940	INJECTION OF EPO, PER 1000 UNITS, AT PATIENT HCT OF 40 OR ABOVE	57	A			D			D
R0070	TRANSPORTATION OF PORTABLE X-RAY EQUIPMENT AND PERSONNEL TO HOME OR NURSING HOME, PER TRIP TO FACILITY OR LOCATION, ONE PATIENT SEEN	13	A			D			N
R0075	TRANSPORTATION OF PORTABLE X-RAY EQUIPMENT AND PERSONNEL TO HOME OR NURSING HOME, PER TRIP TO FACILITY OR LOCATION, MORE THAN ONE PATIENT SEEN	13	A			D			N
R0076	TRANSPORTATION OF PORTABLE EKG TO FACILITY OR LOCATION, PER PATIENT	13	A			D			N
S0009	INJECTION, BUTORPHANOL TARTRATE, 1 MG	00	9			I			D
S0010	INJECTION, SOMATREM, 5 MG	00	9		Q2015	I			N
S0011	INJECTION, SOMATROPIN, 5 MG	00	9		Q2016	I			N
S0012	BUTORPHANOL TARTRATE, NASAL SPRAY, 25 MG	00	9			I			N
S0014	TACRINE HYDROCHLORIDE, 10 MG	00	9			I			N
S0016	INJECTION, AMIKACIN SULFATE, 500 MG	00	9			I			N
S0017	INJECTION, AMINOCAPROIC ACID, 5 GRAMS	00	9			I			N

HCPCS	Long Description	PI	MPI	Statute	X-Ref	Coverage	ASC Pay Grp	ASC Pay Grp Eff Date	Action Code
S0020	INJECTION, BUPIVICAINE HYDROCHLORIDE, 30 ML	00	9			I			N
S0021	INJECTION, CEFOPERAZONE SODIUM, 1 GRAM	00	9			I			N
S0023	INJECTION, CIMETIDINE HYDROCHLORIDE, 300 MG	00	9			I			N
S0024	INJECTION, CIPROFLOXACIN, 200 MG	00	9			I			N
S0028	INJECTION, FAMOTIDINE, 20 MG	00	9			I			N
S0029	INJECTION, FLUCONAZOLE, 400 MG	00	9		J1450	I			N
S0030	INJECTION, METRONIDAZOLE, 500 MG	00	9			I			N
S0032	INJECTION, NAFCILLIN SODIUM, 2 GRAMS	00	9			I			N
S0034	INJECTION, OFLOXACIN, 400 MG	00	9			I			N
S0039	INJECTION, SULFAMETHOXAZOLE AND TRIMETHOPRIM, 10 ML	00	9			I			N
S0040	INJECTION, TICARCILLIN DISODIUM AND CLAVULANATE POTASSIUM, 3.1 GRAMS	00	9			I			N
S0071	INJECTION, ACYCLOVIR SODIUM, 50 MG	00	9			I			N
S0072	INJECTION, AMIKACIN SULFATE, 100 MG	00	9			I			N
S0073	INJECTION, AZTREONAM, 500 MG	00	9			I			N
S0074	INJECTION, CEFOTETAN DISODIUM, 500 MG	00	9			I			N
S0077	INJECTION, CLINDAMYCIN PHOSPHATE, 300 MG	00	9			I			N
S0078	INJECTION, FOSPHENYTOIN SODIUM, 750 MG	00	9			I			N
S0079	INJECTION, OCTREOTIDE ACETATE, 100 MCG (FOR DOSES OVER 1 MG USE J2352 OR C1207)	00	9			I			D
S0080	INJECTION, PENTAMIDINE ISETHIONATE, 300 MG	00	9			I			N
S0081	INJECTION, PIPERACILLIN SODIUM, 500 MG	00	9			I			N
S0085	INJECTION, GATIFLOXACIN, 200 MG	00	9		J1590	I			N
S0086	INJECTION, VERTEPORFIN, 15 MG	00	9		J3395	I			N
S0087	ALEMTUZUMAB INJECTION, 30 MG	00	9		J9010	I			N
S0088	ALEMTUZUMAB INJECTION, 30 MG	00	9			I			N
S0090	SILDENAFIL CITRATE, 25 MG	00	9			I			N
S0091	GRANISETRON HYDROCHLORIDE, 1MG (FOR CIRCUMSTANCES FALLING UNDER THE MEDICARE STATUTE, USE Q0166)	00	9			I			N

HCPCS	Long Description	PTI	MPI	Statute	X-Ref1	Coverage	ASC Pay Grp	ASC Pay Grp Eff Date	Action Code
S0092	INJECTION, HYDROMORPHONE HYDROCHLORIDE, 250 MG (LOADING DOSE FOR INFUSION PUMP)	00	9			I			N
S0093	INJECTION, MORPHINE SULFATE, 500 MG (LOADING DOSE FOR INFUSION PUMP)	00	9			I			N
S0096	INJECTION, ITRACONAZOLE, 200 MG	00	9			I			N
S0097	INJECTION, IBUTILIDE FUMARATE, 1 MG	00	9		J1742	I			N
S0098	INJECTION, SODIUM FERRIC GLUCONATE COMPLEX IN SUCROSE, 62.5 MG	00	9			I			N
S0104	ZIDOVUDINE, ORAL, 100 MG	00	9			I			N
S0106	BUPROPION HCL SUSTAINED RELEASE TABLET, 150 MG, PER BOTTLE OF 60 TABLETS	00	9			I			N
S0107	INJECTION, OMALIZUMAB, 25 MG	00	9			I			A
S0108	MERCAPTOPURINE, ORAL, 50 MG	00	9			I			N
S0112	INJECTION, DARBEPOETIN ALFA, 1 MCG	00	9		J0880	I			N
S0114	INJECTION, TREPROSTINIL SODIUM, 0.5 MG	00	9			I			N
S0115	BORTEZOMIB, 3.5 MG	00	9			I			A
S0122	INJECTION, MENOTROPINS, 75 IU	00	9			I			N
S0124	INJECTION, UROFOLLITROPIN, PURIFIED, 75 IU	00	9			I			D
S0126	INJECTION, FOLLITROPIN ALFA, 75 IU	00	9			I			N
S0128	INJECTION, FOLLITROPIN BETA, 75 IU	00	9			I			N
S0130	INJECTION, CHORIONIC GONADOTROPIN, 5000 UNITS	00	9			I			D
S0132	INJECTION, GANIRELIX ACETATE, 250 MCG	00	9			I			N
S0135	INJECTION, PEGFILGRASTIM, 6 MG	00	9			I			D
S0136	CLOZAPINE, 25 MG	00	9			I			A
S0137	DIDANOSINE (DDI), 25 MG	00	9			I			A
S0138	FINASTERIDE, 5 MG	00	9			I			A
S0139	MINOXIDIL, 10 MG	00	9			I			A
S0140	SAQUINAVIR, 200 MG	00	9			I			A
S0141	ZALCITABINE (DDC), 0.375 MG	00	9			I			A
S0155	STERILE DILUTANT FOR EPOPROSTENOL, 50ML	00	9			I			N
S0156	EXEMESTANE, 25 MG	00	9			I			N
S0157	BECAPLERMIN GEL 0.01%, 0.5 GM	00	9			I			N
S0170	ANASTROZOLE, ORAL, 1MG	00	9			I			N
S0171	INJECTION, BUMETANIDE, 0.5MG	00	9			I			N
S0172	CHLORAMBUCIL, ORAL, 2MG	00	9			I			N

HCPCS	Long Description	PI1	MPI	Statute	X-Ref1	Coverage	ASC Pay Grp	ASC Pay Grp Eff Date	Action Code
S0173	DEXAMETHASONE, ORAL, 4MG	00	9			I			N
S0174	DOLASETRON MESYLATE, ORAL 50MG (FOR CIRCUMSTANCES FALLING UNDER THE MEDICARE STATUTE, USE Q0180)	00	9			I			N
S0175	FLUTAMIDE, ORAL, 125MG	00	9			I			N
S0176	HYDROXYUREA, ORAL, 500MG	00	9			I			N
S0177	LEVAMISOLE HYDROCHLORIDE, ORAL, 50MG	00	9			I			N
S0178	LOMUSTINE, ORAL, 10MG	00	9			I			N
S0179	MEGESTROL ACETATE, ORAL, 20MG	00	9			I			N
S0181	ONDANSETRON HYDROCHLORIDE, ORAL, 4MG (FOR CIRCUMSTANCES FALLING UNDER THE	00	9			I			N
S0181	MEDICARE STATUTE, USE Q0179)								
S0182	PROCARBAZINE HYDROCHLORIDE, ORAL, 50MG	00	9			I			N
S0183	PROCHLORPERAZINE MALEATE, ORAL, 5MG (FOR CIRCUMSTANCES FALLING UNDER THE MEDICARE STATUTE, USE Q0164 - Q0165)	00	9			I			N
S0187	TAMOXIFEN CITRATE, ORAL, 10MG	00	9			I			N
S0189	TESTOSTERONE PELLET, 75MG	00	9			I			N
S0190	MIFEPRISTONE, ORAL, 200 MG	00	9			I			N
S0191	MISOPROSTOL, ORAL, 200 MCG	00	9			I			N
S0193	INJECTION, ALEFACEPT, 7.5 MG (INCLUDES DOSE PACKAGING)	00	9			I			D
S0195	PNEUMOCOCCAL CONJUGATE VACCINE, POLYVALENT, INTRAMUSCULAR, FOR CHILDREN FROM FIVE YEARS TO NINE YEARS OF AGE WHO HAVE NOT PREVIOUSLY RECEIVED THE VACCINE	00	9			I			N
S0199	MEDICALLY INDUCED ABORTION BY ORAL INGESTION OF MEDICATION INCLUDING ALL ASSOCIATED SERVICES AND SUPPLIES (E.G., PATIENT COUNSELING, OFFICE VISITS, CONFIRMATION OF PREGNANCY BY HCG, ULTRASOUND TO CONFIRM DURATION OF PREGNANCY, ULTRASOUND TO CONFIRM COMPLETION OF ABORTION) EXCEPT DRUGS	00	9			I			N
S0201	PARTIAL HOSPITALIZATION SERVICES, LESS THAN 24 HOURS, PER DIEM	00	9			I			N
S0206	PROCEDURE PERFORMED IN SURGERY SUITE IN PHYSICIANS OFFICE (LIST SEPARATELY IN ADDITION TO CODE FOR PRIMARY PROCEDURE TO DENOTE USE OF FACILITY AND EQUIPMENT)	00	9		MODSU	I			N
S0207	PARAMEDIC INTERCEPT, NON-HOSPITAL-BASED ALS SERVICE (NON-VOLUNTARY), NON-TRANSPORT	00	9			I			N
S0208	PARAMEDIC INTERCEPT, HOSPITAL-BASED ALS SERVICE (NON-VOLUNTARY), NON-TRANSPORT	00	9			I			N
S0209	WHEELCHAIR VAN, MILEAGE, PER MILE	00	9			I			N
S0215	NON-EMERGENCY TRANSPORTATION; MILEAGE, PER MILE	00	9			I			N
S0220	MEDICAL CONFERENCE BY A PHYSICIAN WITH INTERDISCIPLINARY TEAM OF HEALTH PROFESSIONALS OR REPRESENTATIVES OF COMMUNITY AGENCIES TO COORDINATE ACTIVITIES OF PATIENT CARE (PATIENT IS PRESENT): APPROXIMATELY 30 MINUTES	00	9			I			N
S0221	MEDICAL CONFERENCE BY A PHYSICIAN WITH INTERDISCIPLINARY TEAM OF HEALTH PROFESSIONALS OR REPRESENTATIVES OF COMMUNITY AGENCIES TO COORDINATE ACTIVITIES OF PATIENT CARE (PATIENT IS PRESENT): APPROXIMATELY 60 MINUTES	00	9			I			N
S0250	COMPREHENSIVE GERIATRIC ASSESSMENT AND TREATMENT PLANNING PERFORMED BY ASSESSMENT TEAM	00	9			I			N
S0255	HOSPICE REFERRAL VISIT (ADVISING PATIENT AND FAMILY OF CARE OPTIONS) PERFORMED BY NURSE, SOCIAL WORKER, OR OTHER DESIGNATED STAFF	00	9			I			N

HCPCS	Long Description	PТ1	MPI	Statute	X-Ref	Coverage	ASC Pay Grp	ASC Pay Grp Eff Date	Action Code
S0260	HISTORY AND PHYSICAL (OUTPATIENT OR OFFICE) RELATED TO SURGICAL PROCEDURE (LIST SEPARATELY IN ADDITION TO CODE FOR APPROPRIATE EVALUATION AND MANAGEMENT SERVICE)	00	9			I			N
S0302	COMPLETED EARLY PERIODIC SCREENING DIAGNOSIS AND TREATMENT (EPSDT) SERVICE (LIST IN ADDITION TO CODE FOR APPROPRIATE EVALUATION AND MANAGEMENT SERVICE)	00	9			I			N
S0310	HOSPITALIST SERVICES (LIST SEPARATELY IN ADDITION TO CODE FOR APPROPRIATE EVALUATION AND MANAGEMENT SERVICE)	00	9			I			N
S0315	DISEASE MANAGEMENT PROGRAM; INITIAL ASSESSMENT AND INITIATION OF THE PROGRAM	00	9			I			N
S0316	FOLLOW-UP/REASSESSMENT	00	9			I			N
S0317	DISEASE MANAGEMENT PROGRAM; PER DIEM	00	9			I			A
S0320	TELEPHONE CALLS BY A REGISTERED NURSE TO A DISEASE MANAGEMENT PROGRAM MEMBER FOR MONITORING PURPOSES; PER MONTH	00	9			I			N
S0340	LIFESTYLE MODIFICATION PROGRAM FOR MANAGEMENT OF CORONARY ARTERY DISEASE, INCLUDING ALL SUPPORTIVE SERVICES; FIRST QUARTER / STAGE	00	9			I			N
S0341	LIFESTYLE MODIFICATION PROGRAM FOR MANAGEMENT OF CORONARY ARTERY DISEASE, INCLUDING ALL SUPPORTIVE SERVICES; SECOND OR THIRD QUARTER / STAGE	00	9			I			N
S0342	LIFESTYLE MODIFICATION PROGRAM FOR MANAGEMENT OF CORONARY ARTERY DISEASE, INCLUDING ALL SUPPORTIVE SERVICES; FOURTH QUARTER / STAGE	00	9			I			N
S0390	ROUTINE FOOT CARE; REMOVAL AND/OR TRIMMING OF CORNS, CALLUSES AND/OR NAILS AND PREVENTIVE MAINTENANCE IN SPECIFIC MEDICAL CONDITIONS (E.G. DIABETES), PER VISIT	00	9			I			N
S0395	IMPRESSION CASTING OF A FOOT PERFORMED BY A PRACTITIONER OTHER THAN THE MANUFACTURER OF THE ORTHOTIC	00	9			I			N
S0400	GLOBAL FEE FOR EXTRACORPOREAL SHOCK WAVE LITHOTRIPSY TREATMENT OF KIDNEY STONE(S)	00	9			I			N
S0500	DISPOSABLE CONTACT LENS, PER LENS	00	9			I			N
S0504	SINGLE VISION PRESCRIPTION LENS (SAFETY, ATHLETIC, OR SUNGLASS), PER LENS	00	9			I			N
S0506	BIFOCAL VISION PRESCRIPTION LENS (SAFETY, ATHLETIC, OR SUNGLASS), PER LENS	00	9			I			N
S0508	TRIFOCAL VISION PRESCRIPTION LENS (SAFETY, ATHLETIC, OR SUNGLASS), PER LENS	00	9			I			N
S0510	NON-PRESCRIPTION LENS (SAFETY, ATHLETIC, OR SUNGLASS), PER LENS	00	9			I			N
S0512	DAILY WEAR SPECIALTY CONTACT LENS, PER LENS	00	9			I			N
S0514	COLOR CONTACT LENS, PER LENS	00	9			I			N
S0516	SAFETY EYEGLASS FRAMES	00	9			I			N
S0518	SUNGLASSES FRAMES	00	9			I			N
S0580	POLYCARBONATE LENS (LIST THIS CODE IN ADDITION TO THE BASIC CODE FOR THE LENS)	00	9			I			N
S0581	NONSTANDARD LENS (LIST THIS CODE IN ADDITION TO THE BASIC CODE FOR THE LENS)	00	9			I			N
S0590	INTEGRAL LENS SERVICE, MISCELLANEOUS SERVICES REPORTED SEPARATELY	00	9			I			N
S0592	COMPREHENSIVE CONTACT LENS EVALUATION	00	9			I			N
S0601	SCREENING PROCTOSCOPY	00	9			I			N
S0605	DIGITAL RECTAL EXAMINATION, ANNUAL	00	9			I			N
S0610	ANNUAL GYNECOLOGICAL EXAMINATION, NEW PATIENT	00	9			I			N
S0612	ANNUAL GYNECOLOGICAL EXAMINATION, ESTABLISHED PATIENT	00	9			I			N

HCPCS	Long Description	PT	MPI	Statute	X-Ref1	Coverage	ASC Pay Grp	ASC Pay Grp Eff Date	Action Code
S0620	ROUTINE OPHTHALMOLOGICAL EXAMINATION INCLUDING REFRACTION; NEW PATIENT	00	9			I			N
S0621	ROUTINE OPHTHALMOLOGICAL EXAMINATION INCLUDING REFRACTION; ESTABLISHED PATIENT	00	9			I			N
S0622	PHYSICAL EXAM FOR COLLEGE, NEW OR ESTABLISHED PATIENT (LIST SEPARATELY IN ADDITION TO APPROPRIATE EVALUATION AND MANAGEMENT CODE)	00	9			I			N
S0630	REMOVAL OF SUTURES; BY A PHYSICIAN OTHER THAN THE PHYSICIAN WHO ORIGINALLY CLOSED THE WOUND	00	9			I			N
S0800	LASER IN SITU KERATOMILEUSIS (LASIK)	00	9			I			N
S0810	PHOTOREFRACTIVE KERATECTOMY (PRK)	00	9			I			N
S0812	PHOTOTHERAPEUTIC KERATECTOMY (PTK)	00	9			I			N
S0820	COMPUTERIZED CORNEAL TOPOGRAPHY, UNILATERAL	00	9			I			N
S0830	ULTRASOUND PACHYMETRY TO DETERMINE CORNEAL THICKNESS, WITH INTERPRETATION AND REPORT, UNILATERAL	00	9			I			N
S1001	DELUXE ITEM, PATIENT AWARE (LIST IN ADDITION TO CODE FOR BASIC ITEM)	00	9			I			N
S1002	CUSTOMIZED ITEM (LIST IN ADDITION TO CODE FOR BASIC ITEM)	00	9			I			N
S1015	IV TUBING EXTENSION SET	00	9			I			N
S1016	NON-PVC (POLYVINYL CHLORIDE) INTRAVENOUS ADMINISTRATION SET, FOR USE WITH DRUGS THAT ARE NOT STABLE IN PVC E.G. PACLITAXEL	00	9			I			N
S1025	INHALED NITRIC OXIDE FOR THE TREATMENT OF HYPOXIC RESPIRATORY FAILURE IN THE NEONATE; PER DIEM	00	9			I			N
S1030	CONTINUOUS NONINVASIVE GLUCOSE MONITORING DEVICE, PURCHASE (FOR PHYSICIAN INTERPRETATION OF DATA, USE CPT CODE)	00	9			I			N
S1031	CONTINUOUS NONINVASIVE GLUCOSE MONITORING DEVICE, RENTAL, INCLUDING SENSOR, SENSOR REPLACEMENT, AND DOWNLOAD TO MONITOR (FOR PHYSICIAN INTERPRETATION OF DATA, USE CPT CODE)	00	9			I			N
S1040	CRANIAL REMOLDING ORTHOSIS, RIGID, WITH SOFT INTERFACE MATERIAL, CUSTOM FABRICATED, INCLUDES FITTING AND ADJUSTMENT(S)	00	9			I			N
S2050	DONOR ENTERECTOMY, WITH PREPARATION AND MAINTENANCE OF ALLOGRAFT; FROM CADAVER DONOR	00	9		44132	I			N
S2052	TRANSPLANTATION OF SMALL INTESTINE ALLOGRAFT (THERE ARE CPT CODES AVAILABLE FOR INTESTINAL ALLOTRANSPLANTATION - 44135 FOR GRAFT FROM CADAVER DONOR OR 44136 FOR GRAFT FROM LIVING DONOR)	00	9			I			N
S2053	TRANSPLANTATION OF SMALL INTESTINE AND LIVER ALLOGRAFTS	00	9			I			N
S2054	TRANSPLANTATION OF MULTIVISCERAL ORGANS	00	9			I			N
S2055	HARVESTING OF DONOR MULTIVISCERAL ORGANS, WITH PREPARATION AND MAINTENANCE OF ALLOGRAFTS; FROM CADAVER DONOR	00	9			I			N
S2060	LOBAR LUNG TRANSPLANTATION	00	9			I			N
S2061	DONOR LOBECTOMY (LUNG) FOR TRANSPLANTATION, LIVING DONOR	00	9			I			N
S2065	SIMULTANEOUS PANCREAS KIDNEY TRANSPLANTATION	00	9			I			N
S2070	CYSTOURETHROSCOPY, WITH URETEROSCOPY AND/OR PYELOSCOPY; WITH ENDOSCOPIC LASER TREATMENT OF URETERAL CALCULI (INCLUDES URETERAL CATHETERIZATION)	00	9			I			A

HCPCS	Long Description	PII	MPI	Statute	X-Ref	Coverage	ASC Pay Grp	ASC Pay Grp Eff Date	Action Code
S2080	LASER-ASSISTED UVULOPALATOPLASTY (LAUP)	00	9			I			N
S2085	LAPAROSCOPY, GASTRIC RESTRICTIVE PROCEDURE, WITH GASTRIC BYPASS FOR MORBID OBESITY, WITH SHORT LIMB (LESS THAN 100 CM) ROUX-EN-Y GASTROENTEROSTOMY	00	9			I			A
S2090	ABLATION, OPEN, ONE OR MORE RENAL TUMOR(S); CRYOSURGICAL	00	9			I			A
S2091	ABLATION, PERCUTANEOUS, ONE OR MORE RENAL TUMOR(S); CRYOSURGICAL	00	9			I			A
S2095	TRANSCATHETER OCCLUSION OR EMBOLIZATION FOR TUMOR DESTRUCTION, PERCUTANEOUS, ANY METHOD, USING YTTRIUM-90 MICROSPHERES	00	9			I			A
S2102	ISLET CELL TISSUE TRANSPLANT FROM PANCREAS; ALLOGENEIC	00	9			I			N
S2103	ADRENAL TISSUE TRANSPLANT TO BRAIN	00	9			I			N
S2107	ADOPTIVE IMMUNOTHERAPY I.E. DEVELOPMENT OF SPECIFIC ANTI-TUMOR REACTIVITY (E.G. TUMOR-INFILTRATING LYMPHOCYTE THERAPY) PER COURSE OF TREATMENT	00	9			I			N
S2109	AUTOLOGOUS CHONDROCYTE TRANSPLANTATION (PREPARATION OF AUTOLOGOUS CULTURED CHONDROCYTES)	00	9		J7330	I			N
S2112	ARTHROSCOPY, KNEE, SURGICAL FOR HARVESTING OF CARTILAGE (CHONDROCYTE CELLS)	00	9			I			N
S2113	ARTHROSCOPY, KNEE, SURGICAL FOR IMPLANTATION OF CULTURED ANALOGOUS CHONDROCYTES	00	9			I			A
S2115	OSTEOTOMY, PERIACETABULAR, WITH INTERNAL FIXATION	00	9			I			N
S2120	LOW DENSITY LIPOPROTEIN (LDL) APHERESIS USING HEPARIN-INDUCED EXTRACORPOREAL LDL PRECIPITATION	00	9			I			N
S2130	ENDOLUMINAL RADIOFREQUENCY ABLATION OF REFLUXING SAPHENOUS VEINS	00	9			I			N
S2135	NEUROLYSIS, BY INJECTION, OF METATARSAL NEUROMA/INTERDIGITAL NEURITIS, ANY INTERSPACE OF THE FOOT	00	9			I			A
S2140	CORD BLOOD HARVESTING FOR TRANSPLANTATION, ALLOGENEIC	00	9			I			N
S2142	CORD BLOOD-DERIVED STEM-CELL TRANSPLANTATION, ALLOGENEIC	00	9			I			N
S2150	BONE MARROW OR BLOOD-DERIVED PERIPHERAL STEM CELL HARVESTING AND TRANSPLANTATION, ALLOGENIC OR AUTOLOGOUS, INCLUDING PHERESIS, HIGH-DOSE CHEMOTHERAPY, AND THE NUMBER OF DAYS OF POST-TRANSPLANT CARE IN THE GLOBAL DEFINITION (INCLUDING DRUGS; HOSPITALIZATION; MEDICAL, SURGICAL, DIAGNOSTIC AND EMERGENCY SERVICES)	00	9			I			C
S2180	DONOR LEUKOCYTE INFUSION (E.G. DLI, DONOR LYMPHOCYTE INFUSION, DONOR BUFFY COAT CELL TRANSFUSION, DONOR PERIPHERAL BLOOD MONOCYTE TRANSFUSION)	00	9		38242	I			N
S2190	SUBCUTANEOUS IMPLANTATION OF MEDICATION PELLET(S)	00	9		11980	I			N
S2202	ECHOSCLEROTHERAPY	00	9			I			N
S2204	TRANSMYOCARDIAL LASER REVASCULARIZATION	00	9		33140	I			N
S2205	MINIMALLY INVASIVE DIRECT CORONARY ARTERY BYPASS SURGERY INVOLVING MINI-THORACOTOMY OR MINI-STERNOTOMY SURGERY, PERFORMED UNDER DIRECT VISION; USING ARTERIAL GRAFT(S), SINGLE CORONARY ARTERIAL GRAFT	00	9			I			N

HCPCS	Long Description	PI	MPI	Statute	X-Ref1	Coverage	ASC Pay Grp	ASC Pay Grp Eff Date	Action Code
S2206	MINIMALLY INVASIVE DIRECT CORONARY ARTERY BYPASS SURGERY INVOLVING MINI-THORACOTOMY OR MINI-STERNOTOMY SURGERY, PERFORMED UNDER DIRECT VISION; USING ARTERIAL GRAFT(S), TWO CORONARY ARTERIAL GRAFTS	00	9			I			N
S2207	MINIMALLY INVASIVE DIRECT CORONARY ARTERY BYPASS SURGERY INVOLVING MINI-THORACOTOMY OR MINI-STERNOTOMY SURGERY, PERFORMED UNDER DIRECT VISION; USING VENOUS GRAFT ONLY, SINGLE CORONARY VENOUS GRAFT	00	9			I			N
S2208	MINIMALLY INVASIVE DIRECT CORONARY ARTERY BYPASS SURGERY INVOLVING MINI-THORACOTOMY OR MINI-STERNOTOMY SURGERY, PERFORMED UNDER DIRECT VISION; USING SINGLE ARTERIAL AND VENOUS GRAFT(S), SINGLE VENOUS GRAFT	00	9			I			N
S2209	MINIMALLY INVASIVE DIRECT CORONARY ARTERY BYPASS SURGERY INVOLVING MINI-THORACOTOMY OR MINI-STERNOTOMY SURGERY, PERFORMED UNDER DIRECT VISION; USING TWO ARTERIAL GRAFTS AND SINGLE VENOUS GRAFT	00	9			I			N
S2210	CRYOSURGICAL ABLATION (IN SITU DESTRUCTION) OF TUMOROUS TISSUE, ONE OR MORE LESIONS; LIVER	00	9			I			N
S2211	TRANSCATHETER PLACEMENT OF INTRAVASCULAR STENT(S), CAROTID ARTERY, PERCUTANEOUS, UNILATERAL (IF PERFORMED BILATERALLY, USE-50 MODIFIER)	00	9			I			N
S2213	IMPLANTATION OF GASTRIC ELECTRICAL STIMULATION DEVICE	00	9			I			A
S2220	THROMBECTOMY, CORONARY; BY MECHANICAL MEANS (E.G. USING RHEOLYTIC CATHETER)	00	9			I			N
S2225	MYRINGOTOMY, LASER-ASSISTED	00	9			I			A
S2230	IMPLANTATION OF MAGNETIC COMPONENT OF SEMI-IMPLANTABLE HEARING DEVICE ON OSSICLES IN MIDDLE EAR	00	9			I			A
S2235	IMPLANTATION OF AUDITORY BRAIN STEM IMPLANT	00	9			I			A
S2250	UTERINE ARTERY EMBOLIZATION FOR UTERINE FIBROIDS	00	9			I			N
S2260	INDUCED ABORTION, 17 TO 24 WEEKS, ANY SURGICAL METHOD	00	9			I			N
S2262	ABORTION FOR MATERNAL INDICATION, 25 WEEKS OR GREATER	00	9			I			N
S2265	ABORTION FOR FETAL INDICATION, 25-28 WEEKS	00	9			I			N
S2266	ABORTION FOR FETAL INDICATION, 29-31 WEEKS	00	9			I			N
S2267	ABORTION FOR FETAL INDICATION, 32 WEEKS OR GREATER	00	9			I			N
S2300	ARTHROSCOPY, SHOULDER, SURGICAL; WITH THERMALLY-INDUCED CAPSULORRHAPHY	00	9			I			N
S2340	CHEMODENERVATION OF ABDUCTOR MUSCLE(S) OF VOCAL CORD	00	9			I			N
S2341	CHEMODENERVATION OF ADDUCTOR MUSCLE(S) OF VOCAL CORD	00	9			I			N
S2342	NASAL ENDOSCOPY FOR POST-OPERATIVE DEBRIDEMENT FOLLOWING FUNCTIONAL ENDOSCOPIC SINUS SURGERY, NASAL AND/OR SINUS CAVITY(S), UNILATERAL OR BILATERAL INCLUDING OSTEOPHYTECTOMY; LUMBAR, SINGLE INTERSPACE	00	9			I			N
S2350	DISKECTOMY, ANTERIOR, WITH DECOMPRESSION OF SPINAL CORD AND/OR NERVE ROOT(S),	00	9			I			N
S2351	DISKECTOMY, ANTERIOR, WITH DECOMPRESSION OF SPINAL CORD AND/OR NERVE ROOT(S), INCLUDING OSTEOPHYTECTOMY; LUMBAR, EACH ADDITIONAL INTERSPACE (LIST SEPARATELY IN ADDITION TO CODE FOR PRIMARY PROCEDURE)	00	9			I			N
S2360	PERCUTANEOUS VERTEBROPLASTY, ONE VERTEBRAL BODY, UNILATERAL OR BILATERAL INJECTION; CERVICAL	00	9			I			N

HCPCS	Long Description	PH	MPI	Statute	X-Ref1	Coverage	ASC Pay Grp	ASC Pay Grp Eff Date	Action Code
S2361	EACH ADDITIONAL CERVICAL VERTEBRAL BODY (LIST SEPARATELY IN ADDITION TO CODE FOR PRIMARY PROCEDURE)	00	9			I			N
S2362	KYPHOPLASTY, ONE VERTEBRAL BODY, UNILATERAL OR BILATERAL INJECTION	00	9			I			A
S2363	KYPHOPLASTY, ONE VERTEBRAL BODY, UNILATERAL OR BILATERAL INJECTION; EACH ADDITIONAL VERTEBRAL BODY (LIST SEPARATELY IN ADDITION TO CODE FOR PRIMARY PROCEDURE)	00	9			I			A
S2370	INTRADISCAL ELECTROTHERMAL THERAPY; SINGLE INTERSPACE	00	9			I			N
S2371	EACH ADDITIONAL INTERSPACE (LIST SEPARATELY IN ADDITION TO CODE FOR PRIMARY PROCEDURE)	00	9			I			N
S2400	REPAIR, CONGENITAL DIAPHRAGMATIC HERNIA IN THE FETUS USING TEMPORARY TRACHEAL OCCLUSION, PROCEDURE PERFORMED IN UTERO	00	9			I			N
S2401	REPAIR, URINARY TRACT OBSTRUCTION IN THE FETUS, PROCEDURE PERFORMED IN UTERO	00	9			I			N
S2402	REPAIR, CONGENITAL CYSTIC ADENOMATOID MALFORMATION IN THE FETUS, PROCEDURE PERFORMED IN UTERO	00	9			I			N
S2403	REPAIR, EXTRALOBAR PULMONARY SEQUESTRATION IN THE FETUS, PROCEDURE PERFORMED IN UTERO	00	9			I			N
S2404	REPAIR, MYELOMENINGOCELE IN THE FETUS, PROCEDURE PERFORMED IN UTERO	00	9			I			N
S2405	REPAIR OF SACROCOCCYGEAL TERATOMA IN THE FETUS, PROCEDURE PERFORMED IN UTERO	00	9			I			N
S2409	REPAIR, CONGENITAL MALFORMATION OF FETUS, PROCEDURE PERFORMED IN UTERO, NOT OTHERWISE CLASSIFIED	00	9			I			N
S2411	FETOSCOPIC LASER THERAPY FOR TREATMENT OF TWIN-TO-TWIN TRANSFUSION SYNDROME	00	9			I			N
S3000	DIABETIC INDICATOR; RETINAL EYE EXAM, DILATED, BILATERAL	00	9			I			A
S3600	STAT LABORATORY REQUEST (SITUATIONS OTHER THAN S3601)	00	9			I			N
S3601	EMERGENCY STAT LABORATORY CHARGE FOR PATIENT WHO IS HOMEBOUND OR RESIDING IN A NURSING FACILITY	00	9			I			N
S3620	NEWBORN METABOLIC SCREENING PANEL, INCLUDES TEST KIT, POSTAGE AND THE LABORATORY TESTS SPECIFIED BY THE STATE FOR INCLUSION IN THIS PANEL (E.G. GALACTOSE; HEMOGLOBIN, ELECTROPHORESIS; HYDROXYPROGESTERONE, 17-D; PHENYLANINE (PKU); AND THYROXINE, TOTAL)	00	9			I			N
S3625	MATERNAL SERUM TRIPLE MARKER SCREEN INCLUDING ALPHA-FETOPROTEIN (AFP), ESTRIOL, AND HUMAN CHORIONIC GONADOTROPIN (HCG)	00	9			I			A
S3630	EOSINOPHIL COUNT, BLOOD, DIRECT	00	9			I			N
S3645	HIV-1 ANTIBODY TESTING OF ORAL MUCOSAL TRANSUDATE	00	9			I			N
S3650	SALIVA TEST, HORMONE LEVEL; DURING MENOPAUSE	00	9			I			N
S3652	SALIVA TEST, HORMONE LEVEL; TO ASSESS PRETERM LABOR RISK	00	9			I			N
S3655	ANTISPERM ANTIBODIES TEST (IMMUNOBEAD)	00	9			I			N
S3700	BLADDER TUMOR-ASSOCIATED ANTIGEN TEST	00	9			I			N
S3701	IMMUNOASSAY FOR NUCLEAR MATRIX PROTEIN 22 (NMP-22), QUANTITATIVE	00	9			I			N
S3708	GASTROINTESTINAL FAT ABSORPTION STUDY	00	9			I			N

HCPCS	Long Description	PII	MPI	Statute	X-Ref†	Coverage	ASC Pay Grp	ASC Pay Grp Eff Date	Action Code
S3818	COMPLETE GENE SEQUENCE ANALYSIS; BRCA1 GENE	00	9			I			N
S3819	COMPLETE GENE SEQUENCE ANALYSIS; BRCA2 GENE	00	9			I			N
S3820	COMPLETE BRCA1 AND BRCA2 GENE SEQUENCE ANALYSIS FOR SUSCEPTIBILITY TO BREAST AND OVARIAN CANCER	00	9			I			A
S3822	SINGLE MUTATION ANALYSIS (IN INDIVIDUAL WITH A KNOWN BRCA1 OR BRCA2 MUTATION IN THE FAMILY) FOR SUSCEPTIBILITY TO BREAST AND OVARIAN CANCER	00	9			I			A
S3823	THREE-MUTATION BRCA1 AND BRCA2 ANALYSIS FOR SUSCEPTIBILITY TO BREAST AND OVARIAN CANCER IN ASHKENAZI INDIVIDUALS	00	9			I			A
S3828	COMPLETE GENE SEQUENCE ANALYSIS; MLH1 GENE	00	9			I			A
S3829	COMPLETE GENE SEQUENCE ANALYSIS; MLH2 GENE	00	9			I			A
S3830	COMPLETE MLH1 AND MLH2 GENE SEQUENCE ANALYSIS FOR HEREDITARY NONPOLYPOSIS COLORECTAL CANCER (HNPCC) GENETIC TESTING	00	9			I			N
S3831	SINGLE-MUTATION ANALYSIS (IN INDIVIDUAL WITH A KNOWN MLH1 AND MLH2 MUTATION IN THE FAMILY) FOR HEREDITARY NONPOLYPOSIS COLORECTAL CANCER (HNPCC) GENETIC TESTING	00	9			I			N
S3833	COMPLETE APC GENE SEQUENCE ANALYSIS FOR SUSCEPTIBILITY TO FAMILIAL ADENOMATOUS POLYPOSIS (FAP) AND ATTENUATED FAP	00	9			I			A
S3834	SINGLE-MUTATION ANALYSIS (IN INDIVIDUAL WITH A KNOWN APC MUTATION IN THE FAMILY) FOR SUSCEPTIBILITY TO FAMILIAL ADENOMATOUS POLYPOSIS (FAP) AND ATTENUATED FAP	00	9			I			A
S3835	COMPLETE GENE SEQUENCE ANALYSIS FOR CYSTIC FIBROSIS GENETIC TESTING	00	9			I			N
S3837	COMPLETE GENE SEQUENCE ANALYSIS FOR HEMOCHROMATOSIS GENETIC TESTING	00	9			I			N
S3840	DNA ANALYSIS FOR GERMLINE MUTATIONS OF THE RET PROTO-ONCOGENE FOR SUSCEPTIBILITY TO MULTIPLE ENDOCRINE NEOPLASIA TYPE 2	00	9			I			A
S3841	GENETIC TESTING FOR RETINOBLASTOMA	00	9			I			A
S3842	GENETIC TESTING FOR VON HIPPEL-LINDAU DISEASE	00	9			I			A
S3843	DNA ANALYSIS OF THE F5 GENE FOR SUSCEPTIBILITY TO FACTOR V LEIDEN THROMBOPHILIA	00	9			I			A
S3844	DNA ANALYSIS OF THE CONNEXIN 26 GENE (GJB2) FOR SUSCEPTIBILITY TO CONGENITAL, PROFOUND DEAFNESS	00	9			I			A
S3845	GENETIC TESTING FOR ALPHA-THALASSEMIA	00	9			I			A
S3846	GENETIC TESTING FOR HEMOGLOBIN E BETA-THALASSEMIA	00	9			I			A
S3847	GENETIC TESTING FOR TAY-SACHS DISEASE	00	9			I			A
S3848	GENETIC TESTING FOR GAUCHER DISEASE	00	9			I			A
S3849	GENETIC TESTING FOR NIEMANN-PICK DISEASE	00	9			I			A
S3850	GENETIC TESTING FOR SICKLE CELL ANEMIA	00	9			I			A
S3851	GENETIC TESTING FOR CANAVAN DISEASE	00	9			I			A
S3852	DNA ANALYSIS FOR APOE EPILSON 4 ALLELE FOR SUSCEPTIBILITY TO ALZHEIMERS DISEASE	00	9			I			A
S3853	GENETIC TESTING FOR MYOTONIC MUSCULAR DYSTROPHY	00	9			I			A
S3900	SURFACE ELECTROMYOGRAPHY (EMG)	00	9			I			N
S3902	BALLISTOCARDIOGRAM	00	9			I			N

HCPCS	Long Description	PTI	MPI	Statute	X-Ref	Coverage	ASC Pay Grp	ASC Pay Grp Eff Date	Action Code
S3904	MASTERS TWO STEP	00	9			I			N
S3906	TRANSFUSION, DIRECT, BLOOD OR BLOOD COMPONENTS	00	9			I			N
S4005	INTERIM LABOR FACILITY GLOBAL (LABOR OCCURRING BUT NOT RESULTING IN DELIVERY)	00	9			I			N
S4011	IN VITRO FERTILIZATION; INCLUDING BUT NOT LIMITED TO IDENTIFICATION AND INCUBATION OF MATURE OOCYTES, FERTILIZATION WITH SPERM, INCUBATION OF EMBRYO(S), AND SUBSEQUENT VISUALIZATION FOR DETERMINATION OF DEVELOPMENT	00	9			I			N
S4013	COMPLETE CYCLE, GAMETE INTRAFALLOPIAN TRANSFER (GIFT), CASE RATE	00	9			I			N
S4014	COMPLETE CYCLE, ZYGOTE INTRAFALLOPIAN TRANSFER (ZIFT), CASE RATE	00	9			I			N
S4015	COMPLETE IN VITRO FERTILIZATION CYCLE, NOT OTHERWISE SPECIFIED, CASE RATE	00	9			I			N
S4016	FROZEN IN VITRO FERTILIZATION CYCLE, CASE RATE	00	9			I			N
S4017	INCOMPLETE CYCLE, TREATMENT CANCELLED PRIOR TO STIMULATION, CASE RATE	00	9			I			N
S4018	FROZEN EMBRYO TRANSFER PROCEDURE CANCELLED BEFORE TRANSFER, CASE RATE	00	9			I			N
S4020	IN VITRO FERTILIZATION PROCEDURE CANCELLED BEFORE ASPIRATION, CASE RATE	00	9			I			N
S4021	IN VITRO FERTILIZATION PROCEDURE CANCELLED AFTER ASPIRATION, CASE RATE	00	9			I			N
S4022	ASSISTED OOCYTE FERTILIZATION, CASE RATE	00	9			I			N
S4023	DONOR EGG CYCLE, INCOMPLETE, CASE RATE	00	9			I			N
S4025	DONOR SERVICES FOR IN VITRO FERTILIZATION (SPERM OR EMBRYO), CASE RATE	00	9			I			N
S4026	PROCUREMENT OF DONOR SPERM FROM SPERM BANK	00	9			I			N
S4027	STORAGE OF PREVIOUSLY FROZEN EMBRYOS	00	9			I			N
S4028	MICROSURGICAL EPIDIDYMAL SPERM ASPIRATION (MESA)	00	9			I			N
S4030	SPERM PROCUREMENT AND CRYOPRESERVATION SERVICES; INITIAL VISIT	00	9			I			N
S4031	SPERM PROCUREMENT AND CRYOPRESERVATION SERVICES; SUBSEQUENT VISIT	00	9			I			N
S4035	STIMULATED INTRAUTERINE INSEMINATION (IUI), CASE RATE	00	9			I			N
S4036	INTRAVAGINAL CULTURE (IVC), CASE RATE	00	9			I			N
S4037	CRYOPRESERVED EMBRYO TRANSFER, CASE RATE	00	9			I			N
S4040	MONITORING AND STORAGE OF CRYOPRESERVED EMBRYOS, PER 30 DAYS	00	9			I			N
S4980	LEVONORGESTREL - RELEASING INTRAUTERINE SYSTEM, EACH	00	9			I			N
S4981	INSERTION OF LEVONORGESTREL-RELEASING INTRAUTERINE SYSTEM	00	9			I			N
S4989	CONTRACEPTIVE INTRAUTERINE DEVICE (E.G. PROGESTACERT IUD), INCLUDING IMPLANTS 'AND SUPPLIES	00	9			I			N
S4990	NICOTINE PATCHES, LEGEND	00	9			I			N
S4991	NICOTINE PATCHES, NON-LEGEND	00	9			I			N

HCPCS	Long Description	PII	MPI	Statute	X-Ref	Coverage	ASC Pay Grp	ASC Pay Grp Eff Date	Action Code
S4993	CONTRACEPTIVE PILLS FOR BIRTH CONTROL	00	9			I			N
S4995	SMOKING CESSATION GUM	00	9			I			N
S5000	PRESCRIPTION DRUG, GENERIC	00	9			I			N
S5001	PRESCRIPTION DRUG, BRAND NAME	00	9			I			N
S5002	FAT EMULSION 10% IN 250 ML, WITH ADMINISTRATION SET	00	9			I			N
S5003	FAT EMULSION 20% IN 250 ML, WITH ADMINISTRATION SET	00	9			I			N
S5010	5% DEXTROSE AND 0.45% NORMAL SALINE, 1000 ML	00	9			I			N
S5011	5% DEXTROSE IN LACTATED RINGERS, 1000 ML	00	9			I			N
S5012	5% DEXTROSE WITH POTASSIUM CHLORIDE, 1000 ML	00	9			I			N
S5013	5% DEXTROSE/0.45% NORMAL SALINE WITH POTASSIUM CHLORIDE AND MAGNESIUM SULFATE, 1000 ML	00	9			I			N
S5014	5% DEXTROSE/0.45% NORMAL SALINE WITH POTASSIUM CHLORIDE AND MAGNESIUM SULFATE, 1500 ML	00	9			I			N
S5016	ANTIBIOTIC ADMINISTRATION SUPPLIES (WITH PUMP), PER DAY	00	9			I			N
S5017	ANTIBIOTIC ADMINISTRATION SUPPLIES (WITHOUT PUMP), PER DAY	00	9			I			N
S5018	PAIN THERAPY ADMINISTRATION SUPPLIES (PCA OR CONTINUOUS), PER DAY	00	9			I			N
S5019	CHEMOTHERAPY ADMINISTRATION SUPPLIES (WITH PUMP), PER DIEM	00	9			I			N
S5020	CHEMOTHERAPY ADMINISTRATION SUPPLIES (WITHOUT PUMP), PER DIEM	00	9			I			N
S5021	HYDRATION THERAPY ADMINISTRATION SUPPLIES, PER DIEM	00	9			I			N
S5022	GROWTH HORMONE THERAPY (E.G., PROTROPIN, HUMATROPE)	00	9			I			N
S5025	INFUSION PUMP RENTAL, PER DIEM	00	9			I			N
S5035	HOME INFUSION THERAPY, ROUTINE SERVICE OF INFUSION DEVICE (E.G. PUMP MAINTENANCE)	00	9			I			N
S5036	HOME INFUSION THERAPY, REPAIR OF INFUSION DEVICE (E.G. PUMP REPAIR)	00	9			I			N
S5100	DAY CARE SERVICES, ADULT; PER 15 MINUTES	00	9			I			N
S5101	DAY CARE SERVICES, ADULT; PER HALF DAY	00	9			I			N
S5102	DAY CARE SERVICES, ADULT; PER DIEM	00	9			I			N
S5105	DAY CARE SERVICES, CENTER-BASED; SERVICES NOT INCLUDED IN PROGRAM FEE, PER DIEM	00	9			I			N
S5108	HOME CARE TRAINING TO HOME CARE CLIENT, PER 15 MINUTES	00	9			I			A

HCPCS	Long Description	PII	MPI	Statute	X-Ref1	Coverage	ASC Pay Grp	ASC Pay Grp Eff Date	Action Code
S5109	HOME CARE TRAINING TO HOME CARE CLIENT, PER SESSION	00	9			I			A
S5110	HOME CARE TRAINING, FAMILY; PER 15 MINUTES	00	9			I			N
S5111	HOME CARE TRAINING, FAMILY; PER SESSION	00	9			I			N
S5115	HOME CARE TRAINING, NON-FAMILY; PER 15 MINUTES	00	9			I			N
S5116	HOME CARE TRAINING, NON-FAMILY; PER SESSION	00	9			I			N
S5120	CHORE SERVICES; PER 15 MINUTES	00	9			I			N
S5121	CHORE SERVICES; PER DIEM	00	9			I			N
S5125	ATTENDANT CARE SERVICES; PER 15 MINUTES	00	9			I			N
S5126	ATTENDANT CARE SERVICES; PER DIEM	00	9			I			N
S5130	HOMEMAKER SERVICE, NOS; PER 15 MINUTES	00	9			I			N
S5131	HOMEMAKER SERVICE, NOS; PER DIEM	00	9			I			N
S5135	COMPANION CARE, ADULT (E.G. IADL/ADL); PER 15 MINUTES	00	9			I			N
S5136	COMPANION CARE, ADULT (E.G. IADL/ADL); PER DIEM	00	9			I			N
S5140	FOSTER CARE, ADULT; PER DIEM	00	9			I			N
S5141	FOSTER CARE, ADULT; PER MONTH	00	9			I			N
S5145	FOSTER CARE, THERAPEUTIC, CHILD; PER DIEM	00	9			I			N
S5146	FOSTER CARE, THERAPEUTIC, CHILD; PER MONTH	00	9			I			N
S5150	UNSKILLED RESPITE CARE, NOT HOSPICE; PER 15 MINUTES	00	9			I			N
S5151	UNSKILLED RESPITE CARE, NOT HOSPICE; PER DIEM	00	9			I			N
S5160	EMERGENCY RESPONSE SYSTEM; INSTALLATION AND TESTING	00	9			I			N
S5161	EMERGENCY RESPONSE SYSTEM; SERVICE FEE, PER MONTH (EXCLUDES INSTALLATION AND TESTING)	00	9			I			N
S5162	EMERGENCY RESPONSE SYSTEM; PURCHASE ONLY	00	9			I			N
S5165	HOME MODIFICATIONS; PER SERVICE	00	9			I			N
S5170	HOME DELIVERED MEALS, INCLUDING PREPARATION; PER MEAL	00	9			I			N

HCPCS	Long Description	PTI	MPI	Statute	X-Refl	Coverage	ASC Pay Grp	ASC Pay Grp Eff Date	Action Code
S5175	LAUNDRY SERVICE, EXTERNAL, PROFESSIONAL; PER ORDER	00	9			I			N
S5180	HOME HEALTH RESPIRATORY THERAPY, INITIAL EVALUATION	00	9			I			N
S5181	HOME HEALTH RESPIRATORY THERAPY, NOS, PER DIEM	00	9			I			N
S5185	MEDICATION REMINDER SERVICE, NON-FACE-TO-FACE; PER MONTH	00	9			I			N
S5190	WELLNESS ASSESSMENT, PERFORMED BY NON-PHYSICIAN	00	9			I			N
S5199	PERSONAL CARE ITEM, NOS, EACH	00	9			I			N
S5497	HOME INFUSION THERAPY, CATHETER CARE / MAINTENANCE, NOT OTHERWISE CLASSIFIED; INCLUDES ADMINISTRATIVE SERVICES, PROFESSIONAL PHARMACY SERVICES, CARE COORDINATION AND ALL NECESSARY SUPPLIES AND EQUIPMENT, (DRUGS AND NURSING VISITS CODED SEPARATELY) PER DIEM	00	9			I			N
S5498	HOME INFUSION THERAPY, CATHETER CARE / MAINTENANCE, SIMPLE (SINGLE LUMEN), INCLUDES ADMINISTRATIVE SERVICES, PROFESSIONAL PHARMACY SERVICES, CARE COORDINATION AND ALL NECESSARY SUPPLIES AND EQUIPMENT, (DRUGS AND NURSING VISITS CODED SEPARATELY) PER DIEM	00	9			I			N
S5501	HOME INFUSION THERAPY, CATHETER CARE / MAINTENANCE, COMPLEX (MORE THAN ONE LUMEN), INCLUDES ADMINISTRATIVE SERVICES, PROFESSIONAL PHARMACY SERVICES, CARE COORDINATION, AND ALL NECESSARY SUPPLIES AND EQUIPMENT (DRUGS AND NURSING VISITS CODED SEPARATELY) PER DIEM	00	9			I			N
S5502	HOME INFUSION THERAPY, CATHETER CARE / MAINTENANCE, IMPLANTED ACCESS DEVICE, INCLUDES ADMINISTRATIVE SERVICES, PROFESSIONAL PHARMACY SERVICES, CARE COORDINATION AND ALL NECESSARY SUPPLIES AND EQUIPMENT, (DRUGS AND NURSING VISITS CODED SEPARATELY), PER DIEM (USE THIS CODE FOR INTERIM MAINTENANCE OF VASCULAR ACCESS NOT CURRENTLY IN USE)	00	9			I			N
S5503	MAINTENANCE OF IMPLANTED VASCULAR ACCESS DEVICE, INCLUDING SUPPLIES; PER DIEM	00	9			I			N
S5517	HOME INFUSION THERAPY, ALL SUPPLIES NECESSARY FOR RESTORATION OF CATHETER PATENCY OR DECLOTTING	00	9			I			N
S5518	HOME INFUSION THERAPY, ALL SUPPLIES NECESSARY FOR CATHETER REPAIR	00	9			I			N
S5520	HOME INFUSION THERAPY, ALL SUPPLIES (INCLUDING CATHETER) NECESSARY FOR A PERIPHERALLY INSERTED CENTRAL VENOUS CATHETER (PICC) LINE INSERTION	00	9			I			N
S5521	HOME INFUSION THERAPY, ALL SUPPLIES (INCLUDING CATHETER) NECESSARY FOR A MIDLINE CATHETER INSERTION	00	9			I			N
S5522	HOME INFUSION THERAPY, INSERTION OF PERIPHERALLY INSERTED CENTRAL VENOUS CATHETER (PICC), NURSING SERVICES ONLY (NO SUPPLIES OR CATHETER INCLUDED)	00	9			I			N
S5523	HOME INFUSION THERAPY, INSERTION OF MIDLINE CENTRAL VENOUS CATHETER, NURSING SERVICES ONLY (NO SUPPLIES OR CATHETER INCLUDED)	00	9			I			N
S5550	INSULIN, RAPID ONSET, 5 UNITS	00	9			I			A
S5551	INSULIN, MOST RAPID ONSET (LISPRO OR ASPART); 5 UNITS	00	9			I			A
S5552	INSULIN, INTERMEDIATE ACTING (NPH OR LENTE); 5 UNITS	00	9			I			A
S5553	INSULIN, LONG ACTING; 5 UNITS	00	9			I			A
S5560	INSULIN DELIVERY DEVICE, REUSABLE PEN; 1.5 ML SIZE	00	9			I			A
S5561	INSULIN DELIVERY DEVICE, REUSABLE PEN; 3 ML SIZE	00	9			I			A

HCPCS	Long Description	PTI	MPI	Statute	X-Refl	Coverage	ASC Pay Grp	ASC Pay Grp Eff Date	Action Code
S5565	INSULIN CARTRIDGE FOR USE IN INSULIN DELIVERY DEVICE OTHER THAN PUMP; 150 UNITS	00	9			I			A
S5566	INSULIN CARTRIDGE FOR USE IN INSULIN DELIVERY DEVICE OTHER THAN PUMP; 300 UNITS	00	9			I			A
S5570	INSULIN DELIVERY DEVICE, DISPOSABLE PEN (INCLUDING INSULIN); 1.5 ML SIZE	00	9			I			A
S5571	INSULIN DELIVERY DEVICE, DISPOSABLE PEN (INCLUDING INSULIN); 3 ML SIZE	00	9			I			A
S8001	RADIOFREQUENCY STIMULATION OF THE THALAMUS FOR TREMOR ACCOMPLISHED BY STEREOTACTIC METHOD, INCLUDING BURR HOLES, LOCALIZING AND RECORDING TECHNIQUES AND PLACEMENT OF THE ELECTRODE(S)	00	9			I			N
S8002	SUPPLY OF DIAGNOSTIC RADIOPHARMACEUTICAL, INDIUM-111	00	9		A9522	I			N
S8003	SUPPLY OF THERAPEUTIC RADIOIMMUNOPHARMACEUTICAL, YTTRIUM-90	00	9		A9523	I			N
S8004	RADIOIMMUNOPHARMACEUTICAL LOCALIZATION OF TARGETED CELLS; WHOLE BODY	00	9			I			N
S8030	SCLERAL APPLICATION OF TANTALUM RING(S) FOR LOCALIZATION OF LESIONS FOR PROTON	00	9			I			N
S8030	BEAM THERAPY								
S8035	MAGNETIC SOURCE IMAGING	00	9			I			N
S8037	MAGNETIC RESONANCE CHOLANGIOPANCREATOGRAPHY (MRCP)	00	9			I			N
S8040	TOPOGRAPHIC BRAIN MAPPING	00	9			I			N
S8042	MAGNETIC RESONANCE IMAGING (MRI), LOW-FIELD	00	9			I			N
S8048	ISOLATED LIMB PERFUSION	00	9		36823	I			N
S8049	INTRAOPERATIVE RADIATION THERAPY (SINGLE ADMINISTRATION)	00	9			I			N
S8055	ULTRASOUND GUIDANCE FOR MULTIFETAL PREGNANCY REDUCTION(S), TECHNICAL COMPONENT (ONLY TO BE USED WHEN THE PHYSICIAN DOING THE REDUCTION PROCEDURE DOES NOT PERFORM THE ULTRASOUND, GUIDANCE IS INCLUDED IN THE CPT CODE FOR MULTIFETAL PREGNANCY REDUCTION - 59866)	00	9			I			N
S8060	SUPPLY OF CONTRAST MATERIAL FOR USE IN ECHOCARDIOGRAPHY (USE IN ADDITION TO ECHOCARDIOGRAPHY CODE)	00	9		A9700	I			N
S8075	COMPUTER ANALYSIS OF FULL-FIELD DIGITAL MAMMOGRAM AND FURTHER PHYSICIAN REVIEW FOR INTERPRETATION, MAMMOGRAPHY (LIST SEPARATELY IN ADDITION TO CODE FOR PRIMARY PROCEDURE)	00	9			I			A
S8080	SCINTIMAMMOGRAPHY (RADIOIMMUNOSCINTIGRAPHY OF THE BREAST), UNILATERAL, INCLUDING SUPPLY OF RADIOPHARMACEUTICAL	00	9			I			N
S8085	FLUORINE-18 FLUORODEOXYGLUCOSE (F-18 FDG) IMAGING USING DUAL-HEAD COINCIDENCE DETECTION SYSTEM (NON-DEDICATED PET SCAN)	00	9			I			N
S8092	ELECTRON BEAM COMPUTED TOMOGRAPHY (ALSO KNOWN AS ULTRAFAST CT, CINE CT)	00	9			I			N
S8095	WIG (FOR MEDICALLY-INDUCED OR CONGENITAL HAIR LOSS)	00	9			I			N
S8096	PORTABLE PEAK FLOW METER	00	9			I			N
S8097	ASTHMA KIT (INCLUDING BUT NOT LIMITED TO PORTABLE PEAK EXPIRATORY FLOW METER, INSTRUCTIONAL VIDEO, BROCHURE, AND/OR SPACER)	00	9			I			N
S8100	HOLDING CHAMBER OR SPACER FOR USE WITH AN INHALER OR NEBULIZER; WITHOUT MASK	00	9			I			N
S8101	HOLDING CHAMBER OR SPACER FOR USE WITH AN INHALER OR NEBULIZER; WITH MASK	00	9			I			N

HCPCS	Long Description	PII	MPI	Statute	X-Ref1	Coverage	ASC Pay Grp	ASC Pay Grp Eff Date	Action Code
S8105	OXIMETER FOR MEASURING BLOOD OXYGEN LEVELS NONINVASIVELY	00	9			I			N
S8110	PEAK EXPIRATORY FLOW RATE (PHYSICIAN SERVICES)	00	9			I			N
S8120	OXYGEN CONTENTS, GASEOUS, 1 UNIT EQUALS 1 CUBIC FOOT	00	9			I			A
S8121	OXYGEN CONTENTS, LIQUID, 1 UNIT EQUALS 1 POUND	00	9			I			A
S8180	TRACHEOSTOMY SHOWER PROTECTOR	00	9			I			D
S8181	TRACHEOSTOMY TUBE HOLDER	00	9			I			D
S8182	HUMIDIFIER, HEATED, USED WITH VENTILATOR, NON-SERVO-CONTROLLED	00	9			I			N
S8183	HUMIDIFIER, HEATED, USED WITH VENTILATOR, DUAL SERVO-CONTROLLED WITH TEMPERATURE MONITORING	00	9			I			N
S8185	FLUTTER DEVICE	00	9			I			N
S8186	SWIVEL ADAPTOR	00	9			I			N
S8189	TRACHEOSTOMY SUPPLY, NOT OTHERWISE CLASSIFIED	00	9			I			N
S8190	ELECTRONIC SPIROMETER (OR MICROSPIROMETER)	00	9			I			N
S8200	CHEST COMPRESSION VEST	00	9		E0483	I			N
S8205	CHEST COMPRESSION SYSTEM GENERATOR AND HOSES (FOR USE WITH CHEST COMPRESSION VEST - S8200)	00	9		E0483	I			N
S8210	MUCUS TRAP	00	9			I			N
S8260	ORAL ORTHOTIC FOR TREATMENT OF SLEEP APNEA, INCLUDES FITTING, FABRICATION, AND MATERIALS	00	9			I			N
S8262	MANDIBULAR ORTHOPEDIC REPOSITIONING DEVICE, EACH	00	9			I			N
S8265	HABERMAN FEEDER FOR CLEFT LIP/PALATE	00	9			I			N
S8300	SACRAL NERVE STIMULATION TEST LEAD KIT	00	9			I			N
S8400	INCONTINENCE PANTS, EACH	00	9			I			N
S8401	CHILD-SIZE INCONTINENCE GARMENT, DIAPER, EACH	00	9		A4529,30	I			N
S8402	DIAPERS, EACH	00	9			I			N
S8403	ADULT-SIZED INCONTINENCE GARMENT, DISPOSABLE, PULL-UP BRIEF, EACH	00	9		A4525-8	I			N
S8404	CHILD-SIZE INCONTINENCE GARMENT, DISPOSABLE, PULL-UP BRIEF, EACH	00	9		A4531-2	I			N
S8405	DISPOSABLE LINER/SHIELD FOR INCONTINENCE, EACH	00	9		A4535	I			N
S8415	SUPPLIES FOR HOME DELIVERY OF INFANT	00	9			I			N
S8420	GRADIENT PRESSURE AID (SLEEVE AND GLOVE COMBINATION), CUSTOM MADE	00	9			I			N
S8421	GRADIENT PRESSURE AID (SLEEVE AND GLOVE COMBINATION), READY MADE	00	9			I			N
S8422	GRADIENT PRESSURE AID (SLEEVE), CUSTOM MADE, MEDIUM WEIGHT	00	9			I			N
S8423	GRADIENT PRESSURE AID (SLEEVE), CUSTOM MADE, HEAVY WEIGHT	00	9			I			N
S8424	GRADIENT PRESSURE AID (SLEEVE), READY MADE	00	9			I			N
S8425	GRADIENT PRESSURE AID (GLOVE), CUSTOM MADE, MEDIUM WEIGHT	00	9			I			N

HCPCS	Long Description	PII	MPI	Statute	X-Ref1	Coverage	ASC Pay Grp	ASC Pay Grp Eff Date	Action Code
S8426	GRADIENT PRESSURE AID (GLOVE), CUSTOM MADE, HEAVY WEIGHT	00	9			I			N
S8427	GRADIENT PRESSURE AID (GLOVE), READY MADE	00	9			I			N
S8428	GRADIENT PRESSURE AID (GAUNTLET), READY MADE	00	9			I			N
S8429	GRADIENT PRESSURE EXTERIOR WRAP	00	9			I			N
S8430	PADDING FOR COMPRESSION BANDAGE, ROLL	00	9			I			N
S8431	COMPRESSION BANDAGE, ROLL	00	9			I			N
S8433	SKIN SUPPORT FOR BREAST PROSTHESIS, EACH	00	9		A4280	I			N
S8450	SPLINT, PREFABRICATED, DIGIT (SPECIFY DIGIT BY USE OF MODIFIER)	00	9			I			N
S8451	SPLINT, PREFABRICATED, WRIST OR ANKLE	00	9			I			N
S8452	SPLINT, PREFABRICATED, ELBOW	00	9			I			N
S8460	CAMISOLE, POST-MASTECTOMY	00	9			I			A
S8470	POSITIONING DEVICE, STANDER, FOR USE BY PATIENT WHO IS UNABLE TO STAND	00	9			I			D
S8490	INSULIN SYRINGES (100 SYRINGES, ANY SIZE)	00	9			I			N
S8945	PHYSICAL MEDICINE TREATMENT (CONSTANT ATTENDANCE BY PROVIDER) TO ONE AREA, INITIAL 30 MINUTES, EACH VISIT; PHONOPHORESIS	00	9			I			D
S8948	APPLICATION OF A MODALITY (REQUIRING CONSTANT PROVIDER ATTENDANCE) TO ONE OR MORE AREAS; LOW-LEVEL LASER; EACH 15 MINUTES	00	9			I			A
S8950	COMPLEX LYMPHEDEMA THERAPY, EACH 15 MINUTES	00	9			I			N
S8990	PHYSICAL OR MANIPULATIVE THERAPY PERFORMED FOR MAINTENANCE RATHER THAN RESTORATION	00	9			I			A
S8999	RESUSCITATION BAG (FOR USE BY PATIENT ON ARTIFICIAL RESPIRATION DURING POWER FAILURE OR OTHER CATASTROPHIC EVENT)	00	9			I			N
S9001	HOME UTERINE MONITOR WITH OR WITHOUT ASSOCIATED NURSING SERVICES	00	9			I			N
S9007	ULTRAFILTRATION MONITOR	00	9			I			N
S9015	AUTOMATED EEG MONITORING	00	9			I			N
S9022	DIGITAL SUBTRACTION ANGIOGRAPHY (USE IN ADDITION TO CPT CODE FOR THE PROCEDURE FOR FURTHER IDENTIFICATION)	00	9			I			N
S9023	XENON REGIONAL CEREBRAL BLOOD FLOW STUDIES	00	9			I			N
S9024	PARANASAL SINUS ULTRASOUND	00	9			I			N
S9025	OMNICARDIOGRAM/CARDIOINTEGRAM	00	9			I			N
S9033	GAIT ANALYSIS	00	9		95979,86	I			N
S9034	EXTRACORPOREAL SHOCKWAVE LITHOTRIPSY FOR GALL STONES (IF PERFORMED WITH ERCP, USE 43265)	00	9			I			N
S9035	MEDICAL EQUIPMENT OR SUPPLIES DISTRIBUTED BY HOME CARE PROVIDER WITHOUT PROFESSIONAL NURSING INTERVENTION, PER DAY	00	9			I			N

HCPCS	Long Description	PII	MPI	Statute	X-Ref1	Coverage	ASC Pay Grp	ASC Pay Grp Eff Date	Action Code
S9055	PROCUREN OR OTHER GROWTH FACTOR PREPARATION TO PROMOTE WOUND HEALING	00	9			I			N
S9056	COMA STIMULATION PER DIEM	00	9			I			N
S9061	HOME ADMINISTRATION OF AEROSOLIZED DRUG THERAPY (E.G., PENTAMIDINE);	00	9			I			N
S9061	ADMINISTRATIVE SERVICES, PROFESSIONAL PHARMACY SERVICES, CARE COORDINATION, ALL NECESSARY SUPPLIES AND EQUIPMENT (DRUGS AND NURSING VISITS CODED SEPARATELY), PER DIEM								
S9075	SMOKING CESSATION TREATMENT	00	9			I			N
S9083	GLOBAL FEE URGENT CARE CENTERS	00	9			I			N
S9085	MENISCAL ALLOGRAFT TRANSPLANTATION	00	9			I			N
S9088	SERVICES PROVIDED IN AN URGENT CARE CENTER (LIST IN ADDITION TO CODE FOR SERVICE)	00	9			I			N
S9090	VERTEBRAL AXIAL DECOMPRESSION, PER SESSION	00	9			I			N
S9092	CANOLITH REPOSITIONING, PER VISIT	00	9			I			N
S9098	HOME VISIT, PHOTOTHERAPY SERVICES (E.G. BILI-LITE), INCLUDING EQUIPMENT RENTAL, NURSING SERVICES, BLOOD DRAW, SUPPLIES, AND OTHER SERVICES, PER DIEM	00	9			I			N
S9109	CONGESTIVE HEART FAILURE TELEMONITORING, EQUIPMENT RENTAL, INCLUDING TELESCALE, COMPUTER SYSTEM AND SOFTWARE, TELEPHONE CONNECTIONS, AND MAINTENANCE, PER MONTH	00	9			I			N
S9117	BACK SCHOOL, PER VISIT	00	9			I			N
S9122	HOME HEALTH AIDE OR CERTIFIED NURSE ASSISTANT, PROVIDING CARE IN THE HOME; PER HOUR	00	9			I			N
S9123	NURSING CARE, IN THE HOME; BY REGISTERED NURSE, PER HOUR (USE FOR GENERAL NURSING CARE ONLY, NOT TO BE USED WHEN CPT CODES 99500-99602 CAN BE USED)	00	9			I			C
S9124	NURSING CARE, IN THE HOME; BY LICENSED PRACTICAL NURSE, PER HOUR	00	9			I			N
S9125	RESPITE CARE, IN THE HOME, PER DIEM	00	9			I			N
S9126	HOSPICE CARE, IN THE HOME, PER DIEM	00	9			I			N
S9127	SOCIAL WORK VISIT, IN THE HOME, PER DIEM	00	9			I			N
S9128	SPEECH THERAPY, IN THE HOME, PER DIEM	00	9			I			N
S9129	OCCUPATIONAL THERAPY, IN THE HOME, PER DIEM	00	9			I			N
S9131	PHYSICAL THERAPY; IN THE HOME, PER DIEM	00	9			I			N
S9140	DIABETIC MANAGEMENT PROGRAM, FOLLOW-UP VISIT TO NON-MD PROVIDER	00	9			I			N
S9141	DIABETIC MANAGEMENT PROGRAM, FOLLOW-UP VISIT TO MD PROVIDER	00	9			I			N
S9145	INSULIN PUMP INITIATION, INSTRUCTION IN INITIAL USE OF PUMP (PUMP NOT INCLUDED)	00	9			I			N
S9150	EVALUATION BY OCULARIST	00	9			I			N
S9200	NURSING SERVICES AND ALL NECESSARY SUPPLIES (INCLUDING PCA PUMP RENTAL) FOR HOME ADMINISTRATION OF PATIENT CONTROLLED ANALGESIA (PCA) PER DIEM (DRUGS NOT INCLUDED)	00	9			I			N

HCPCS	Long Description	PH	MPI	Statute	X-Ref1	Coverage	ASC Pay Grp	ASC Pay Grp Eff Date	Action Code
S9208	HOME MANAGEMENT OF PRETERM LABOR, INCLUDING ADMINISTRATIVE SERVICES, PROFESSIONAL PHARMACY SERVICES, CARE COORDINATION, AND ALL NECESSARY SUPPLIES OR EQUIPMENT (DRUGS AND NURSING VISITS CODED SEPARATELY), PER DIEM (DO NOT USE THIS CODE WITH ANY HOME INFUSION PER DIEM CODE)	00	9			I			N
S9209	HOME MANAGEMENT OF PRETERM PREMATURE RUPTURE OF MEMBRANES (PPROM), INCLUDING ADMINISTRATIVE SERVICES, PROFESSIONAL PHARMACY SERVICES, CARE COORDINATION, AND ALL NECESSARY SUPPLIES OR EQUIPMENT (DRUGS AND NURSING VISITS CODED SEPARATELY), PER DIEM (DO NOT USE THIS CODE WITH ANY HOME INFUSION PER DIEM CODE)	00	9			I			N
S9210	NURSING SERVICES AND ALL NECESSARY EQUIPMENT AND SUPPLIES FOR CONTINUOUS, UNINTERRUPTED INFUSION OF EPOPROSTENOL (INCLUDES VENOUS ACCESS DEVICE, INFUSION PUMP, BACK UP PUMP, ICE PACKS FOR CASSETTES, BATTERIES, ALL RELATED SUPPLIES, AND ALL NURSING SERVICES INCLUDING FOLLOW-UP VISITS, TELEPHONE MONITORING, 24 HOUR/7 DAY A WEEK AVAILABILITY, AND ALL EDUCATION TO PATIENT AND CARE GIVERS); PER DIEM	00	9			I			N
S9211	HOME MANAGEMENT OF GESTATIONAL HYPERTENSION, INCLUDES ADMINISTRATIVE SERVICES, PROFESSIONAL PHARMACY SERVICES, CARE COORDINATION AND ALL NECESSARY SUPPLIES AND EQUIPMENT (DRUGS AND NURSING VISITS CODED SEPARATELY); PER DIEM (DO NOT USE THIS CODE WITH ANY HOME INFUSION PER DIEM CODE)	00	9			I			N
S9212	HOME MANAGEMENT OF POSTPARTUM HYPERTENSION, INCLUDES ADMINISTRATIVE SERVICES, PROFESSIONAL PHARMACY SERVICES, CARE COORDINATION, AND ALL NECESSARY SUPPLIES AND EQUIPMENT (DRUGS AND NURSING VISITS CODED SEPARATELY), PER DIEM (DO NOT USE THIS CODE WITH ANY HOME INFUSION PER DIEM CODE)	00	9			I			N
S9213	HOME MANAGEMENT OF PREECLAMPSIA, INCLUDES ADMINISTRATIVE SERVICES, PROFESSIONAL PHARMACY SERVICES, CARE COORDINATION, AND ALL NECESSARY SUPPLIES AND EQUIPMENT (DRUGS AND NURSING SERVICES CODED SEPARATELY); PER DIEM (DO NOT USE THIS CODE WITH ANY HOME INFUSION PER DIEM CODE)	00	9			I			N
S9214	HOME MANAGEMENT OF GESTATIONAL DIABETES, INCLUDES ADMINISTRATIVE SERVICES, PROFESSIONAL PHARMACY SERVICES, CARE COORDINATION, AND ALL NECESSARY SUPPLIES AND EQUIPMENT (DRUGS AND NURSING VISITS CODED SEPARATELY); PER DIEM (DO NOT USE THIS CODE WITH ANY HOME INFUSION PER DIEM CODE)	00	9			I			N
S9216	NURSING SERVICES AND ALL NECESSARY EQUIPMENT AND SUPPLIES FOR GESTATIONAL HYPERTENSION PROGRAM (INCLUDES MATERNAL ASSESSMENT AS NEEDED, TELEPHONIC COLLECTION OF BLOOD PRESSURE, URINE PROTEIN, WEIGHT AND FETAL MOVEMENT COUNTING VIA A HOME DATA COLLECTION SYSTEM, PATIENT STATUS REPORTS, 24 HOUR/7 DAY A WEEK NURSING SUPPORT, AND ALL EDUCATION TO THE PATIENT AND CAREGIVER); PER DIEM	00	9		S9211	I			N
S9217	NURSING SERVICES AND ALL NECESSARY EQUIPMENT AND SUPPLIES FOR POSTPARTUM HYPERTENSION PROGRAM (INCLUDES MATERNAL ASSESSMENT AS NEEDED, TELEPHONIC COLLECTION OF BLOOD PRESSURE, URINE PROTEIN, WEIGHT, COMPLIANCE MANAGEMENT SUPPORT, PATIENT STATUS REPORTS, 24 HOUR/7 DAY A WEEK NURSING SUPPORT, AND ALL EDUCATION TO THE PATIENT AND CAREGIVER); PER DIEM	00	9		S9212	I			N
S9218	NURSING SERVICES AND ALL NECESSARY EQUIPMENT AND SUPPLIES FOR PREECLAMPSIA PROGRAM (INCLUDES MATERNAL ASSESSMENT AS NEEDED, TELEPHONIC COLLECTION OF BLOOD PRESSURE, URINE PROTEIN, WEIGHT AND DAILY FETAL MOVEMENT COUNTS VIA A HOME DATA COLLECTION SYSTEM, COMPLIANCE MANAGEMENT SUPPORT, PATIENT STATUS REPORTS, 24 HOUR/7 DAY A WEEK NURSING SUPPORT, AND ALL EDUCATION TO THE PATIENT AND CAREGIVER); PER DIEM	00	9		S9213	I			N
S9220	NURSING SERVICES AND ALL NECESSARY EQUIPMENT AND SUPPLIES FOR HOME ADMINISTRATION OF CONTROLLED RATE INTRAVENOUS INFUSION (E.G. DOBUTAMINE) REQUIRING PROLONGED ATTENDANCE BY THE NURSE, PER DIEM (DRUGS NOT INCLUDED)	00	9			I			N
S9225	NURSING SERVICES AND ALL NECESSARY EQUIPMENT AND SUPPLIES FOR HOME ADMINISTRATION OF INTRAVENOUS TOCOLYTIC THERAPY, PER DIEM - USE NEW CPT CODE	00	9			I			N

HCPCS	Long Description	PII	MPI	Statute	X-Ref	Coverage	ASC Pay Grp	ASC Pay Grp Eff Date	Action Code
S9230	NURSING SERVICES AND ALL NECESSARY EQUIPMENT AND SUPPLIES FOR HOME ADMINISTRATION OF HEPARIN, PER DIEM	00	9			I			N
S9300	NURSING SERVICES AND ALL NECESSARY SUPPLIES FOR HOME ENTERAL FEEDING BY GRAVITY, PER DIEM (ENTERAL FORMULA NOT INCLUDED)	00	9			I			N
S9308	NURSING SERVICES AND ALL NECESSARY SUPPLIES FOR HOME ENTERAL FEEDING BY PUMP, INCLUDING PUMP RENTAL, PER DIEM (ENTERAL FORMULA NOT INCLUDED)	00	9			I			N
S9310	NURSING SERVICES AND ALL NECESSARY SUPPLIES FOR HOME PARENTERAL NUTRITION WITHOUT LIPIDS, INCLUDING PUMP RENTAL, PER DIEM (PARENTERAL SOLUTIONS NOT INCLUDED)	00	9			I			N
S9325	HOME INFUSION THERAPY, PAIN MANAGEMENT INFUSION; ADMINISTRATIVE SERVICES, PROFESSIONAL PHARMACY SERVICES, CARE COORDINATION, AND ALL NECESSARY SUPPLIES AND EQUIPMENT, (DRUGS AND NURSING VISITS CODED SEPARATELY), PER DIEM (DO NOT USE THIS CODE WITH S9326, S9327 OR S9328)	00	9			I			N
S9326	HOME INFUSION THERAPY, CONTINUOUS (TWENTY-FOUR HOURS OR MORE) PAIN MANAGEMENT INFUSION; ADMINISTRATIVE SERVICES, PROFESSIONAL PHARMACY SERVICES, CARE COORDINATION AND ALL NECESSARY SUPPLIES AND EQUIPMENT (DRUGS AND NURSING VISITS CODED SEPARATELY), PER DIEM	00	9			I			N
S9327	HOME INFUSION THERAPY, INTERMITTENT (LESS THAN TWENTY-FOUR HOURS) PAIN MANAGEMENT INFUSION; ADMINISTRATIVE SERVICES, PROFESSIONAL PHARMACY SERVICES, CARE COORDINATION, AND ALL NECESSARY SUPPLIES AND EQUIPMENT (DRUGS AND NURSING VISITS CODED SEPARATELY), PER DIEM	00	9			I			N
S9328	HOME INFUSION THERAPY, IMPLANTED PUMP PAIN MANAGEMENT INFUSION; ADMINISTRATIVE SERVICES, PROFESSIONAL PHARMACY SERVICES, CARE COORDINATION, AND ALL NECESSARY SUPPLIES AND EQUIPMENT (DRUGS AND NURSING VISITS CODED SEPARATELY), PER DIEM	00	9			I			N
S9329	HOME INFUSION THERAPY, CHEMOTHERAPY INFUSION; ADMINISTRATIVE SERVICES, PROFESSIONAL PHARMACY SERVICES, CARE COORDINATION, AND ALL NECESSARY SUPPLIES AND EQUIPMENT (DRUGS AND NURSING VISITS CODED SEPARATELY), PER DIEM (DO NOT USE THIS CODE WITH S9330 OR S9331)	00	9			I			N
S9330	HOME INFUSION THERAPY, CONTINUOUS (TWENTY-FOUR HOURS OR MORE) CHEMOTHERAPY INFUSION; ADMINISTRATIVE SERVICES, PROFESSIONAL PHARMACY SERVICES, CARE COORDINATION, AND ALL NECESSARY SUPPLIES AND EQUIPMENT (DRUGS AND NURSING VISITS CODED SEPARATELY), PER DIEM	00	9			I			N
S9331	HOME INFUSION THERAPY, INTERMITTENT (LESS THAN TWENTY-FOUR HOURS) CHEMOTHERAPY INFUSION; ADMINISTRATIVE SERVICES, PROFESSIONAL PHARMACY SERVICES, CARE COORDINATION, AND ALL NECESSARY SUPPLIES AND EQUIPMENT (DRUGS AND NURSING VISITS CODED SEPARATELY), PER DIEM	00	9			I			N
S9335	HOME THERAPY, HEMODIALYSIS; ADMINISTRATIVE SERVICES, PROFESSIONAL PHARMACY SERVICES, CARE COORDINATION, AND ALL NECESSARY SUPPLIES AND EQUIPMENT (DRUGS AND NURSING SERVICES CODED SEPARATELY) PER DIEM	00	9			I			A
S9336	HOME INFUSION THERAPY, CONTINUOUS ANTICOAGULANT INFUSION THERAPY (E.G. HEPARIN), ADMINISTRATIVE SERVICES, PROFESSIONAL PHARMACY SERVICES, CARE COORDINATION AND ALL NECESSARY SUPPLIES AND EQUIPMENT (DRUGS AND NURSING VISITS CODED SEPARATELY) PER DIEM	00	9			I			N
S9338	HOME INFUSION THERAPY, IMMUNOTHERAPY, ADMINISTRATIVE SERVICES, PROFESSIONAL PHARMACY SERVICES, CARE COORDINATION, AND ALL NECESSARY SUPPLIES AND EQUIPMENT (DRUGS AND NURSING VISITS CODED SEPARATELY) PER DIEM	00	9			I			N
S9339	HOME THERAPY; PERITONEAL DIALYSIS, ADMINISTRATIVE SERVICES, PROFESSIONAL PHARMACY SERVICES, CARE COORDINATION AND ALL NECESSARY SUPPLIES AND EQUIPMENT (DRUGS AND NURSING VISITS CODED SEPARATELY) PER DIEM	00	9			I			N
S9340	HOME THERAPY; ENTERAL NUTRITION; ADMINISTRATIVE SERVICES, PROFESSIONAL PHARMACY SERVICES, CARE COORDINATION, AND ALL NECESSARY SUPPLIES AND EQUIPMENT (ENTERAL FORMULA AND NURSING VISITS CODED SEPARATELY), PER DIEM	00	9			I			N

HCPCS	Long Description	PTI	MPI	Statute	X-Ref1	Coverage	ASC Pay Grp	ASC Pay Grp Eff Date	Action Code
S9341	HOME THERAPY; ENTERAL NUTRITION VIA GRAVITY; ADMINISTRATIVE SERVICES, PROFESSIONAL PHARMACY SERVICES, CARE COORDINATION, AND ALL NECESSARY SUPPLIES AND EQUIPMENT (ENTERAL FORMULA AND NURSING VISITS CODED SEPARATELY), PER DIEM	00	9			I			N
S9342	HOME THERAPY; ENTERAL NUTRITION VIA PUMP; ADMINISTRATIVE SERVICES, PROFESSIONAL PHARMACY SERVICES, CARE COORDINATION, AND ALL NECESSARY SUPPLIES AND EQUIPMENT (ENTERAL FORMULA AND NURSING VISITS CODED SEPARATELY), PER DIEM	00	9			I			N
S9343	HOME THERAPY; ENTERAL NUTRITION VIA BOLUS; ADMINISTRATIVE SERVICES, PROFESSIONAL PHARMACY SERVICES, CARE COORDINATION, AND ALL NECESSARY SUPPLIES AND EQUIPMENT (ENTERAL FORMULA AND NURSING VISITS CODED SEPARATELY), PER DIEM	00	9			I			N
S9345	HOME INFUSION THERAPY, ANTI-HEMOPHILIC AGENT INFUSION THERAPY (E.G. FACTOR VIII); ADMINISTRATIVE SERVICES, PROFESSIONAL PHARMACY SERVICES, CARE COORDINATION, AND ALL NECESSARY SUPPLIES AND EQUIPMENT (DRUGS AND NURSING VISITS CODED SEPARATELY), PER DIEM	00	9			I			N
S9346	HOME INFUSION THERAPY, ALPHA-1-PROTEINASE INHIBITOR (E.G., PROLASTIN); ADMINISTRATIVE SERVICES, PROFESSIONAL PHARMACY SERVICES, CARE COORDINATION, AND ALL NECESSARY SUPPLIES AND EQUIPMENT (DRUGS AND NURSING VISITS CODED SEPARATELY), PER DIEM	00	9			I			N
S9347	HOME INFUSION THERAPY, UNINTERRUPTED, LONG-TERM, CONTROLLED RATE INTRAVENOUS OR SUBCUTANEOUS INFUSION THERAPY (E.G. EPOPROSTENOL); ADMINISTRATIVE SERVICES, PROFESSIONAL PHARMACY SERVICES, CARE COORDINATION, AND ALL NECESSARY SUPPLIES AND EQUIPMENT (DRUGS AND NURSING VISITS CODED SEPARATELY), PER DIEM	00	9			I			N
S9348	HOME INFUSION THERAPY, SYMPATHOMIMETIC/INOTROPIC AGENT INFUSION THERAPY (E.G., DOBUTAMINE); ADMINISTRATIVE SERVICES, PROFESSIONAL PHARMACY SERVICES, CARE COORDINATION, ALL NECESSARY SUPPLIES AND EQUIPMENT (DRUGS AND NURSING VISITS CODED SEPARATELY) PER DIEM	00	9			I			N
S9349	HOME INFUSION THERAPY, TOCOLYTIC INFUSION THERAPY; ADMINISTRATIVE SERVICES, PROFESSIONAL PHARMACY SERVICES, CARE COORDINATION, AND ALL NECESSARY SUPPLIES AND EQUIPMENT (DRUGS AND NURSING VISITS CODED SEPARATELY), PER DIEM	00	9			I			N
S9351	HOME INFUSION THERAPY, CONTINUOUS ANTI-EMETIC INFUSION THERAPY; ADMINISTRATIVE SERVICES, PROFESSIONAL PHARMACY SERVICES, CARE COORDINATION, ALL NECESSARY SUPPLIES AND EQUIPMENT (DRUGS AND NURSING VISITS CODED SEPARATELY), PER DIEM	00	9			I			N
S9353	HOME INFUSION THERAPY, CONTINUOUS INSULIN INFUSION THERAPY; ADMINISTRATIVE SERVICES, PROFESSIONAL PHARMACY SERVICES, CARE COORDINATION, AND ALL NECESSARY SUPPLIES AND EQUIPMENT (DRUGS AND NURSING VISITS CODED SEPARATELY), PER DIEM	00	9			I			N
S9355	HOME INFUSION THERAPY, CHELATION THERAPY; ADMINISTRATIVE SERVICES, PROFESSIONAL PHARMACY SERVICES, CARE COORDINATION, AND ALL NECESSARY SUPPLIES AND EQUIPMENT (DRUGS AND NURSING VISITS CODED SEPARATELY), PER DIEM	00	9			I			N
S9357	HOME INFUSION THERAPY, ENZYME REPLACEMENT INTRAVENOUS THERAPY; (E.G. IMIGLUCERASE); ADMINISTRATIVE SERVICES, PROFESSIONAL PHARMACY SERVICES, CARE COORDINATION, AND ALL NECESSARY SUPPLIES AND EQUIPMENT (DRUGS AND NURSING VISITS CODED SEPARATELY) PER DIEM	00	9			I			N
S9359	HOME INFUSION THERAPY, ANTI-TUMOR NECROSIS FACTOR INTRAVENOUS THERAPY; (E.G. INFLIXIMAB); ADMINISTRATIVE SERVICES, PROFESSIONAL PHARMACY SERVICES, CARE COORDINATION, AND ALL NECESSARY SUPPLIES AND EQUIPMENT (DRUGS AND NURSING VISITS CODED SEPARATELY) PER DIEM	00	9			I			N
S9361	HOME INFUSION THERAPY, DIURETIC INTRAVENOUS THERAPY; ADMINISTRATIVE SERVICES, PROFESSIONAL PHARMACY SERVICES, CARE COORDINATION, AND ALL NECESSARY SUPPLIES AND EQUIPMENT (DRUGS AND NURSING VISITS CODED SEPARATELY), PER DIEM	00	9			I			N

HCPCS	Long Description	PII	MPI	Statute	X-Ref	Coverage	ASC Pay Grp	ASC Pay Grp Eff Date	Action Code
S9363	HOME INFUSION THERAPY, ANTI-SPASMOTIC INTRAVENOUS THERAPY; ADMINISTRATIVE SERVICES, PROFESSIONAL PHARMACY SERVICES, CARE COORDINATION, AND ALL NECESSARY SUPPLIES AND EQUIPMENT (DRUGS AND NURSING VISITS CODED SEPARATELY), PER DIEM	00	9			I			N
S9364	HOME INFUSION THERAPY, TOTAL PARENTERAL NUTRITION (TPN); ADMINISTRATIVE SERVICES, PROFESSIONAL PHARMACY SERVICES, CARE COORDINATION, AND ALL NECESSARY SUPPLIES AND EQUIPMENT INCLUDING STANDARD TPN FORMULA (LIPIDS, SPECIALTY AMINO ACID FORMULAS, DRUGS OTHER THAN IN STANDARD FORMULA AND NURSING VISITS CODED SEPARATELY), PER DIEM (DO NOT USE WITH HOME INFUSION CODES S9365-S9368 USING DAILY VOLUME SCALES)	00	9			I			N
S9365	HOME INFUSION THERAPY, TOTAL PARENTERAL NUTRITION (TPN); ONE LITER PER DAY, ADMINISTRATIVE SERVICES, PROFESSIONAL PHARMACY SERVICES, CARE COORDINATION, AND ALL NECESSARY SUPPLIES AND EQUIPMENT INCLUDING STANDARD TPN FORMULA (LIPIDS, SPECIALTY AMINO ACID FORMULAS, DRUGS OTHER THAN IN STANDARD FORMULA AND NURSING VISITS CODED SEPARATELY), PER DIEM	00	9			I			N
S9366	HOME INFUSION THERAPY, TOTAL PARENTERAL NUTRITION (TPN); MORE THAN ONE LITER BUT NO MORE THAN TWO LITERS PER DAY, ADMINISTRATIVE SERVICES, PROFESSIONAL PHARMACY SERVICES, CARE COORDINATION, AND ALL NECESSARY SUPPLIES AND EQUIPMENT INCLUDING STANDARD TPN FORMULA (LIPIDS, SPECIALTY AMINO ACID FORMULAS, DRUGS OTHER THAN IN STANDARD FORMULA AND NURSING VISITS CODED SEPARATELY), PER DIEM	00	9			I			N
S9367	HOME INFUSION THERAPY, TOTAL PARENTERAL NUTRITION (TPN); MORE THAN TWO LITERS BUT NO MORE THAN THREE LITERS PER DAY, ADMINISTRATIVE SERVICES, PROFESSIONAL PHARMACY SERVICES, CARE COORDINATION, AND ALL NECESSARY SUPPLIES AND EQUIPMENT INCLUDING STANDARD TPN FORMULA (LIPIDS, SPECIALTY AMINO ACID FORMULAS, DRUGS OTHER THAN IN STANDARD FORMULA AND NURSING VISITS CODED SEPARATELY), PER DIEM	00	9			I			N
S9368	HOME INFUSION THERAPY, TOTAL PARENTERAL NUTRITION (TPN); MORE THAN THREE LITERS PER DAY, ADMINISTRATIVE SERVICES, PROFESSIONAL PHARMACY SERVICES, CARE COORDINATION, AND ALL NECESSARY SUPPLIES AND EQUIPMENT INCLUDING STANDARD TPN FORMULA (LIPIDS, SPECIALTY AMINO ACID FORMULAS, DRUGS OTHER THAN IN STANDARD FORMULA AND NURSING VISITS CODED SEPARATELY), PER DIEM	00	9			I			N
S9370	HOME THERAPY, INTERMITTENT ANTI-EMETIC INJECTION THERAPY; ADMINISTRATIVE SERVICES, PROFESSIONAL PHARMACY SERVICES, CARE COORDINATION, AND ALL NECESSARY SUPPLIES AND EQUIPMENT (DRUGS AND NURSING VISITS CODED SEPARATELY), PER DIEM	00	9			I			N
S9372	HOME THERAPY; INTERMITTENT ANTICOAGULANT INJECTION THERAPY (E.G. HEPARIN); ADMINISTRATIVE SERVICES, PROFESSIONAL PHARMACY SERVICES, CARE COORDINATION, AND ALL NECESSARY SUPPLIES AND EQUIPMENT (DRUGS AND NURSING VISITS CODED SEPARATELY), PER DIEM (DO NOT USE THIS CODE FOR FLUSHING OF INFUSION DEVICES WITH HEPARIN TO MAINTAIN PATENCY)	00	9			I			N
S9373	HOME INFUSION THERAPY, HYDRATION THERAPY; ADMINISTRATIVE SERVICES, PROFESSIONAL PHARMACY SERVICES, CARE COORDINATION, AND ALL NECESSARY SUPPLIES AND EQUIPMENT (DRUGS AND NURSING VISITS CODED SEPARATELY), PER DIEM (DO NOT USE WITH HYDRATION THERAPY CODES S9374-S9377 USING DAILY VOLUME SCALES)	00	9			I			N
S9374	HOME INFUSION THERAPY, HYDRATION THERAPY; ONE LITER PER DAY, ADMINISTRATIVE SERVICES, PROFESSIONAL PHARMACY SERVICES, CARE COORDINATION, AND ALL NECESSARY SUPPLIES AND EQUIPMENT (DRUGS AND NURSING VISITS CODED SEPARATELY), PER DIEM	00	9			I			N
S9375	HOME INFUSION THERAPY, HYDRATION THERAPY; MORE THAN ONE LITER BUT NO MORE THAN TWO LITERS PER DAY, ADMINISTRATIVE SERVICES, PROFESSIONAL PHARMACY SERVICES, CARE COORDINATION, AND ALL NECESSARY SUPPLIES AND EQUIPMENT (DRUGS AND NURSING VISITS CODED SEPARATELY), PER DIEM	00	9			I			N

HCPCS	Long Description	PB	MPI	Statute	X-Ref	Coverage	ASC Pay Grp	ASC Pay Grp Eff Date	Action Code
S9376	HOME INFUSION THERAPY, HYDRATION THERAPY; MORE THAN TWO LITERS BUT NO MORE THAN THREE LITERS PER DAY, ADMINISTRATIVE SERVICES, PROFESSIONAL PHARMACY SERVICES, CARE COORDINATION, AND ALL NECESSARY SUPPLIES AND EQUIPMENT (DRUGS AND NURSING VISITS CODED SEPARATELY) PER DIEM	00	9			I			N
S9377	HOME INFUSION THERAPY, HYDRATION THERAPY; MORE THAN THREE LITERS PER DAY, ADMINISTRATIVE SERVICES, PROFESSIONAL PHARMACY SERVICES, CARE COORDINATION, AND ALL NECESSARY SUPPLIES (DRUGS AND NURSING VISITS CODED SEPARATELY), PER DIEM	00	9			I			N
S9379	HOME INFUSION THERAPY, INFUSION THERAPY, NOT OTHERWISE CLASSIFIED; ADMINISTRATIVE SERVICES, PROFESSIONAL PHARMACY SERVICES, CARE COORDINATION, AND ALL NECESSARY SUPPLIES AND EQUIPMENT (DRUGS AND NURSING VISITS CODED SEPARATELY), PER DIEM	00	9			I			N
S9381	DELIVERY OR SERVICE TO HIGH RISK AREAS REQUIRING ESCORT OR EXTRA PROTECTION, PER VISIT	00	9			I			N
S9395	NURSING SERVICES AND ALL NECESSARY SUPPLIES AND ADDITIVES FOR HOME IV HYDRATION (VIA GRAVITY OR PUMP), PER DIEM (HYDRATION SOLUTION AND DRUGS NOT INCLUDED)	00	9			I			N
S9401	ANTICOAGULATION CLINIC, INCLUSIVE OF ALL SERVICES EXCEPT LABORATORY TESTS, PER SESSION	00	9			I			N
S9420	NURSING SERVICES AND ALL NECESSARY SUPPLIES FOR INTERIM HOME MAINTENANCE OF IMPLANTED VASCULAR ACCESS PORT/CATHETER/RESERVOIR, PER DIEM	00	9			I			N
S9423	NURSING SERVICES, PATIENT ASSESSMENT AND EDUCATION, FOLLOW-UP VISITS, ELECTRONIC PROGRAMMER AND EQUIPMENT (USE OF COMPUTER), PROGRAMMING OF THE PUMP, ALL NECESSARY SUPPLIES, PRODUCTS OR SERVICES FOR INTRATHECAL DRUG INFUSION, PER DIEM	00	9			I			N
S9425	NURSING SERVICES AND ALL NECESSARY SUPPLIES AND ADDITIVES FOR HOME IV CHEMOTHERAPY (VIA IV PUSH, GRAVITY DRIP, STATIONARY PUMP, AMBULATORY BELT PUMP), PER DIEM (HYDRATION SOLUTION AND DRUGS NOT INCLUDED)	00	9			I			N
S9430	PHARMACY COMPOUNDING AND DISPENSING SERVICES	00	9			I			N
S9434	MODIFIED SOLID FOOD SUPPLEMENTS FOR INBORN ERRORS OF METABOLISM	00	9			I			A
S9435	MEDICAL FOODS FOR INBORN ERRORS OF METABOLISM	00	9			I			N
S9436	CHILDBIRTH PREPARATION/LAMAZE CLASSES, NON-PHYSICIAN PROVIDER, PER SESSION	00	9			I			N
S9437	CHILDBIRTH REFRESHER CLASSES, NON-PHYSICIAN PROVIDER, PER SESSION	00	9			I			N
S9438	CESAREAN BIRTH CLASSES, NON-PHYSICIAN PROVIDER, PER SESSION	00	9			I			N
S9439	VBAC (VAGINAL BIRTH AFTER CESAREAN) CLASSES, NON-PHYSICIAN PROVIDER, PER SESSION	00	9			I			N
S9441	ASTHMA EDUCATION, NON-PHYSICIAN PROVIDER, PER SESSION	00	9			I			N
S9442	BIRTHING CLASSES, NON-PHYSICIAN PROVIDER, PER SESSION	00	9			I			N
S9443	LACTATION CLASSES, NON-PHYSICIAN PROVIDER, PER SESSION	00	9			I			N
S9444	PARENTING CLASSES, NON-PHYSICIAN PROVIDER, PER SESSION	00	9			I			N
S9445	PATIENT EDUCATION, NOT OTHERWISE CLASSIFIED, NON-PHYSICIAN PROVIDER, INDIVIDUAL, PER SESSION	00	9			I			N
S9446	PATIENT EDUCATION, NOT OTHERWISE CLASSIFIED, NON-PHYSICIAN PROVIDER, GROUP, PER SESSION	00	9			I			N
S9447	INFANT SAFETY (INCLUDING CPR) CLASSES, NON-PHYSICIAN PROVIDER, PER SESSION	00	9			I			N
S9449	WEIGHT MANAGEMENT CLASSES, NON-PHYSICIAN PROVIDER, PER SESSION	00	9			I			N
S9451	EXERCISE CLASSES, NON-PHYSICIAN PROVIDER, PER SESSION	00	9			I			N
S9452	NUTRITION CLASSES, NON-PHYSICIAN PROVIDER, PER SESSION	00	9			I			N

HCPCS	Long Description	PH	MPI	Statute	X-Ref	Coverage	ASC Pay Grp	ASC Pay Grp Eff Date	Action Code
S9453	SMOKING CESSATION CLASSES, NON-PHYSICIAN PROVIDER, PER SESSION	00	9			I			N
S9454	STRESS MANAGEMENT CLASSES, NON-PHYSICIAN PROVIDER, PER SESSION	00	9			I			N
S9455	DIABETIC MANAGEMENT PROGRAM, GROUP SESSION	00	9			I			N
S9460	DIABETIC MANAGEMENT PROGRAM, NURSE VISIT	00	9			I			N
S9465	DIABETIC MANAGEMENT PROGRAM, DIETITIAN VISIT	00	9			I			N
S9470	NUTRITIONAL COUNSELING, DIETITIAN VISIT	00	9			I			N
S9472	CARDIAC REHABILITATION PROGRAM, NON-PHYSICIAN PROVIDER, PER DIEM	00	9			I			N
S9473	PULMONARY REHABILITATION PROGRAM, NON-PHYSICIAN PROVIDER, PER DIEM	00	9			I			N
S9474	ENTEROSTOMAL THERAPY BY A REGISTERED NURSE CERTIFIED IN ENTEROSTOMAL THERAPY, PER DIEM	00	9			I			N
S9475	AMBULATORY SETTING SUBSTANCE ABUSE TREATMENT OR DETOXIFICATION SERVICES, PER DIEM	00	9			I			N
S9476	VESTIBULAR REHABILITATION PROGRAM, NON-PHYSICIAN PROVIDER, PER DIEM	00	9			I			A
S9480	INTENSIVE OUTPATIENT PSYCHIATRIC SERVICES, PER DIEM	00	9			I			N
S9484	CRISIS INTERVENTION MENTAL HEALTH SERVICES, PER HOUR	00	9			I			N
S9485	CRISIS INTERVENTION MENTAL HEALTH SERVICES, PER DIEM	00	9			I			N
S9490	HOME INFUSION THERAPY, CORTICOSTEROID INFUSION; ADMINISTRATIVE SERVICES, PROFESSIONAL PHARMACY SERVICES, CARE COORDINATION, AND ALL NECESSARY SUPPLIES AND EQUIPMENT (DRUGS AND NURSING VISITS CODED SEPARATELY), PER DIEM	00	9			I			N
S9494	HOME INFUSION THERAPY, ANTIBIOTIC, ANTIVIRAL, OR ANTIFUNGAL THERAPY; ADMINISTRATIVE SERVICES, PROFESSIONAL PHARMACY SERVICES, CARE COORDINATION, AND ALL NECESSARY SUPPLIES AND EQUIPMENT (DRUGS AND NURSING VISITS CODED SEPARATELY, PER DIEM) (DO NOT USE THIS CODE WITH HOME INFUSION CODES FOR HOURLY DOSING SCHEDULES S9497-S9504)	00	9			I			N
S9497	HOME INFUSION THERAPY, ANTIBIOTIC, ANTIVIRAL, OR ANTIFUNGAL THERAPY; ONCE EVERY 3 HOURS; ADMINISTRATIVE SERVICES, PROFESSIONAL PHARMACY SERVICES, CARE COORDINATION, AND ALL NECESSARY SUPPLIES AND EQUIPMENT (DRUGS AND NURSING VISITS CODED SEPARATELY), PER DIEM	00	9			I			N
S9500	HOME INFUSION THERAPY, ANTIBIOTIC, ANTIVIRAL, OR ANTIFUNGAL THERAPY; ONCE EVERY 24 HOURS; ADMINISTRATIVE SERVICES, PROFESSIONAL PHARMACY SERVICES, CARE COORDINATION, AND ALL NECESSARY SUPPLIES AND EQUIPMENT (DRUGS AND NURSING VISITS CODED SEPARATELY), PER DIEM	00	9			I			N
S9501	HOME INFUSION THERAPY, ANTIBIOTIC, ANTIVIRAL, OR ANTIFUNGAL THERAPY; ONCE EVERY 12 HOURS; ADMINISTRATIVE SERVICES, PROFESSIONAL PHARMACY SERVICES, CARE COORDINATION, AND ALL NECESSARY SUPPLIES AND EQUIPMENT (DRUGS AND NURSING VISITS CODED SEPARATELY), PER DIEM	00	9			I			N

HCPCS	Long Description	PII	MPI	Statute	X-Ref	Coverage	ASC Pay Grp	ASC Pay Grp Eff Date	Action Code
S9502	HOME INFUSION THERAPY, ANTIBIOTIC, ANTIVIRAL, OR ANTIFUNGAL THERAPY; ONCE EVERY 8 HOURS, ADMINISTRATIVE SERVICES, PROFESSIONAL PHARMACY SERVICES, CARE COORDINATION, AND ALL NECESSARY SUPPLIES AND EQUIPMENT (DRUGS AND NURSING VISITS CODED SEPARATELY) PER DIEM	00	9			I			N
S9503	HOME INFUSION THERAPY, ANTIBIOTIC, ANTIVIRAL, OR ANTIFUNGAL; ONCE EVERY 6 HOURS; ADMINISTRATIVE SERVICES, PROFESSIONAL PHARMACY SERVICES, CARE COORDINATION, AND ALL NECESSARY SUPPLIES AND EQUIPMENT (DRUGS AND NURSING VISITS CODED SEPARATELY) PER DIEM	00	9			I			N
S9504	HOME INFUSION THERAPY, ANTIBIOTIC, ANTIVIRAL, OR ANTIFUNGAL; ONCE EVERY 4 HOURS; ADMINISTRATIVE SERVICES, PROFESSIONAL PHARMACY SERVICES, CARE COORDINATION, AND ALL NECESSARY SUPPLIES AND EQUIPMENT (DRUGS AND NURSING VISITS CODED SEPARATELY) PER DIEM	00	9			I			N
S9524	NURSING SERVICES RELATED TO HOME IV THERAPY, PER DIEM	00	9			I			D
S9526	SKILLED NURSING VISITS FOR BLOOD PRODUCT ADMINISTRATION, INCLUDING PUMP AND ALL RELATED SUPPLIES; PER SERVICE	00	9			I			N
S9527	INSERTION OF A PERIPHERALLY INSERTED CENTRAL VENOUS CATHETER (PICC), INCLUDING NURSING SERVICES AND ALL SUPPLIES	00	9			I			N
S9528	INSERTION OF MIDLINE CENTRAL VENOUS CATHETER, INCLUDING NURSING SERVICES AND ALL SUPPLIES	00	9			I			N
S9529	ROUTINE VENIPUNCTURE FOR COLLECTION OF SPECIMEN(S), SINGLE HOME BOUND, NURSING HOME, OR SKILLED NURSING FACILITY PATIENT	00	9			I			N
S9533	PAIN MANAGEMENT, INTRAVENOUS, EPIDURAL OR SUBCUTANEOUS, INCLUDING SOLUTION, EQUIPMENT RENTAL, NURSING CARE, AND SUPPLIES; DAILY (DRUGS NOT INCLUDED)	00	9			I			N
S9535	ADMINISTRATION OF HEMATOPOIETIC HORMONES (E.G. ERYTHROPOIETIN, G-CSF, GM-CSF) OR PLATELETS, INTRAVENOUSLY, IN THE HOME SETTING, INCLUDING ALL NURSING CARE, EQUIPMENT, AND SUPPLIES; PER DIEM	00	9			I			N
S9537	HOME THERAPY; HEMATOPOIETIC HORMONE INJECTION THERAPY (E.G.ERYTHROPOIETIN, G-CSF, GM-CSF); ADMINISTRATIVE SERVICES, PROFESSIONAL PHARMACY SERVICES, CARE COORDINATION, AND ALL NECESSARY SUPPLIES AND EQUIPMENT (DRUGS AND NURSING VISITS CODED SEPARATELY) PER DIEM	00	9			I			N
S9538	HOME TRANSFUSION OF BLOOD PRODUCT(S); ADMINISTRATIVE SERVICES, PROFESSIONAL PHARMACY SERVICES, CARE COORDINATION AND ALL NECESSARY SUPPLIES AND EQUIPMENT (BLOOD PRODUCTS, DRUGS, AND NURSING VISITS CODED SEPARATELY), PER DIEM	00	9			I			N
S9539	ADMINISTRATION OF ANTIBIOTICS, INTRAVENOUSLY, IN THE HOME SETTING, INCLUDING ALL NURSING CARE, EQUIPMENT, AND SUPPLIES; PER DIEM	00	9			I			N
S9542	HOME INJECTABLE THERAPY, NOT OTHERWISE CLASSIFIED, INCLUDING ADMINISTRATIVE SERVICES, PROFESSIONAL PHARMACY SERVICES, CARE COORDINATION, AND ALL NECESSARY SUPPLIES AND EQUIPMENT (DRUGS AND NURSING VISITS CODED SEPARATELY), PER DIEM	00	9			I			N
S9543	ADMINISTRATION OF MEDICATION, INTRAMUSCULARLY, EPIDURALLY OR SUBCUTANEOUSLY, IN THE HOME SETTING, INCLUDING ALL NURSING CARE, EQUIPMENT, AND SUPPLIES; PER DIEM	00	9			I			N
S9545	ADMINISTRATION OF IMMUNE GLOBULIN, INTRAVENOUSLY, IN THE HOME SETTING, INCLUDING ALL NURSING CARE, EQUIPMENT, AND SUPPLIES; PER DIEM	00	9			I			N
S9546	HOME INFUSION OF BLOOD PRODUCTS, NURSING SERVICES, PER VISIT	00	9			I			D
S9550	HOME IV THERAPY, HYDRATION FLUIDS AND ELECTROLYTES, INCLUDING ALL NURSING CARE, EQUIPMENT, AND SUPPLIES; PER DIEM	00	9			I			N
S9555	ADDITIONAL HOME INFUSION THERAPY, INCLUDING ALL NURSING CARE, EQUIPMENT, AND SUPPLIES; EACH THERAPY, PER DIEM (S9555 SHOULD BE USED IN ADDITION TO THE CODE FOR THE PRIMARY THERAPY)	00	9			I			N

HCPCS	Long Description	PH	MPI	Statute	X-Ref	Coverage	ASC Pay Grp	ASC Pay Grp Eff Date	Action Code
S9558	HOME INJECTABLE THERAPY; GROWTH HORMONE, INCLUDING ADMINISTRATIVE SERVICES, PROFESSIONAL PHARMACY SERVICES, CARE COORDINATION, AND ALL NECESSARY SUPPLIES AND EQUIPMENT (DRUGS AND NURSING VISITS CODED SEPARATELY), PER DIEM	00	9			I			N
S9559	HOME INJECTABLE THERAPY, INTERFERON, INCLUDING ADMINISTRATIVE SERVICES, PROFESSIONAL PHARMACY SERVICES, CARE COORDINATION, AND ALL NECESSARY SUPPLIES AND EQUIPMENT (DRUGS AND NURSING VISITS CODED SEPARATELY), PER DIEM	00	9			I			N
S9560	HOME INJECTABLE THERAPY; HORMONAL THERAPY (E.G.; LEUPROLIDE, GOSERELIN), INCLUDING ADMINISTRATIVE SERVICES, PROFESSIONAL PHARMACY SERVICES, CARE COORDINATION, AND ALL NECESSARY SUPPLIES AND EQUIPMENT (DRUGS AND NURSING VISITS CODED SEPARATELY), PER DIEM	00	9			I			N
S9562	HOME INJECTABLE THERAPY, PALIVIZUMAB, INCLUDING ADMINISTRATIVE SERVICES, PROFESSIONAL PHARMACY SERVICES, CARE COORDINATION, AND ALL NECESSARY SUPPLIES AND EQUIPMENT (DRUGS AND NURSING VISITS CODED SEPARATELY), PER DIEM	00	9			I			N
S9590	HOME THERAPY, IRRIGATION THERAPY (E.G. STERILE IRRIGATION OF AN ORGAN OR ANATOMICAL CAVITY); INCLUDING ADMINISTRATIVE SERVICES, PROFESSIONAL PHARMACY SERVICES, CARE COORDINATION, AND ALL NECESSARY SUPPLIES AND EQUIPMENT (DRUGS AND NURSING VISITS CODED SEPARATELY), PER DIEM	00	9			I			N
S9800	HOME THERAPY; PROVISION OF INFUSION, SPECIALTY DRUG ADMINISTRATION, AND/OR ASSOCIATED NURSING SERVICES AND PROCEDURES, BY HIGHLY TECHNICAL R.N., PER HOUR (DO NOT USE THIS CODE WITH S9524)	00	9		S9802-3	I			N
S9802	HOME INFUSION/SPECIALTY DRUG ADMINISTRATION, NURSING SERVICES; PER VISIT (UP TO 2 HOURS)	00	9			I			D
S9803	HOME INFUSION/SPECIALTY DRUG ADMINISTRATION, NURSING SERVICES; EACH ADDITIONAL HOUR (LIST SEPARATELY IN ADDITION TO CODE S9802)	00	9			I			D
S9806	RN SERVICES IN THE INFUSION SUITE OF THE IV THERAPY PROVIDER, PER VISIT	00	9			I			D
S9810	HOME THERAPY; PROFESSIONAL PHARMACY SERVICES FOR PROVISION OF INFUSION, SPECIALTY DRUG ADMINISTRATION, AND/OR DISEASE STATE MANAGEMENT, NOT OTHERWISE CLASSIFIED, PER HOUR (DO NOT USE THIS CODE WITH ANY PER DIEM CODE)	00	9			I			N
S9900	SERVICES BY AUTHORIZED CHRISTIAN SCIENCE PRACTITIONER FOR THE PROCESS OF HEALING, PER DIEM; NOT TO BE USED FOR REST OR STUDY; EXCLUDES IN-PATIENT SERVICES	00	9			I			N
S9970	HEALTH CLUB MEMBERSHIP, ANNUAL	00	9			I			N
S9975	TRANSPLANT RELATED LODGING, MEALS AND TRANSPORTATION, PER DIEM	00	9			I			N
S9981	MEDICAL RECORDS COPYING FEE, ADMINISTRATIVE	00	9			I			N
S9982	MEDICAL RECORDS COPYING FEE, PER PAGE	00	9			I			N
S9986	NOT MEDICALLY NECESSARY SERVICE (PATIENT IS AWARE THAT SERVICE NOT MEDICALLY NECESSARY)	00	9			I			N
S9989	SERVICES PROVIDED OUTSIDE OF THE UNITED STATES OF AMERICA (LIST IN ADDITION TO CODE(S) FOR SERVICES(S))	00	9			I			N
S9990	SERVICES PROVIDED AS PART OF A PHASE II CLINICAL TRIAL	00	9			I			N
S9991	SERVICES PROVIDED AS PART OF A PHASE III CLINICAL TRIAL	00	9			I			N
S9992	TRANSPORTATION COSTS TO AND FROM TRIAL LOCATION AND LOCAL TRANSPORTATION COSTS (E.G., FARES FOR TAXICAB OR BUS) FOR CLINICAL TRIAL PARTICIPANT AND ONE CAREGIVER/COMPANION	00	9			I			N
S9994	LODGING COSTS (E.G., HOTEL CHARGES) FOR CLINICAL TRIAL PARTICIPANT AND ONE CAREGIVER/COMPANION	00	9			I			N

HCPCS	Long Description	PH	MPI	Statute	X-Ref1	Coverage	ASC Pay Grp	ASC Pay Grp Eff Date	Action Code
S9996	MEALS FOR CLINICAL TRIAL PARTICIPANT AND ONE CAREGIVER/COMPANION	00	9			I			N
S9999	SALES TAX	00	9			I			N
T1000	PRIVATE DUTY / INDEPENDENT NURSING SERVICE(S) - LICENSED, UP TO 15 MINUTES	00	9			I			N
T1001	NURSING ASSESSMENT / EVALUATION	00	9			I			N
T1002	RN SERVICES, UP TO 15 MINUTES	00	9			I			N
T1003	LPN/LVN SERVICES, UP TO 15 MINUTES	00	9			I			N
T1004	SERVICES OF A QUALIFIED NURSING AIDE, UP TO 15 MINUTES	00	9			I			N
T1005	RESPITE CARE SERVICES, UP TO 15 MINUTES	00	9			I			N
T1006	ALCOHOL AND/OR SUBSTANCE ABUSE SERVICES, FAMILY/COUPLE COUNSELING	00	9			I			N
T1007	ALCOHOL AND/OR SUBSTANCE ABUSE SERVICES, TREATMENT PLAN DEVELOPMENT AND/OR MODIFICATION	00	9			I			N
T1008	DAY TREATMENT FOR INDIVIDUAL ALCOHOL AND/OR SUBSTANCE ABUSE SERVICES	00	9			I			D
T1009	CHILD SITTING SERVICES FOR CHILDREN OF THE INDIVIDUAL RECEIVING ALCOHOL AND/OR SUBSTANCE ABUSE SERVICES	00	9			I			N
T1010	MEALS FOR INDIVIDUALS RECEIVING ALCOHOL AND/OR SUBSTANCE ABUSE SERVICES (WHEN MEALS NOT INCLUDED IN THE PROGRAM)	00	9			I			N
T1011	ALCOHOL AND/OR SUBSTANCE ABUSE SERVICES, NOT OTHERWISE CLASSIFIED	00	9			I			D
T1012	ALCOHOL AND/OR SUBSTANCE ABUSE SERVICES, SKILLS DEVELOPMENT	00	9			I			N
T1013	SIGN LANGUAGE OR ORAL INTERPRETIVE SERVICES, PER 15 MINUTES	00	9			I			N
T1014	TELEHEALTH TRANSMISSION, PER MINUTE, PROFESSIONAL SERVICES BILL SEPARATELY	00	9			I			N
T1015	CLINIC VISIT/ENCOUNTER, ALL-INCLUSIVE	00	9			I			N
T1016	CASE MANAGEMENT, EACH 15 MINUTES	00	9			I			N
T1017	TARGETED CASE MANAGEMENT, EACH 15 MINUTES	00	9			I			N
T1018	SCHOOL-BASED INDIVIDUALIZED EDUCATION PROGRAM (IEP) SERVICES, BUNDLED	00	9			I			N
T1019	PERSONAL CARE SERVICES, PER 15 MINUTES, NOT FOR AN INPATIENT OR RESIDENT OF A HOSPITAL, NURSING FACILITY, ICF/MR OR IMD, PART OF THE INDIVIDUALIZED PLAN OF TREATMENT (CODE MAY NOT BE USED TO IDENTIFY SERVICES PROVIDED BY HOME HEALTH AIDE OR CERTIFIED NURSE ASSISTANT)	00	9			I			N
T1020	PERSONAL CARE SERVICES, PER DIEM, NOT FOR AN INPATIENT OR RESIDENT OF A HOSPITAL, NURSING FACILITY, ICF/MR OR IMD, PART OF THE INDIVIDUALIZED PLAN OF TREATMENT (CODE MAY NOT BE USED TO IDENTIFY SERVICES PROVIDED BY HOME HEALTH AIDE OR CERTIFIED NURSE ASSISTANT)	00	9			I			N
T1021	HOME HEALTH AIDE OR CERTIFIED NURSE ASSISTANT, PER VISIT	00	9			I			N

HCPCS	Long Description	PII	MPI	Statute	X-Ref1	Coverage	ASC Pay Grp	ASC Pay Grp Eff Date	Action Code
T1022	CONTRACTED HOME HEALTH AGENCY SERVICES, ALL SERVICES PROVIDED UNDER CONTRACT, PER DAY	00	9			I			N
T1023	SCREENING TO DETERMINE THE APPROPRIATENESS OF CONSIDERATION OF AN INDIVIDUAL FOR PARTICIPATION IN A SPECIFIED PROGRAM, PROJECT OR TREATMENT PROTOCOL, PER ENCOUNTER	00	9			I			N
T1024	EVALUATION AND TREATMENT BY AN INTEGRATED, SPECIALTY TEAM CONTRACTED TO PROVIDE COORDINATED CARE TO MULTIPLE OR SEVERELY HANDICAPPED CHILDREN, PER ENCOUNTER	00	9			I			N
T1025	INTENSIVE, EXTENDED MULTIDISCIPLINARY SERVICES PROVIDED IN A CLINIC SETTING TO CHILDREN WITH COMPLEX MEDICAL, PHYSICAL, MENTAL AND PSYCHOSOCIAL IMPAIRMENTS, PER DIEM	00	9			I			N
T1026	INTENSIVE, EXTENDED MULTIDISCIPLINARY SERVICES PROVIDED IN A CLINIC SETTING TO CHILDREN WITH COMPLEX MEDICAL, PHYSICAL, MEDICAL AND PSYCHOSOCIAL IMPAIRMENTS, PER HOUR	00	9			I			N
T1027	FAMILY TRAINING AND COUNSELING FOR CHILD DEVELOPMENT, PER 15 MINUTES	00	9			I			N
T1028	ASSESSMENT OF HOME, PHYSICAL AND FAMILY ENVIRONMENT, TO DETERMINE SUITABILITY TO MEET PATIENTS MEDICAL NEEDS	00	9			I			N
T1029	COMPREHENSIVE ENVIRONMENTAL LEAD INVESTIGATION, NOT INCLUDING LABORATORY ANALYSIS, PER DWELLING	00	9			I			N
T1030	NURSING CARE, IN THE HOME, BY REGISTERED NURSE, PER DIEM	00	9			I			N
T1031	NURSING CARE, IN THE HOME, BY LICENSED PRACTICAL NURSE, PER DIEM	00	9			I			N
T1500	DIAPER/INCONTINENT PANT, REUSABLE/WASHABLE, ANY SIZE, EACH	00	9			I			N
T1502	ADMINISTRATION OF ORAL, INTRAMUSCULAR AND/OR SUBCUTANEOUS MEDICATION BY HEALTH CARE AGENCY/PROFESSIONAL, PER VISIT	00	9			I			N
T1999	MISCELLANEOUS THERAPEUTIC ITEMS AND SUPPLIES, RETAIL PURCHASES, NOT OTHERWISE CLASSIFIED; IDENTIFY PRODUCT IN "REMARKS"	00	9			I			N
T2001	NON-EMERGENCY TRANSPORTATION; PATIENT ATTENDANT/ESCORT	00	9			I			N
T2002	NON-EMERGENCY TRANSPORTATION; PER DIEM	00	9			I			N
T2003	NON-EMERGENCY TRANSPORTATION; ENCOUNTER/TRIP	00	9			I			N
T2004	NON-EMERGENCY TRANSPORT; COMMERCIAL CARRIER, MULTI-PASS	00	9			I			N
T2005	NON-EMERGENCY TRANSPORTATION; NON-AMBULATORY STRETCHER VAN	00	9			I			N
T2006	AMBULANCE RESPONSE AND TREATMENT, NO TRANSPORT	00	9			I			N
T2007	TRANSPORTATION WAITING TIME, AIR AMBULANCE AND NON-EMERGENCY VEHICLE, ONE-HALF (1/2) HOUR INCREMENTS	00	9			I			N
T2010	PREADMISSION SCREENING AND RESIDENT REVIEW (PASRR) LEVEL I IDENTIFICATION SCREENING, PER SCREEN	00	9			I			A
T2011	PREADMISSION SCREENING AND RESIDENT REVIEW (PASRR) LEVEL II EVALUATION, PER EVALUATION	00	9			I			A
T2012	HABILITATION, EDUCATIONAL; WAIVER, PER DIEM	00	9			I			A
T2013	HABILITATION, EDUCATIONAL, WAIVER; PER HOUR	00	9			I			A
T2014	HABILITATION, PREVOCATIONAL, WAIVER; PER DIEM	00	9			I			A
T2015	HABILITATION, PREVOCATIONAL, WAIVER; PER HOUR	00	9			I			A
T2016	HABILITATION, RESIDENTIAL, WAIVER; PER DIEM	00	9			I			A

HCPCS	Long Description	PTI	MPI	Statute	X-Ref1	Coverage	ASC Pay Grp	ASC Pay Grp Eff Date	Action Code
T2017	HABILITATION, RESIDENTIAL, WAIVER; 15 MINUTES	00	9			I			A
T2018	HABILITATION, SUPPORTED EMPLOYMENT, WAIVER; PER DIEM	00	9			I			A
T2019	HABILITATION, SUPPORTED EMPLOYMENT, WAIVER; PER 15 MINUTES	00	9			I			A
T2020	DAY HABILITATION, WAIVER; PER DIEM	00	9			I			A
T2021	DAY HABILITATION, WAIVER; PER 15 MINUTES	00	9			I			A
T2022	CASE MANAGEMENT, PER MONTH	00	9			I			A
T2023	TARGETED CASE MANAGEMENT; PER MONTH	00	9			I			A
T2024	SERVICE ASSESSMENT/PLAN OF CARE DEVELOPMENT, WAIVER	00	9			I			A
T2025	WAIVER SERVICES; NOT OTHERWISE SPECIFIED (NOS)	00	9			I			A
T2026	SPECIALIZED CHILDCARE, WAIVER; PER DIEM	00	9			I			A
T2027	SPECIALIZED CHILDCARE, WAIVER; PER 15 MINUTES	00	9			I			A
T2028	SPECIALIZED SUPPLY, NOT OTHERWISE SPECIFIED, WAIVER	00	9			I			A
T2029	SPECIALIZED MEDICAL EQUIPMENT, NOT OTHERWISE SPECIFIED, WAIVER	00	9			I			A
T2030	ASSISTED LIVING, WAIVER; PER MONTH	00	9			I			A
T2031	ASSISTED LIVING; WAIVER, PER DIEM	00	9			I			A
T2032	RESIDENTIAL CARE, NOT OTHERWISE SPECIFIED (NOS), WAIVER; PER MONTH	00	9			I			A
T2033	RESIDENTIAL CARE, NOT OTHERWISE SPECIFIED (NOS), WAIVER; PER DIEM	00	9			I			A
T2034	CRISIS INTERVENTION, WAIVER; PER DIEM	00	9			I			A
T2035	UTILITY SERVICES TO SUPPORT MEDICAL EQUIPMENT AND ASSISTIVE TECHNOLOGY/DEVICES, WAIVER	00	9			I			A
T2036	THERAPEUTIC CAMPING, OVERNIGHT, WAIVER; EACH SESSION	00	9			I			A
T2037	THERAPEUTIC CAMPING, DAY, WAIVER; EACH SESSION	00	9			I			A
T2038	COMMUNITY TRANSITION, WAIVER; PER SERVICE	00	9			I			A
T2039	VEHICLE MODIFICATIONS, WAIVER; PER SERVICE	00	9			I			A
T2040	FINANCIAL MANAGEMENT, SELF-DIRECTED, WAIVER; PER 15 MINUTES	00	9			I			A
T2041	SUPPORTS BROKERAGE, SELF-DIRECTED, WAIVER; PER 15 MINUTES	00	9			I			A

HCPCS	Long Description	PII	MPI	Statute	X-Ref1	Coverage	ASC Pay Grp	ASC Pay Grp Eff Date	Action Code
T2042	HOSPICE ROUTINE HOME CARE; PER DIEM	00	9			I			A
T2043	HOSPICE CONTINUOUS HOME CARE; PER HOUR	00	9			I			A
T2044	HOSPICE INPATIENT RESPITE CARE; PER DIEM	00	9			I			A
T2045	HOSPICE GENERAL INPATIENT CARE; PER DIEM	00	9			I			A
T2046	HOSPICE LONG TERM CARE, ROOM AND BOARD ONLY; PER DIEM	00	9			I			A
T2048	BEHAVIORAL HEALTH; LONG-TERM CARE RESIDENTIAL (NON-ACUTE CARE IN A RESIDENTIAL TREATMENT PROGRAM WHERE STAY IS TYPICALLY LONGER THAN 30 DAYS), WITH ROOM AND BOARD, PER DIEM	00	9			I			A
T2101	HUMAN BREAST MILK PROCESSING, STORAGE AND DISTRIBUTION ONLY	00	9			I			A
T5001	POSITIONING SEAT FOR PERSONS WITH SPECIAL ORTHOPEDIC NEEDS, FOR USE IN VEHICLES	00	9			I			A
T5999	SUPPLY, NOT OTHERWISE SPECIFIED	00	9			I			A
V2020	FRAMES, PURCHASES	38	A			D			T
V2025	DELUXE FRAME	00	9			M			T
V2100	SPHERE, SINGLE VISION, PLANO TO PLUS OR MINUS 4.00, PER LENS	38	A			C			T
V2101	SPHERE, SINGLE VISION, PLUS OR MINUS 4.12 TO PLUS OR MINUS 7.00D, PER LENS	38	A			C			T
V2102	SPHERE, SINGLE VISION, PLUS OR MINUS 7.12 TO PLUS OR MINUS 20.00D, PER LENS	38	A			C			T
V2103	SPHEROCYLINDER, SINGLE VISION, PLANO TO PLUS OR MINUS 4.00D SPHERE, .12 TO 2.00D CYLINDER, PER LENS	38	A			C			T
V2104	SPHEROCYLINDER, SINGLE VISION, PLANO TO PLUS OR MINUS 4.00D SPHERE, 2.12 TO 4.00D CYLINDER, PER LENS	38	A			C			T
V2105	SPHEROCYLINDER, SINGLE VISION, PLANO TO PLUS OR MINUS 4.00D SPHERE, 4.25 TO 6.00D CYLINDER, PER LENS	38	A			C			T
V2106	SPHEROCYLINDER, SINGLE VISION, PLANO TO PLUS OR MINUS 4.00D SPHERE, OVER 6.00D CYLINDER, PER LENS	38	A			C			T
V2107	SPHEROCYLINDER, SINGLE VISION, PLUS OR MINUS 4.25 TO PLUS OR MINUS 7.00 SPHERE, .12 TO 2.00D CYLINDER, PER LENS	38	A			C			T
V2108	SPHEROCYLINDER, SINGLE VISION, PLUS OR MINUS 4.25D TO PLUS OR MINUS 7.00D SPHERE, 2.12 TO 4.00D CYLINDER, PER LENS	38	A			C			T
V2109	SPHEROCYLINDER, SINGLE VISION, PLUS OR MINUS 4.25 TO PLUS OR MINUS 7.00D SPHERE, 4.25 TO 6.00D CYLINDER, PER LENS	38	A			C			T
V2110	SPHEROCYLINDER, SINGLE VISION, PLUS OR MINUS 4.25 TO 7.00D SPHERE, OVER 6.00D CYLINDER, PER LENS	38	A			C			T
V2111	SPHEROCYLINDER, SINGLE VISION, PLUS OR MINUS 7.25 TO PLUS OR MINUS 12.00D SPHERE, .25 TO 2.25D CYLINDER, PER LENS	38	A			C			T
V2112	SPHEROCYLINDER, SINGLE VISION, PLUS OR MINUS 7.25 TO PLUS OR MINUS 12.00D SPHERE, 2.25D TO 4.00D CYLINDER, PER LENS	38	A			C			T
V2113	SPHEROCYLINDER, SINGLE VISION, PLUS OR MINUS 7.25 TO PLUS OR MINUS 12.00D SPHERE, 4.25 TO 6.00D CYLINDER, PER LENS	38	A			C			T
V2114	SPHEROCYLINDER, SINGLE VISION, SPHERE OVER PLUS OR MINUS 12.00D, PER LENS	38	A			C			T

HCPCS	Long Description	PII	MPI	Statute	X-Refl	Coverage	ASC Pay Grp	ASC Pay Grp Eff Date	Action Code
V2115	LENTICULAR, (MYODISC), PER LENS, SINGLE VISION	38	A			C			T
V2116	LENTICULAR LENS, NONASPHERIC, PER LENS, SINGLE VISION	38	A			C			D
V2117	LENTICULAR, ASPHERIC, PER LENS, SINGLE VISION	38	A			C			D
V2118	ANISEIKONIC LENS, SINGLE VISION	38	A			C			T
V2121	LENTICULAR LENS, PER LENS, SINGLE	38	A			D			A
V2199	NOT OTHERWISE CLASSIFIED, SINGLE VISION LENS	46	A			C			T
V2200	SPHERE, BIFOCAL, PLANO TO PLUS OR MINUS 4.00D, PER LENS	38	A			C			T
V2201	SPHERE, BIFOCAL, PLUS OR MINUS 4.12 TO PLUS OR MINUS 7.00D, PER LENS	38	A			C			T
V2202	SPHERE, BIFOCAL, PLUS OR MINUS 7.12 TO PLUS OR MINUS 20.00D, PER LENS	38	A			C			T
V2203	SPHEROCYLINDER, BIFOCAL, PLANO TO PLUS OR MINUS 4.00D SPHERE, .12 TO 2.00D CYLINDER, PER LENS	38	A			C			T
V2204	SPHEROCYLINDER, BIFOCAL, PLANO TO PLUS OR MINUS 4.00D SPHERE, 2.12 TO 4.00D CYLINDER, PER LENS	38	A			C			T
V2205	SPHEROCYLINDER, BIFOCAL, PLANO TO PLUS OR MINUS 4.00D SPHERE, 4.25 TO 6.00D CYLINDER, PER LENS	38	A			C			T
V2206	SPHEROCYLINDER, BIFOCAL, PLANO TO PLUS OR MINUS 4.00D SPHERE, OVER 6.00D CYLINDER, PER LENS	38	A			C			T
V2207	SPHEROCYLINDER, BIFOCAL, PLUS OR MINUS 4.25 TO PLUS OR MINUS 7.00D SPHERE, .12 TO 2.00D CYLINDER, PER LENS	38	A			C			T
V2208	SPHEROCYLINDER, BIFOCAL, PLUS OR MINUS 4.25 TO PLUS OR MINUS 7.00D SPHERE, 2.12 TO 4.00D CYLINDER, PER LENS	38	A			C			T
V2209	SPHEROCYLINDER, BIFOCAL, PLUS OR MINUS 4.25 TO PLUS OR MINUS 7.00D SPHERE, 4.25 TO 6.00D CYLINDER, PER LENS	38	A			C			T
V2210	SPHEROCYLINDER, BIFOCAL, PLUS OR MINUS 4.25 TO PLUS OR MINUS 7.00D SPHERE, OVER 6.00D CYLINDER, PER LENS	38	A			C			T
V2211	SPHEROCYLINDER, BIFOCAL, PLUS OR MINUS 7.25 TO PLUS OR MINUS 12.00D SPHERE, .25 TO 2.25D CYLINDER, PER LENS	38	A			C			T
V2212	SPHEROCYLINDER, BIFOCAL, PLUS OR MINUS 7.25 TO PLUS OR MINUS 12.00D SPHERE, 2.25 TO 4.00D CYLINDER, PER LENS	38	A			C			T
V2213	SPHEROCYLINDER, BIFOCAL, PLUS OR MINUS 7.25 TO PLUS OR MINUS 12.00D SPHERE, 4.25 TO 6.00D CYLINDER, PER LENS	38	A			C			T
V2214	SPHEROCYLINDER, BIFOCAL, SPHERE OVER PLUS OR MINUS 12.00D, PER LENS	38	A			C			T
V2215	LENTICULAR (MYODISC), PER LENS, BIFOCAL	38	A			C			T
V2216	LENTICULAR, NONASPHERIC, PER LENS, BIFOCAL	38	A			C			D
V2217	LENTICULAR, ASPHERIC LENS, BIFOCAL	38	A			C			D

HCPCS	Long Description	PII	MPI	Statute	X-Ref	Coverage	ASC Pay Grp	ASC Pay Grp Eff Date	Action Code
V2218	ANISEIKONIC, PER LENS, BIFOCAL	38	A			C			T
V2219	BIFOCAL SEG WIDTH OVER 28MM	38	A			C			T
V2220	BIFOCAL ADD OVER 3.25D	38	A			C			T
V2221	LENTICULAR LENS, PER LENS, BIFOCAL	38	A			D			A
V2299	SPECIALTY BIFOCAL (BY REPORT)	46	A			C			T
V2300	SPHERE, TRIFOCAL, PLANO TO PLUS OR MINUS 4.00D, PER LENS	38	A			C			T
V2301	SPHERE, TRIFOCAL, PLUS OR MINUS 4.12 TO PLUS OR MINUS 7.00D, PER LENS	38	A			C			T
V2302	SPHERE, TRIFOCAL, PLUS OR MINUS 7.12 TO PLUS OR MINUS 20.00, PER LENS	38	A			C			T
V2303	SPHEROCYLINDER, TRIFOCAL, PLANO TO PLUS OR MINUS 4.00D SPHERE, .12-2.00D CYLINDER, PER LENS	38	A			C			T
V2304	SPHEROCYLINDER, TRIFOCAL, PLANO TO PLUS OR MINUS 4.00D SPHERE, 2.25-4.00D CYLINDER, PER LENS	38	A			C			T
V2305	SPHEROCYLINDER, TRIFOCAL, PLANO TO PLUS OR MINUS 4.00D SPHERE, 4.25 TO 6.00 CYLINDER, PER LENS	38	A			C			T
V2306	SPHEROCYLINDER, TRIFOCAL, PLANO TO PLUS OR MINUS 4.00D SPHERE, OVER 6.00D CYLINDER, PER LENS	38	A			C			T
V2307	SPHEROCYLINDER, TRIFOCAL, PLUS OR MINUS 4.25 TO PLUS OR MINUS 7.00D SPHERE, .12 TO 2.00D CYLINDER, PER LENS	38	A			C			T
V2308	SPHEROCYLINDER, TRIFOCAL, PLUS OR MINUS 4.25 TO PLUS OR MINUS 7.00D SPHERE, 2.12 TO 4.00D CYLINDER, PER LENS	38	A			C			T
V2309	SPHEROCYLINDER, TRIFOCAL, PLUS OR MINUS 4.25 TO PLUS OR MINUS 7.00D SPHERE, 4.25 TO 6.00D CYLINDER, PER LENS	38	A			C			T
V2310	SPHEROCYLINDER, TRIFOCAL, PLUS OR MINUS 4.25 TO PLUS OR MINUS 7.00D SPHERE, OVER 6.00D CYLINDER, PER LENS	38	A			C			T
V2311	SPHEROCYLINDER, TRIFOCAL, PLUS OR MINUS 7.25 TO PLUS OR MINUS 12.00D SPHERE, .25 TO 2.25D CYLINDER, PER LENS	38	A			C			T
V2312	SPHEROCYLINDER, TRIFOCAL, PLUS OR MINUS 7.25 TO PLUS OR MINUS 12.00D SPHERE, 2.25 TO 4.00D CYLINDER, PER LENS	38	A			C			T
V2313	SPHEROCYLINDER, TRIFOCAL, PLUS OR MINUS 7.25 TO PLUS OR MINUS 12.00D SPHERE, 4.25 TO 6.00D CYLINDER, PER LENS	38	A			C			T
V2314	SPHEROCYLINDER, TRIFOCAL, SPHERE OVER PLUS OR MINUS 12 .00D, PER LENS	38	A			C			T
V2315	LENTICULAR, (MYODISC), PER LENS, TRIFOCAL	38	A			C			T
V2316	LENTICULAR NONASPHERIC, PER LENS, TRIFOCAL	38	A			C			D
V2317	LENTICULAR, ASPHERIC LENS, TRIFOCAL	38	A			C			D
V2318	ANISEIKONIC LENS, TRIFOCAL	38	A			C			T
V2319	TRIFOCAL SEG WIDTH OVER 28 MM	38	A			C			T

HCPCS	Long Description	PTI	MPI	Statute	X-Ref	Coverage	ASC Pay Grp	ASC Pay Grp Eff Date	Action Code
V2320	TRIFOCAL ADD OVER 3.25D	38	A			C			T
V2321	LENTICULAR LENS, PER LENS, TRIFOCAL	38	A			D			A
V2399	SPECIALTY TRIFOCAL (BY REPORT)	46	A			C			T
V2410	VARIABLE ASPHERICITY LENS, SINGLE VISION, FULL FIELD, GLASS OR PLASTIC, PER LENS	38	A			C			T
V2430	VARIABLE ASPHERICITY LENS, BIFOCAL, FULL FIELD, GLASS OR PLASTIC, PER LENS	38	A			C			T
V2499	VARIABLE SPHERICITY LENS, OTHER TYPE	46	A			C			T
V2500	CONTACT LENS, PMMA, SPHERICAL, PER LENS	38	A			C			T
V2501	CONTACT LENS, PMMA, TORIC OR PRISM BALLAST, PER LENS	38	A			C			T
V2502	CONTACT LENS PMMA, BIFOCAL, PER LENS	38	A			C			T
V2503	CONTACT LENS, PMMA, COLOR VISION DEFICIENCY, PER LENS	38	A			C			T
V2510	CONTACT LENS, GAS PERMEABLE, SPHERICAL, PER LENS	38	A			C			T
V2511	CONTACT LENS, GAS PERMEABLE, TORIC, PRISM BALLAST, PER LENS	38	A			C			T
V2512	CONTACT LENS, GAS PERMEABLE, BIFOCAL, PER LENS	38	A			C			T
V2513	CONTACT LENS, GAS PERMEABLE, EXTENDED WEAR, PER LENS	38	A			C			T
V2520	CONTACT LENS, HYDROPHILIC, SPHERICAL, PER LENS	38	A			D			T
V2521	CONTACT LENS, HYDROPHILIC, TORIC, OR PRISM BALLAST, PER LENS	38	A			D			T
V2522	CONTACT LENS, HYDROPHILLIC, BIFOCAL, PER LENS	38	A			D			T
V2523	CONTACT LENS, HYDROPHILIC, EXTENDED WEAR, PER LENS	38	A			D			T
V2530	CONTACT LENS, SCLERAL, GAS IMPERMEABLE, PER LENS (FOR CONTACT LENS MODIFICATION, SEE 92325)	38	A			C			T
V2531	CONTACT LENS, SCLERAL, GAS PERMEABLE, PER LENS (FOR CONTACT LENS MODIFICATION, SEE 92325)	38	A			D			T
V2599	CONTACT LENS, OTHER TYPE	46	A			C			T
V2600	HAND HELD LOW VISION AIDS AND OTHER NONSPECTACLE MOUNTED AIDS	46	A			C			T
V2610	SINGLE LENS SPECTACLE MOUNTED LOW VISION AIDS	46	A			C			T
V2615	TELESCOPIC AND OTHER COMPOUND LENS SYSTEM, INCLUDING DISTANCE VISION TELESCOPIC, NEAR VISION TELESCOPES AND COMPOUND MICROSCOPIC LENS SYSTEM	46	A			C			T
V2623	PROSTHETIC EYE, PLASTIC, CUSTOM	38	A			D			T
V2624	POLISHING/RESURFACING OF OCULAR PROSTHESIS	38	A			C			T

HCPCS	Long Description	PII	MPI	Statute	X-Ref	Coverage	ASC Pay Grp	ASC Pay Grp Eff Date	Action Code
V2625	ENLARGEMENT OF OCULAR PROSTHESIS	38	A			C			T
V2626	REDUCTION OF OCULAR PROSTHESIS	38	A			C			T
V2627	SCLERAL COVER SHELL	38	A			D			T
V2628	FABRICATION AND FITTING OF OCULAR CONFORMER	38	A			C			T
V2629	PROSTHETIC EYE, OTHER TYPE	46	A			C			T
V2630	ANTERIOR CHAMBER INTRAOCULAR LENS	52	A			D			T
V2631	IRIS SUPPORTED INTRAOCULAR LENS	52	A			D			T
V2632	POSTERIOR CHAMBER INTRAOCULAR LENS	52	A			D			T
V2700	BALANCE LENS, PER LENS	38	A			C			T
V2710	SLAB OFF PRISM, GLASS OR PLASTIC, PER LENS	38	A			C			T
V2715	PRISM, PER LENS	38	A			C			T
V2718	PRESS-ON LENS, FRESNELL PRISM, PER LENS	38	A			C			T
V2730	SPECIAL BASE CURVE, GLASS OR PLASTIC, PER LENS	38	A			C			T
V2740	TINT, PLASTIC, ROSE 1 OR 2 PER LENS	38	A			D			D
V2741	TINT, PLASTIC, OTHER THAN ROSE 1-2, PER LENS	38	A			D			D
V2742	TINT, GLASS ROSE 1 OR 2, PER LENS	38	A			D			D
V2743	TINT, GLASS OTHER THAN ROSE 1 OR 2, PER LENS	38	A			D			D
V2744	TINT, PHOTOCHROMATIC, PER LENS	38	A			D			T
V2745	ADDITION TO LENS, TINT, ANY COLOR, SOLID, GRADIENT OR EQUAL, EXCLUDES PHOTOCHROATIC, ANY LENS MATERIAL, PER LENS	38	A			D			A
V2750	ANTI-REFLECTIVE COATING, PER LENS	38	A			D			T
V2755	U-V LENS, PER LENS	38	A			D			T
V2756	EYE GLASS CASE	00	9			I			A
V2760	SCRATCH RESISTANT COATING, PER LENS	38	A			C			T
V2761	MIRROR COATING, ANY TYPE, SOLID, GRADIENT OR EQUAL, ANY LENS MATERIAL, PER LENS	38	A			D			A
V2762	POLARIZATION, ANY LENS MATERIAL, PER LENS	38	A			D			A
V2770	OCCLUDER LENS, PER LENS	38	A			C			T
V2780	OVERSIZE LENS, PER LENS	38	A			C			T
V2781	PROGRESSIVE LENS, PER LENS	00	9			C			T
V2782	LENS, INDEX 1.54 TO 1.65 PLASTIC OR 1.60 TO 1.79 GLASS, EXCLUDES POLYCARBONATE, PER LENS	38	A			D			A
V2783	LENS, INDEX GREATER THAN OR EQUAL TO 1.66 PLASTIC OR GREATER THAN OR EQUAL TO '1.80 GLASS, EXCLUDES POLYCARBONATE, PER LENS	38	A			D			A
V2783									

HCPCS	Long Description	PTI	MPI	Statute	X-Ref	Coverage	ASC Pay Grp	ASC Pay Grp Eff Date	Action Code
V2784	LENS, POLYCARBONATE OR EQUAL, ANY INDEX, PER LENS	38	A			D			A
V2785	PROCESSING, PRESERVING AND TRANSPORTING CORNEAL TISSUE	46	A			C			T
V2786	SPECIALTY OCCUPATIONAL MULTIFOCAL LENS, PER LENS	38	A			D			A
V2790	AMNIOTIC MEMBRANE FOR SURGICAL RECONSTRUCTION, PER PROCEDURE	57	A			C			T
V2797	VISION SUPPLY, ACCESSORY AND/OR SERVICE COMPONENT OF ANOTHER HCPCS VISION CODE	00	9			C			A
V2799	VISION SERVICE, MISCELLANEOUS	46	A			C			T
V5008	HEARING SCREENING	00	9			M			N
V5010	ASSESSMENT FOR HEARING AID	00	9	1862A7		S			N
V5011	FITTING/ORIENTATION/CHECKING OF HEARING AID	00	9	1862A7		S			N
V5014	REPAIR/MODIFICATION OF A HEARING AID	00	9	1862A7		S			N
V5020	CONFORMITY EVALUATION	00	9	1862A7		S			N
V5030	HEARING AID, MONAURAL, BODY WORN, AIR CONDUCTION	00	9	1862A7		S			N
V5040	HEARING AID, MONAURAL, BODY WORN, BONE CONDUCTION	00	9	1862A7		S			N
V5050	HEARING AID, MONAURAL, IN THE EAR	00	9	1862A7		S			N
V5060	HEARING AID, MONAURAL, BEHIND THE EAR	00	9	1862A7		S			N
V5070	GLASSES, AIR CONDUCTION	00	9	1862A7		S			N
V5080	GLASSES, BONE CONDUCTION	00	9	1862A7		S			N
V5090	DISPENSING FEE, UNSPECIFIED HEARING AID	00	9	1862A7		S			N
V5095	SEMI-IMPLANTABLE MIDDLE EAR HEARING PROSTHESIS	00	9	1862A7		S			N
V5100	HEARING AID, BILATERAL, BODY WORN	00	9	1862A7		S			N
V5110	DISPENSING FEE, BILATERAL	00	9	1862A7		S			N
V5120	BINAURAL, BODY	00	9	1862A7		S			N
V5130	BINAURAL, IN THE EAR	00	9	1862A7		S			N
V5140	BINAURAL, BEHIND THE EAR	00	9	1862A7		S			N
V5150	BINAURAL, GLASSES	00	9	1862A7		S			N
V5160	DISPENSING FEE, BINAURAL	00	9	1862A7		S			N
V5170	HEARING AID, CROS, IN THE EAR	00	9	1862A7		S			N

HCPCS	Long Description	PII	MPI	Statute	X-Ref	Coverage	ASC Pay Grp	ASC Pay Grp Eff Date	Action Code
V5180	HEARING AID, CROS, BEHIND THE EAR	00	9	1862A7		S			N
V5190	HEARING AID, CROS, GLASSES	00	9	1862A7		S			N
V5200	DISPENSING FEE, CROS	00	9	1862A7		S			N
V5210	HEARING AID, BICROS, IN THE EAR	00	9	1862A7		S			N
V5220	HEARING AID, BICROS, BEHIND THE EAR	00	9	1862A7		S			N
V5230	HEARING AID, BICROS, GLASSES	00	9	1862A7		S			N
V5240	DISPENSING FEE, BICROS	00	9	1862A7		S			N
V5241	DISPENSING FEE, MONAURAL HEARING AID, ANY TYPE	00	9	1862A7		S			N
V5242	HEARING AID, ANALOG, MONAURAL, CIC (COMPLETELY IN THE EAR CANAL)	00	9	1862A7		S			N
V5243	HEARING AID, ANALOG, MONAURAL, ITC (IN THE CANAL)	00	9	1862A7		S			N
V5244	HEARING AID, DIGITALLY PROGRAMMABLE ANALOG, MONAURAL, CIC	00	9	1862A7		S			N
V5245	HEARING AID, DIGITALLY PROGRAMMABLE, ANALOG, MONAURAL, ITC	00	9	1862A7		S			N
V5246	HEARING AID, DIGITALLY PROGRAMMABLE ANALOG, MONAURAL, ITE (IN THE EAR)	00	9	1862A7		S			N
V5247	HEARING AID, DIGITALLY PROGRAMMABLE ANALOG, MONAURAL, BTE (BEHIND THE EAR)	00	9	1862A7		S			N
V5248	HEARING AID, ANALOG, BINAURAL, CIC	00	9	1862A7		S			N
V5249	HEARING AID, ANALOG, BINAURAL, ITC	00	9	1862A7		S			N
V5250	HEARING AID, DIGITALLY PROGRAMMABLE ANALOG, BINAURAL, CIC	00	9	1862A7		S			N
V5251	HEARING AID, DIGITALLY PROGRAMMABLE ANALOG, BINAURAL, ITC	00	9	1862A7		S			N
V5252	HEARING AID, DIGITALLY PROGRAMMABLE, BINAURAL, ITE	00	9	1862A7		S			N
V5253	HEARING AID, DIGITALLY PROGRAMMABLE, BINAURAL, BTE	00	9	1862A7		S			N
V5254	HEARING AID, DIGITAL, MONAURAL, CIC	00	9	1862A7		S			N
V5255	HEARING AID, DIGITAL, MONAURAL, ITC	00	9	1862A7		S			N
V5256	HEARING AID, DIGITAL, MONAURAL, ITE	00	9	1862A7		S			N
V5257	HEARING AID, DIGITAL, MONAURAL, BTE	00	9	1862A7		S			N
V5258	HEARING AID, DIGITAL, BINAURAL, CIC	00	9	1862A7		S			N
V5259	HEARING AID, DIGITAL, BINAURAL, ITC	00	9	1862A7		S			N
V5260	HEARING AID, DIGITAL, BINAURAL, ITE	00	9	1862A7		S			N
V5261	HEARING AID, DIGITAL, BINAURAL, BTE	00	9	1862A7		S			N
V5262	HEARING AID, DISPOSABLE, ANY TYPE, MONAURAL	00	9	1862A7		S			N
V5263	HEARING AID, DISPOSABLE, ANY TYPE, BINAURAL	00	9	1862A7		S			N
V5264	EAR MOLD/INSERT, NOT DISPOSABLE, ANY TYPE	00	9	1862A7		S			N

HCPCS	Long Description	PTI	MPI	Statute	X-Ref	Coverage	ASC Pay Grp	ASC Pay Grp Eff Date	Action Code
V5265	EAR MOLD/INSERT, DISPOSABLE, ANY TYPE	00	9	1862A7		S			N
V5266	BATTERY FOR USE IN HEARING DEVICE	00	9	1862A7		S			N
V5267	HEARING AID SUPPLIES / ACCESSORIES	00	9	1862A7		S			N
V5268	ASSISTIVE LISTENING DEVICE, TELEPHONE AMPLIFIER, ANY TYPE	00	9	1862A7		S			N
V5269	ASSISTIVE LISTENING DEVICE, ALERTING, ANY TYPE	00	9	1862A7		S			N
V5270	ASSISTIVE LISTENING DEVICE, TELEVISION AMPLIFIER, ANY TYPE	00	9	1862A7		S			N
V5271	ASSISTIVE LISTENING DEVICE, TELEVISION CAPTION DECODER	00	9	1862A7		S			N
V5272	ASSISTIVE LISTENING DEVICE, TDD	00	9	1862A7		S			N
V5273	ASSISTIVE LISTENING DEVICE, FOR USE WITH COCHLEAR IMPLANT	00	9	1862A7		S			N
V5274	ASSISTIVE LISTENING DEVICE, NOT OTHERWISE SPECIFIED	00	9	1862A7		S			N
V5275	EAR IMPRESSION, EACH	00	9	1862A7		S			N
V5298	HEARING AID, NOT OTHERWISE CLASSIFIED	00	9	1862A7		S			N
V5299	HEARING SERVICE, MISCELLANEOUS	13	A			D			N
V5336	REPAIR/MODIFICATION OF AUGMENTATIVE COMMUNICATIVE SYSTEM OR DEVICE (EXCLUDES ADAPTIVE HEARING AID)	00	9	1862A7		S			N
V5362	SPEECH SCREENING	00	9	42cfr41062		S			F
V5363	LANGUAGE SCREENING	00	9	42cfr41062		S			F
V5364	DYSPHAGIA SCREENING	00	9	42cfr41062		S			F

2004 Alpha-Numeric Index

A

Abciximab, J0130

Abdomen
    dressing holder/binder, A4462
    pad, low profile, L1270
    supports, pendulous, L0920, L0930

Abduction control, each, L2624

Abduction rotation bar, foot, L3140-L3170

Absorption dressing, A6251-A6256

Access system, A4301

Accessories
    ambulation devices, E0153-E0159
    artificial kidney and machine (see also ESRD), E1510-E1699
    beds, E0271-E0280, E0300-E0326
    wheelchairs, E0950-E1030, E1050-E1298, E2300-E2399, K0001-K0109

Acetazolamide sodium, J1120

Acetylcysteine, inhalation solution, J7608

Acyclovir, Q4075

Adenosine, J0150, J0152

Adhesive, A4364
    disc or foam pad, A5126
    remover, A4365, A4455
    support, breast prosthesis, A4280
    tape, A4454, A6265

Administrative, Miscellaneous and Investigational, A9000-A9999

Adrenalin, J0170

Aerosol
    compressor, E0571, E0572
    compressor filter, K0178-K0179
    mask, K0180

AFO, E1815, E1830, L1900-L1990, L4392, L4396

Aggrastat, J3245

A-hydroCort, J1710

Air ambulance (see also Ambulance), A0030, A0040

Air bubble detector, dialysis, E1530

Air fluidized bed, E0194

Air pressure pad/mattress, E0176, E0186, E0197

Air travel and nonemergency transportation, A0140

Alarm, pressure, dialysis, E1540

Alatrofloxacin mesylate, J0200

Albumin, human, P9041, P9042

Albuterol, all formulations, inhalation solution, concentrated, J7618

Albuterol, all formulations, inhalation solution, unit dose, J7619

Albuterol, all formulations, inhalation solution, J7621

Alcohol, A4244

Alcohol wipes, A4245

Aldesleukin (IL2), J9015

Alefacept, J0215

Alemtuzumab, J9010

Alert device, A9280

Alginate dressing, A6196-A6199

Alglucerase, J0205

Alpha-1-proteinase inhibitor, human, J0256

Alprostadil, injection, J0270

Alprostadil, urethral supposity, J0275

Alteplase recombinant, J2997

Alternating pressure mattress/pad, A4640, E0180, E0181, E0277

Alveoloplasty, D7310-D7320

Amalgam dental restoration, D2110-D2161

Ambulance, A0021-A0999
    air, A0430, A0431, A0435, A0436
    disposable supplies, A0382-A0398
    oxygen, A0422

Ambulation device, E0100-E0159

Aminolevulinic acid HCl, J7308

Aminophylline, J0280

Amiodarone Hcl, J0282

Amitriptyline HCI, J1320

Ammonia N-13, A9526

Ammonia test paper, A4774

Amniotic membrane, V2790

Amobarbital, J0300

Amphotericin B, J0285

Amphotericin B Lipid Complex, J0287-J0289

Ampicillin sodium, J0290

Ampicillin sodium/sulbactam sodium, J0295

Amputee
    adapter, wheelchair, E0959
    prosthesis, L5000-L7510, L7520, L7900, L8400-L8465
    stump sock, L8470-L8490
    wheelchair, E1170-E1190, E1200, K0100

Amygdalin, J3570

Analgesia, dental, D9230

Anesthesia
    dental, D7110-D7130, D7210-D7250, D9210-D9240
    dialysis, A4735

Anistreplase, J0350

Ankle splint, recumbent, K0126-K0130

Ankle-foot orthosis (AFO), L1900-L1990, L2106-L2116, L4392, L4396

Anterior-posterior-lateral orthosis, L0520, L0550-L0565, L0700, L0710

Anterior-posterior-lateral-rotary orthosis, L0340-L0440

Anterior-posterior orthosis, L0320, L0330, L0530

Anti-emetic, oral, Q0163-Q0181

Anti-hemophilic factor (Factor VIII), J7190-J7192

Anti-inhibitors, per I.U., J7198

Anti-neoplastic drug, NOC, J9999

Antithrombin III, J7197

Antral fistula closure, oral, D7260

Apexification, dental, D3351-D3353

Apicoectomy, D3410-D3426

Apnea monitor, E0608

Appliance
    cleaner, A5131
    pneumatic, E0655-E0673

Aprotinin, Q2003

Aqueous

shunt, L8612
sterile, J7051
Arbutamine HCl, J0395
Arch support, L3040-L3100
Intralesional, J3302
Arm, wheelchair, E0973
Arsenic trioxide, J9017
Artificial
kidney machines and accessories (see also Dialysis), E1510-E1699
larynx, L8500
Asparaginase, J9020
Assessment
audiologic, V5008-V5020
cardiac output, M0302
speech, V5362-V5364
Astramorph, J2275
Atropine, inhalation solution, concentrated, J7635
Atropine, inhalation solution, unit dose, J7636
Atropine sulfate, J0460
Audiologic assessment, V5008-V5020
Auricular prosthesis, D5914, D5927
Aurothioglucose, J2910
Azathioprine, J7500, J7501
Azithromycin injection, J0456

B

Back supports, L0500-L0960
Baclofen, J0475, J0476
Bacterial sensitivity study, P7001
Bag
drainage, A4357
irrigation supply, A4398
urinary, A5112, A4358
Bandage, A4441-A4456
Basiliximab, Q2019
Bathtub
chair, E0240
stool or bench, E0245, E0247-E0248
transfer rail, E0246
wall rail, E0241, E0242
Battery, K0082-K0087, L7360, L7364-L7368
charger, E1066, K0088, K0089, L7362, L7366
replacement for blood glucose monitor, A4254
replacement for TENS, A4630
ventilator, A4611-A4613
wheelchair, A4631
BCG live, intravesical, J9031
Beclomethasone inhalation solution, J7622
Bed
air fluidized, E0194
cradle, any type, E0280
drainage bag, bottle, A4357, A5102
hospital, E0250-E0270, E0298-E0301
pan, E0275, E0276
rail, E0305, E0310

safety enclosure frame/canopy, E0316
Below knee suspension sleeve, L5674, L5675
Belt
    extremity, E0945
    ostomy, A4367
    pelvic, E0944
    safety, K0031
    wheelchair, E0978, E0979
Bench, bathtub (see also Bathtub), E0245
Benefix, see Factor IX, Q0161
Benesch boot, L3212-L3214
Benztropine, J0515
Betadine, A4246, A4247
Betameth, J0704
Betamethasone inhalation solution, J7624
Betamethasone acetate and betamethasone sodium phosphate, J0702
Betamethasone sodium phosphate, J0704
Bethanechol chloride, J0520
Bicarbonate dialysate, A4705
Bicuspid (excluding final restoration), D3320
    retreatment, by report, D3347
    surgery, first root, D3421
Bifocal, glass or plastic, V2200-V2299
Bilirubin (phototherapy) light, E0202
Binder, A4465
Biofeedback device, E0746
Bioimpedance, electrical, cardiac output, M0302
Biperiden lactate, J0190
Bitewing, D0270-D0274
Bitolterol mesylate, inhalation solution, concentrated, J7628
Bitolterol mesylate, inhalation solution, unit dose, J7629
Bivalirudin, J0583
Bladder calculi irrigation solution, Q2004
Bladder capacity test, ultrasound, G0050
Bleaching tooth, D3960
Bleomycin sulfate, J9040
Blood
    Congo red, P2029
    fresh frozen plasma, P9017
    glucose monitor, E0607, E2100, E2101
    glucose test, A4253
    granulocytes, pheresis, P9050
    leak detector, dialysis, E1560
    leukocyte poor, P9016
    mucoprotein, P2038
    platelets, P9019
    platelets, irradiated, P9032
    platelets, leukocytes reduced, P9031
    platelets, leukocytes reduced, irradiated, P9033
    platelets, pheresis, P9034
    platelets, pheresis, irradiated, P9036
    platelets, pheresis, leukocytes reduced, P9035
    platelets, pheresis, leukocytes reduced, irradiated, P9037
    pressure monitor, A4660, A4663, A4670
    pump, dialysis, E1620

red blood cells, deglycerolized, P9039
red blood cells, irradiated, P9038
red blood cells, leukocytes reduced, P9016
red blood cells, leukocytes reduced, irradiated, P9040
red blood cells, washed, P9022
strips, A4253
supply, P9010-P9022
testing supplies, A4770
tubing, A4750, A4755
Blood collection devices accessory, A4257, E0620
Body jacket
lumbar-sacral orthosis (spinal), L0500-L0565, L0600, L0610
scoliosis, L1300, L1310
Body sock, L0984
Bond or cement, ostomy skin, A4364
Bone mineral density study, G0062, G0063
Boot
pelvic, E0944
surgical, ambulatory, L3260
Botulinum toxin type A, J0585
Botulinum toxin type B, J0587
Brachytherapy radioelements, Q3001
Brachytherapy source, A9670
Breast prosthesis, L8000-L8035, L8600
Breast prosthesis, adhesive skin support, A4280
Breast pump
accessories, A4281-A4286
electric, any type, E0603
heavy duty, hospital grade, E0604
manual, any type, E0602
Breathing circuit, A4618
Bridge
recement, D6930
repair, by report, D6980
Brompheniramine maleate, J0945
Budesonide inhalation solution, J7626, J7633
Buprenorphine hydrochloride, J0592
Bus, nonemergency transportation, A0110
Butorphanol tartrate, J0595

C

Cabergoline, oral, Q2001
Caffeine citrate, J0706
Calcitriol, J0636
Calcitonin-salmon, J0630
Calcium disodium edetate, J0600
Calcium gluconate, J0610
Calcium glycerophosphate and calcium lactate, J0620
Calcium lactate and calcium glycerophosphate, J0620
Calcium leucovorin, J0640
Calibrator solution, A4256
Cane, E0100, E0105
accessory, A4636, A4637
Canister, disposable, used with suction pump, A7000
Canister, non-disposable, used with suction pump, A7001

Cannula, nasal, A4615
Capecitabine, oral, J8520, J8521
Carbon filter, A4680
Carboplatin, J9045
Cardia Event, recorder, implantable, E0616
Cardiokymography, Q0035
Cardiovascular services, M0300-M0302
Carmustine, J9050
Caries susceptibility test, D0425
Case management, T1016, T1017
Caspofungin acetate, J0637
Cast
    diagnostic, dental, D0470
    hand restoration, L6900-L6915
    materials, special, A4590
    plaster, L2102, L2122
    supplies, A4580, A4590, Q4001-Q4051
    synthetic, L2104, L2124
    thermoplastic, L2106, L2126
Caster, front, for power wheelchair, K0099
Caster, wheelchair, E0997, E0998
Catheter, A4300-A4365
    anchoring device, A5200, A4333, A4334
    cap, disposable (dialysis), A4860
    external collection device, A4327-A4330, A4347, K0410, K0411
    implanted, A7042, A7043
    indwelling, A4338-A4346
    indwelling, insertion of, G0002
    insertion tray, A4354
    intermittent with insertion supplies, A4353
    irrigation supplies, A4355, K0409
    male external, A4324, A4325, A4348
    oropharyngeal suction, A4628
    starter set, A4329
    trachea (suction), A4609, A4610, A4624
    transtracheal oxygen, A4608
Catheterization, specimen collection, P9612, P9615
Cefazolin sodium, J0690
Cefepime HCl, J0692
Cefotaxime sodium, J0698
Ceftazidime, J0713
Ceftizoxime sodium, J0715
Ceftriaxone sodium, J0696
Cefuroxime sodium, J0697
CellCept, K0412
Cellular therapy, M0075
Cement, ostomy, A4364
Centrifuge, A4650
Cephalin Floculation, blood, P2028
Cephalothin sodium, J1890
Cephapirin sodium, J0710
Cervical
    halo, L0810-L0830
    head harness/halter, E0942
    orthosis, L0100-L0200

pillow, E0943
traction, E0855
Cervical cap contraceptive, A4261
Cervical-thoracic-lumbar-sacral orthosis (CTLSO), L0700, L0710
Chair
    adjustable, dialysis, E1570
    commode with seat lift, E0169
    lift, E0627
    rollabout, E1031
    sitz bath, E0160-E0162
Chelation therapy, M0300
Chemical endarterectomy, M0300
Chemistry and toxicology tests, P2028-P3001
Chemotherapy
    administration, Q0083-Q0085 (hospital reporting only)
    drug, oral, not otherwise classified, J8999
    drugs (see also drug by name), J9000-J9999
Chest shell (cuirass), E0457
Chest Wall Oscillation System, E0483
    hose, replacement, A7026
    vest, replacement, A7025
Chest wrap, E0459
Chin cup, cervical, L0150
Chin strap (for positive airway pressure device), K0186
Chloramphenicol sodium succinate, J0720
Chlordiazepoxide HCl, J1990
Chloromycetin Sodium Succinate, J0720
Chloroprocaine HCl, J2400
Chloroquine HCl, J0390
Chlorothiazide sodium, J1205
Chlorpromazine HCl, J3230
Chorionic gonadotropin, J0725
Chromic phosphate P32 suspension, Q3011
Cidofovir, J0740
Cilastatin sodium, imipenem, J0743
Ciprofloxacin, for intravenous infusion, J0744
Cisplatin, J9060, J9062
Cladribine, J9065
Clamp
    dialysis, A4910, A4918, A4920
    external urethral, A4356
Cleanser, wound, A6260
Cleansing agent, dialysis equipment, A4790
Clonidine, J0735
Clotting time tube, A4771
Clubfoot wedge, L3380
Cochlear prosthetic implant, L8614
    replacement, L8619
Codeine phosphate, J0745
Colchicine, J0760
Colistimethate sodium, J0770
Collagen
    skin test, G0025
    urinary tract implant, L8603
    wound dressing, A6020-A6024

non-contact wound warming cover, and accessory, A6000, E0231, E0232

specialty absorptive dressing, A6251-A6256

CPAP (continuous positive airway pressure) device, E0601

chin strap, K0186

compressor, K0269

filter, K0188, K0189

headgear, K0185

humidifier, A7046, K0193, K0268

intermittent assist, E0452, K0194

nasal application accessories, K0183, K0184

tubing, K0187

Cradle, bed, E0280

Crib, E0300

Cromolyn sodium, inhalation solution, unit dose, J7631

Crowns, D2710-D2810, D2930-D2933, D4249, D6720-D6792

Crutches, E0110-E0118

accessories, A4635-A4637, K0102

Cryoprecipitate, each unit, P9012

CTLSO, L1000-L1120, L0700, L0710

Cuirass, E0457

Culture sensitivity study, P7001

Cushion, wheelchair, E0962-E0965, E0977

Cyanocobalamin Cobalt C057, Q3012

Cycler dialysis machine, E1594

Cyclophosphamide, J9070-J9092

Cyclophosphamide, lyophilized, J9093-J9097

Cyclophosphamide, oral, J8530

Cyclosporine, J7502, J7515, J7516

Cylinder tank carrier, K0104

Cytarabine, J9110

Cytarabine liposome, J9098

Cytomegalovirus immune globulin (human), J0850

D

Dacarbazine, J9130, J9140

Daclizumab, J7513

Dactinomycin, J9120

Dalalone, J1100

Dalteparin sodium, J1645

Darbepoetin Alfa, J0880, Q0137, Q4054

Daunorubicin Citrate, J9151

Daunorubicin HCl, J9150

DaunoXome, see Daunorubicin citrate

Decubitus care equipment, E0176-E0199

Deferoxamine mesylate, J0895

Defibrillator, external, E0617, K0606

battery, K0607

electrode, K0609

garment, K0608

Deionizer, water purification system, E1615

Delivery/set-up/dispensing, A9901

Denileukin diftitox, J9160

Dental procedures

adjunctive general services, D9000-D9999

Diaper, T1500, T1501
Diaper, adult incontinence garment, A4360
Diazepam, J3360
Diazoxide, J1730
Dicyclomine HCl, J0500
Diethylstilbestrol diphosphate, J9165
Digoxin, J1160
Digoxin immune fab (ovine), Q2006
Dihydroergotamine mesylate, J1110
Dimenhydrinate, J1240
Dimercaprol, J0470
Dimethyl sulfoxide (DMSO), J1212
Diphenhydramine HCl, J1200
Dipyridamole, J1245
Disarticulation
    lower extremities, prosthesis, L5000-L5999
    upper extremities, prosthesis, L6000-L6692
Disposable supplies, ambulance, A0382, A0384, A0392- A0398
Distilled water (for nebulizer), K0182
DMSO, J1212
Dobutamine HCl, J1250
Docetaxel, J9170
Dolasetron mesylate, J1260
Dome and mouthpiece (for nebulizer), A7016
Dopamine HCl, Q4076
Dornase alpha, inhalation solution, unit dose form, J7639
Doxercalciferol, J1270
Doxil, J9001
Doxorubicin HCl, J9000, J9001
Drainage
    bag, A4347, A4357, A4358
    board, postural, E0606
    bottle, A5102
Dressing (see also Bandage), A6020-A6406
    alginate, A6196-A6199
    collagen, A6020-A6024
    composite, A6200-A6205
    contact layer, A6206-A6208
    foam, A6209-A6215
    gauze, A6216-A6230, A6402-A6406
    holder/binder, A4462
    hydrocolloid, A6234-A6241
    hydrogel, A6242-A6248
    specialty absorptive, A6251-A6256
    tape, A4454, A6265
    transparent film, A6257-A6259
    tubular, K0620
Droperidol, J1790
    and fentanyl citrate, J1810
Dropper, A4649
Drugs (see also Table of Drugs)
    administered through a metered dose inhaler, J3535
    chemotherapy, J8500-J9999
    dispensing fee for DME drugs, E0590
    disposable delivery system, 5 ml or less per hour, A4306

disposable delivery system, 50 ml or greater per hour, A4305
immunosuppressive, J7500-J7599
infusion supplies, A4230-A4232, A4221, A4222
inhalation solutions, J7608-J7699
not otherwise classified, J3490, J7599, J7699, J7799, J8499, J8999, J9999
prescription, oral, J8499, J8999
Dry pressure pad/mattress, E0179, E0184, E0199
Durable medical equipment (DME), E0100-E1830, K Codes
Duraclon, see Clonidine
Dyphylline, J1180

E

Ear mold, V5264
Echocardiography injectable contrast material, A9700
Edetate calcium disodium, J0600
Edetate disodium, J3520
Eggcrate dry pressure pad/mattress, E0179, E0184, E0199
Elastic
    bandage, A4460
    gauze, A6263, A6405
Elbow
    disarticulation, endoskeletal, L6450
    orthosis (EO), E1800, L3700-L3740, L3760
    protector, E0191
Electrical work, dialysis equipment, A4870
Electrocardiogram strips,
    monitoring, G0004-G0007
    physician interpretation, G0016
    tracing, G0015
    transmission, G0015, G0016
Electrodes, per pair, A4556
Elevating leg rest, K0195
Elliotts b solution, Q2002
EMG, E0746
Eminase, J0350
Endarterectomy, chemical, M0300
Endodontic procedures, D3000-D3999
    periapical services, D3410-D3470
    pulp capping, D3110, D3120
    root canal therapy, D3310-D3353
Endoscope sheath, A4270
Endoskeletal system, addition, L5848, L5925
Enoxaparin sodium, J1650
Enteral
    feeding supply kit (syringe) (pump) (gravity), B4034-B4036
    formulae, B4150-B4156
    nutrition infusion pump (with alarm) (without), B9000, B9002
Epinephrine, J0170
Epirubicin HCl, J9178
Epoetin alpha, for non ESRD use, Q0136, Q4055
Epoprostenol, J1325
Ergonovine maleate, J1330
Ertapenem sodium, J1335
Erythromycin lactobionate, J1364
ESRD (End Stage Renal Disease; see also Dialysis)

machines and accessories, E1500-E1699
plumbing, A4870
supplies, A4651-A4929
Estrogen conjugated, J1410
Estrone (5, Aqueous), J1435
Ethanolamine oleate, Q2007
Etidronate disodium, J1436
Etoposide, J9181, J9182
Etoposide, oral, J8560
Examination, oral, D0120-D0160
Exercise equipment, A9300
External
ambulatory infusion pump, E0781, E0784
power, battery components, L7360-L7499
power, elbow, L7160-L7191
urinary supplies, A4356-A4359
Extractions (see also Dental procedures), D7110-D7130, D7250
Extraoral films, D0250, D0260
Extremity belt/harness, E0945
Eye
case, V2756
lens (contact) (spectacle), V2100-V2615
pad, A4610-A4612
prosthetic, V2623, V2629
service (miscellaneous), V2700-V2799

F

Faceplate, ostomy, A4361, K0428
Face tent, oxygen, A4619
Factor VIII, anti-hemophilic factor, J7190-J7192
Factor IX, J7193, J7194, J7195
Family Planning Education, H1010
Fecal leukocyte examination, G0026
Fentanyl citrate, J3010
Fentanyl citrate and droperidol, J1810
Fern test, Q0114
Filgrastim (G-CSF), J1440, J1441
Filler, wound
alginate dressing, A6199
foam dressing, A6215
hydrocolloid dressing, A6240, A6241
hydrogel dressing, A6248
not elsewhere classified, A6261, A6262
Film, transparent (for dressing), A6257-A6259
Filter
aerosol compressor, A7014
CPAP device, K0188, K0189
dialysis carbon, A4680
ostomy, A4368
tracheostoma, A4481
ultrasonic generator, A7014
Fistula cannulation set, A4730
Flowmeter, E0440, E0555, E0580
Floxuridine, J9200
Fluconazole, injection, J1450

Fludarabine phosphate, J9185
Fluid barrier, dialysis, E1575
Flunisolide inhalation solution, J7641
Fluoride treatment, D1201-D1205
Fluorouracil, J9190
Foam dressing, A6209-A6215
Foam pad adhesive, A5126
Folding walker, E0135, E0143
Foley catheter, A4312-A4316, A4338-A4346
Fomepizole, Q2008
Fomivirsen sodium intraocular, J1452
Fondaparinux sodium, J1652
Footdrop splint, L4398
Footplate, E0175, E0970, L3031
Footwear, orthopedic, L3201-L3265
Forceps, dialysis, A4910
Forearm crutches, E0110, E0111
Foscarnet sodium, J1455
Fosphenytoin, Q2009
Fracture
    bedpan, E0276
    frame, E0920, E0930, E0946-E0948
    orthosis, L2102-L2136, L3980-L3986
    orthotic additions, L2180-L2192, L3995
Fragmin, see Dalteparin sodium
Frames (spectacles), V2020, V2025
Fulvestrant, J9395
Furosemide, J1940

G
Gadolinium, A4647
Gallium Ga67, Q3002
Gamma globulin, J1460-J1561
Ganciclovir, implant, J7310
Ganciclovir sodium, J1570
Garamycin, J1580
Gas system
    compressed, E0424, E0425
    gaseous, E0430, E0431, E0441, E0443
    liquid, E0434-E0440, E0442, E0444
Gastrostomy/jejunostomy tubing, B4084
Gastrostomy tube, B4085
Gatifloxacin, J1590
Gauze (see also Bandage)
    elastic, A6263, A6405
    impregnated, A6222-A6230, A6231-A6233, A6266
    nonelastic, A6264, A6406
    nonimpregnated, A6216-A6221, A6402-A6404
Gel
    conductive, A4558
    pressure pad, E0178, E0185, E0196
Gemcitabine HCl, J9201
Gemtuzumab ozogamicin, J9300
Generator
    implantable neurostimulator, E0751

ultrasonic with nebulizer, E0574
Gentamicin (Sulfate), J1580
Gingival procedures, D4210-D4240
Glasses
    air conduction, V5070
    binaural, V5120-V5150
    bone conduction, V5080
    frames, V2020, V2025
    hearing aid, V5230
Glatiramer acetate, Q2010
Gloves, A4927
Glucagon HCl, J1610
Glucose monitor with integrated lancing/blood sample collection, E2101
Glucose monitor with integrated voice synthesizer, E2100
Glucose test strips, A4253, A4772
Gluteal pad, L2650
Glycopyrrolate, inhalation solution, concentrated, J7642
Glycopyrrolate, inhalation solution, unit dose, J7643
Gold foil dental restoration, D2410-D2430
Gold sodium thiomalate, J1600
Gomco drain bottle, A4912
Gonadorelin HCl, J1620
Goserelin acetate implant (see also Implant), J9202
Grab bar, trapeze, E0910, E0940
Grade-aid, wheelchair, E0974
Granisetron HCl, J1626
Gravity traction device, E0941
Gravlee jet washer, A4470

H

Hair analysis (excluding arsenic), P2031
Hallus-Valgus dynamic splint, L3100
Hallux prosthetic implant, L8642
Haloperidol, J1630
    decanoate, J1631
Halo procedures, L0810-L0860
Halter, cervical head, E0942
Hand finger orthosis, prefabricated, L3923
Hand restoration, L6900-L6915
    partial prosthesis, L6000-L6020
    orthosis (WHFO), E1805, E1825, L3800-L3805, L3900-L3954
    rims, wheelchair, E0967
Handgrip (cane, crutch, walker), A4636
Harness, E0942, E0944, E0945
Harvard pressure clamp, dialysis, A4920
Headgear (for positive airway pressure device), K0185
Hearing devices, V5000-V5299, L8614
Heat
    application, E0200-E0239
    lamp, E0200, E0205
    infrared heating pad system, A4639, E0221
    pad, E0210, E0215, E0237, E0238, E0249
Heater (nebulizer), E1372
Heel
    elevator, air, E0370

protector, E0191
shoe, L3430-L3485
stabilizer, L3170
Helicopter, ambulance (see also Ambulance)
Helmet, cervical, L0100, L0110
Helmet, head, E0701
Hemin, Q2011
Hemi-wheelchair, E1083-E1086
Hemipelvectomy prosthesis, L5280, L5340
Hemodialysis
kit, A4820
machine, E1590
Hemodialyzer, portable, E1635
Hemofil M, J7190
Hemoglobin, Q0116
Hemophilia clotting factor, J7190-J7198
Hemophilia clotting factor, NOC, J7199
Hemostats, A4850
Hemostix, A4773
Heparin infusion pump, dialysis, E1520
Heparin lock flush, J1642
Heparin sodium, A4800, J1644
Hepatitis B vaccine, Q3021-Q3023
Hep-Lock (U/P), J1642
Hexalite, A4590
Hip
disarticulation prosthesis, L5250, L5270, L5330
orthosis (HO), L1600-L1690
Hip-knee-ankle-foot orthosis (HKAFO), L2040-L2090
Histrelin acetate, Q2020
HKAFO, L2040-L2090
Home Health Agency Services, T0221
Hot water bottle, E0220
Humidifier, A7046, E0550-E0562
Hyaluronate, sodium, J7316
Hyaluronidase, J3470
Hydralazine HCl, J0360
Hydraulic patient lift, E0630
Hydrocollator, E0225, E0239
Hydrocolloid dressing, A6234-A6241
Hydrocortisone
acetate, J1700
sodium phosphate, J1710
sodium succinate, J1720
Hydrogel dressing, A6242-A6248, A6231-A6233
Hydromorphone, J1170
Hydroxyzine HCl, J3410
Hylan G-F 20, J7320
Hyoscyamine Sulfate, J1980
Hyperbaric oxygen chamber, topical, A4575
Hypertonic saline solution, J7130

I

Ibutilide Fumarate, J1742
Ice

cap, E0230
collar, E0230
Idarubicin HCl, J9211
Ifosfamide, J9208
Imiglucerase, J1785
Immune globulin intravenous, J1563-J1564
Immunosuppressive drug, not otherwise classified, J7599
Implant
    access system, A4301
    aqueous shunt, L8612
    breast, L8600
    cochlear, L8614, L8619
    collagen, urinary tract, L8603
    contraceptive, A4260
    ganciclovir, J7310
    hallux, L8642
    urinary tract, L8603, L8606
    indium III-in Pentetreotide, Q3008
    infusion pump, programmable, E0783, E0786
    joint, L8630, L8641, L8658
    lacrimal duct, A4262, A4263
    maintenance procedures, D6080
    maxillofacial, D5913-D5937
    metacarpophalangeal joint, L8630
    metatarsal joint, L8641
    neurostimulator electrode, E0752
    neurostimulator pulse generator, E0756
    neurostimulator radiofrequency receiver, E0757
    not otherwise specified, L8699
    ocular, L8610
    ossicular, L8613
    osteogenesis stimulator, E0749
    percutaneous access system, A4301
    removal, dental, D6100
    repair, dental, D6090
    replacement implantable intraspinal catheter, E0785
    synthetic, urinary, L8606
    vascular graft, L8670
Impregnated gauze dressing, A6222-A6230, K0535-K0537
Incontinence
    appliances and supplies, A4310-A4355, A4356-A4360, A5071-A5075, A5102-A5114, K0280, K0281
    products, A4521-A4538
    treatment system, E0740
Indium in 111 carpromab pendetide, A9507
Indwelling catheter insertion, G0002
Infliximab injection, J1745
Infusion
    pump, ambulatory, with administrative equipment, E0781
    pump, heparin, dialysis, E1520
    pump, implantable, E0782, E0783
    pump, implantable, refill kit, A4220
    pump, insulin, E0784
    pump, mechanical, reusable, E0779, E0780
    pump, uninterrupted infusion of Epiprostenol, K0455

271

J

scoliosis, L1300, L1310
Jenamicin, J1580
Joint supportive device/garment, A4464

K

Kanamycin sulfate, J1840, J1850
Kartop patient lift, toilet or bathroom (see also Lift), E0625
Ketorolac thomethamine, J1885
Kidney
    ESRD supply, A4650-A4927
    system, E1510
    wearable artificial, E1632
Kits
    continuous ambulatory peritoneal dialysis (CAPD), A4900
    continuous cycling peritoneal dialysis (CCPD), A4901
    dialysis, A4910
    enteral feeding supply (syringe) (pump) (gravity), B4034-B4036
    fistula cannulation (set), A4730
    intermittent peritoneal dialysis (IPD) supply, A4905
    parenteral nutrition, B4220-B4224
    surgical dressing (tray), A4550
    tracheostomy, A4625
Knee
    disarticulation, prosthesis, L5150, L5160
    joint, miniature, L5826
    orthosis (KO), E1810, L1800-L1885
Knee-ankle-foot orthosis (KAFO), L2000-L2039, L2126-L2136
Knee-ankle-foot orthosis (KAFO) addition, high strength, lightweight material, L2755
Kutapressin, J1910
Kyphosis pad, L1020, L1025

L

Laboratory tests
    chemistry, P2028-P2038
    microbiology, P7001
    miscellaneous, P9010-P9615, Q0111-Q0115
    toxicology, P3000-P3001, Q0091
Lacrimal duct implant
    permanent, A4263
    temporary, A4262
Lactated Ringer's infusion, J7120
Laetrile, J3570
Lancet, A4258, A4259
Larynx, artificial, L8500
Laser blood collection device and accessory, E0620, A4257
Lead investigation, T1029
Lead wires, per pair, A4557
Leg
    bag, A4358, A5105, A5112
    extensions for walker, E0158
    rest, elevating, K0195
    rest, wheelchair, E0990
    strap, replacement, A5113-A5114
Legg Perthes orthosis, L1700-L1755

Lens
    aniseikonic, V2118, V2318
    contact, V2500-V2599
    eye, V2100-V2615, V2700-V2799
    intraocular, V2630-V2632
    low vision, V2600-V2615
    progressive, V2781
Lepirudin, Q2021
Leucovorin calcium, J0640
Leukocyte examination, fecal, G0026
Leukocyte poor blood, each unit, P9016
Leuprolide acetate, J9217, J9218, J9219, J1950
Levocarnitine, J1955
Levofloxacin, J1956
Levonorgestrel, (contraceptive), implants and supplies, A4260
Levorphanol tartrate, J1960
Lidocaine HCl, J2001
Lift
    patient (includes seat lift), E0621-E0635
    shoe, L3300-L3334
Lincomycin HCl, J2010
Linezolid, J2020
Liquid barrier, ostomy, A4363
Lodging, recipient, escort nonemergency transport, A0180, A0200
Lorazepam, J2060
LSO, L0500-L0565
Lubricant, A4402, A4332
Lumbar flexion, L0540
Lumbar-sacral orthosis (LSO), L0500-L0565
Lymphocyte immune globulin, J7504, J7511

M

Magnesium sulphate, J3475
Maintenance contract, ESRD, A4890
Manipulation of spine, chiropractic, A2000
Mannitol, J2150
Mask
    aerosol, K0180
    oxygen, A4620, A4621
Mastectomy
    bra, L8000
    form, L8020
    prosthesis, L8030, L8600
    sleeve, L8010
Mattress
    air pressure, E0186
    alternating pressure, E0277
    dry pressure, E0184
    gel pressure, E0196
    hospital bed, E0271, E0272
    non-powered, pressure reducing, E0373
    overlay, E0371-E0372
    powered, pressure reducing, E0277
    water pressure, E0187
Measuring cylinder, dialysis, A4921

274

Mechlorethamine HCl, J9230
Medical and surgical supplies, A4206-A8999
Medroxyprogesterone acetate, J1051, J1055
Medroxyprogesterone acetate/estradiol cypionate, J1056
Melphalan HCl, J9245
Melphalan, oral, J8600
Meperidine, J2175
Meperidine and promethazine, J2180
Mepivacaine HCl, J0670
Meropenem, J2185
Mesna, J9209
Metabolically active tissue, Q0184
Metabolically active D/E tissue, Q0185
Metacarpophalangeal joint, prosthetic implant, L8630, L8631
Metaproterenol sulfate, inhalation solution, concentrated, J7668
Metaproterenol sulfate, inhalation solution, unit dose, J7669
Metaraminol bitartrate, J0380
Metatarsal joint, prosthetic implant, L8641
Meter, bath conductivity, dialysis, E1550
Methadone HCl, J1230
Methocarbamol, J2800
Methotrexate, oral, J8610
Methotrexate sodium, J9250, J9260
Methyldopate HCl, J0210
Methylergonovine maleate, J2210
Methylprednisolone
    acetate, J1020-J1040
    oral, J7509
    sodium succinate, J2920, J2930
Metoclopramide HCl, J2765
Microbiology test, P7001
Midazolam HCl, J2250
Mileage, ambulance, A0380, A0390
Mini-bus, nonemergency transportation, A0120
Milrinone lactate, J2260
Mitomycin, J9280-J9291
Mitoxantrone HCl, J9293
Modalities, with office visit, M0005-M0008
Moisture exchanger for use with invasive mechanical ventilation, A4483
Moisturizer, skin, A6250
Monitor
    apnea, E0608
    blood glucose, E0607, E0609
    blood pressure, A4670
    pacemaker, E0610, E0615
Monitoring and recording, EKG, G0004-G0007
Monoclonal antibodies, J7505
Mononine, Q0160
Morphine sulfate, J2270, J2271
    sterile, preservative-free, J2275
Mouthpiece (for respiratory equipment), A4617
    and dome (for nebulizer), K0181
Moxifloxacin, J2280
MRI contrast material, A4643
Mucoprotein, blood, P2038

Multiaxial ankle, L5986
Multidisciplinary services, H2000-H2001, T1023-T1028
Multiple post collar, cervical, L0180-L0200
Multi-Podus type AFO, L4396
Muromonab-CD3, J7505
Mycophenolate mofetil, J7517

N

Nalbuphine HCl, J2300
Naloxone HCl, J2310
Nandrolone
    decanoate, J2320-J2322
Narrowing device, wheelchair, E0969
Nasal application device, K0183
Nasal pillows/seals (for nasal application device), K0184
Nasal vaccine inhalation, J3530
Nasogastric tubing, B4081, B4082
Nebulizer, E0570-E0585
    aerosol compressor, E0571
    aerosol mask, A7015
    corrugated tubing, disposable, A7010
    corrugated tubing, non-disposable, A7011
    distilled water, K0182
    drug dispensing fee, E0590
    filter, disposable, A7013
    filter, non-disposable, A7014
    heater, E1372
    large volume, disposable, prefilled, A7008
    large volume, disposable, unfilled, A7007
    not used with oxygen, durable, glass, A7017
    pneumatic, administration set, A7003, A7005, A7006
    pneumatic, nonfiltered, A7004
    portable, E0570
    small volume, A7003-A7005
    ultrasonic, E0575
    ultrasonic, dome and mouthpiece, A7016
    ultrasonic, reservoir bottle, non-disposable, A7009
    water collection device, large volume nebulizer, A7012
Needle, A4215
    dialysis, A4655
    non-coring, A4212
    with syringe, A4206-A4209
Negative pressure wound therapy pump, E2402
    accessories, A6550-A6551
Neonatal transport, ambulance, base rate, A0225
Neostigmine methylsulfate, J2710
Nerve stimulator with batteries, E0765
Nesiritide injection, J2324
Neuromuscular stimulator, E0745
Neurostimulator
    electrodes, E0753
    programmer, E0754
    pulse generator, E0756
    receiver, E0757
    transmitter, 0758

Nonchemotherapy drug, oral, NOS, J8499
Noncovered services, A9270
Nonelastic gauze, A6264, A6406
Nonemergency transportation, A0080-A0210
Nonimpregnated gauze dressing, A6216-A6221, A6402-A6404
Nonmetabolic active tissue, Q0183
Nonprescription drug, A9150
Not otherwise classified drug, J3490, J7599, J7699, J7799, J8499, J8999, J9999, Q0181
NPH, J1820
NTIOL category 1, Q1001
NTIOL category 2, Q1002
NTIOL category 3, Q1003
NTIOL category 4, Q1004
NTIOL category 5, Q1005
Nursing care, T1030-T1031
Nutrition
    counseling, dental, D1310, D1320
    enteral infusion pump, B9000, B9002
    parenteral infusion pump, B9004, B9006
    parenteral solution, B4164-B5200

O

Obturator prosthesis
    definitive, D5932
    interim, D5936
    surgical, D5931
Occipital/mandibular support, cervical, L0160
Octreotide acetate, J2353, J2354
Ocular prosthetic implant, L8610
Ondansetron HCl, J2405
One arm, drive attachment, K0101
Oprelvekin, J2355
O & P supply/accessory/service, L9900
Oral and maxillofacial surgery, D7000-D7999
Oral examination, D0120-D0160
Oropharyngeal suction catheter, A4628
Orphenadrine, J2360
Orthodontics, D8000-D8999
Orthopedic shoes
    arch support, L3040-L3100
    footwear, L3201-L3265
    insert, L3000-L3030
    lift, L3300-L3334
    miscellaneous additions, L3500-L3595
    positioning device, L3140-L3170
    transfer, L3600-L3649
    wedge, L3340-L3420
Orthotic additions
    carbon graphite lamination, L2755
    fracture, L2180-L2192, L3995
    halo, L0860
    lower extremity, L2200-L2999, L4320
    ratchet lock, L2430
    scoliosis, L1010-L1120, L1210-L1290
    shoe, L3300-L3595, L3649

Oximeter devices, E0454, A4609
Oxygen
    ambulance, A0422
    catheter, transtracheal, A7018
    chamber, hyperbaric, topical, A4575
    concentrator, E1390-E1391
    mask, A4620, A4621
    medication supplies, A4611-A4627
    rack/stand, E1355
    regulator, E1353
    respiratory equipment/supplies, A4611-A4627, E0424-E0480
    supplies and equipment, E0425-E0444, E0455
    tent, E0455
    tubing, A4616
    water vapor enriching system, E1405, E1406
Oxymorphone HCl, J2410
Oxytetracycline HCl, J2460
Oxytocin, J2590

P

Pacemaker monitor, E0610, E0615
Paclitaxel, J9265
Pad
    gel pressure, E0178, E0185, E0196
    heat, E0210, E0215, E0217, E0238, E0249
    orthotic device interface, E1820
    sheepskin, E0188, E0189
    water circulating cold with pump, E0218
    water circulating heat with pump, E0217
    water circulating heat unit, E0249
    Wheelchair, low pressure & positioning, E0192
Pail, for use with commode chair, E0167
Palate, prosthetic implant, L8618
Pamidronate disodium, J2430
Pan, for use with commode chair, E0167
Papanicolaou (Pap) screening smear, P3000, P3001, Q0091
Papaverine HCl, J2440
Paraffin, A4265
Paraffin bath unit, E0235
Paramagnetic contrast material, (Gadolinium), A4647
Paramedic intercept, rural, Q0186
Parenteral nutrition
    administration kit, B4224
    pump, B9004, B9006
    solution, B4164-B5200
    supply kit, B4220, B4222
Paricalcitol, J2501
Parking fee, nonemergency transport, A0170
Paste, conductive, A4558
Patella, prosthetic implant, L8640
Pathology and laboratory tests, miscellaneous, P9010-P9615
Patient support system, E0636
PEFR, peak expiratory flow rate meter, A4614
Pegademase bovine, Q2012
Pegaspargase, J9266

Pegfilgrastim, J2505
Pelvic belt/harness/boot, E0944
Penicillin
  G benzathine/G benzathine and penicillin G procaine, J0530-J0580
  G potassium, J2540
  G procaine, aqueous, J2510
Pentamidine isethionate, J2545
Pentastarch, 10% solution, Q2013
Pentazocine HCl, J3070
Pentobarbital sodium, J2515
Pentostatin, J9268
Percussor, E0480
Percutaneous access system, A4301
Periapical service, D3410-D3470
Periodontal procedures, D4000-D4999
Peroneal strap, L0980
Peroxide, A4244
Perphenazine, J3310
Personal care services, T1019-T1021
Personal comfort item, A9190
Pessary, A4561, A4562
PET myocardial perfusion imaging, G0030-G0047
Phenobarbital sodium, J2560
Phentolamine mesylate, J2760
Phenylephrine HCl, J2370
Phenytoin sodium, J1165
Phisohex solution, A4246
Photofrin, see Porfimer sodium
Phototherapy light, E0202
Phytonadione, J3430
Pillow, cervical, E0943
Pin retention (per tooth), D2951
Pinworm examination, Q0113
Plasma
  protein fraction, P9018
  single donor, fresh frozen, P9017
  multiple donor, pooled, frozen, P9023
Plastazote, L3002, L3252, L3253, L3265, L5654-L5658
Platelet
  concentrate, each unit, P9019
  rich plasma, each unit, P9020
Platform attachment
  forearm crutch, E0153
  walker, E0154
Plicamycin, J9270
Plumbing, for home ESRD equipment, A4870
Pneumatic
  appliance, E0655-E0673, L4350-L4380
  compressor, E0650-E0652
  splint, L4350-L4380
  tire, wheelchair, E0953
Pneumatic nebulizer
  administration set, small volume, filtered, A7006
  administration set, small volume, nonfiltered, A7003
  administration set, small volume, nonfiltered, non-disposable, A7005

maxillofacial, provided by a non-physician, L8040-L8048
miscellaneous service, L8499
obturator, D5931-D5933, D5936
ocular, V2623-V2629
repair of, L7520, L8049
socks (shrinker, sheath, stump sock), L8400-L8485
taxes, orthotic/prosthetic/other, L9999
tracheo-esophageal, L8507-L8509
upper extremity, L6000-L6999
vacuum erection system, L7900
voice amplifier, E1904
Prosthetic additions
lower extremity, L5610-L5999
upper extremity, L6600-L7274
Prosthodontic procedure
fixed, D6200-D6999
removable, D5000-D5899
Protamine sulfate, J2720
Protectant, skin, A6250
Protector, heel or elbow, E0191
Protirelin, J2725
Pulp capping, D3110, D3120
Pulpotomy, D3220
vitality test, D0460
Pulse generator, E2120
Pump
alternating pressure pad, E0182
ambulatory infusion, E0781
ambulatory insulin, E0784
blood, dialysis, E1620
breast, E0602-E0604
enteral infusion, B9000, B9002
external infusion, E0779
heparin infusion, E1520
implantable infusion, E0782, E0783
implantable infusion, refill kit, A4220
infusion, supplies, A4230, A4232, K0110-K0111
negative pressure wound therapy, K0538
parenteral infusion, B9004, B9006
suction, portable, E0600
suction, supplies, K0190-K0192
water circulating pad, E0236
Purification system, A4880, E1610, E1615
Pyridoxine HCl, J3415

Q
Quad cane, E0105
Quinupristin/dalfopristin, J2770

R
Rack/stand, oxygen, E1355
Radial head, prosthetic implant, L8620
Radioelements for brachytherapy, Q3001
Radiofrequency transmitter, E0758, E0759

Radiograph, dental, D0210-D0340
Radiology service, R0070-R0076
Radiopharmaceutical diagnostic imaging agent, A4641, A4642, A9500-A9507, A9512-A9532, Q3002-Q3004
Radiopharmaceutical, therapeutic, A9600, A9605
Rail
    bathtub, E0241, E0242, E0246
    bed, E0305, E0310
    toilet, E0243
Rasburicase, J2783
Recement
    crown, D2920
    inlay, D2910
Reciprocating peritoneal dialysis system, E1630
Red blood cells, P9021, P9022
Reduction pneumoplasty, G0061
Regular insulin, J1820
Regulator, oxygen, E1353
Repair
    contract, ESRD, A4890
    durable medical equipment, E1340
    maxillofacial prosthesis, L8049
    orthosis, L4000-L4130
    prosthetic, L7500, L7510, K0285
Replacement
    battery, A4254, A4630, A4631
    components, ESRD machine, E1640
    pad (alternating pressure), A4640
    tanks, dialysis, A4880
    tip for cane, crutches, walker, A4637
    underarm pad for crutches, A4635
Reservoir bottle (for ultrasonic nebulizer), K0174
Resin dental restoration, D2330-D2387
RespiGam, see Respiratory syncytial virus immune globulin
Respiratory
    Heated humidifier used with PAP, K0531
    Invasive assist with backup, K0534
    Noninvasive assist with backup, K0533
    Noninvasive assist without backup, K0532
Respiratory syncytial virus immune globulin, J1565
Restorative dental procedure, D2000-D2999
Restraint, any type, E0710
Reteplase, J2993
Rho(D) immune globulin, human, J2788, J2790, J2792
Rib belt, thoracic, A4572, L0210, L0220
Ringers lactate infusion, J7120
Ring, ostomy, A4404
Rituximab, J9310
Robin-Aids, L6000, L6010, L6020, L6855, L6860
Rocking bed, E0462
Rollabout chair, E1031
Root canal therapy, D3310-D3353
Ropivacaine HCl, J2795
Rubidium Rb-82, Q3000

S

bond or cement, ostomy, A4364

    sealant, protectant, moisturizer, A6250

    test, collagen, G0025

Sling, A4565

    patient lift, E0621, E0630, E0635

Social worker, nonemergency transport, A0160

Sock

    body sock, L0984

    prosthetic sock, L8420-L8435, L8470, L8480, L8485

    stump sock, L8470-L8485

Sodium

    chloride injection, J2912

    ferric gluconate complex in sucrose, J2916

    hyaluronate, J7315, J7317

    phosphate P32, Q3007

    succinate, J1720

Solution,

    calibrator, A4256

    dialysate, A4700, A4705, A4760

    elliotts b, Q2002

    enteral formulae, B4150-B4156

    irrigation, A4323

    parenteral nutrition, B4164-B5200

Somatrem, J2940

Somatropin, J2941

Sorbent cartridge, ESRD, E1636

Specialty absorptive dressing, A6251-A6256

Spectinomycin HCl, J3320

Speech assessment, V5362-V5364

Speech generating device, E2500-E2599

Spinal orthosis,

    anterior-posterior, L0320, L0330, L0530

    anterior-posterior-lateral, L0520, L0550-L0565

    anterior-posterior-lateral-rotary, L0340-L0440

    cervical, L0100-L0200

    cervical-thoracic-lumbar-sacral (CTLSO), L0700, L0710

    DME, K0112-K0116

    halo, L0810-L0830

    lumbar flexion, L0540

    lumbar-sacral (LSO), L0500-L0565

    multiple post collar, L0180-L0200

    sacroiliac, L0600-L0620

    scoliosis, L1000-L1499

    torso supports, L0900-L0960

Splint, A4570, L3100, L4350-L4380

    ankle, L4390-L4398

    dynamic, E1800, E1805, E1810, E1815, E1825, E1830, E1840

    footdrop, L4398

Spoke protectors, each, K0065

Static progressive stretch, E1801, E1806, E1811, E1816, E1818, E1821

Sterile cefuroxime sodium, J0697

Sterile water, A4216-A4217

Stimulators

    neuromuscular, E0744, E0745

    osteogenesis, electrical, E0747-E0749

Temozolmide, oral, J8700
Temporomandibular joint, D0320, D0321
Tenecteplase, J3100
Teniposide, Q2017
TENS, A4595, E0720-E0749
Tent, oxygen, E0455
Terbutaline sulfate, J3105
Terbutaline sulfate, inhalation solution, concentrated, J7680
Terbutaline sulfate, inhalation solution, unit dose, J7681
Terminal devices, L6700-L6895
Testosterone
    aqueous, J3140
    cypionate and estradiol cypionate, J1060
    enanthate, J3120, J3130
    enanthate and estradiol valerate, J0900
    propionate, J3150
    suspension, J3140
Tetanus immune globulin, human, J1670
Tetracycline, J0120
Thallous Chloride TL 201, A9505
Theophylline, J2810
Therapeutic lightbox, A4634, E0203
Therapy
    activity, Q0082
    occupational, H5300
    physical (evaluation/treatment), Q0086
Thermometer, A4931-A4932
Thermometer, dialysis, A4910
Thiamine HCl, J3411
Thiethylperazine maleate, J3280
Thiotepa, J9340
Thoracic-hip-knee-ankle (THKAO), L1500-L1520
Thoracic-lumbar-sacral orthosis (TLSO)
    scoliosis, L1200-L1290
    spinal, K0618-K0619, L0300-L0440
Thoracic orthosis, L0210
Thymol turbidity, blood, P2033
Thyrotropin Alfa, J3240
Tinzarparin sodium, J1655
Tip (cane, crutch, walker) replacement, A4637
Tire, wheelchair, E0996, E0999, E1000
Tissue-based surgical dressings, Q0183-Q0185
Tissue of human origin, J7340, J7342, J7350
TLSO, L0300-L0440, L1200-L1290
Tobramycin, inhalation solution, unit dose, J7682
Tobramycin sulfate, J3260
Toilet accessories, E0167-E0179, E0243, E0244, E0625
Tolazoline HCl, J2670
Toll, non emergency transport, A0170
Tomographic radiograph, dental, D0322
Tool kit, dialysis, A4910
Topical hyperbaric oxygen chamber, A4575
Topotecan, J9350
Torsemide, J3265
Torso support, L0900-L0960

Tourniquet, dialysis, A4910
Tracheostoma heat moisture exchange system, A7501-A7509
Tracheostomy
    care kit, A4629
    filter, A4481
    speaking valve, L8501
    supplies, A4623, A4629, A7523-A7524
    tube, A7520-A7522
Tracheotomy mask or collar, A7525-A7526
Traction device, ambulatory, E0830
Traction equipment, E0840-E0948
Transcutaneous electrical nerve stimulator (TENS), E0720-E0749
Transducer protector, dialysis, E1575
Transfer board or device, E0972
Transfer (shoe orthosis), L3600-L3640
Transfer system with seat, E1035
Transparent film (for dressing), A6257-A6259
Transportation
    ambulance, A0021-A0999, Q3019, Q3020
    corneal tissue, V2785
    EKG (portable), R0076
    handicapped, A0130
    non emergency, A0080-A0210, T2001-T2005
    service, including ambulance, A0021-A0999, T2006
    taxi, non emergency, A0100
    toll, non emergency, A0170
    volunteer, non emergency, A0080, A0090
    x-ray (portable), R0070, R0075
Transtracheal oxygen catheter, A7018
Trapeze bar, E0910, E0940
Trapezium, prosthetic implant, L8625
Tray
    insertion, A4310-A4316
    irrigation, A4320
    surgical (see also kits), A4550
    wheelchair, E0950
Triamcinolone, J3301-J3303
    acetonide, J3301
    diacetate, J3302
    hexacetonide, J3303
    inhalation solution, concentrated, J7683
    inhalation solution, unit dose, J7684
Triflupromazine HCl, J3400
Trifocal, glass or plastic, V2300-V2399
Trigeminal division block anesthesia, D9212
Trimethobenzamide HCl, J3250
Trimetrexate glucuoronate, J3305
Triptorelin pamoate, J3315
Trismus appliance, D5937
Truss, L8300-L8330
Tube/Tubing
    anchoring device, A5200
    blood, A4750, A4755
    corrugated, for nebulizer, K0175, K0176
    CPAP device, K0187

drainage extension, A4331
gastrostomy, B4084, B4085, B4086
irrigation, A4355
larynectomy, A4622
nasogastric, B4081, B4082
oxygen, A4616
serum clotting time, A4771
stomach, B4083
suction pump, each, A7002
tire, K0064, K0068, K0078, K0091, K0093, K0095, K0097
tracheostomy, A4622
urinary drainage, K0280

U

Ultrasonic nebulizer, E0575
Ultrasonic nebulizer reservoir bottle, K0174
Ultrasound bladder capacity test, G0050
Ultrasound bone mineral study, G0133
Ultraviolet cabinet, E0690
Ultraviolet light therapy system, A4633, E0691-E0694
Unclassified drug, J3490
Unipuncture control system, dialysis, E1580
Upper extremity addition, locking elbow, L6693
Upper extremity fracture orthosis, L3980-L3999
Upper limb prosthesis, L6000-L7499
Urea, J3350
Ureterostomy supplies, A4454-A4590
Urethral suppository, Alprostadil, J0275
Urinal, E0325, E0326
Urinary
    catheter, A4338-A4346, A4351-A4353, K0410, K0411
    collection and retention (supplies), A4310-A4359, K0407,K0408, K0410, K0411
    tract implant, collagen, L8603
    tract implant, snythetic, L8606
Urine
    sensitivity study, P7001
    tests, A4250
Urofollitropin, Q2018
Urokinase, J3364, J3365
U-V lens, V2755

V

Vabra aspirator, A4480
Vaccination, administration
    hepatitis B, G0010
    influenza virus, G0008
    pneumococcal, G0009
Vancomycin HCl, J3370
Vaporizer, E0605
Vascular
    catheter (appliances and supplies), A4300-A4306
    graft material, synthetic, L8670
Vasoxyl, J3390
Venipuncture, routine specimen collection, G0001

Venous pressure clamp, dialysis, A4918
Ventilator
    battery, A4611-A4613
    moisture exchanger, disposable, A4483
    negative pressure, E0460
    volume, stationary or portable, E0450, E0461
Verteporfin, J3395
Vest, safety, wheelchair, E0980
Vinblastine sulfate, J9360
Vincristine sulfate, J9370-J9380
Vinorelbine tartrate, J9390
Vision service, V2020-V2799
Vitamin B-12 cyanocobalamin, J3420
Vitamin K, J3430
Voice amplifier, L8510
Voice prosthesis, L8511-L8514
Voriconazole, J3465

W

Waiver, T2012-T2050
Walker, E0130-E0149
    accessories, A4636, A4637
    attachments, E0153-E0159
Walking splint, L4386
Water
    collection device (for nebulizer), K0177
    distilled (for nebulizer), A7018
    pressure pad/mattress, E0177, E0187, E0198
    purification system (ESRD), E1610, E1615
    softening system (ESRD), E1625
    sterile, A4712, A4714, A4319
    tanks (dialysis), A4880
Wedges, shoe, L3340-L3420
Wet mount, Q0111
Wheel attachment, rigid pickup walker, E0155
Wheelchair, E0950-E1298, K0001-K0108
    accessories, E0192, E0950-E1030, E1065-E1069, E2300-E2399
    amputee, E1170-E1200
    back, fully reclining, manual, E1226
    battery, A4631
    component or accessory, not otherwise specified, K0108
    motorized, E1210-E1213
    narrowing device, E0969
    power add-on, E0983-E0984
    shock absorber, E1015-E1018
    specially sized, E1220, E1230
    stump support system, K0551
    tire, E0996, E0999, E1000,
    transfer board or device, E0972
    tray, K0107
    van, nonemergency, A0130
    youth, E1091
WHFO with inflatable air chamber, L3807
WHO, wrist extension, L3914
Whirlpool equipment, E1300-E1310

X

Z

2004 Table of Drugs

IA - Intra-arterial administration
IV - Intravenous administration
IM - Intramuscular administration
IT - Intrathecal
SC - Subcutaneous administration
INH - Administration by inhaled solution
VAR - Various routes of administration
OTH - Other routes of administration
ORAL - Administered orally

Intravenous administration includes all methods, such as gravity infusion, injections, and timed pushes. The 'VAR' posting denotes various routes of administration and is used for drugs that are commonly administered into joints, cavities, tissues, or topical applications, in addition to other parenteral administrations. Listings posted with 'OTH' indicate other administration methods, such as suppositories or catheter injections.

A

Abbokinase, see Urokinase			
Abbokinase, Open Cath, see Urokinase			
Abciximab	10 mg	IV	J0130
Abelcet, see Amphotericin B Lipid Complex			
ABLC, see Amphotericin B			
Acetazolamide sodium	up to 500 mg	IM, IV	J1120
Acetylcysteine, unit dose form	per gram	INH	J7608
Achromycin, see Tetracycline			
ACTH, see Corticotropin			
Acthar, see Corticotropin			
Actimmune, see Interferon gamma 1-B			
Activase, see Alteplase recombinant			
Acyclovir	5 mg		Q4075
Adenocard, see Adenosine			
Adenoscan, see Adenosine			
Adenosine	6 mg	IV	J0150
Adenosine	30 mg	IV	J0152
Adrenalin Chloride, see Adrenalin, epinephrine			
Adrenalin, epinephrine	up to 1 ml ampule	SC, IM	J0170
Adriamycin PFS, see Doxorubicin HCl			
Adriamycin RDF, see Doxorubicin HCl			
Adrucil, see Fluorouracil			
Aggrastat, see Tirofiban hydrochloride			
A-hydroCort, see Hydrocortisone sodium phosphate			
Akineton, see Biperiden			
Alatrofloxacin mesylate, injection	100 mg	IV	J0200
Albuterol	up to 5 mg	INH	J7621
Albuterol, concentrated form	per mg	INH	J7618
Albuterol, unit dose form	per mg	INH	J7619
Aldesleukin	per single use vial	IM, IV	J9015
Aldomet, see Methyldopa HCl			
Alefacept	0.5 mg		J0215
Alemtuzumab	10 mg		J9010
Alferon N, see Interferon alfa-n3			

Alglucerase	per 10 units	IV	J0205
Alkaban-AQ, see Vinblastine sulfate			
Alkeran, see Melphalan, oral			
Alpha 1-proteinase inhibitor, human	10 mg	IV	J0256
Alprostadil, injection	1.25 mcg	OTH	J0270
Alprostadil, urethral suppository		OTH	J0275
Alteplase recombinant	1 mg	IV	J2997
Alupent, see Metaproterenol sulfate or Metaproterenol, compounded			
Amcort, see Triamcinolone diacetate			
A-methaPred, see Methylprednisolone sodium succinate			
Amgen, see Interferon alphacon-1			
Amifostine	500 mg	IV	J0207
Aminolevalinic acid Hcl	unit dose (354 mg)	OTH	J7308
Aminophylline/Aminophyllin	up to 250 mg	IV	J0280
Amiodarone HCl	30 mg	IV	J0282
Amitriptyline HCl	up to 20 mg	IM	J1320
Amobarbital	up to 125 mg	IM, IV	J0300
Amphocin, see Amphotericin B			
Amphotericin B	50 mg	IV	J0285
Amphotericin B, lipid complex	10 mg	IV	J0287-9
Ampicillin sodium	up to 500 mg	IM, IV	J0290
Ampicillin sodium/sulbactam sodium	per 1.5 gm	IM, IV	J0295
Amygdalin, see Laetrile, Amygdalin, vitamin B-17			
Amytal, see Amobarbital			
Anabolin LA 100, see Nandrolone decanoate			
Ancef, see Cefazolin sodium			
Andrest 90-4, see Testosterone enanthate and estradiol valerate			
Andro-Cyp, see Testosterone cypionate			
Andro-Cyp 200, see Testosterone cypionate			
Andro L.A. 200, see Testosterone enanthate			
Andro-Estro 90-4, see Testosterone enanthate and estradiol valerate			
Andro/Fem, see Testosterone cypionate and estradiol cypionate			
Androgyn L.A., see Testosterone enanthate and estradiol valerate			
Androlone-50, see Nandrolone phenpropionate			
Androlone-D 100, see Nandrolone decanoate			
Andronaq-50, see Testosterone suspension			
Andronaq-LA, see Testosterone cypionate			
Andronate-200, see Testosterone cypionate			
Andronate-100, see Testosterone cypionate			
Andropository 100, see Testosterone enanthate			
Andryl 200, see Testosterone enanthate			
Anectine, see Succinylcholine chloride			
Anergan 25, see Promethazine HCl			
Anergan 50, see Promethazine HCl			
Anistreplase	30 units	IV	J0350
Anti-Inhibitor	per IU	IV	J7198
Antispas, see Dicyclomine HCl			
Antithrombin III (human)	per IU	IV	J7197
Anzemet, see Dolasetron mesylate injection			
A.P.L., see Chorionic gonadotropin			
Apresoline, see Hydralazine HCl			
Aprotinin	10,000 kiu		Q2003
AquaMEPHYTON, see Vitamin K			
Aralen, see Chloroquine HCl			
Aramine, see Metaraminol			

Aranesp, see Darbepoetin Alfa			
Arbutamine	1 mg	IV	J0395
Aredia, see Pamidronate disodium			
Arfonad, see Trimethaphan camsylate			
Aristocort Forte, see Triamcinolone diacetate			
Aristocort Intralesional, see Triamcinolone diacetate			
Aristospan Intra-Articular, see Triamcinolone hexacetonide			
Aristospan Intralesional, see Triamcinolone hexacetonide			
Arrestin, see Trimethobenzamide HCl			
Arsenic trioxide	1 mg	IV	J9017
Asparaginase	10,000 units	IV, IM	J9020
Astramorph PF, see Morphine sulfate			
Atgam, see Lymphocyte immune globulin			
Ativan, see Lorazepam			
Atropine, concentrated form	per mg	INH	J7635
Atropine, unit dose form	per mg	INH	J7636
Atropine sulfate	up to 0.3 mg	IV, IM, SC	J0460
Atrovent, see Ipratropium bromide			
Aurothioglucose	up to 50 mg	IM	J2910
Autologous cultured chondrocytes implant			J7330
Autoplex T, see Hemophilia clotting factors			
Avonex, see Interferon beta-1a			
Azathioprine	50 mg	ORAL	J7500
Azathioprine, parenteral	100 mg	IV	J7501
Azithromycin, dihydrate	1 gm	ORAL	Q0144
Azithromycin, injection	500 mg	IV	J0456

B

Baclofen	10 mg	IT	J0475
Baclofen for intrathecal trial	50 mcg	OTH	J0476
Bactocill, see Oxacillin sodium			
BAL in oil, see Dimercaprol			
Banflex, see Orphenadrine citrate			
Basiliximab	20 mg		Q2019
BCG (Bacillus Calmette and Guérin), live			
	per vial instillation	IV	J9031
Beclomethasone inhalation solution, unit dose form per mg		INH	J7622
Bena-D 10, see Diphenhydramine HCl			
Bena-D 50, see Diphenhydramine HCl			
Benadryl, see Diphenhydramine HCl			
Benahist 10, see Diphenhydramine HCl			
Benahist 50, see Diphenhydramine HCl			
Ben-Allergin-50, see Diphenhydramine HCl			
Benefix, see Factor IX, recombinant			
Benoject-10, see Diphenhydramine HCl			
Benoject-50, see Diphenhydramine HCl			
Bentyl, see Dicyclomine			
Benztropine mesylate	per 1 mg	IM, IV	J0515
Berubigen, see Vitamin B-12 cyanocobalamin			
Betalin 12, see Vitamin B-12 cyanocobalamin			
Betameth, see Betamethasone sodium phosphate			
Betamethasone acetate			
& betamethasone sodium phosphate 3 mg of ea		IM	J0702
Betamethasone inhalation solution, unit dose form per mg		INH	J7624
Betamethasone sodium phosphate	4 mg	IM, IV	J0704

Betaseron, see Interferon beta-1b

Bethanechol chloride	up to 5 mg	SC	J0520

Bicillin L-A, see Penicillin G benzathine

Bicillin C-R 900/300, see Penicillin G procaine and penicillin G benzathine

Bicillin C-R, see Penicillin G benzathine and penicillin G procaine

BiCNU, see Carmustine

Biperiden lactate	per 5 mg	IM, IV	J0190
Bitolterol mesylate,concentrated form	per mg	INH	J7628
Bitolterol mesylate,unit dose form	per mg	INH	J7629
Bivalirudin	1 mg		J0583

Blenoxane, see Bleomycin sulfate

Bleomycin sulfate	15 units	IM, IV, SC	J9040
Botulinum toxin type A	per unit	IM	J0585
Botulinum toxin type B	per 100 units	IM	J0587

Brethine, see Terbutaline sulfate or Terbutaline, compounded

Bricanyl Subcutaneous, see Terbutaline sulfate

Brompheniramine maleate	per 10 mg	IM, SC, IV	J0945

Bronkephrine, see Ethylnorepinephrine HCl

Bronkosol, see Isoetharine HCl

Budesonide inhalation solution, concentrated form 0.25 mg		INH	J7633
Budesonide inhalation solution, unit dose form	0.25 mg	INH	J7626
Buprenorphine Hydrochloride	0.1 mg		J0592
Busulfan	2 mg	ORAL	J8510
Butorphanol tartrate	2 mg		J0595

C

Cabergoline	0.5 mg	ORAL	Q2001

Cafcit, see Caffeine citrate

Caffeine citrate	5 mg	IV	J0706

Caine-1, see Lidocaine Hcl

Caine-2, see Lidocaine HCl

Calcijex, see Calcitriol

Calcimar, see Calcitonin-salmon

Calcitonin-salmon	up to 400 units	SC, IM	J0630
Calcitriol	0.1 mcg	IM	J0636

Calcium Disodium Versenate, see Edetate calcium disodium

Calcium gluconate	per 10 ml	IV	J0610
Calcium glycerophosphate & calcium lactate per 10 ml		IM, SC	J0620

Calphosan, see Calcium glycerophosphate and calcium lactate

Camptosar, see Irinotecan

Capecitabine	150 mg	ORAL	J8520
Capecitabine	500 mg	ORAL	J8521

Carbocaine with Neo-Cobefrin, see Mepivacaine

Carbocaine, see Mepivacaine

Carboplatin	50 mg	IV	J9045
Carmustine	100 mg	IV	J9050

Carnitor, see Levocarnitine

Carticel, see Autologous cultured chondrocytes

Caspofungin acetate	5 mg	IV	J0637

Cefadyl, see Cephapirin Sodium

Cefazolin sodium	up to 500 mg	IV, IM	J0690
Cefepime hydrochloride	500 mg	IV	J0692

Cefizox, see Ceftizoxime sodium

Cefotaxime sodium	per 1 g	IV, IM	J0698
Cefoxitin sodium	1 g	IV, IM	J0694

Ceftazidime	per 500 mg	IM, IV	J0713
Ceftizoxime sodium	per 500 mg	IV, IM	J0715
Ceftriaxone sodium	per 250 mg	IV, IM	J0696
Cefuroxime sodium, sterile	per 750 mg	IM, IV	J0697
Celestone Phosphate, see Betamethasone sodium phosphate			
Celestone Soluspan, see Betamethasone acetate			
and betamethasone sodium phosphate			
CellCept, see Mycophenolate mofetil			
Cel-U-Jec, see Betamethasone sodium phosphate			
Cenacort Forte, see Triamcinolone diacetate			
Cenacort A-40, see Triamcinolone acetonide			
Cephalothin sodium	up to 1 g	IM, IV	J1890
Cephapirin sodium	up to 1 g	IV, IM	J0710
Ceredase, see Alglucerase			
Cerezyme, see Imiglucerase			
Cerubidine, see Daunorubicin HCl			
Chealamide, see Endrate ethylenediamine-tetra-acetic acid			
Chloramphenicol sodium succinate	up to 1 g	IV	J0720
Chlordiazepoxide HCl	up to 100 mg	IM, IV	J1990
Chloromycetin Sodium Succinate, see Chloramphenicol sodium succinate			
Chloroprocaine HCl	per 30 ml	VAR	J2400
Chlorpromazine HCl, oral	10 mg	ORAL	Q0171
	25 mg	ORAL	Q0172
Chloroquine HCl	up to 250 mg	IM	J0390
Chlorothiazide sodium	per 500 mg	IV	J1205
Chlorpromazine HCl	up to 50 mg	IM, IV	J3230
Chorex-5, see Chorionic gonadotropin			
Chorex-10, see Chorionic gonadotropin			
Chorignon, see Chorionic gonadotropin			
Chorionic gonadotropin	per 1,000 USP units	IM	J0725
Choron 10, see Chorionic gonadotropin			
Cidofovir	375 mg	IV	J0740
Cilastatin sodium, imipenem	per 250 mg	IV, IM J0743	
Cipro IV, see Ciprofloxacin			
Ciprofloxacin	200 mg	IV	J0706
Cisplatin, powder or solution	per 10 mg	IV	J9060
Cisplatin	50 mg	IV	J9062
Cladribine	per mg	IV	J9065
Claforan, see Cefotaxime sodium			
Clonidine Hydrochloride	1 mg	epidural	J0735
Cobex, see Vitamin B-12 cyanocobalamin			
Codeine phosphate	per 30 mg	IM, IV, SC	J0745
Codimal-A, see Brompheniramine			
Cogentin, see Benztropine mesylate			
Colchicine	per 1 mg	IV	J0760
Colistimethate sodium	up to 150 mg	IM, IV	J0770
Coly-Mycin M, see Colistimethate sodium			
Compa-Z, see Prochlorperazine			
Compazine, see Prochlorperazine			
Cophene-B, see Brompheniramine maleate			
Copper contraceptive, intrauterine		OTH	J7300
Cordarone, see Amiodarone HCl			
Corgonject-5, see Chorionic gonadotropin			
Corticorelin ovine triflutate	per dose		Q2005
Corticotropin	up to 40 units	IV, IM, SC	J0800

Cortrosyn, see Cosyntropin
Cosmegen, see Dactinomycin

Cosyntropin	per 0.25 mg	IM, IV	J0835

Cotranzine, see Prochlorperazine

Cromolyn sodium, unit dose form	per 10 mg	INH	J7631

Crysticillin 300 A.S., see Penicillin G procaine
Crysticillin 600 A.S., see Penicillin G procaine

Cyclophosphamide	100 mg	IV	J9070
	200 mg	IV	J9080
	500 mg	IV	J9090
	1 g	IV	J9091
	2 g	IV	J9092
Cyclophosphamide, lyophilized	100 mg	IV	J9093
	200 mg	IV	J9094
	500 mg	IV	J9095
	1 g	IV	J9096
	2 g	IV	J9097
Cyclophosphamide, oral	25 mg	ORAL	J8530
Cyclosporine, oral	25 mg	ORAL	J7515
	100 mg	ORAL	J7502
Cyclosporine, parenteral	250 mg	IV	J7516
Cytarabine	100 mg	SC, IV	J9100
Cytarabine	500 mg	SC, IV	J9110
Cytarabine liposome	10 mg		J9098
Cytomegalovirus immune globulin intravenous(human)			
	per vial	IV	J0850

Cytosar-U, see Cytarabine
Cytovene, see Ganciclovir sodium
Cytoxan, see Cyclophosphamide; cyclophosphamide, lyophilized; and
cyclophosphamide, oral

D

D-5-W, infusion	1000 cc	IV	J7070
Dacarbazine	100 mg	IV	J9130
	200 mg	IV	J9140
Daclizumab	25 mg	IV	J7513
Dactinomycin	0.5 mg	IV	J9120

Dalalone, see Dexamethasone sodium phosphate
Dalalone L.A., see Dexamethasone acetate

Dalteparin sodium	per 2500	IU SC	J1645
Darbepoetin Alfa	1 mcg		Q4054
	5 mcg		J0880
	1000 units		Q0137
Daunorubicin citrate, liposomal formulation			
	10 mg	IV	J9151
Daunorubicin HCl	10 mg	IV	J9150

Daunoxome, see Daunorubicin citrate
DDAVP, see Desmopressin acetate
Decadron Phosphate, see Dexamethasone sodium phosphate
Decadron, see Dexamethasone sodium phosphate
Decadron-LA, see Dexamethasone acetate
Deca-Durabolin, see Nandrolone decanoate
Decaject, see Dexamethasone sodium phosphate
Decaject-L.A., see Dexamethasone acetate
Decolone-50, see Nandrolone decanoate

Decolone-100, see Nandrolone decanoate

De-Comberol, see Testosterone cypionate and estradiol cypionate

Deferoxamine mesylate	500 mg	IM, SC, IV	J0895

Dehist, see Brompheniramine maleate

Deladumone OB, see Testosterone enanthate and estradiol valerate

Deladumone, see Testosterone enanthate and estradiol valerate

Delatest, see Testosterone enanthate

Delatestadiol, see Testosterone enanthate and estradiol valerate

Delatestryl, see Testosterone enanthate

Delta-Cortef, see Prednisolone, oral

Delestrogen, see Estradiol valerate

Demadex, see Torsemide

Demerol HCl, see Meperidine HCl

Denileukin diftitox	300 mcg		J9160

DepAndro 100, see Testosterone cypionate

DepAndro 200, see Testosterone cypionate

DepAndrogyn, see Testosterone cypionate and estradiol cypionate

DepGynogen, see Depo-estradiol cypionate

DepMedalone 40, see Methylprednisolone acetate

DepMedalone 80, see Methylprednisolone acetate

Depo-estradiol cypionate	up to 5 mg	IM	J1000

Depogen, see Depo-estradiol cypionate

Depoject, see Methyprednisolone acetate

Depo-Medrol, see Methylprednisolone acetate

Depopred-40, see Methylprednisolone acetate

Depopred-80, see Methylprednisolone acetate

Depo-Provera, see Medroxyprogesterone acetate

Depotest, see Testosterone cypionate

Depo-Testadiol, see Testosterone cypionate and estradiol cypionate

Depotestogen, see Testosterone cypionate and estradiol cypionate

Depo-Testosterone, see Testosterone cypionate

Desferal Mesylate, see Deferoxamine mesylate

Desmopressin acetate	1 mcg	IV, SC	J2597

Dexacen LA-8, see Dexamethasone acetate

Dexacen-4, see Dexamethasone sodium phosphate

Dexamethasone, concentrated form	per mg	INH	J7637
Dexamethasone, unit form	per mg	INH	J7638
Dexamethasone acetate	1 mg	IM	J1094
Dexamethasone sodium phosphate	1 mg	IM, IV, OTH	J1100

Dexasone, see Dexamethasone sodium phosphate

Dexasone L.A., see Dexamethasone acetate

Dexferrum, see Iron Dextran

Dexone, see Dexamethasone sodium phosphate

Dexone LA, see Dexamethasone acetate

Dexrazoxane hydrochloride	250 mg	IV	J1190
Dextran 40	500 ml	IV	J7100
Dextran 75	500 ml	IV	J7110
Dextrose 5%/normal saline solution,	500 ml = 1 unit	IV	J7042
Dextrose/water (5%)	500 ml = 1 unit	IV	J7060

D.H.E. 45, see Dihydroergotamine

Diamox, see Acetazolamide sodium

Diazepam	up to 5 mg	IM, IV	J3360
Diazoxide	up to 300 mg	IV	J1730

Dibent, see Dicyclomine HCl

Dicyclomine HCl	up to 20 mg	IM	J0500

Didronel, see Etidronate disodium			
Diethylstilbestrol diphosphate	250 mg	IV	J9165
Diflucan, see Fluconazole			
Digoxin	up to 0.5 mg	IM, IV	J1160
Digoxin immune fab (ovine)	per vial		Q2006
Dihydrex, see Diphenhydramine Hcl			
Dihydroergotamine mesylate	per 1 mg	IM, IV	J1110
Dilantin, see Phenytoin sodium			
Dilaudid, see Hydromorphone HCl			
Dilocaine, see Lidocaine HCl			
Dilomine, see Dicyclomine HCl			
Dilor, see Dyphylline			
Dimenhydrinate	up to 50 mg	IM, IV	J1240
Dimercaprol	per 100 mg	IM	J0470
Dimethyl sulfoxide, see DMSO, Dimethylsulfoxide			
Dinate, see Dimenhydrinate			
Dioval, see Estradiol valerate			
Dioval 40, see Estradiol valerate			
Dioval XX, see Estradiol valerate			
Diphenacen-50, see Diphenhydramine HCl			
Diphenhydramine HCl, injection	up to 50 mg	IV, IM	J1200
Diphenhydramine HCl, oral	50 mg	ORAL	Q0163
Dipyridamole	per 10 mg	IV	J1245
Disotate, see Endrate ethylenediamine-tetra-acetic acid			
Di-Spaz, see Dicyclomine HCl			
Ditate-DS, see Testosterone enanthate and estradiol valerate			
Diuril Sodium, see Chlorothiazide sodium			
D-Med 80, see Methylprednisolone acetate			
DMSO, Dimethyl sulfoxide 50%,	50 ml	OTH	J1212
Dobutamine HCl	per 250 mg	IV	J1250
Dobutrex, see Dobutamine Hcl			
Docetaxel	20 mg	IV	J9170
Dolasetron mesylate, injection	10 mg	IV	J1260
Dolasetron mesylate, tablets	100 mg	ORAL	Q0180
Dolophine HCl, see Methadone Hcl			
Dommanate, see Dimenhydrinate			
Dopamine HCl	40 mg		Q4076
Dornase alpha, unit dose form	per mg	INH	J7639
Doxercalciferol	1 mcg	IV	J1270
Doxil, see Doxorubicin HCL, lipid			
Doxorubicin HCL	10 mg	IV	J9000
Doxorubicin HCL, all lipid	10 mg	IV	J9001
Dramamine, see Dimenhydrinate			
Dramanate, see Dimenhydrinate			
Dramilin, see Dimenhydrinate			
Dramocen, see Dimenhydrinate			
Dramoject, see Dimenhydrinate			
Dronabinol, oral	2.5 mg	ORAL	Q0167
Dronabinol, oral	5 mg	ORAL	Q0168
Droperidol up to	5 mg	IM, IV	J1790
Drug administered through a metered dose inhaler		INH	J3535
Droperidol and fentanyl citrate	up to 2 ml ampule	IM, IV	J1810
DTIC-Dome, see Dacarbazine			
Dua-Gen L.A., see Testosterone enanthate and estradiol valerate cypionate			
Duoval P.A., see Testosterone enanthate and estradiol valerate			

Durabolin, see Nandrolone phenpropinate
Duraclon, see Clonidine Hydrochloride
Dura-Estrin, see Depo-estradiol cypionate
Duracillin A.S., see Penicillin G procaine
Duragen-10, see Estradiol valerate
Duragen-20, see Estradiol valerate
Duragen-40, see Estradiol valerate
Duralone-40, see Methylprednisolone acetate
Duralone-80, see Methylprednisolone acetate
Duralutin, see Hydroxyprogesterone Caproate
Duramorph, see Morphine sulfate
Duratest-100, see Testosterone cypionate
Duratest-200, see Testosterone cypionate
Duratestrin, see Testosterone cypionate and estradiol cypionate
Durathate-200, see Testosterone enanthate
Dymenate, see Dimenhydrinate

Dyphylline up to	500 mg	IM	J1180

E

Edetate calcium disodium	up to 1000 mg	IV, SC, IM	J0600
Edetate disodium	per 150 mg	IV	J3520
Elavil, see Amitriptyline HCl			
Ellence, see Epirubicin HCl			
Elliotts b solution	per ml	OTH	Q2002

Elspar, see Asparaginase
Emete-Con, see Benzquinamide
Eminase, see Anistreplase
Enbrel, see Etanercept
Endrate ethylenediamine-tetra-acetic acid, see Edetate disodium
Enovil, see Amitriptyline HCl

Enoxaparin sodium	10 mg	SC	J1650
Epinephrine, adrenalin	up to 1 ml amp	SC, IM	J0170
Epirubicin hydrochloride	2 mg		J9178
Epoetin alfa	1000 units		Q4055
Epoprostenol	0.5 mg	IV	J1325
Eptifibatide, injection	5 mg	IM, IV	J1327
Ergonovine maleate	up to 0.2 mg	IM, IV	J1330
Ertapenem sodium	500 mg		J1335
Erythromycin lactobionate	500 mg	IV	J1364

Estra-D, see Depo-estradiol cypionate
Estra-L 20, see Estradiol valerate
Estra-L 40, see Estradiol valerate
Estra-Testrin, see Testosterone enanthate and estradiol valerate
Estradiol Cypionate, see Depo-estradiol cypionate
Estradiol L.A., see Estradiol valerate
Estradiol L.A. 20, see Estradiol valerate
Estradiol L.A. 40, see Estradiol valerate

Estradiol valerate	up to 10 mg	IM	J1380
	up to 20 mg	IM	J1390
	up to 40 mg	IM	J0970

Estro-Cyp, see Depo-estradiol cypionate

Estrogen, conjugated	per 25 mg	IV, IM	J1410

Estroject L.A., see Depo-estradiol cypionate

Estrone	per 1 mg	IM	J1435

Estrone 5, see Estrone

Estrone Aqueous, see Estrone
Estronol, see Estrone
Estronol-L.A., see Depo-estradiol cypionate

Etanercept, injection	25 mg	IM, IV	J1438
Ethanolamine	100 mg		Q2007

Ethyol, see Amifostine

Etidronate disodium	per 300 mg	IV	J1436

Etopophos, see Etoposide

Etoposide	10 mg	IV	J9181
	100 mg	IV	J9182
Etoposide, oral	50 mg	ORAL	J8560

Everone, see Testosterone Enanthate

F

Factor VIIa (coagulation factor, recombinant)			
	per mg	IV	Q0187
Factor VIII (anti-hemophilic factor, human)			
	per IU	IV	J7190
Factor VIII (anti-hemophilic factor, porcine)			
	per IU	IV	J7191
Factor VIII (anti-hemophilic factor, recombinant)			
	per IU	IV	J7192
Factor IX (anti-hemophilic factor, purified, non-recombinant)			
	per IU	IV	Q0160
Factor IX (anti-hemophilic factor, recombinant)			
	per IU	IV	Q0161
Factor IX, complex	per IU	IV	J7194
Factors, other hemophilia clotting	per IU	IV	J7196

Factrel, see Gonadorelin HCl
Feiba VH Immuno, see Factors, other hemophilia clotting

Fentanyl citrate	0.1 mg	IM, IV	J3010

Ferrlecit, see Sodium ferricgluconate complex in sucrose injection

Filgrastim (G-CSF)	300 mcg	SC, IV	J1440
	480 mcg	SC, IV	J1441

Flexoject, see Orphenadrine citrate
Flexon, see Orphenadrine citrate
Flolan, see Epoprostenol

Floxuridine	500 mg	IV	J9200
Fluconazole	200 mg	IV	J1450

Fludara, see Fludarabine phosphate

Fludarabine phosphate	50 mg	IV	J9185
Flunisolide inhalation solution, unit dose form			
	per mg	INH	J7641
Fluorouracil	500 mg	IV	J9190

Folex, see Methotrexate sodium
Folex PFS, see Methotrexate sodium
Follutein, see Chorionic gonadotropin

Fomepizole	1.5 mg		Q2008
Fomivirsen sodium	1.65 mg	Intraocular	J1452
Fondaparinux sodium	0.5 mg		J1652

Fortaz, see Ceftazidime

Foscarnet sodium	per 1,000 mg	IV	J1455

Foscavir, see Foscarnet sodium

Fosphenytoin	50 mg		Q2009

FUDR, see Floxuridine

Fulvestrant	25 mg		J9395
Fungizone Intravenous, see Amphotericin B			
Furomide M.D., see Furosemide			
Furosemide	up to 20 mg	IM, IV	J1940

G

Gamastan, see Gamma globulin and Immune globulin			
Gamma globulin	1 cc	IM	J1460
	2 cc	IM	J1470
	3 cc	IM	J1480
	4 cc	IM	J1490
	5 cc	IM	J1500
	6 cc	IM	J1510
	7 cc	IM	J1520
	8 cc	IM	J1530
	9 cc	IM	J1540
	10 cc	IM	J1550
	over 10 cc	IM	J1560
Gammar, see Gamma globulin and Immune globulin			
Gammar-IV, see Immune globulin intravenous (human)			
Gamulin RH, see Rho(D) immune globulin			
Ganciclovir, implant	4.5 mg	OTH	J7310
Ganciclovir sodium	500 mg	IV	J1570
Garamycin, gentamicin	up to 80 mg	IM, IV	J1580
Gatifloxacin	10 mg	IV	J1590
Gesterol 50, see Progesterone			
Glatiramer Acetate	20 mg		J1595
Glucagon Hcl	per 1 mg	SC, IM, IV	J1610
Glukor, see Chorionic gonadotropin			
Glycopyrrolate, concentrated form	per 1 mg	INH	J7642
Glycopyrrolate, unit dose form	per 1 mg	INH	J7643
Gold sodium thiomalate	up to 50 mg	IM	J1600
Gonadorelin HCl	per 100 mcg	SC, IV	J1620
Gonic, see Chorionic gonadotropin			
Goserelin acetate implant	per 3.6 mg	SC	J9202
Granisetron HCl, injection	100 mcg	IV	J1626
Granisetron HCl, oral	1 mg	ORAL	Q0166
Gynogen L.A. A10,@ see Estradiol valerate			
Gynogen L.A. A20,@ see Estradiol valerate			
Gynogen L.A. A40,@ see Estradiol valerate			

H

Haldol, see Haloperidol			
Haloperidol	up to 5 mg	IM, IV	J1630
Haloperidol decanoate	per 50 mg	IM	J1631
Hectoral, see Doxercalciferol			
Hemin per	1 mg		Q2011
Hemofil M, see Factor VIII			
Hemophilia clotting factors(e.g., anti-inhibitors)			
	per IU	IV	J7198
Hemophilia clotting factors, NOC	per IU	IV	J7199
Hepatitis B vaccine			Q3021-23
Hep-Lock, see Heparin sodium (heparin lock flush)			
Hep-Lock U/P, see Heparin sodium (heparin lock flush)			

Drug	Amount	Route	Code
Heparin sodium	1,000 units	IV, SC	J1644
Heparin sodium (heparin lock flush)	10 units	IV	J1642
Herceptin, see Trastuzumab			
Hexadrol Phosphate, see Dexamethasone sodium phosphate			
Histaject, see Brompheniramine maleate			
Histerone 50, see Testosterone suspension			
Histerone 100, see Testosterone suspension			
Histrelin acetate	10 mg		Q2020
Hyalgan, see Sodium Hyaluronate			
Hyaluronidase	up to 150 units	SC, IV	J3470
Hyate:C, see Factor VIII (anti-hemophilic factor (porcine))			
Hybolin Improved, see Nandrolone phenpropionate			
Hybolin Decanoate, see Nandrolone decanoate			
Hycamtin, see Topotecan			
Hydralazine HCl	up to 20 mg	IV, IM	J0360
Hydrate, see Dimenhydrinate			

I

Drug	Amount	Route	Code
Ibutilide fumarate	1 mg	IV	J1742
Idamycin, see Idarubicin HCl			
Idarubicin HCl	5 mg	IV	J9211
Ifex, see Ifosfamide			
Ifosfamide	per 1 g	IV	J9208
Ilotycin, see Erythromycin gluceptate			
Imferon, see Iron dextran			
Imiglucerase	per unit	IV	J1785
Imitrex, see Sumatriptan succinate			
Immune globulin	per 500 mg	IV	J1561
Immune globulin, anti-thymocyte globulin	25 mg	IV	J7504
Immune globulin, intravenous	1 gm	IV	J1563
Immune globulin, intravenous	10 mg	IV	J1564
Immunosuppressive drug, not otherwise classified			J7599
Imuran, see Azathioprine			
Inapsine, see Droperidol			
Inderal, see Propranolol HCl			
Infed, see Iron Dextran			
Infergen, see Interferon alfa-1			
Infliximab, injection	10 mg	IM, IV	J1745
Innohep, see Tinzarparin			
Innovar, see Droperidol with fentanyl citrate			
Insulin	5 units	SC	J1815
Insulin lispro	50 units	SC	J1817
Intal, see Cromolyn sodium or Cromolyn sodium, compounded			
Integrilin, injection, see Eptifibatide			
Interferon alphacon-1, recombinant	1 mcg	SC	J9212
Interferon alfa-2a, recombinant	3 million units	SC, IM	J9213
Interferon alfa-2b, recombinant	1 million units	SC, IM	J9214
Interferon alfa-n3 (human leukocyte derived)	250,000 IU	IM	J9215
Interferon beta-1a	33 mcg	IM	J1825
Interferon beta-1a	11 mcg	IM	Q3025
Interferon beta-1a	11 mcg	SC	Q3026
Interferon beta-1b	0.25 mg	SC	J1830
Interferon gamma-1b	3 million units	SC	J9216

Intrauterine copper contraceptive, see Copper contraceptive, intrauterine

Ipratropium bromide, unit dose form	per mg	INH	J7644
Irinotecan	20 mg	IV	J9206
Iron dextran	50 mg	IV, IM	J1750
Iron sucrose	1 mg	IV	J1756
Irrigation solution for Tx of bladder calculi			
	per 50 ml	OTH	Q2004

Isocaine HCl, see Mepivacaine

Isoetharine HCl, concentrated form	per mg	INH	J7648
Isoetharine Hcl, unit dose form	per mg	INH	J7649
Isoproterenol HCl, concentrated form	per mg	INH	J7658
Isoproterenol Hcl, unit dose form	per mg	INH	J7659

Isuprel, see Isoproterenol HCl

Itraconazole	50 mg	IV	J1835

J

Jenamicin, see Garamycin, gentamicin

K

Kabikinase, see Streptokinase

Kaleinate, see Calcium gluconate

Kanamycin sulfate	up to 75 mg	IM, IV	J1850
Kanamycin sulfate	up to 500 mg	IM, IV	J1840

Kantrex, see Kanamycin sulfate

Keflin, see Cephalothin sodium

Kefurox, see Cufuroxime sodium

Kefzol, see Cefazolin sodium

Kenaject-40, see Triamcinolone acetonide

Kenalog-10, see Triamcinolone acetonide

Kenalog-40, see Triamcinolone acetonide

Kestrone 5, see Estrone

Ketorolac tromethamine	per 15 mg	IM, IV	J1885

Key-Pred 25, see Prednisolone acetate

Key-Pred 50, see Prednisolone acetate

Key-Pred-SP, see Prednisolone sodium phosphate

K-Flex, see Orphenadrine citrate

Klebcil, see Kanamycin sulfate

Koate-HP, see Factor VIII

Kogenate, see Factor VIII

Konakion, see Vitamin K, phytonadione, etc.

Konyne-80, see Factor IX, complex

Kutapressin	up to 2 ml	SC, IM	J1910

Kytril, see Granisetron HCl

L

L.A.E. 20, see Estradiol valerate

Laetrile, Amygdalin, vitamin B-17			J3570

Lanoxin, see Digoxin

Largon, see Propiomazine HCl

Lasix, see Furosemide

L-Caine, see Lidocaine HCl

Lepirudin	50 mg		Q2021
Leucovorin calcium	per 50 mg	IM, IV	J0640

Leukine, see Sargramostim (GM-CSF)
Leuprolide acetate (for depot suspension)

	3.75 mg	IM	J1950
	7.5 mg	IM	J9217
Leuprolide acetate	per 1 mg	IM	J9218
Leuprolide acetate implant	65 mg		J9219

Leustatin, see Cladribine

Levalbuterol Hcl, concentrated form	0.5 mg	INH	J7618
Levalbuterol Hcl, unit form	0.5 mg	INH	J7619

Levaquin I.U., see Levofloxacin

Levocarnitine	per 1 gm	IV	J1955

Levo-Dromoran, see Levorphanol tartrate

Levofloxacin	250 mg	IV	J1956

Levonorgestrel releasing intrauterin contraceptive

	52 mg	OTH	J7302
Levorphanol tartrate	up to 2 mg	SC, IV	J1960

Levsin, see Hyoscyamine sulfate
Levulan Kerastick, see Aminolevulinic acid HCl
Librium, see Chlordiazepoxide HCl

Lidocaine HCl	10 mg	IV	J2001

Lidoject-1, see Lidocaine HCl
Lidoject-2, see Lidocaine HCl
Lincocin, see Lincomycin HCl

Lincomycin HCl	up to 300 mg	IV	J2010
Linezolid	200 mg	IV	J2020

Liquaemin Sodium, see Heparin sodium
Lioresal, see Baclofen
LMD (10%), see Dextran 40
Lovenox, see Enoxaparin sodium Lorazepam

	2 mg	IM, IV	J2060

Lufyllin, see Dyphylline
Luminal Sodium, see Phenobarbitol sodium
Lunelle, see Medroxyprogesterone acetate/estradiol cypionate
Lupron, see Leuprolide acetate
Lymphocyte immune globulin,

anti-thymocyte globulin, equine	250 mg	IV	J7504
anti-thymocyte globulin, rabbit	25 mg	IV	J7511

Lyophilized, see Cyclophosphamide, lyophilized

M

Magnesium sulfate	500 mg		J3475
Mannitol 25%	in 50 ml	IV	J2150

Marmine, see Dimenhydrinate
Maxipime, see Cefepime hydrochloride
Mechlorethamine HCl (nitrogen mustard), HN2

	10 mg	IV	J9230

Medralone 40, see Methylprednisolone acetate
Medralone 80, see Methylprednisolone acetate
Medrol, see Methylprednisolone

Medroxyprogesterone acetate	50 mg	IM	J1051
	150 mg	IM	J1055

Medroxyprogesterone acetate/estradiol cypionate

	5 mg/25 mg	IM	J1056

Mefoxin, see Cefoxitin sodium

Melphalan HCl	50 mg	IV	J9245

Melphalan, oral	2 mg	ORAL	J8600

Menoject LA, see Testosterone cypionate and estradiol cypionate
Mepergan Injection, see Meperdinc and promethazine HCl

Meperidine HCl	per 100 mg	IM, IV, SC	J2175
Meperidine and promethazine HCl	up to 50 mg	IM, IV	J2180
Mepivacaine HCL	per 10 ml	VAR	J0670
Meropenem	100 mg		J2185
Mesna	200 mg	IV	J9209

Mesnex, see Mesna
Metaprel, see Metaproterenol sulfate
Metaproterenol sulfate, concentrated form

	per 10 mg	INH	J7668

Metaproterenol sulfate, unit dose form per

	10 mg	INH	J7669
Metaraminol bitartrate	per 10 mg	IV, IM, SC	J0380

Metastron, see Strontium-89 chloride

Methadone HCl	up to 10 mg	IM, SC	J1230

Methergine, see Methylergonovine maleate

Methocarbamol	up to 10 ml	IV, IM	J2800
Methotrexate, oral	2.5 mg	ORAL	J8610
Methotrexate sodium	5 mg	IV, IM, IT, IA	J9250

Methotrexate LPF, see Methotrexate sodium

Methylergonovine maleate	up to 0.2 mg	IM, IV	J2210
Methyldopate HCl	up to 250 mg	IV	J0210
Methylergonovine maleate	up to 0.2 mg		J2210
Methylprednisolone, oral	per 4 mg	ORAL	J7509
Methylprednisolone acetate	20 mg	IM	J1020
	40 mg	IM	J1030
	80 mg	IM	J1040
Methylprednisolone sodium succinate	up to 40 mg	IM, IV	J2920
	up to 125 mg	IM, IV	J2930
Metoclopramide HCl	up to 10 mg	IV	J2765

Miacalcin, see Calcitonin-salmon

Midazolam HCl	per 1 mg	IM, IV	J2250
Milrinone lactate	5 mg	IV	J2260

Mirena, see Levonorgestrel releasing intrauterine contraceptive
Mithracin, see Plicamycin

Mitomycin	5 mg	IV	J9280
	20 mg	IV	J9290
	40 mg	IV	J9291
Mitoxantrone HCl	per 5 mg	IV	J9293

Monocid, see Cefonicic sodium
Monoclate-P, see Factor VIII

Monoclonal antibodies, parenteral	5 mg	IV	J7505

Mononine, see Factor IX, purified, non-recombinant

Morphine sulfate	up to 10 mg	IM, IV, SC	J2270
	100 mg	IM, IV, SC	J2271
Morphine sulfate, preservative-free	per 10 mg	SC, IM, IV	J2275
Moxifloxacin	100 mg		J2280

M-Prednisol-40, see Methylprednisolone acetate
M-Prednisol-80, see Methylprednisolone acetate
Mucomyst, see Acetylcysteine or Acetylcysteine, compounded
Mucosol, see Acetylcysteine

Muromonab-CD3	5 mg	IV	J7505

Muse, see Alprostadil

Mustargen, see Mechlorethamine HCl
Mutamycin, see Mitomycin

Mycophenolate Mofetil	250 mg	ORAL	J7517

Myleran, see Busulfan
Mylotarg, see Gemtuzumab ozogamicin
Myobloc, see Botulinum toxin type B
Myochrysine, see Gold sodium thiomalate
Myolin, see Orphenadrine citrate

N

Nalbuphine HCl	per 10 mg	IM, IV, SC	J2300
Naloxone HCl	per 1 mg	IM, IV, SC	J2310

Nandrobolic L.A., see Nandrolone decanoate

Nandrolone decanoate	up to 50 mg	IM	J2320
	up to 100 mg	IM	J2321
	up to 200 mg	IM	J2322

Narcan, see Naloxone HCl
Naropin, see Ropivacaine HCl
Nasahist B, see Brompheniramine maleate

Nasal vaccine inhalation		INH	J3530

Navane, see Thiothixene
Navelbine, see Vinorelbine tartrate
ND Stat, see Brompheniramine maleate
Nebcin, see Tobramycin sulfate
NebuPent, see Pentamidine isethionate
Nembutal Sodium Solution, see Pentobarbital sodium
Neocyten, see Orphenadrine citrate
Neo-Durabolic, see Nandrolone decanoate
Neoquess, see Dicyclomine HCl
Neosar, see Cyclophosphamide

Neostigmine methylsulfate	up to 0.5 mg	IM, IV, SC	J2710

Neo-Synephrine, see Phenylephrine HCl
Nervocaine 1%, see Lidocaine HCl
Nervocaine 2%, see Lidocaine HCl
Nesacaine, see Chloroprocaine HCL
Nesacaine-MPF, see Chloroprocaine HCl

Nesiritide	0.5 mg		J2324

Neumega, see Oprelvekin
Neupogen, see Filgrastim (G-CSF)
Neutrexin, see Trimetrexate glucuronate
Nipent, see Pentostatin
Nordryl, see Diphenhydramine HCl
Norflex, see Orphenadrine citrate
Norzine, see Thiethylperazine maleate

Not otherwise classified drugs			J3490
Not otherwise classified drugs other than administered thru DME		INH	J7799
Not otherwise classified drugs administered thru DME		INH	J7699
Not otherwise classified drugs, anti-neoplastic			J9999
Not otherwise classified drugs, chemotherapeutic		ORAL	J8999
Not otherwise classified drugs, immunosuppressive			J7599
Not otherwise classified drugs, nonchemotherapeutic		ORAL	J8499

Novantrone, see Mitoxantrone HCl

Novo Seven, see Factor VIIa
NPH, see Insulin
Nubain, see Nalbuphine HCl
Nulicaine, see Lidocaine HCl
Numorphan, see Oxymorphone HCl
Numorphan H.P., see Oxymorphone HCl

O

Octreotide Acetate, injection	1 mg	IM	J2353
	25 mcg	IV,SQ	J2354
Oculinum, see Botulinum toxin type A			
O-Flex, see Orphenadrine citrate			
Omnipen-N, see Ampicillin			
Oncaspar, see Pegaspargase			
Oncovin, see Vincristine sulfate			
Ondansetron HCl	1 mg	IV	J2405
Ondansetron HCl, oral	8 mg	ORAL	Q0179
Oprelvekin	5 mg	SC	J2355
Oraminic II, see Brompheniramine maleate			
Ormazine, see Chlorpromazine HCl			
Orphenadrine citrate	up to 60 mg	IV, IM	J2360
Orphenate, see Orphenadrine citrate			
Or-Tyl, see Dicyclomine			
Oxacillin sodium	up to 250 mg	IM, IV	J2700
Oxaliplatin	0.5 mg		J9263
Oxymorphone HCl	up to 1 mg	IV, SC, IM	J2410
Oxytetracycline HCl	up to 50 mg	IM	J2460
Oxytocin	up to 10 units	IV, IM	J2590

P

Paclitaxel	30 mg	IV	J9265
Pamidronate disodium	per 30 mg	IV	J2430
Papaverine HCl	up to 60 mg	IV, IM	J2440
Paragard T 380 A, see Copper contraceptive, intrauterine			
Paraplatin, see Carboplatin			
Paricalcitol, injection	1 mcg	IV, IM	J2501
Pegademase bovine	25 iu		Q2012
Pegaspargase	per single dose vial	IM, IV	J9266
Pegfilgrastim	6 mg		J2505
Penicillin G benzathine	up to 600,000 units	IM	J0560
	up to 1,200,000 units	IM	J0570
	up to 2,400,000 units	IM	J0580
Penicillin G benzathine and penicillin G procaine			
	22 up to 600,000 units	IM	J0530
	up to 1,200,000 units	IM	J0540
	up to 2,400,000 units	IM	J0550
Penicillin G potassium	up to 600,000 units	IM, IV	J2540
Penicillin G procaine, aqueous	up to 600,000 units	IM, IV	J2510
Pentamidine isethionate	per 300 mg	INH	J2545
Pentastarch, 10% per	100 ml		Q2013
Pentazocine HCl	up to 30 mg	IM, SC, IV	J3070
Pentobarbital sodium	per 50 mg	IM, IV, OTH	J2515
Pentostatin	per 10 mg	IV	J9268
Permapen, see Penicillin G benzathine			

Perphenazine, injection	up to 5 mg	IM, IV	J3310
Perphenazine, tablets	4 mg	ORAL	Q0175
	8 mg	ORAL	Q0176
Persantine IV, see Dipyridamole			
Pfizerpen, see Penicillin G potassium			
Pfizerpen A.S., see Penicillin G procaine			
Phenazine 25, see Promethazine HCl			
Phenazine 50, see Promethazine HCl			
Phenergan, see Promethazine HCl			
Phenobarbital sodium	up to 120 mg	IM, IV	J2560
Phentolamine mesylate	up to 5 mg	IM, IV	J2760
Phenylephrine HCl	up to 1 ml	SC, IM, IV	J2370
Phenytoin sodium	per 50 mg	IM, IV	J1165
Photofrin, see Porfimer sodium			
Phytonadione (Vitamin K)	per 1 mg	IM, SC, IV	J3430
Piperacillin/Tazobactam Sodium, injection 1.			
	125 g	IV	J2543
Pitocin, see Oxytocin			
Plantinol AQ, see Cisplatin			
Plas+SD, see Plasma, pooled multiple donor			
Plasma, cryoprecipitate reduced each unit			P9044
Plasma, pooled multiple donor, frozen, each unit		IV	P9023
Platinol, see Cisplatin			
Plicamycin	2,500 mcg	IV	J9270
Polocaine, see Mepivacaine			
Polycillin-N, see Ampicillin			
Porfimer Sodium	75 mg	IV	J9600
Potassium chloride	per 2 mEq	IV	J3480
Pralidoxime chloride	up to 1 g	IV, IM, SC	J2730
Predalone-50, see Prednisolone acetate			
Predcor-25, see Prednisolone acetate			
Predcor-50, see Prednisolone acetate			
Predicort-50, see Prednisolone acetate			
Prednisone	per 5 mg	ORAL	J7506
Prednisolone,	oral 5 mg	ORAL	J7510
Prednisolone acetate	up to 1 ml	IM	J2650
Predoject-50, see Prednisolone acetate			
Pregnyl, see Chorionic gonadotropin			
Premarin Intravenous, see Estrogen, conjugated			
Prescription,chemotherapeutic,not otherwise specified		ORAL	J8999
Prescription,nonchemotherapeutic,not otherwise specified		ORAL	J8499
Primacor, see Milrinone lactate			
Primaxin I.M., see Cilastatin sodium, imipenem			
Primaxin I.V., see Cilastatin sodium, imipenem			
Priscoline HCl, see Tolazoline HCl			
Pro-Depo, see Hydroxyprogesterone Caproate			
Procainamide HCl	up to 1 g	IM, IV	J2690
Prochlorperazine	up to 10 mg	IM, IV	J0780
Prochlorperazine maleate, oral	5 mg	ORAL	Q0164
	10 mg	ORAL	Q0165
Profasi HP, see Chorionic gonadotropin			
Profilnine Heat-Treated, see Factor IX			
Progestaject, see Progesterone			
Progesterone	per 50 mg		J2675
Prograf, see Tacrolimus, oral or parenteral			

Prokine, see Sargramostim (GM-CSF)
Prolastin, see Alpha 1-proteinase inhibitor, human
Proleukin, see Aldesleukin
Prolixin Decanoate, see Fluphenazine decanoate

Promazine HCl	up to 25 mg	IM	J2950
Promethazine HCl, injection	up to 50 mg	IM, IV	J2550
Promethazine HCl, oral	12.5 mg	ORAL	Q0169
	25 mg	ORAL	Q0170

Pronestyl, see Procainamide HCl
Proplex T, see Factor IX
Proplex SX-T, see Factor IX

Propranolol HCl	up to 1 mg	IV	J1800

Prorex-25, see Promethazine HCl
Prorex-50, see Promethazine HCl
Prostaphlin, see Procainamide HCl
Prostigmin, see Neostigmine methylsulfate

Protamine sulfate	per 10 mg	IV	J2720
Protirelin	per 250 mcg	IV	J2725

Prothazine, see Promethazine HCl
Protopam Chloride, see Pralidoxime chloride
Proventil, see Albuterol sulfate, compounded
Prozine-50, see Promazine HCl
Pulmicort Respules, see Budesonide

Pyridoxine HCl	100 mg		J3415

Q

Quelicin, see Succinylcholine chloride Quinupristin/dalfopristin

	500 mg(150/350)	IV	J2770

R

Ranitidine HCL, injection	25 mg	IV, IM	J2780

Rapamune, see Sirolimus

Rasburicase	0.5 mg		J2783

Recombinate, see Factor VIII
Redisol, see Vitamin B-12 cyanocobalamin
Regitine, see Phentolamine mesylate
Reglan, see Metoclopramide HCl
Regular, see Insulin
Relefact TRH, see Protirelin
Remicade, see Infliximab, injection
Reo Pro, see Abciximab
Rep-Pred 40, see Methylprednisolone acetate
Rep-Pred 80, see Methylprednisolone acetate
RespiGam, see Respiratory Syncytial Virus
Respiratory Syncytial Virus Immuneglobulin

	50 mg	IV	J1565

Retavase, see Reteplase

Reteplase	18.8 mg	IV	J2993

Retrovir, see Zidovudine
Rheomacrodex, see Dextran 40
Rhesonativ, see Rho(D) immune globulin, human
Rheumatrex Dose Pack, see Methotrexate, oral

Rho(D) immune globulin, human 1 dose package,			
	300 mcg	IM	J2790
	50 mcg	IM	J2798
Rho(D)immune globulin, human,solvent detergent			
	100 IU	IV	J2792
RhoGAM, see Rho(D) immune globulin, human			
Ringers lactate infusion	up to 1,000 cc	IV	J7120
Rituxan, see Rituximab			
Rituximab	100 mg	IV	J9310
Robaxin, see Methocarbamol			
Rocephin, see Ceftriaxone sodium			
Roferon-A, see Interferon alfa-2A, recombinant			
Ropivacaine Hydrochloride	1 mg		J2795
Rubex, see Doxorubicin HCl			
Rubramin PC, see Vitamin B-12 cyanocobalamin			

S

Saline solution 5% dextrose,	500 ml	IV	J7042
	infusion, 250 cc	IV	J7050
	infusion, 1,000 cc	IV	J7030
Saline solution, sterile	500 ml = 1 unit	IV, OTH	J7040
	up to 5 cc	IV, OTH	J7051
Sandimmune, see Cyclosporine			
Sandoglobulin, see Immune globulin intravenous (human)			
Sandostatin Lar Depot, see Octreotide			
Sargramostim (GM-CSF)	50 mcg	IV	J2820
Secobarbital sodium	up to 250 mg	IM, IV	J2860
Seconal, see Secobarbital sodium			
Selestoject, see Betamethasone sodium phosphate			
Sermorelin acetate	0.5 mg		Q2014
Sinusol-B, see Brompheniramine maleate			
	per 2 ml	IV	J2912
Sirolimus	1 mg	Oral	J7520
Sodium chloride, 0.9%	per 2 ml		J2912
Sodium ferricgluconate in sucrose	12.5 mg		J2916
Sodium hyaluronate	5 mg	OTH	J7316
Solganal, see Aurothioglucose			
Solu-Cortef, see Hydrocortisone sodium phosphate (J1710)			
Solu-Medrol, see Methylprednisolone sodium succinate			
Solurex, see Dexamethasone sodium phosphate			
Solurex LA, see Dexamethasone acetate			
Somatrem	1 mg		J2940
Somatropin	1 mg		J2941
Sparine, see Promazine Hcl			
Spasmoject, see Dicyclomine HCl			
Spectinomycin HCl	up to 2 g	IM	J3320
Sporanox, see Itraconazole			
Staphcillin, see Methicillin sodium			
Stilphostrol, see Diethylstilbestrol diphosphate			
Streptase, see Streptokinase			
Streptokinase	per 250,000 IU	IV	J2995
Streptomycin Sulfate, see Streptomycin			
Streptomycin	up to 1 g	IM	J3000
Streptozocin	1 gm	IV	J9320
Strontium-89 chloride	per 10 ml	IV	J3005

Sublimaze, see Fentanyl citrate

Succinylcholine chloride	up to 20 mg	IV, IM	J0330
Sumatriptan succinate	6 mg	SC	J3030

Supartz, see Sodium hyaluronate

Surostrin, see Succinycholine chloride

Sus-Phrine, see Adrenalin, epinephrine

Synercid, see Quinupristin/dalfopristin

Synkavite, see Vitamin K, phytonadione, etc.

Syntocionon, see Oxytocin

Synvisc, see Hylan G-F 20

Sytobex, see Vitamin B-12 cyanocobalamin

T

Tacrolimus, oral	per 1 mg	ORAL	J7507
Tacrolimus, parenteral	5 mg		J7515

Talwin, see Pentazocine Hcl

Taractan, see Chlorprothixene

Taxol, see Paclitaxel

Taxotere, see Docetaxel

Tazidime, see Ceftazidime Technetium TC Sestambi

	per dose		A9500

TEEV, see Testosterone enanthate and estradiol valerate

Temozolmide	5 mg	ORAL	J8700
Tenecteplase	50 mg		J3100
Teniposide	50 mg		Q2017

Tequin, see Gatifloxacin

Terbutaline sulfate	up to 1 mg	SC, IV	J3105
Terbutaline sulfate, concentrated form	per 1 mg	INH	J7680
Terbutaline sulfate, unit dose form	per 1 mg	INH	J7681

Terramycin IM, see Oxytetracycline Hcl

Testa-C, see Testosterone cypionate

Testadiate, see Testosterone enanthate and estradiol valerate

Testadiate-Depo, see Testosterone cypionate

Testaject-LA, see Testosterone cypionate

Testaqua, see Testosterone suspension

Test-Estro Cypionates, see Testosterone cypionate and estradiol cypionate

Test-Estro-C, see Testosterone cypionate and estradiol cypionate

Testex, see Testosterone propionate

Testoject-50, see Testosterone suspension

Testoject-LA, see Testosterone cypionate

Testone LA 200, see Testosterone enanthate

Testone LA 100, see Testosterone enanthate

Testosterone Aqueous, see Testosterone suspension

Testosterone enanthate and estradiol valerate

	up to 1 cc	IM	J0900
Testosterone enanthate	up to 100 mg	IM	J3120
	up to 200 mg	IM	J3130
Testosterone cypionate	up to 100 mg	IM	J1070
	1 cc, 200 mg	IM	J1080

Testosterone cypionate and estradiol cypionate

	up to 1 ml	IM	J1060
Testosterone propionate	up to 100 mg	IM	J3150
Testosterone suspension	up to 50 mg	IM	J3140

Testradiol 90/4, see Testosterone enanthate and estradiol valerate

Testrin PA, see Testosterone enanthate

Tetanus immune globulin, human	up to 250 units	IM	J1670
Tetracycline	up to 250 mg	IM, IV	J0120
Thallous Chloride TL 201	per MCI		A9505
Theelin Aqueous, see Estrone			
Theophylline	per 40 mg	IV	J2810
TheraCys, see BCG live			
Thiamine HCl	100 mg		J3411
Thiethylperazine maleate, injection	up to 10 mg	IM	J3280
Thiethylperazine maleate, oral	10 mg	ORAL	Q0174
Thiotepa	15 mg	IV	J9340
Thorazine, see Chlorpromazine HCl			
Thymoglobulin, see Immune globulin, anti-thymocyte			
Thypinone, see Protirelin			
Thyrogen, see Thyrotropin Alfa			
Thyrotropin Alfa, injection	0.9 mg	IM, SC	J3240
Tice BCG, see BCG live			
Ticon, see Trimethobenzamide HCl			
Tigan, see Trimethobenzamide HCl			
Tiject-20, see Trimethobenzamide HCl			
Tinzarparin	1000 IU	SC	J1655
Tirofiban Hydrochloride, injection	12.5 mg	IM, IV	J3245
TNKase, see Tenecteplase			
Tobi, see Tobramycin, inhalation solution			
Tobramycin, inhalation solution	300 mg	INH	J7682
Tobramycin sulfate	up to 80 mg	IM, IV	J3260
Tofranil, see Imipramine HCl			
Tolazoline HCl	up to 25 mg	IV	J2670
Topotecan	4 mg	IV	J9350
Toradol, see Ketorolac tromethamine			
Torecan, see Thiethylperazine maleate			
Tornalate, see Bitolterol mesylate			
Torsemide	10 mg/ml	IV	J3265
Totacillin-N, see Ampicillin			
Trastuzumab	10 mg	IV	J9355
Treprostinil	1 mg		Q4077
Tri-Kort, see Triamcinolone acetonide			
Triam-A, see Triamcinolone acetonide			
Triamcinolone, concentrated form	per 1 mg	INH	J7683
Triamcinolone, unit dose	per 1 mg	INH	J7684
Triamcinolone acetonide	per 10 mg	IM	J3301
Triamcinolone diacetate	per 5 mg	IM	J3302
Triamcinolone hexacetonide	per 5 mg	VAR	J3303
Triflupromazine HCl	up to 20 mg	IM, IV	J3400
Trilafon, see Perphenazine			
Trilog, see Triamcinolone acetonide			
Trilone, see Triamcinolone diacetate			
Trimethobenzamide HCl, injection	up to 200 mg	IM	J3250
Trimethobenzamide HCl, oral	250 mg	ORAL	Q0173
Trimetrexate glucuronate	per 25 mg	IV	J3305
Triptorelin Pamoate	3.75 mg		J3315
Trisenox, see Arsenic trioxide			
Trobicin, see Spectinomycin HCl			
Trovan, see Alatrofloxacin mesylate			

U

Ultrazine-10, see Prochlorperazine
Unasyn, see Ampicillin sodium/sulbactam sodium

Unclassified drugs (see also Not elsewhere classified)			J3490
Unspecified oral antiemetic			Q0181
Urea	up to 40 g	IV	J3350
Ureaphil, see Urea			
Urecholine, see Bethanechol chloride			
Urofollitropin	75 iu		Q2018
Urokinase	5,000 IU vial	IV	J3364
	250,000 IU vial	IV	J3365

V

V-Gan 25, see Promethazine HCl
V-Gan 50, see Promethazine HCl
Valergen 10, see Estradiol valerate
Valergen 20, see Estradiol valerate
Valergen 40, see Estradiol valerate
Valertest No. 1, see Testosterone enanthate and estradiol valerate
Valertest No. 2, see Testosterone enanthate and estradiol valerate
Valium, see Diazepam

Valrubicin, intravesical	200 mg	OTH	J9357
Valstar, see Valrubicin			
Vancocin, see Vancomycin HCl			
Vancoled, see Vancomycin HCl			
Vancomycin HCl	up to 500 mg	IV, IM	J3370
Vasoxyl, see Methoxamine HCl			
Velban, see Vinblastine sulfate			
Velsar, see Vinblastine sulfate			
Venofer, see Iron sucrose			
Ventolin, see Albuterol sulfate			
VePesid, see Etoposide and Etoposide, oral			
Versed, see Midazolam HCl			
Verteporfin	15 mg	IV	J3395
Vesprin, see Triflupromazine HCl			
Viadur, see Leuprolide acetate implant			
Vinblastine sulfate	1 mg	IV	J9360
Vincasar PFS, see Vincristine sulfate			
Vincristine sulfate	1 mg	IV	J9370
	2 mg	IV	J9375
	5 mg	IV	J9380
Vinorelbine tartrate	per 10 mg	IV	J9390
Vistaject-25, see Hydroxyzine HCl			
Vistaril, see Hydroxyzine HCl			
Vistide, see cidofovir			
Visudyne, see Verteporfin			
Vitamin K, phytonadione, menadione, menadiol sodium diphosphate	per 1 mg	IM, SC, IV	J3430
Vitamin B-12 cyanocobalamin	up to 1,000 mcg	IM, SC	J3420
Von Willebrand Factor Complex, human		per IU	IV
	Q2022		
Voriconazole	10 mg		J3465

W

Wehamine, see Dimenhydrinate
Wehdryl, see Diphenhydramine HCl
Wellcovorin, see Leucovorin calcium
Win Rho SD, see Rho(D)immuglobulin, human, solvent detergent
Wyamine Sulfate, see Mephentermine sulfate
Wycillin, see Penicillin G procaine
Wydase, see Hyaluronidase

X

Xeloda, see Capecitabine
Xopenex, see Albuterol
Xylocaine HCl, see Lidocaine HCl

Z

Zanosar, see Streptozocin
Zantac, see Ranitidine HCL
Zemplar, see Paricalcitol
Zenapax, see Daclizumab
Zetran, see Diazepam

Zidovudine	10 mg	IV	J3485

Zinacef, see Cefuroxime sodium

Ziprasidone Mesylate	10 mg		J3486

Zithromax, see Azithromycin dihydrate
Zithromax I.V., see Azithromycin, injection
Zofran, see Ondansetron HCl

Zoladex, see Goserelin acetate implant Zoledronic Acid	J3487

Zolicef, see Cefazolin sodium
Zosyn, see Piperacillin
Zyvox, see Linezolid

Printed in the United States
15863LVS00001B/138